Serology and Immunology
A Clinical Approach

Serology and Immunology
A Clinical Approach

WILLIAM D. STANSFIELD
California Polytechnic State University

Macmillan Publishing Co., Inc.
New York

Collier Macmillan Publishers
London

COPYRIGHT © 1981, WILLIAM D. STANSFIELD

PRINTED IN THE UNITED STATES OF AMERICA

All rights reserved. No part of this book may be reproduced or transmitted in any form or by any means, electronic or mechanical, including photocopying, recording, or any information storage and retrieval system, without permission in writing from the Publisher.

MACMILLAN PUBLISHING CO., INC.
866 Third Avenue, New York, New York 10022

COLLIER MACMILLAN CANADA, LTD.

Library of Congress Cataloging in Publication Data

 Stansfield, William D (date)
  Serology and immunology.

  Bibliography: p.
  Includes index.
   1. Serology. 2. Immunology. 3. Immunodiagnosis.
 I. Title. [DNLM: 1. Allergy and immunology.
2. Serology. QW570 S791s]
 RB46.5.S7   616.07'9   80-13671
 ISBN 0-02-415740-6

Printing: 1 2 3 4 5 6 7 8   Year: 1 2 3 4 5 6 7 8

To My Children, Lorrie, Lynn, and Bill

PREFACE

This text is primarily directed toward providing an introduction to the various disciplines of immunology (serology, immunity, immunopathology, immunochemistry, etc.) for students and practitioners in the human health professions. Special emphasis is given to the immunodiagnostic tests performed by medical laboratory technologists. The book should also provide a firm foundation for those interested in using serological techniques in research projects outside the field of immunology. Although human medicine is the main focus, the basic immunological principles are general enough to be useful to veterinarians and others concerned with the health of animals. Indeed, much of our knowledge about the workings of the human immune system have been obtained by using laboratory animals as models. For example, much more is known about the major histocompatibility complex (MHC) of mice than of humans, and for this reason the MHC of mice must be discussed in detail.

Immunology is seldom offered as a lower division course in colleges or universities because it is a discipline that requires a rather broad scientific background. There simply is not time in a quarter or semester immunology course to teach the fundamentals of subjects such as bacteriology, protein chemistry, Mendelian genetics, cytology, anatomy and physiology that are needed to understand many immunological principles. This book assumes that the reader has gained the required degree of sophistication in these basic sciences.

An attempt has been made to marry the theoretical and practical aspects of immunology wherever possible. Immunology is such a rapidly expanding field of science that some of the modern theories discussed herein may soon be obsolete. Nevertheless, it is hoped that the presentation of these ephemeral theories will serve to stimulate the reader to try to keep abreast of new developments in this exciting field.

Modern theories of immunology are but tips on the icebergs of fundamental knowledge accumulated largely since the time of Louis Pasteur, and we should remember that we are "standing on the shoulders of giants." However, no attempt has been made in this book to provide a historical frame of reference for modern theories, largely because of space limitations. For example, template theories of antibody production are not discussed because everything we presently know about protein synthesis renders these theories untenable. Likewise, other outmoded concepts will not be found in this volume, except perhaps for some archaic terms likely to be encountered in reading classical papers.

Heavy emphasis is given to the burgeoning vocabulary of immunology so that one may be equipped to launch into journal articles with a high degree of comprehension following mastery of the material in this book. As new terms are introduced and defined in the text, they appear in boldface. Likewise, the boldface citation of a term in the index is the location of its definition. In this way, the index can also function as a glossary. It has become common practice among professionals to freely use acronyms in communication (oral and written) with one another. One cannot hope to comprehend these discussions unless the language (terms and acronyms) is known. An unusual feature of this book is its glossary of immunological acronyms widely used in the clinical laboratory.

For each type of diagnostic test, a thorough explanation is given of the basic principles, the controls that need to be run simultaneously, the interpretation of the results, and the pitfalls in performing and interpreting the tests. This is the kind of knowledge required of modern medical technologists to obtain licensure and for professional performance of daily tasks in the clinical laboratory. Furthermore, the mechanical and mathematical aspects of quality control are extremely important for the assurance of reliable test results. For this reason, an appendix has been added to the ten basic chapters that introduces the clinician to the mathematics of quality control.

An attempt has also been made to provide ample illustrations to help visualize abstract immunological processes. Careful study of these illustrations together with the detailed explanations in the text should aid in fixing the basic ideas in one's mind for long-term retention.

A self-evaluation section is included at the end of each chapter to provide the student with some immediate feedback on the degree of mastery of the subject matter. Three kinds of objective questions are available (terms, multiple choice, and true-false). There are 300 such items in this text, and collectively they and their answers should allow the student to gain a fairly accurate assessment of the need for restudy.

I especially wish to acknowledge the many helpful suggestions provided by my colleague David Grady. Thanks are also due to Cynthia Sommer and Duane Sears for their work in reviewing the manuscript. I would appreciate being informed of errors (both of commission and of omission) so that they may be corrected in any subsequent editions.

W. D. STANSFIELD

Biological Sciences Department
California Polytechnic State University
San Luis Obispo, CA 93407

CONTENTS

CHAPTER

1 Basic Principles — 1

2 Antigens and Antibodies — 30

3 Immunohematology Part I — 67
   The ABO and Rh Blood Group Systems

4 Immunohematology Part II — 103
   Minor Blood Group Systems, Compatibility Test, Antibody Identification, and Quality Controls

5 Precipitation — 135

6 Agglutination — 168

7 Complement and Cytotoxicity — 200

8 Tagged Reagents — 239

9 Immunopathology — 277

10 Transplantation and Oncoimmunology — 315

   APPENDIX: Quality Control in Serological Testing — 347

   Acronyms — 354

   References — 361

   Answers — 365

   Index — 369

Basic Principles

CHAPTER 1

CHAPTER OUTLINE

Nonsusceptibility
Three Lines of Defense
  Integumentary System
  Reticuloendothelial System
  Immune System
    "Humoral" Immunity
    "Cellular" Immunity
Types of Immunity
  "Vaccines" and "Vaccinations"
  Typical Responses of the
Immunologically Competent
  Individual
  Immune Responses of the Newborn
  The End of Smallpox
Phylogeny of the Immune System
Ontogeny of the Immune System
  Clonal Selection Theory
  Plasma Cells
Immunocytology
  Cellular Interactions
Self-evaluation

Immunology is that branch of vertebrate zoology concerned with the specific responses made by lymphocytes to foreign substances. **Serology** is a subdivision of immunology concerned with *in vitro* ("in the test tube"; extraorganismal) antigen-antibody reactions. Antibodies are found in the fluid portion of blood and in other fluids of the body. Approximately half of whole blood is cells (most are red blood cells called **erythrocytes;** some are white blood cells called **leukocytes**). The other half of blood is a fluid called **plasma.** The fluid remaining after blood clots in a test tube is called **serum.** The main difference between plasma and serum is that serum does not contain the protein fibrinogen. Serum is more commonly used than plasma in serological tests because serum will not clot when other materials are added to it. An **antigen** is any substance that can trigger specific responses from lymphocytes or that can react specifically with antibody. An **antibody** or functional **immunoglobulin** is a humoral (referring to body fluids) protein that is produced by a lymphocyte in response to an antigenic stimulus and that is capable of reacting specifically with that same antigen. **Immunity** is another subdivision of immunology involved with responses of lymphocytes that benefit the organism, as in prophylaxis (prevention) and therapeutics (treatment) of diseases caused by microorganisms. **Hypersensitivity** is a term that may be applied to lymphocyte reactions harmful to the body, as in allergies and graft rejections. Loose usage of the term "immune response" has been variously applied to either the beneficial or the detrimental aspects of immunology. Indeed, there are some instances where an immune response is neither completely beneficial nor detrimental. For example, invasion of host cells by certain viruses results in the appearance of new antigens on the cell membranes. Lymphocytes responding specifically to these new, foreign antigens may cause the destruction of virus-infected cells, limiting viral release and spread to uninfected cells. This activity produces some of the symptoms associated with the viral disease. Virally stimulated lymphocytes may also produce antiviral substances, such as antibodies and interferons, that prevent attachment of viruses to host cells or inhibit replication of viruses within infected cells. Thus, the total effect of the immune response may be partly destructive and partly protective.

In the broad sense that includes hypersensitivity and immunity, the "immune response" of vertebrate animals can be defined as the acquired, transferable capacity of lymphocytes to react with specificity and memory to foreign substances. From this definition, it can be seen that true immune and hypersensitivity reactions have the following properties.

1. They are lymphocyte-mediated by products called antibodies and lymphokines.
2. These reactions are acquired only after contact between lymphocytes and the inciting antigen.
3. The response is directed specifically only at the inciting antigen. Antibodies combine with antigens as complementary molecular complexes analogous to the lock-and-key models of enzyme-substrate interactions.
4. They can be transferred from one individual to another via sensitized lymphocytes and/or antibodies.
5. Subsequent contacts with the inciting antigen produce more vigorous memory responses.
6. Self-components are distinguished from nonself-molecules so that these responses normally are made only to foreign substances. Autoallergies are an exception to the rule.

Nonsusceptibility

There are many communicable diseases that do not affect any member of a given species. Dogs, for example, do not suffer from measles, and humans do not contract canine distemper. **Nonsusceptibility** is the term that will be applied in this book to natural refractoriness of a species to infection by specific microorganisms. Although it has been common practice to refer to nonsusceptibility as nonspecific immunity, innate immunity, constitutional immunity, or genetic immunity, it is the opinion of the author that the word "immunity" should be restricted to the specific acquired activities of lymphocytes.

It is seldom known precisely why certain diseases are species-specific. Ultimately, genotypic differences between species must be held accountable, but this tells us nothing of the specific mechanisms involved. One of the best examples of how one kind of nonsusceptibility works was provided by Louis Pasteur in the nineteenth century. Anthrax is a disease found naturally only in mammals. Pasteur found that he could induce anthrax bacilli to infect chickens by artificially lowering their body temperatures from their normal 106°F down to the normal of many mammals (approximately 100°F). The genotype of the bird establishes a higher metabolic rate and consequently a higher body temperature. The anthrax bacillus can multiply *in vitro* at 42° to 43°C (108° to 110°F), but probably loses virulence *in vivo* (in the living organism) because one or more enzymes required for capsule production are denatured (loss of native three-dimensional molecular shape) at these slightly higher temperatures. Encapsulated bacteria are generally more resistant to phagocytosis than unencapsulated forms of the same organism.

Nonsusceptibility provides complete protection (under normal conditions) for every member of the species without previously contacting the specific microorganism. Immunity, on the other hand, is acquired only after lymphocyte contact with an antigen (microorganism, foreign protein, etc.). Protection by immunity is variable from one individual to another within the species and from one time to another within the same individual. Even high levels of antimicrobial antibodies may not provide complete protection. The immune defenses can be overwhelmed by a sufficiently large inoculum of a pathogen so that clinical disease (or possibly death) ensues.

Three Lines of Defense

INTEGUMENTARY SYSTEM

The vertebrate body has, in addition to its immune response, two other major lines of defense against invasion by foreign substances. The first line of defense against pathogenic microorganisms includes the skin (integument) and the mucous membranes and their secretions. Most microorganisms cannot multiply *in vivo* and cause disease unless they can breach the barrier of the epithelial layers of these tissues. **Infection** is the result of microbial growth and/or multiplication at the expense of the host. Infecting microbes usually harm their hosts in one or more of three major ways: (1) by competing with host cells for essential nutrients, (2) by the elaboration of products that are toxic to host cells, and (3) by microbial products that promote the spread and persistence of pathogens without being directly toxic to host cells. These latter products, called **aggressins,** are exemplified by enzymes such as hyaluronidase, coagulase, collagenases, and fibinolysins.

The dry, thick, dead, cornified layer of the skin is normally an effective nonspecific barrier to the entry of most microorganisms. The moister, thinner epithelial linings of the mucous membranes found in the nasopharyngeal, gastrointestinal, and urogenital tracts would seem to provide a relatively easy route for microbial entry into the body. The gastrointestinal (GI) tract normally contains a massive microbial flora, but these bacteria are usually unable to infect the body because of the impermeable mucous layer covering the epithelial cells of the GI tract. The enzyme **lysozyme** is secreted by the nasal mucosa (also found in tears and sweat). Lysozyme digests some acetyl-amino sugars from the cell walls of many bacteria, weakening them and causing microbial death. Several other nonspecific antimicrobial substances are known to be present in blood and tissue fluids. A sticky coat of mucus tends to entrap foreign substances entering the nasopharyngeal passages. This layer of mucus is moved by ciliary action of epithelial cells to the throat and is usually swallowed. In the stomach, the action of hydrochloric acid and pepsin (a proteolytic enzyme) usually degrades accessible proteins on bacterial and viral surfaces.

RETICULOENDOTHELIAL SYSTEM

The second line of defense against microbes is the nonspecific **reticuloendothelial system** (RES), a group of cells in various tissues and organs with only one major property in common, viz., phagocytosis. **Phagocytes** are cells that engulf and digest foreign substances (such as microbes). They may be fixed (immobilized) as cells lining the sinusoids of "filtering organs" (liver, spleen, and lymph nodes), or they may be ameboid wandering cells in the tissue spaces (macrophages, histiocytes). How phagocytes recognize foreign materials is not well known, but their response is apparently nonspecific, attacking india ink particles as readily as microbes on first encounter. In both vertebrates and invertebrates, some phagocytes appear to exhibit specific responses in "experienced individuals" (i.e., those that have previously contacted the same antigen). This specificity could be partly acquired by phagocytes from the immune system of vertebrates via antibodies or lymphokines, but other explanations must be sought for this phenomenon in animals devoid of a lymphoid system.

Bacteria and injured tissues are thought to release chemicals that attract phagocytes. Such substances are called **chemotaxins.** These scavenger cells engulf bacteria and debris by surrounding the particles with pseudopod "arms" formed by sol-gel transformations of the cytoplasm. The enclosed phagocytic vacuole then coalesces with one or more lysosomes to form a **phagolysosome.** Digestion of the ingested particles is accomplished by activated lysosomal proteolytic enzymes. It is currently believed that singlet oxygen ($^1O_2$) generated by phagocytes is a more potent bactericidal agent than lysosomal enzymes. Singlet oxygen might be produced by decomposition of the superoxide radical (O_2^-) as a consequence of oxidation of reduced pyridine nucleotides or by other conceivable pathways. Carotenoid pigments are known to inactivate singlet oxygen, so that bacteria possessing these pigments tend to be protected against being killed within phagocytes. Many pathogenic bacteria of the genera *Mycobacterium* and *Brucella* are resistant to phagocytosis and are actually transported throughout the body by phagocytes, being thus protected from the immune system as long as they remain sequestered within the phagocytic cell. Bacteria possessing a polysaccharide capsule are commonly resistant to destruction by phagocytes. Still other bacteria such as the pyogenic (pus-forming) streptococci and staphylococci produce **leukocidins** that kill white blood cells (leukocytes) and the wandering tissue phagocytes called macrophages.

If a break should occur in the skin or mucous membranes, microbes may penetrate past the first line of defense. If not attacked by wandering phagocytes near the point of entry, they would likely be swept by either the bloodstream or the lymphatic system to and through the "filtering organs" where they would encounter the fixed phagocytes. The first and second lines of defense collectively constitute what is called **resistance.** Note that resistance mechanisms are nonspecific and that their strength in repelling invading microorganisms is quite variable. It is a well-known fact that when we fail to get enough sleep, fail to get adequate nutrition, suffer anxiety or depression, etc., we are more likely to succumb to colds and other common contagious diseases. We say that our resistance is low. This poorly defined physiological state implies that the nonspecific mechanisms of the first and second lines of defense are subnormal. Resistance does not require prior contact with the antigens and is operative at various levels of effectiveness throughout our lives. Some immunologists use the term "specific resistance" or "acquired resistance" synonymously with "immunity," but the author of this text prefers to include only nonspecific protective mechanisms in the term "resistance."

IMMUNE SYSTEM

Should the invading microbes escape destruction by the second line of defense, there is still a chance that they can be destroyed by the action of the immune system, the third line of defense. The immune response involves interactions between antigens and lymphocytes and/or antibodies. There are three major limbs of the immune response (Figure 1.1). The **afferent limb** constitutes all of the functions involved in processing and delivery of antigens to the lymphoid tissues. The **central limb** comprises all of the changes that lymphocytes incur, as a consequence of the antigenic stimulus, to become transformed into effector cells and the subsequent release of effector substances called antibodies or lymphokines. Certain lymphoid cells become **primed** or specifically activated by an antigen and thereafter are referred to as **committed cells** or committed lymphocytes; these cells are destined to a particular line of development such as antibody production, immunologic memory, etc. The **efferent limb** of the immune response encompasses all of the processes that occur after the release of effectors. This involves specific interaction of lymphocytes or antibodies with inciting antigen that may, in turn, activate other cells or chemicals (such as macrophages and complement proteins) that tend to exacerbate or amplify the immune response. Table 1.1 summarizes the major differences between nonsusceptibility, resistance, and immunity.

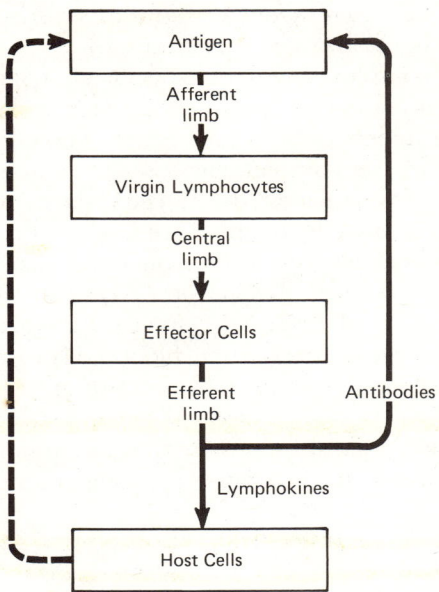

FIGURE 1.1. Three major limbs of the immune response.

Serology and Immunology

Table 1.1 Distinguishing Features of Three Major Types of Protection Against Pathogenic Organisms

Type of Protection	Responsible Agents	Requiring Prior Contact	Degree of Specificity	Degree of Protection
Nonsusceptibility	Heredity common to the species	No	High	Absolute
Resistance	Skin and mucous membranes; phagocytes	No	Low	Variable
Immunity	Antibodies, lymphokines	Yes	High	Variable

"Humoral" Immunity. Immunity in vertebrates depends on the cooperation of lymphocytes and phagocytes. Macrophages usually prepare or process antigens in ways that render them capable of binding to those lymphocytes that bear homologous cell-surface receptors. This antigenic stimulus causes certain immature lymphocytes (immunoblasts) to differentiate into mature antibody-producing immunocytes called **plasma cells.** Before antigenic stimulation, the antibodies made by a plasma cell are attached to the cell membrane, forming the antigen receptor sites. After stimulation by macrophage-processed antigen fragments, the plasma cell begins to release antibodies into the body fluids or "humors." Antibody-mediated immunity is therefore sometimes referred to as **humoral immunity.**

If the animal is encountering microbial antigens for the first time, some of its lymphocytes may be stimulated to produce antibodies. The interval from invasion to the time that specific antibodies can be detected in the serum commonly varies from a few days to a few weeks. Once these antibodies are released into the bloodstream, they can aid in the disposal of those same kinds of microbes by one or more of several mechanisms (lysis, agglutination, toxin neutralization, opsonization).

Antigen-antibody complexes may nonspecifically trigger activation of a series of normal serum enzymes known collectively as **complement** (Chapter 7). Although the mechanism is imprecisely known, it seems that the proteins at the end of the complement cascade (sequence of interacting complement components) is activated with the capacity to produce holes in the membranes of certain cells to which antibodies and complement have attached. Substances normally restricted from entry into cells may then flow through these holes and cause dissolution or **lysis** of the cell. Antibodies that can thus cause lysis of bacterial cells are called **bacteriolysins;** antibodies that can thus cause foreign red blood cells to rupture are called **hemolysins.** Some activated complement proteins are chemotactic, attracting lymphocytes and other white blood cells toward the site. The activities of these cells may contribute substantially to some inflammatory reactions, but not all inflammations are mediated by antigen-antibody-complement complexes.

Antibodies may cause **agglutination** or clumping of microbes, inhibiting their spread through the body and making phagocytic cells more efficient by allowing groups of microbes to be engulfed by a single psuedopodic movement of the cell membrane. The antigens involved in agglutination reactions are known as **agglutinogens;** the corresponding antibodies are **agglutinins.** If agglutinating antibodies activate the complement system, cells such as gram-negative bacteria, foreign leukocytes, and erythrocytes can be lysed. However, many gram-positive bacteria, molds and yeasts, and most plant and foreign mammalian cells are resistant to complement-mediated cytolysis and might be agglutinated *in vivo*.

Antibodies may neutralize (render harmless) certain poisons and viruses. **Antitoxins** are antibodies that neutralize toxic bacterial products. **Antivenoms** are antibodies that neutralize the poisons of certain reptiles (mainly snakes) and certain arthopods such as spiders and scorpions. The diseases of diphtheria, tetanus, and botulism poisoning are apparently caused exclusively by the secreted toxic products of specific bacteria. One theory of antitoxin activity is that the attachment of antibody to the toxin occurs at a site other than the active site. Interaction of antitoxin with this other site (the **allosteric site**) causes a conformational change in the toxin molecule, altering either its toxic site and/or the site by which it attaches to and gains entry into the target cell (Figure 1.2). According to another theory, neutralization occurs by **steric hindrance.** If an antibody attaches at or near the toxic site, effective contact of the toxin molecule with the target cell is prohibited. In analogous but more complicated ways, antibodies may neutralize viruses by combining with their coat proteins whereby the viruses would normally attach to receptor sites on host cells. By either steric hindrance and/or allosteric transformation the antibody renders the virus unable to recognize or contact the receptors, and hence it becomes unable to infect the host cell (Figure 1.3).

Antibodies may enhance phagocytosis by poorly understood mechanisms other than agglutination. It seems that the attachment of antibodies to microbial cells tends to render them "sticky," perhaps by nullification of an electrostatic charge identical to that of the phagocytic cell. The name **opso-**

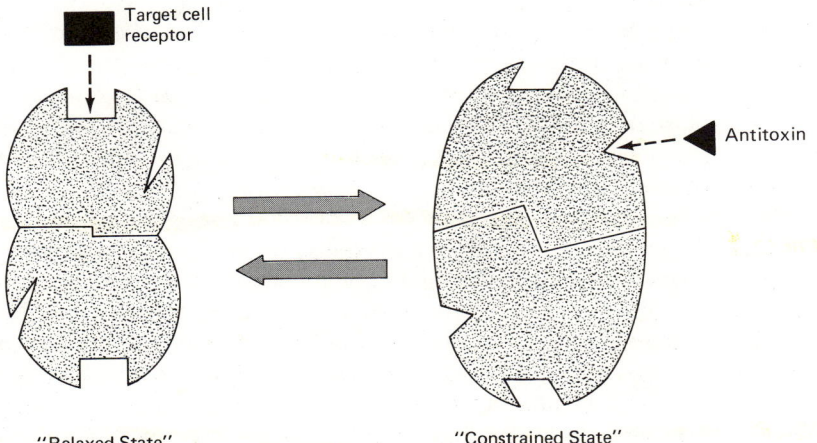

FIGURE 1.2. Model of an allosteric protein. If a protein consists of two identical subunits, it is inferred that an axis of symmetry exists. This model proposes that the protein may alternate between two structural states in which symmetry is preserved. In the "relaxed state," it can bind to target cells. In the "constrained state," it can bind antitoxin. Having bound antitoxin, the protein can no longer bind to the target cell receptor.

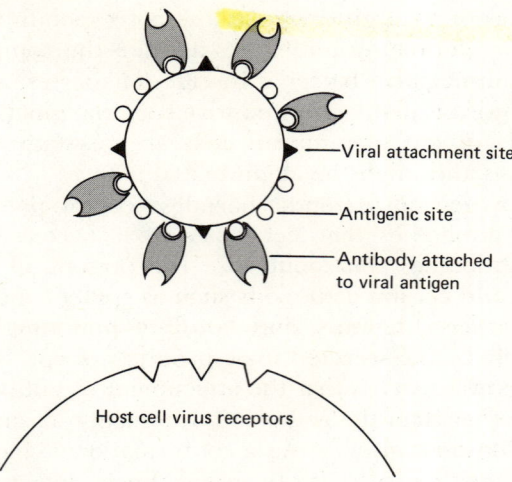

FIGURE 1.3. Diagram illustrating how an antibody complexed with a viral antigen near a viral attachment site prevents the virus from contacting receptors on a host cell by steric hindrance.

nin or opsonic antibody is given to antibodies that facilitate phagocytosis. The opsonic activity of a given antiserum can be quantitated by either an *in vitro* or an *in vivo* test. A **phagocytic index** can be calculated that expresses the average number of bacteria or inert particles ingested per phagocytic cell during a given time period. When this index is applied to bacteria subjected to prior treatment with an **antiserum** (a serum containing specific antibodies), an **opsonic index** can be obtained and compared with a replicate experiment in which the bacteria are not treated with an antiserum. The difference in the two experiments, if performed under the same conditions, is attributed to the enhancement of phagocytosis contributed by the opsonic antibodies.

After recovery from the infection, the animal has a reserve of antibodies ready to react with the antigens of that same kind of pathogenic microorganism. This is why subsequent infection with the same pathogen produces either no disease or a milder form of the disease, depending on such factors as the quantity or titer of specific antibodies present at the time of infection, the dosage of the pathogen, etc.

All antibodies are proteins having the molecular structure of immunoglobulins. The immunoglobulins are presently divided into five classes designated IgG, IgM, IgA, IgE, and IgD. The most common class of antibody (immunoglobulin G or IgG) consists of four polypeptide chains (Figure 1.4). Two of these chains, called heavy chains or H chains, are about twice as long as the other two, called light chains or L chains. These four chains are associated into a tetrameric or tetrapeptide structure that resembles the letter "Y." The arms of the Y-shaped antibody function in antigen recognition and binding; the tail of the immunoglobulin has effector functions that depend on the class to which it belongs. For example, antibodies of classes IgM and IgG can bind complement, those of class IgG can pass the placenta, etc. Antibodies of class IgM and some of class IgA exist as multiples of this basic tetrameric, Y-shaped structure. Further details of antibody structure, classification, and function are given in Chapter 2.

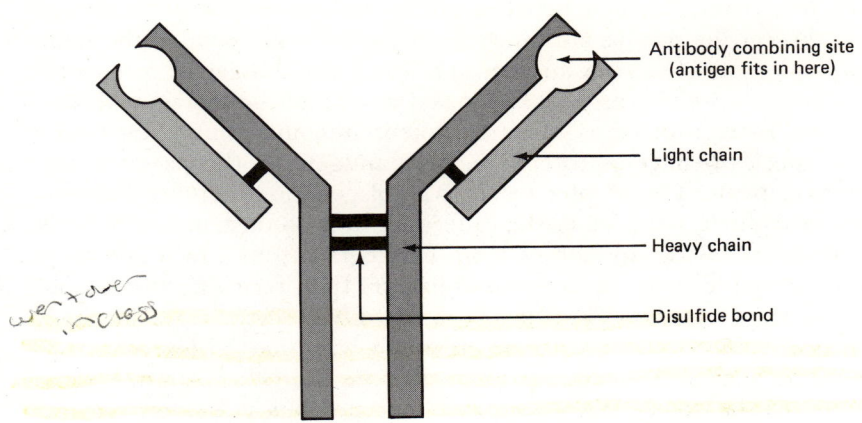

FIGURE 1.4. Model of a common immunoglobulin of class G (IgG).

"Cellular" Immunity. Some kinds of lymphocytes do not make an antibody response to antigens, but rather release chemicals called **lymphokines** that activate cells of the host. Some of these lymphokines cause mitotic activity in other lymphocytes; others attract macrophages or lymphocytes. Still other lymphokines cause the destruction of virally infected cells, etc. The protection afforded by these kinds of lymphocytes is sometimes called "cellular" immunity. This aspect of the immune system will be discussed in greater detail in Chapters 9 and 10. Each lymphocyte involved in either humoral or cellular immunity appears to respond specifically to one kind of antigen or to the molecular variants of an antigen that are nearly identical.

Types of Immunity

If the individual develops his own antibodies, he is said to have **active immunity.** If he receives antibodies or immune cells from another individual, this is **passive immunity.** Both forms of immunity may be attained **naturally** or **artificially.** Natural active immunity is developed when an immunologically competent individual contacts the antigen in his environment, as when he steps on a rusty nail or ingests microorganisms with his food. Natural passive immunity develops in mammals by one or two routes, both from the mother. Some antibodies may cross the placenta (only those of class IgG can do this), and some secretory antibodies of class IgA may cross the epithelium of the mammary ducts and be present in the mother's milk (especially in colostrum) and subsequently are absorbed by the newborn from its gastrointestinal (GI) tract. Artificial active immunity results from, for example, vaccination against smallpox (variola virus) by the purposeful introduction of cross-reacting cowpox (vaccinia) virus into the patient. Cowpox is probably the naturally occurring ancestor of human vaccinia virus. Artificial passive immunity can be conferred on an individual that receives specific antibodies in the serum from another individual of the same (homologous) or different (heterologous) species. For example, heterologous antitetanus antibodies made in a horse or goat or (preferably, if available) in a human should probably be administered to a person who has a puncture wound and who has not been immunized to tetanus within the past five years. A major problem for an immunologically competent individual receiving passive immunity from another individual of the same species (and especially from another species) is the danger of a harmful systemic hypersensitivity response acquired as a result of contact with foreign serum. Foreign proteins are often potent antigens; antibodies from a different species behave as foreign protein antigens in the passively immunized recipient. The greater the degree of genetic difference between the two individuals, the greater the difference in protein structure is likely to be. Thus, receiving antibodies from members of one's own species is much more desirable for passive immunization than receiving them from another species. Furthermore, passive immunity is short-lived. Passively derived antibodies are degraded exponentially with time within the recipient, so that after several weeks or months the individual is once again susceptible to the disease and retains no "immunological memory" of the first encounter with the antigen. Table 1.2 summarizes the major attributes of active and passive immunities.

Table 1.2 Comparison of Active and Passive Immunities

	Type of Immunity	
	Active	Passive
Source of Ab	Self	Non-self
Immunizing agent	Antigen	Immune serum (antibodies)
Relative effectiveness in:		
Newborn	Low	Moderate to high
Adult	High	Moderate to low
Relative effective dosage required	Small	Large
Latent period (approximate time from immunization until it becomes effective)	5 days to 2 weeks	None (immediately effective)
Relative length of immunity	Long but variable (may be lifelong)	Short (up to 2 or 3 months)
Usual route of injection	Intramuscular or intradermal	Intravenous
Function	Prophylactic	Therapeutic and/or prophylactic
Undesirable effects attending:		
Natural immunity	Disease*	Usually none†
Artificial immunity	Usually none‡	Serum sickness (systemic hypersensitivity reaction)

* Most common infections are subclinical and detected only retrospectively in serological screening "field" studies.
† Rh disease (q.v.), antiplatelet antibodies and other exceptions are known.
‡ Some patients may develop a local hypersensitivity reaction to the foreign proteins of the animal in which a virus is grown (e.g., chicken egg proteins). Some vaccinations (e.g., typhoid, cholera) may be painful (due to presence of endotoxin lipopolysaccharide in antigen) at the injection site. This may cause nausea, generalized aches, fatigue, etc. With some infectious ("live") virus vaccines, generalized disease due to dissemination of the immunizing virus can occur in immunologically "compromised" (deficient) individuals.

"VACCINES" AND "VACCINATIONS"

Technically, the term "vaccine" should only be applied to cowpox virus when used as an antigen to stimulate immunity to the cross-reacting smallpox virus (the Latin word "vacca" refers to "cow"). In general usage, however, vaccination is often employed synonymously with immunization. A **vaccine,** therefore, is an antigen preparation designed to stimulate a favorable immune response. There are various ways to render microorganisms or their toxic products harmless. Microorganisms that are unable to cause disease are said to be **avirulent** or **nonpathogenic.** One way is to kill or inactivate them with heat, radiation, or chemicals. The Salk polio vaccine is prepared by chemically inactivating all three strains or "antigenic types" of the virus with formaldehyde. Diphtheria and tetanus toxins are also rendered harmless, yet retain their antigenicity, by treatment with formaldehyde. These latter preparations are called **toxoids.** Vaccines may also utilize **attenuated** (weakened) microorganisms as antigens. Pathogens may be artifically attenuated by judicious use of heat, chemicals, desiccation, growth in tissue culture, and serial passages through unnatural hosts. Louis Pasteur discovered that vaccines made from dried spinal cords of rabid animals could safely induce immunity to rabies. He also discovered that inoculation of aged cultures of chicken cholera organisms conferred immunity to this disease in poultry. Furthermore, he found that attenuated cultures of anthrax bacilli grown at 42°C could be used to induce immunity in sheep to normally virulent inoculations of 37°C cultures of the organism. Albert Sabin developed an attenuated polio vaccine by growing the viruses in tissue cultures. The Sabin vaccine is pleasantly administered orally by ingesting the attenuated viruses seeded on a sugar cube. These weakened viruses can multiply in the salivary glands and other parts of the digestive tract, but have lost the capacity to invade nerve tissue. A fundamental difference between a living attenuated virus vaccine and a "killed" (inactivated) vaccine is that the latter must supply all of the antigen required for immunization. A much smaller dose of attenuated virus can be administered as a vaccine because of the great amplification of antigen that occurs as a result of viral replication. Whether there is any difference in the degree of immunity conferred by the Sabin and the Salk vaccines is still a subject of debate.

Antigens entering the body via the mucous membranes, as is true of the Sabin preparation, are more likely to stimulate secretory antibodies of class IgA, but other classes of immunoglobulins are also produced. IgA antibodies are less likely to be produced in response to intramuscular injections of the Salk vaccine. Many immunologists now tend to favor the use of vaccines that mimic subclinical infections of natural diseases. Indeed, the currently used vaccines against smallpox, measles, mumps, rubella, and yellow fever all contain living attentuated viruses. One potential disadvantage of live virus vaccines is the remote possibility of mutations that could restore virulence to an otherwise attenuated culture. If there were no difference in the safety and immunogenicity of inactivated vs. attenuated vaccines, then economics alone would probably favor the use of the latter. Historically, however, inadequate methods of vaccine preparation on occasion have failed to completely inactivate viruses, causing active disease in

Serology and Immunology

some of the recipients. There have also been some unfortunate repercussions from the use of viruses grown in cell cultures later shown to be carriers of oncogenic ("tumor-producing") simian RNA viruses.

Weakly antigenic substances can sometimes be made more immunogenic by mixing them with other materials. Any material that enhances the antigenicity of another substance is called an **adjuvant**. A very popular adjuvant for experimental animals is Freund's adjuvant. Incomplete Freund's adjuvant consists of mineral oil and an emulsifying agent. Complete Freund's adjuvant also contains dead mycobacteria. An aqueous solution of antigen is mixed vigorously with the adjuvant, producing a water-in-oil emulsion. It is hypothesized that injection of such a relatively insoluble mixture either subcutaneously or intramuscularly forms a depot from which antigen is released slowly over a prolonged period of time. It is a well-known principle of immunology that repeated contact with antigen, rather than the amount of antigen per se, is important in the production of high antibody titers. Thus, the Freund's adjuvant-antigen mixture persists much longer than would soluble antigen, providing continuous "boosting" doses as it is gradually released from the depot at the site of inoculation. Freund's adjuvant causes a granuloma or sterile abscess to form at the injection site; this reaction is exacerbated by mycobacteria. These granulomas contain large numbers of marcophages that are known to be instrumental in antigen processing and stimulation of antibody production by lymphocytes. Granuloma formation is an undesirable side effect that makes Freund's adjuvant unacceptable for use in humans.

Particulate antigens are generally more efficiently phagocytosed than are soluble antigens. Therefore, coupling soluble antigens to any of a variety of particulate "carriers" such as alum, bentonite, latex, or calcium phosphate may enhance their immunogenic capacity. When protein antigens are mixed with aluminum compounds, they are adsorbed and form a precipitate. When injected subcutaneously or intramuscularly, these mixtures may facilitate slow release of antigen, thereby enhancing phagocytosis and stimulating lymphocyte activity. Alum-precipitated antigens do not induce the intense local granulomatous reactions of Freund's adjuvant and therefore are more useful for stimulating immunity in humans. Alum-precipitated toxoids (APT) are commonly used for vaccinating against diphtheria and tetanus. Adjuvants are widely used in vaccines for two major reasons. One reason is because a single dose of an adjuvated antigen may elicit the same immune response as several separate "booster doses" of unadjuvated antigen. This minimizes trauma to the patient, eliminates the need for repeated visits by the patient to the clinic, and reduces the costs of materials and professional labor. A second reason is because a smaller amount of adjuvated antigen may be used, thus allowing more doses to be prepared from a single batch of highly purified and costly antigen.

Exposure to antigens may occur in a number of ways. The term **antigenization** is noncommittal, implying only that the individual is exposed to an antigen. It does not necessarily imply that the exposure will result in or is intended for beneficial aspects of stimulating the immune system, as is the case with the term **immunization.** Antigens may gain entry into the body by various routes. They may be accidently introduced by cuts or scarifications in the skin, by animal bites or stings, or by being inhaled or ingested. They may be artificially introduced into the body by injections (e.g., "vaccinations") into the skin (intradermal, intracutaneous), under the skin (SC = subcutaneous), into the muscle (IM = intramuscular), into the bloodstream by way of the veins (IV = intravenous), etc. Antigens may also be artificially introduced into the body via the GI tract, as is done with the Sabin oral vaccine for poliomyelitis. Polio viruses normally gain entry into the body by this route and multiply in the nasopharynx and/or lining of the GI tract before dissemination via the lymphatic system into nerve tissue where they may ultimately cause paralysis. Other mucous membranes offer sites for antigenization, as commonly occurs naturally with respiratory disease organisms. The nasopharynx is commonly used to immunize cattle against herpes virus of infectious bovine rhinotracheitis (IBR), and the conjunctiva of the eye is used to immunize chickens against the viruses of laryngotracheitis and bronchitis. The venereal contact diseases of syphilis and gonorrhea are caused by pathogens that invade the mucous membranes of the urogenital tract, but effective vaccines for these diseases have not yet been produced. A few microorganisms are capable of entering the fetus from the mother across the placenta (i.e., syphilis).

TYPICAL RESPONSES OF THE IMMUNOLOGICALLY COMPETENT INDIVIDUAL

The immune system develops gradually during the embryological period. By a mysterious process near the time of birth, the infant gains most of its ability to distinguish foreign substances from self-molecules. Additional immunological capabilities are gradually gained during the postnatal period, reaching maturity in the late teens or early adult years. The functional capacity of the immune system then declines progressively with old age.

Once the individual has attained **immunological maturity** or **competence** (i.e., the ability to respond to a given antigenic stimulus), the general response to that antigen is fairly predictable. A period of several days to about two weeks usually elapses from the time that the individual is exposed to the antigen until the time that specific antibodies can be detected in the serum, depending on many variables such as the resolution limit of the serological test. This initial phase is called **latent period.** Following the latent period, antibody titers rise rapidly for several weeks, peak, and then begin a slow decline. This is the **primary response** (Figure 1.5). Without further antigenic stimulation, the level of antibodies may remain low for a prolonged period of time or disappear altogether. There is great variation in this respect from one antigen to another and from one individual to another. In some cases, a single immunization appears sufficient to induce lifelong immunity, as happens with smallpox vaccination. In other cases, immunization may induce immunity for only a season, as happens with various strains of influenza viruses. If a booster dose of the same antigen is given during the "decay" or "decline" phase of the primary response, there may be an immediate drop in the level of detectable circulating free antibody in the patient's serum. This would be attributed to antibodies of the primary response complexing with the newly introduced antigen, thus leaving less free antibody in circulation. In only a few days, however, the titer of

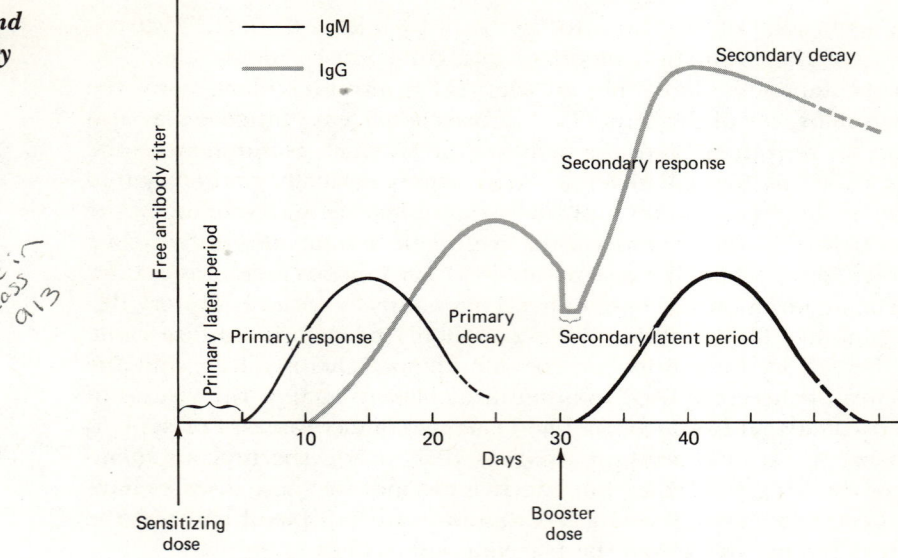

FIGURE 1.5. Diagram of a typical immune response.

antibodies should begin to rapidly increase in what is called the **secondary** or **anamnestic response.** The secondary latent period is shorter than the primary latent period. The slope of the anamnestic response curve is steeper, and the antibody level attained in the secondary response is generally higher and decays slower than that of the primary response.

The term "anamnestic" literally means "not forgetting," hence "remembering." This memory response, which is both faster and more exaggerated than the primary response, is attributed largely to two facts. In the first place, primary stimulation has produced by division a large number of committed immunoblast memory cells (members of a clone), all with the capacity to react with one and the same antigen. In the second place, each memory cell has undergone partial differentiation toward becoming a plasma cell. Hence, secondary contact with homologous antigen requires less time for the memory cell to convert to antibody production.

Antibodies of class IgM are about six times the molecular weight of those of class IgG. The initial primary immune response is usually IgM, but later in the primary response IgG production predominates. The secondary immune reaction simultaneously produces a relatively feeble IgM response by "virgin" lymphocytes that have not previously contacted antigen and a strong IgG response by "experienced" lymphocytes that have partially differentiated as a consequence of previous antigenic stimulation. Because of their large size, IgM molecules generally make good serological agglutinins. IgG molecules, on the other hand, are often too small to act as serological agglutinins unless special conditions are provided in the test tube. Since most commercial antisera used in the clinical laboratory are derived from hyperimmunized ("boosted") animals, antibodies for serological tests are commonly IgG.

IMMUNE RESPONSES OF THE NEWBORN

Because of the newborn's relative immunological incompetence or immaturity, its capacity to respond to antigens is restricted, but not completely so. Most of the newborn's antibodies are not self-made, but rather are of maternal origin and are transmitted to the offspring across the placenta and/or by way of the early milk, colostrum. As the maternal antibodies of class IgG in the baby become catabolized over the first few weeks to months of life, the infant's own immune system gains functional capacity to partially compensate for the progressive loss of specific protection formerly afforded only by the maternal antibodies. There is a crucial period in the life of a child when immunization should not be attempted for two main reasons. First, the level of maternal antibodies may still be so high that they combine with and "neutralize" the antigen before it can reach the lymphoid tissues, and thus the antigen fails to stimulate the infant's immune system. Second, the baby's own immune system may still be so immature that a good response is not obtained on exposure to a specific antigen.

Physicians are aware that during the critical first few months of life the baby is almost totally dependent on maternal antibodies for defense against certain diseases such as diphtheria, tetanus, measles, polioviruses, and coxsackieviruses. Yet they dare not wait too long to immunize the baby for fear of infection by a pathogen and subsequent disease after maternal antibodies have disappeared. Many physicians therefore begin DPT (diphtheria, pertussis, tetanus) immunizations at about one to two months of age, and follow it with subsequent immunizations, or booster doses, at about four months and six months. Table 1.3 summarizes the current immunization recommendations against some of the major communicable diseases. Most states now require that all children entering grade school at about five years of age be immunized against diphtheria, whooping cough (pertussis), tetanus, measles, polio, and rubella.

THE END OF SMALLPOX

The last natural outbreak of variola major occurred October 26, 1977, in Merka, Somalia. In October 1979, the World Health Organization (WHO) officially announced that the world was free of smallpox. This is the first instance of an infectious disease being eradicated from the earth. Because the virus has bred remarkably true and does not mutate to new antigenic types (as with influenza virus) every few years, it is improbable that a mutant variety will suddenly appear. It is still not known if the virus exists in animals. Diligent search for animal reservoirs has not disclosed any. WHO plans to recommend that member countries stop all vaccinations against smallpox. Travelers will no longer need smallpox certificates. This will save the world community about a billion dollars a year that can be diverted to solving other health problems. The use of "live" virus vaccines is not completely free of risk. For example, if cowpox vaccine is given to an individual who is deficient in cell-mediated immunity, that person may not be able to arrest the multiplication of the virus and is likely to succumb to a generalized vaccinia.

Table 1.3 RECOMMENDED IMMUNIZATION SCHEDULE

Disease	Immunizing Agent	Primary Immunization Interval(s)	Booster Doses
Diphtheria Tetanus Pertussis	Diphtheria and tetanus immunogens available as monovalent toxoids or combined with pertussis antigen (DPT)	Three IM injections at 4–8 weeks; fourth IM injection at 1 year	One IM booster at 3–6 years, preferably at time of school entrance. Over 6 years booster every 10 years for life
Influenza	Inactivated (killed) polyvalent, bivalent, or monovalent influenza virus vaccine (grown in chick embryo tissue)	6–35 months, two IM or SC doses; 3–5 years, two doses; 6 years and older, one dose	Seasonally for high-risk groups (the elderly and those with chronic illness)
Measles (rubeola)	*Active:* Attenuated (live) measles virus vaccine. Various combinations of measles-mumps-rubella vaccines are available *Passive:* Measles immune serum globulin or standard immune serum globulin	*Active:* One SC injection at 15 months or older *Passive:* One IM injection within 6 days of exposure at any age if not actively immunized, especially if in high-risk groups (the immunologically deficient and infants)	No boosters required. Older children who received measles vaccines prior to 1968 may need boosters if (a) they received a killed measles vaccine, (b) vaccine was given before 1 year of age, (c) measles vaccine given with an uncertain dose of measles immune globulin
Mumps	Attenuated (live) mumps virus vaccine	One SC injection at 12 months or older	No boosters required
Poliomyelitis	Sabin agent = attenuated (live) oral trivalent (types 1, 2, 3 combined) poliovirus vaccine	At least three oral doses must be given for effectiveness beginning at 2 months of age; 6–8 weeks should elapse between doses 1 and 2, 8–12 months between doses 2 and 3	Preschool and when traveling to endemic areas
	Salk agent = inactive (killed) trivalent (types 1, 2, 3 combined) poliovirus vaccine	Four IM injections beginning at 2 months of age; 4 weeks should elapse between doses 1 and 2, 2 and 3; 6–12 months between doses 3 and 4	Regular booster doses every few (?) years

Table 1.3 (*Continued*)

Disease	Immunizing Agent	Primary Immunization Interval(s)	Booster Doses
Rubella	Attenuated (live) rubella virus vaccine	One SC injection at 12 months or older. MUST NOT BE GIVEN DURING PREGNANCY! Women of childbearing age may be considered for immunization if advised of the necessity to avoid pregnancy for at least two months following vaccine administration	No boosters required

(SOURCE: October 1977 State of California Department of Health, Infectious Disease Section)

Phylogeny of the Immune System

The immune system reaches its highest development in the "warm-blooded" or homeothermic vertebrates such as birds and mammals. Both specific cellular and humoral responses are present in all vertebrates. Even some of the most primitive jawless (agnathan) vertebrates exhibit these responses in the absence of a thymus and other definitive lymphoid tissues. All jawed vertebrates or gnathostomes possess a primary lymphoid organ called the thymus and specialized secondary lymphoid organs such as lymph nodes and spleen. Immunologically incompetent stem cells of the immune system arise in blood-forming or hematopoietic tissues such as bone marrow, embryonic yolk sac, fetal liver, and spleen. From there, the stem cells migrate to the thymus or the bursa of Fabricius in birds (or its equivalent in other animals) and divide to produce populations of immunologically competent lymphocytes. Some of these lymphocytes will remain in the primary lymphoid organs; others will travel to the secondary lymphoid organs where the final stage in lymphocyte differentiation occurs. After contacting antigen, lymphocytes possessing homologous cell-surface receptors divide to produce a clone of cells, some becoming effector cells and others functioning as memory cells. The major difference between the mitotic activity of lymphocytes in the primary and secondary lymphoid tissues is that the former is antigen-independent whereas the latter is antigen-driven.

Nonimmunoglobulin agglutinins and lysins are known to exist in many invertebrates. These humoral substances function to sequester foreign materials and are sometimes referred to as "protoimmunoglobulins." Immunoglobulins and certain proteins of the classical complement pathway have not been found in invertebrates. The only immunoglobulin found in agnathans such as the lamprey is IgM. Presumably IgM is the most primitive class of immunoglobulin, but the phylogenetic origin of the other classes is unresolved. All higher vertebrates have a complete complement system. By contrast, cell-mediated immunity is widely represented among invertebrates by cells that resemble lymphocytes (hemocytes, coelomocytes), but that may originate from sources different from those in vertebrates and possibly possess abilities to differentiate along completely different lines. The most primitive cells of the immune system are phagocytes exhibiting the ability to distinguish self from foreign components. Even single-celled protozoans exhibit this self-recognition phenomenon. Phagocytosis in these lowly animals most obviously functions in acquisition of food. Some phagocytic cells of higher animals evolved as scavenger cells to remove foreign debris without necessarily contributing to the nutritional needs of the organism. Phagocytic cells generally lack specificity and/or memory and usually fail to be mitotically stimulated by contact with specific antigens. Rejection of foreign tissue grafts is a hallmark of cell-mediated immunity and is demonstrable in some of the lowliest metazoans (multicellular animals) such as the coelenterates (corals, hydroids, etc.). In comparison with vertebrates, the cell-mediated immunity of invertebrates tends to be more restrictive in the range of "foreignness" recognized by its histocompatibility system. Graft rejection is slower and memory is shorter. The anamnestic response may be poor or absent because of limited antigen-stimulated cellular proliferation on first contact with the antigen. Because of these limitations, some immunologists refer to the defensive capabilities of invertebrates against foreign materials as "protoimmune responses" or "quasi-immune responses."

The ability to discriminate between foreign molecules and self components has undoubtedly been an important component of biological fitness in the evolution of the immune system. Those organisms that could recognize and destroy invading microorganisms would have an adaptive advantage in the "struggle for existence," and their genes would be represented in proportionately greater numbers in succeeding generations. If an organism dies of cancer before maturity (reproductive age), the individual will have no fitness (leaves no progeny). New antigens (neoantigens) tend to appear on many kinds of cancerous cells. Therefore, the ability to recognize and destroy cells bearing these "foreign" markers would also be selectively advantageous. **Immunological surveillance** is the term given to that function of the immune system concerned with the recognition and destruction of neoplastic (cancer) cells.

There has been a long evolutionary history in the development of the highly complex vertebrate immune system, and it is therefore not surprising to find some immune capabilities in the lower animals. Elements of the older "immune" responses have not been discarded in the evolution of the higher forms, but have been retained and become a highly integrated and regulated system involving macrophages, lymphocytes, antibodies, lymphokines, and complement.

Ontogeny of the Immune System

Lymphocytes are produced from stem cells in the bone marrow. In the chicken, lymphocytes released from the bone marrow may mature in either of two organs. There is a saclike structure that opens into the cloaca, called the **bursa of Fabricius** (Figure 1.6). If lymphocytes mature in the bursa they become capable of producing antibodies in response to the correct

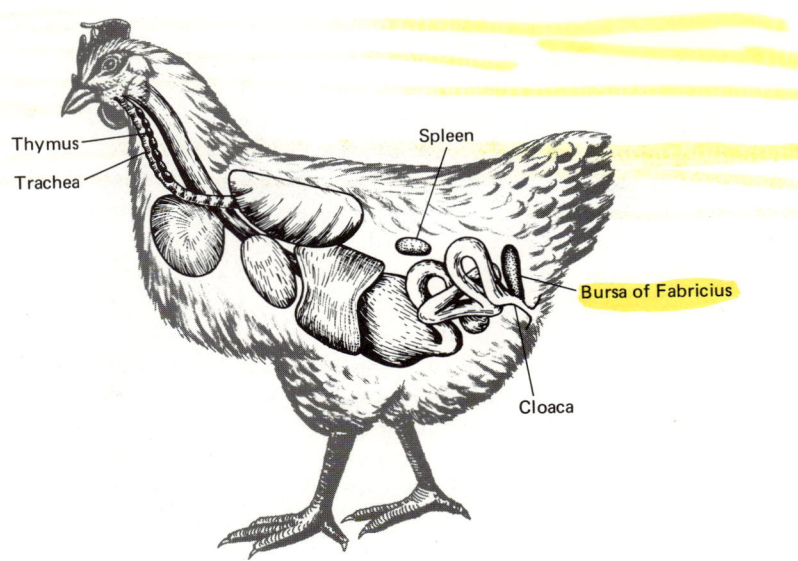

FIGURE 1.6. Diagram of the immune system of the chicken. The bird's thymus consists of seven pairs of lobes in the neck region. The bursa of Fabricius is a saclike structure associated with the terminal portion of the gut.

antigenic stimulus. These are called **B lymphocytes** or **B cells** (B, for bursa). In their mature state as plasma cells, they are responsible for the production of antibodies and humoral immunity. A second organ, found in the neck region of the chicken, is the **thymus.** The human thymus is a bilobed organ in the front of the chest just behind the top of the sternum. It generally increases in proportion with growth of the individual until eight or ten years of age. Thereafter, it begins to atrophy. For technical reasons, the thymus of experimental animals has been much more thoroughly studied than that of humans. The mouse thymus reaches its peak of activity within a few days after birth. Early removal of the thymus renders the mouse more susceptible to certain infectious agents and unable to reject tissue grafts from genetically dissimilar donors later in life. These neonatally thymectomized mice grow slowly and usually die within a few months as runts. During this early period, the thymus is thought to supply the other lymphoid tissues with uncommitted lymphocytes. It also liberates one or more hormones that enhance the maturation of certain thymic lymphocytes or **thymocytes** and that of the disseminated lymphocytes in lymph nodes, spleen, and other lymphoid tissues. Once these functions have been performed, the thymus is no longer an essential organ and usually begins to atrophy. Several protein thymic hormones have been found in calf thymus (calf thymus and/or pancreas are called "sweetbread") and given names such as thymosin, thymopoietin, thymic humoral factor, and lymphocyte-stimulating hormones. These hormones have been variously implicated in such activities as helping stimulate antibody-producing cells, maturation of thymocytes, increasing graft-vs.-host reactions, increasing thymocyte numbers, protecting thymectomized mice against runting disease, and enhancing skin transplant rejection. Most of these functions will be discussed more fully in later chapters.

Serology and Immunology

If lymphocytes mature in the thymus, they become **T lymphocytes** or **T cells** (T, for thymus), responsible for cellular immunity, immunological surveillance, tissue graft rejection, and delayed hypersensitivity reactions. T cells respond to specific antigens by the release of various low molecular weight polypeptides called **lymphokines.** These substances usually cause responses in other cells of the host rather than reacting with antigen the way that antibodies do. Some lymphokines play important roles in the inflammatory process by attracting phagocytic cells to the region of T cell–antigen interaction. Other lymphokines induce uncommitted T lymphocytes (ones not directly stimulated by antigen) to undergo several division cycles to produce a **clone** of descendants, all genetically identical through mitosis and with the physiological capacity to react specifically with the same antigen. When this clone of cells also pours out lymphokines, there is a tremendous biological amplification of the immune response initiated by the original T cell–antigen interaction. T and B lymphocytes have many other distinguishing characteristics, most of which are summarized in Table 1.4.

Mammals have a thymus gland, but do not possess a bursa of Fabricius. Where in mammals do B lymphocytes originate? They are predominantly found in the medullary regions of lymph nodes throughout the body, but they may arise in various dispersed **gut-associated lymphoid tissues** (GALT) as the analog of the compact bursa of the chicken. These GALT include the appendix, Peyer's patches of the intestinal mucosa, tonsils, and other lymphoid structures of the alimentary canal.

The most fundamental rule of immunology is that the body does not mount an immunological response to its own normal constituents that are accessible to lymphocytes. This principle, recognized long ago by Paul Ehrlich, prompted his dictum of "horror autotoxicus," which literally means that the body abhors poisoning itself. How the body can recognize and mount an attack against only foreign chemicals and not self molecules is still one of the greatest mysteries of immunology.

Before birth, the immune system of mammals generally has not yet completely matured to learn self from nonself. By the time of birth, however, gradual recognition of self antigens has been made, and soon thereafter the immune system generally responds only to "foreign" substances, i.e., those molecular structures not present in the individual as the ability to recognize "self" constituents developed. It is possible to introduce into a fetal mammal or some newborn mammals many substances or tissues that would be foreign and antigenic at a later stage in its life. A substance of this nature would probably be recognized as self, and when challenged later in life by the same antigen the animals would not be expected to mount an immune response to it. This phenomenon of specific **immune tolerance** is now a well-established principle of immunology. Immunological tolerance has also been reported to occur naturally in **dizygotic** (two-egg, hence genetically nonidentical) cattle twins. In this species, placental vascular anastomoses between twins is very common. Stem cells from each twin are exchanged early in embryological development, and each individual becomes a **chimera,** harboring some cells with the genotype and antigens of its twin. As adults, these twins are mutually immunologically tolerant of blood transfusions or tissue transplantations. The sharing of common blood vessels between twins in other species appears to be rare or nonexistent.

Table 1.4 DISTINGUISHING CHARACTERISTICS OF B AND T LYMPHOCYTES

Attributes	B Lymphocyte	T Lymphocyte
Site of maturation	Bursa of Fabricius (birds) or bursal equivalent (mammals)	Thymus
Mature stage of differentiation (transformation)	Plasma cell	T_H, T_C, T_D, T_A, T_S
Products	Antibodies	Lymphokines
Major immune functions	Bacterial opsonization and lysis through complement activation	Antiviral; antifungal; tumor and transplant rejection
Portion of conjugated antigen to which reactivity is primarily directed	Hapten	Carrier
Relative concentration in peripheral blood	Low (1–15%)	High (75–85%)
Relative sensitivity to immunosuppression	High	Low
Relative ease of induction of immune tolerance	Low	High
Relative response to antilymphocyte serum (ALS)	Low	High
Relative lifespan	Short	Long
Nylon wool column	Adhere	Pass through
Surface antigens present (mice)	β or B	Thy 1 (θ or T)
Surface receptors present		
Immunoglobulins	Yes	No
Fc receptors (for IgG tails)	Yes	No (?)
Complement receptors	Yes (for C3)	No
Ia antigens (mouse)	Yes	No (?)
Antigen receptors	Yes (through surface immunoglobulins)	Yes (mechanism unknown)
Transformation response to mitogens	*Human* *Mouse*	*Human* *Mouse*
Concanavallin A (conA)	No No	Yes Yes
Phytohemagglutinin (PHA)	No No	Yes Yes
Purified protein derivative (tuberculin PPD)	No Yes	No No
Pokeweed mitogen (PWM)	Yes Yes	Yes Yes
Dextran or dextran sulfate	No Yes	No No
Lipopolysaccharides (LPS) from gram-negative bacteria (also known as endotoxin)	No Yes	No No

CLONAL SELECTION THEORY

The currently most useful theory of antibody production can also be extended to explain specific immune tolerance and the maturation of the immune system itself. This theory is called the **clonal selection theory.** It appears that subpopulations (clones) of "virgin" or inexperienced lymphocytes are generated during embryological development, each with the capacity to recognize and respond to a different antigenic determinant. The mechanisms that generate this diversity are unknown at present. As the capacity for self-recognition develops, it is hypothesized that all lymphocytes that have complexed with self components or foreign substances present at that time are somehow destroyed. This leaves only lymphocytes with the capacity to recognize new foreign antigenic determinants as survivors of this "selection process." After the period of self-recognition has passed in embryological development, a B lymphocyte subsequently encountering a foreign substance, to which it is programmed to respond via its specific cell-surface receptors, would be stimulated to divide and form a clone of cells, all with the capacity to respond to one and the same antigenic determinant. The term **homologous** or **cognate** antigen indicates that it is the same or identical antigen used to elicit the antibodies with which it now reacts. Thus, an antigen "selects" one or more of the cells from a clone of homologous virgin lymphocytes and specifically triggers their mitotic activity. Some of the antigen-selected cells of the clone begin to differentiate to plasma cells and antibody production. Evidence of this can be seen in electron micrographs of maturing B lymphocytes showing large amounts of endoplasmic reticulum and ribosomes for protein synthesis.

PLASMA CELLS

Mature B lymphocytes synthesizing antibody are called plasma cells. They are rich in ribosomal RNA and therefore "love pyronin" stain (pyroninophilic). Pyronin is a basic dye commonly used to stain cells rich in ribonucleic acid. Plasma cells are derived from small lymphocytes by a process of differentiation. A small lymphocyte characteristically has a centrally placed spherical or slightly indented nucleus with dense coarse chromatin (heterochromatin) and a thin rim of cytoplasm containing few organelles. This is probably the earliest stage capable of responding to antigenic stimulation and is variously termed a virgin immunocompetent cell, progenitor cell, or target cell. After antigenic stimulation, a small lymphocyte undergoes transformation into a larger cell with a more diffuse (euchromatic) nucleus and a greater cytoplasm/nucleus ratio, called an immunoblast or plasmablast. This cell has well-developed, rough endoplasmic reticulum, stains with pyronin, and is capable of limited antibody synthesis. An immunoblast may possess immunological memory and may be capable of replicating other memory cells without further antigenic stimulation. Alternatively, an immunoblast may continue differentiation and become a mature plasma cell. A plasma cell is characterized by an eccentric nucleus, a large centrosome or cytocentrum, abundant rough endoplasmic reticulum, and large Golgi vessicles filled with antibody. These antibody aggregates readily stain with eosin or other anionic (acid) dyes and are called **Russell bodies.** Fully differentiated plasma cells do not divide and are thought to be relatively short-lived, perhaps surviving only a few weeks. Because many memory cells, partly differentiated toward becoming antibody-releasing plasma cells, have been produced by the initial contact with antigen, a second contact with homologous antigen allows greater and more rapid antibody production typical of the booster response. Progenitor cells, immunoblasts, and mature plasma cells have been called X, Y, and Z cells, respectively. Figure 1.7 diagrams the major steps in B lymphocyte maturation.

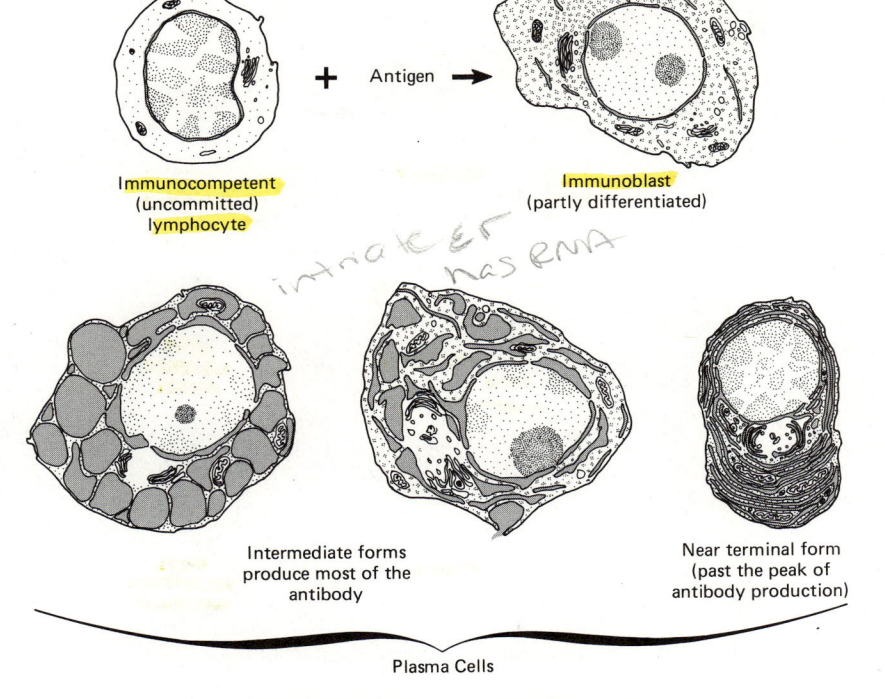

FIGURE 1.7. Major steps in B lymphocyte maturation.

Immunocytology

Bone marrow is the site from which all blood cells are derived. Undifferentiated stem cells give rise to five major blood cell lines: (1) erythrocytes (red blood cells), (2) lymphocytes, (3) monocytes (and their tissue counterparts, macrophages), (4) granulocytes (including neutrophils, basophils, and eosinophils), and (5) megakaryocytes (from which platelets are derived). All blood cells other than erythrocytes are classified as leukocytes (white blood cells).

Granulocytes are sometimes called **polymorphonuclear** (PMN) **leukocytes** because their nuclei are multilobed, giving the false impression that several nuclei are present (Figure 1.8) The cytoplasm of all three kinds of PMN cells contain granules that stain differentially. Granules of neutrophils do not take up acidic or basic dyes strongly, hence their name meaning "loves neither." These granules contain lysosomal enzymes. Neutrophils are actively phagocytic and respond to chemotactic stimuli. They are the most numerous of the leukocytes and constitute the major cell in acute inflammatory lesions. Eosinophils ("loves eosin") have large granules containing basic chemicals that stain dark red with the acidic dye eosin. The function of these cells is not well understood. They appear to be associated with antibody-mediated hypersensitivities (e.g., allergies) and with certain parasitic infestations such as nematode worms. Basophils ("loves basic

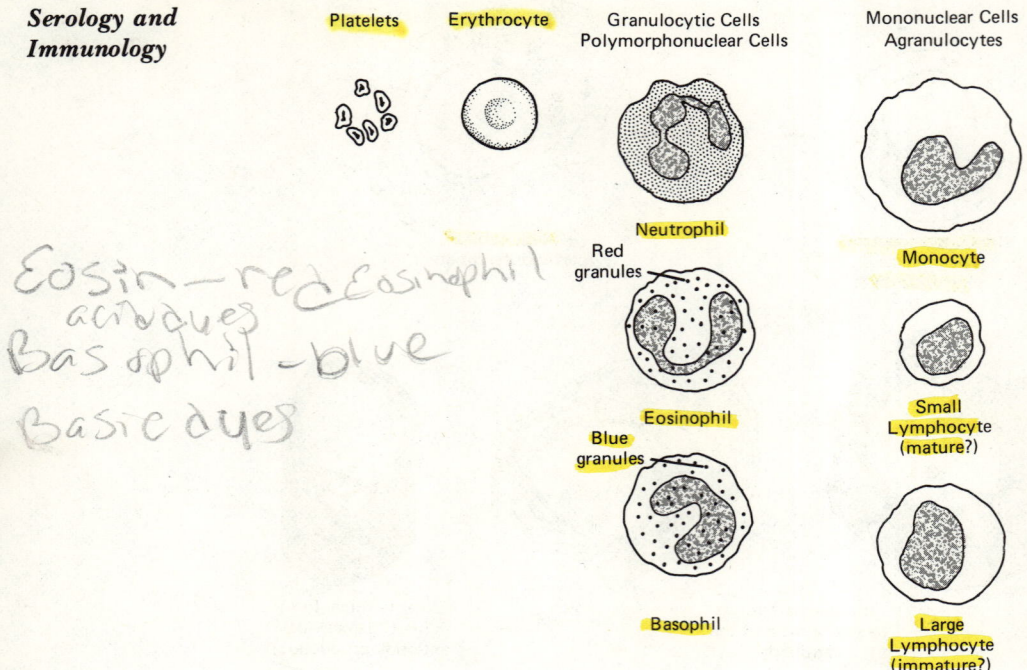

FIGURE 1.8. Diagrams of typical human blood cells.

dyes") and their tissue counterparts called mast cells possess large cytoplasmic granules that take up basic dyes. These granules are believed to contain histamine and other vasoactive amines (substances containing amino groups that cause peripheral dilation and increased capillary permeability of small blood vessels). The plasma membrane of the basophil has receptor sites for the tail end of the Y-shaped antibodies of immunoglobulin class IgE (the antibodies associated with classical allergies). The granules of eosinophils and basophils do not contain lysosomal enzymes. Wright's stain is widely used to stain blood smears for making differential leukocyte counts. It contains both the acidic dye eosin and the basic dye methylene blue. Table 1.5 lists the normal counts and percentages of these various cell types in normal human blood.

Monocytes and lymphocytes are **mononuclear leukocytes,** so called because the nucleus of each cell is a singluar globular entity. Monocytes are the largest of all circulating leukocytes. They stay in the bloodstream for a relatively short period of time and then migrate through the endothelial lining of capillaries into various tissues by a process called **diapedesis** ("leaping through") where they become **macrophages** or "big eaters." They are called histiocytes in connective tissues, Kupffer's cells in the liver, microglial cells in the nervous system, alveolar macrophages in the lung, etc. Macrophages possess receptor sites for immunoglobulins of class IgG. Any antibody that nonspecifically attaches to immunoglobulin receptors on macrophages is called a **cytophilic antibody.** The tail end of the antibody molecule attaches to the plasma membrane of the macrophage, leaving its arms free to bind antigen. This serves to facilitate phagocytosis of the anti-

Table 1.5 NORMAL CELLULAR COMPOSITION OF ADULT HUMAN BLOOD

Cell Type	No. of cells per mm³ (Microliter)	Approximate % (leukocytes)
Leukocytes (white cells)*	4,500–9,000	
Granulocytes		
Neutrophils	3,000–6,750	59 ± 15
Basophils	25–90	<1 (0.5)
Eosinophils	100–360	2 to 4
Mononuclear cells		
Lymphocytes	1,000–2,700	34 ± 10
Monocytes	150–170	3 to 8
Platelets	145,000–375,000	
Erythrocytes (red cells)	Men = 4.2–5.4 × 10⁶	
	Women = 3.6–5.0 × 10⁶	

* There is currently a trend in hematology to report results in terms of numbers of cells per liter (e.g., $4.5–9 \times 10^9/L$) rather than as cells/cubic millimeter (microliter).

gen. Phagocytic cells also possess receptors for one of the activated complement proteins (C3b). When C3b is bound to antigen-antibody compexes, they behave as though they were sticky and become easily attached to erythrocytes and other cells (including phagocytic cells) or to endothelium and other surfaces. This phenomenon, known as **immune adherence,** also enhances phagocytosis. When opsonic antibodies (cytophilic or otherwise) bind antigen, they may "fix" or activate complement, and the antigen-antibody-complement complex may then become attached to C3b receptors on phagocytic cells by immune adherence. Neutrophils and monocytes (blood macrophages) are the only blood cells considered to be highly phagocytic. Macrophages are so named because they are so much larger than neutrophils, the latter sometimes being referred to as **microphages** ("little eaters").

Immature lyphocytes that have neither the beta nor theta cell-surface antigens are called **null lymphocytes.** Those that mature in the thymus develop the theta antigen and become T cells; those that mature in the bursa of Fabricius of the chicken (or its analog in other vertebrates) develop the beta antigen and become B cells. Both B and T lymphocytes have specific surface receptors for antigens. Each cell presumably has receptors for only one kind of antigenic determinant. The receptors on virgin B lymphocytes are IgM; the IgM-like receptors on T cells have not been proven to be immunoglobulins, but are nontheless tentatively designated IgT. Some antigens (usually synthetic repeating polymers presenting an array of identical determinants and lipopolysaccharides associated with the cell walls of gram-negative bacteria) can apparently stimulate B lymphocytes without the aid of T lymphocytes. These antigens are called **thymus-independent antigens** (T-independent antigens). Antibodies of class IgM are commonly produced by T-independent antigens, and memory B cells are not produced. The existence of such antigens is easily demonstrated in animals that develop without a thymus. The nude mouse is such an animal. Homozygosity for an autosomal recessive gene (*nu*) not only produces a "hairless" phenotype, but also results in a congenital absence of a thymus.

Most natural antigens, however, fail to stimulate maturation of B lymphocytes unless T lymphocytes are also present. Such antigens are termed **thymus-dependent antigens** (T-dependent antigens). Most antigens that present a variety of antigenic determinants (e.g., natural proteins) are thymus-dependent. They generate memory cells and tend to stimulate IgG antibodies.

CELLULAR INTERACTIONS

Several theories have been proposed to explain how "helper" T lymphocytes (T_H cells) are involved in antibody production by B lymphocytes. Some of the models postulate a two-cell interaction of T_H and B lymphocytes. Other models propose a three-cell interaction involving T_H and B lymphocytes as well as macrophages and possibly other accessory cells such as dendritic reticular cells.

Interaction with T_H cells is required by B cells in order to mature into plasma cells with the capacity to liberate antibodies of classes IgG, IgA, and IgE. Small molecules that can react specifically with antibodies but cannot by themselves stimulate the immune system are called **incomplete antigens** or **haptens.** However, haptens that are artificially coupled or conjugated to larger "carrier" molecules such as proteins can stimulate antibody production. T lymphocytes tend to respond better to antigens of the carrier in such a conjugate, whereas B lymphocytes tend to respond more favorably to the added haptenic groups. According to one theory (Figure 1.9a), a T_H cell may react with antigenic determinants of the carrier molecule and concentrate the haptens into an array that is stimulatory to a B cell. Immunoglobulin receptors on B cell membranes are highly mobile. On contact with a multivalent antigen, these receptors are capable of congregating into several patches and then into a single large cluster at one position or pole on the cell surface. This phenomenon is termed **capping.** When immunoglobulin receptors on the capped B lymphocyte cross-link to the haptenic array presented to it by the T_H cell, this may provide the stimulus that activates the B cell. Capping requires the cell to expend energy in contraction of microfilaments. This, in turn, may be involved in transmission of a signal from the plasma membrane to the nucleus. The events by which this signal activates or derepresses only certain genes are not known. A stimulated B lymphocyte usually first becomes mitotically active to produce a clone of descendants, each member of which is committed to respond only to that same antigenic determinant. Later, some members of the clone differentiate into plasma cells and liberate the homologous antibody. Other cells of the clone remain as relatively long-lived memory cells. What causes some cells of the clone to differentiate into short-lived plasma cells and others to remain as long-lived memory cells is not known.

A second model to explain the helper activity of T cells proposes that when T_H cells contact antigen, they release factors that stimulate division **(mitogens)** of B cells, provided that antigen is also bound by B cells (Figure 1.9b). A third hypothesis (Figure 1.9c) involves an accessory cell, such as a macrophage, to concentrate antigen in such a way that effective contact is made between T_H and B lymphocytes. According to a fourth possibility (Figure 1.9d), after antigen is bound to a specific T-cell receptor (IgT), the

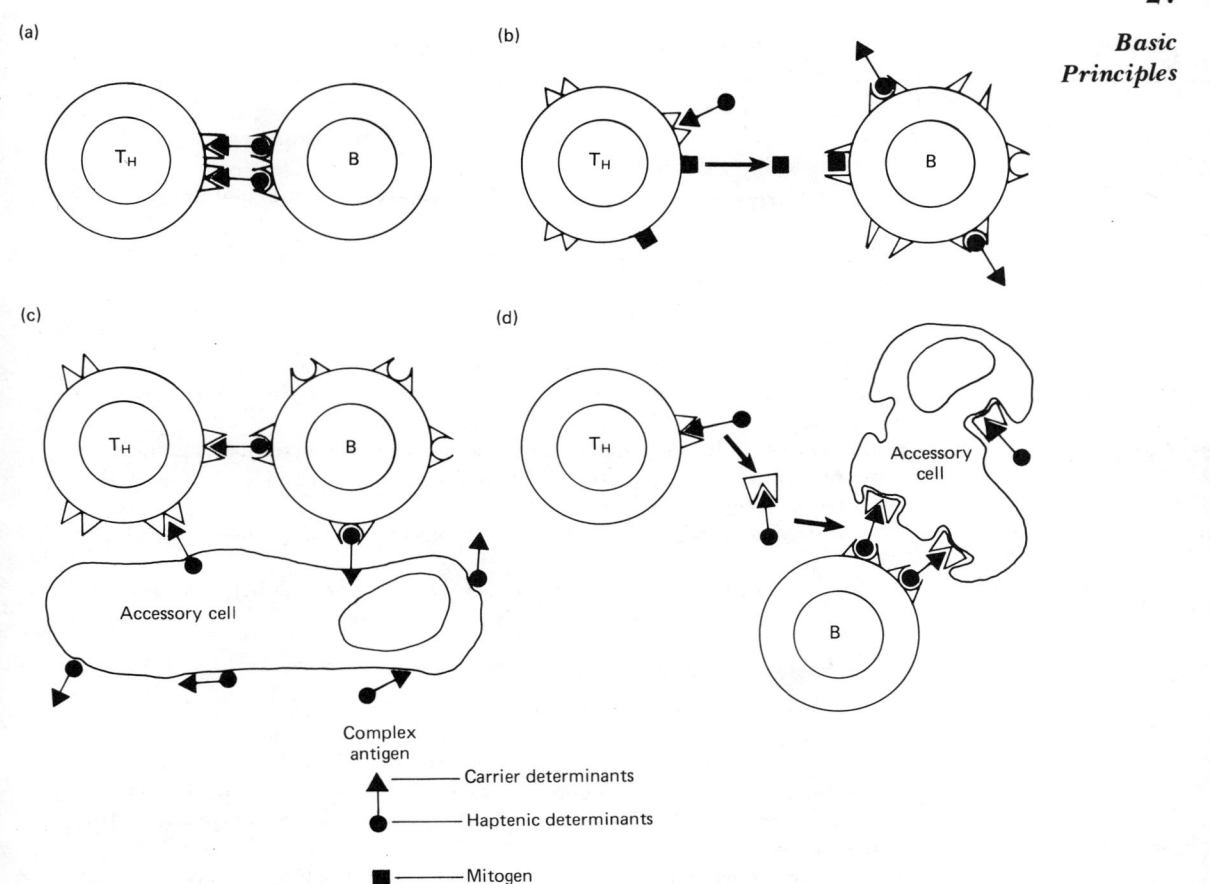

FIGURE 1.9. Four models of T cell–B cell interactions. Models *a* and *b* involve two-cell interactions; models *c* and *d* are three-cell interactions. Models *a* and *c* employ antigen bridging between the cells; models *b* and *d* propose that factors are released from T_H cells that stimulate B cells. (See text.)

IgT-antigen complex is liberated. Accessory cells would have receptors for the IgT-antigen complex and concentrate the antigen in an array that becomes stimulatory to B cells.

Several classes of lymphocytes that have effector functions other than helping stimulate B cells are known. Suppressor T (T_S) cells inhibit antibody production by B cells. In contrast to T_H cells, T_S cells are produced in response to repeating antigenic determinants. It is not known if they act on antigen-complexed accessory cells, on B cells, or on T_H cells. Neither is it known if the interaction involves soluble factors or cell-surface components. It is known, however, that B cell activities are subject to both positive and negative controls by T_H and T_S cells, respectively. There are also cytotoxic or killer T cells (T_C) that cause lysis of specific antigenic target cells, T cells that are responsible for the specific local chronic inflammatory response of delayed hypersensitivities such as those of the tuberculin skin test (T_D cells), and T cells that amplify killer T cell differentiation and proliferation (T_A cells).

SELF-EVALUATION

Terms

1. Any substance that can trigger specific responses from lymphocytes or that can react specifically with antibody.
2. A subdivision of immunology concerned with *in vitro* antigen-antibody reactions.
3. A group of cells in various organs and tissues sharing the property of phagocytosis. (2 words)
4. A term that includes the nonspecific responses of the first and second lines of defense against foreign substances, including infectious microorganisms.
5. Antibodies that are involved in clumping of particulate antigens.
6. A group of serum proteins that become activated by certain antigen-antibody complexes.
7. Antibodies that enhance phagocytosis whether they are cytophilic or not.
8. A type of immunity acquired by an individual that has received antibodies or immune cells from another individual.
9. An immunological organ in the chicken responsible for maturation of B cells. (3 words)
10. A failure or depression of specific lymphocyte response following exposure to an antigen in fetal or early postnatal life. (1 or 2 words)

Multiple Choice. Choose the one best answer.

1. Which of the following is not one of the hallmarks of the vertebrate immune response? (a) lymphocyte-mediated (b) an innate responsiveness of one's genotype apart from antigenic stimulation (c) response is directed only at the inciting antigen (d) subsequent contacts with the inciting antigen produce more vigorous responses (e) can sometimes be transferred from one individual to another via antibodies
2. Which of the following is not considered to be part of the first or second lines of defense against pathogenic microorganisms? (a) lysozyme (b) macrophage (c) antibody (d) mucus (e) pepsin
3. Mature antibody-producing cells are called (a) immunoblasts (b) histiocytes (c) T cells (d) neutrophils (e) plasma cells
4. Which of the following is not considered to be an organ or tissue containing immunologically competent cells? (a) thyroid (b) lymph node (c) spleen (d) appendix (e) Payer's patches
5. According to current practice, against which of the following diseases is a preschool child least likely to be artificially immunized? (a) measles (b) pertussis (c) polio (d) smallpox (e) diphtheria
6. Which of the following is not characteristic of a typical immune response? (a) the primary latent period is longer than the secondary latent period (b) the antibody titer of the secondary response is higher than the primary response (c) the secondary response tends to be longer-lasting than the primary response (d) the first antibody to appear is usually IgG (e) more than one of the above is not characteristic of a typical immune response
7. A vaccine labeled APT would most likely be used to immunize against (a) diphtheria (b) smallpox (c) measles (d) whooping cough (e) anthrax
8. Which of the following is characteristic of T cells? (a) they possess surface immunoglobulins (b) they mature in lymph nodes (c) they secrete lymphokines (d) they respond primarily to the haptenic component of a hapten-carrier complex (e) more than one of these choices is correct
9. Which of the following treatments is not used in the production of vaccines? (a) heat (b) formaldehyde (c) growth in tissue culture (d) desiccation (e) sonication

10. Which of the following is not associated with an enhanced immune response to microorganisms or their products? (a) bacteriolysins (b) antibiotics (c) agglutinins (d) opsonins (e) antitoxins

True-False

1. Immune responses can unequivocally be classified as either harmful or beneficial.
2. Nonsusceptibility is an innate refractoriness to a potential pathogen.
3. B cells respond to most natural antigens only by interaction with certain T cells.
4. Antibodies are produced by all animals possessing a circulatory system.
5. Pyronin is an acidic dye commonly used to stain antibody proteins in plasma cells.
6. It is generally conceded that each B lymphocyte can respond to the full range of antigens to which the host organism in total reacts.
7. Dizygotic cattle twins share a common blood supply and hence become immunologically tolerant of one another's antigens.
8. Babies should be vaccinated against infectious diseases before the titer of maternal antibodies begins to wane.
9. Passive and active immunities generally have about the same longevity.
10. Phagocytic cells generally react nonspecifically toward antigens.

CHAPTER 2
Antigens and Antibodies

CHAPTER OUTLINE

Antigens
   Characteristics of Antigens
   Haptens
   Immunological Valence
   Antigenic Determinants
Fractionation of Serum
Structure of Immunoglobulin G
Immunoglobulin Classification
   Immunoglobulin G
   Immunoglobulin M
   Immunoglobulin A

Immunoglobulin D
Immunoglobulin E
Antibody Production By Single Cells
Genetic Control of Antibody Diversity
The Antibody-combining Site
Preparation of Purified Serological Reagents
Serological Tests
   Specificity-Sensitivity
Self-evaluation

Antigens

CHARACTERISTICS OF ANTIGENS

An antigen or immunogen is any substance that elicits specific activation of lymphocytes. Generally, the most potent antigens are proteins. Polysaccharides are usually weaker antigens by themselves, but are highly antigenic coupled to proteins. Lipopolysaccharides (LPS) of gram-negative bacteria are also potent antigens. The least potent antigens are pure lipids and nucleic acids, but anti-DNA and anti-RNA antibodies are produced in some autoimmune disease states. In general, larger-molecular-weight proteins are likely to have more amino acids with reactive side groups that furnish multiple immunological **determinant sites** (antigenic sites, reactive sites) for activating lymphocytes. Usually substances must be over 10,000 daltons in molecular weight to be good antigens. Low-molecular-weight substances such as insulin (5,700 daltons), histones (6,000 daltons), and glucagon (4,600 daltons) are poor antigens.

In addition to molecular size, molecular complexity is also an important attribute of antigenicity. Proteins are polypeptides made from twenty species of amino acids. Different proteins have different compositions of amino acids, different lengths and shapes, and different chemical side groups (radicals) available as reactive antigenic determinants. The sequence of amino acids in a polypeptide chain constitutes the primary structure of the protein. This, in turn, determines its secondary structure (alpha helix) and tertiary structure (folding into globular, ellipsoidal, or other shapes). Some proteins function only when two or more polypeptides (identical or different chains) associate into a quarternary structure. Each level of complexity may contribute to antigenicity. A single amino acid substitution may produce a new antigenic specificity in the protein and also may profoundly alter the secondary and higher structural levels of organization. Such restructured proteins can exhibit different biological properties. They may partly or completely lose biological functions (e.g., loss of catalytic activity as enzymes), and/or their antigenicity or serological reactivity may be altered. A polysaccharide seldom consists of more than four or five different sugars. Because they can form branching structures, polysaccharides are capable of greater sequence diversity than proteins. Deoxyribonucleic acid (DNA) consists of only four basic units (nucleotides) in a regular double helix. It is the largest known biopolymer, but it is usually a poor antigen because most of its chemically reactive groups in each chain are hidden internally. RNA molecules, being single-stranded, usually have some unpaired nucleotides that can function as antigenic determinants.

Certain amino acids tend to be more frequently found in antigenic sites than others; they are called **immunodominant** groups. Basic or acidic amino acids enhance antigenicity. If immunodominant groups reside within the interior of a protein molecule, they can neither stimulate an immune response nor react with homologous antibodies. Therefore, accessibility of determinant groups on the surface of the molecule is another important aspect of antigenicity.

Perhaps one of the most important attributes of an antigen is its ability to be partly digested by phagocytic cells. It appears that macrophage processing of high-molecular-weight antigens releases hydrolytic products that are the immunogenic units rather than the intact antigen molecules themselves. Inexplicably, the antigen is not degraded completely by lysosomal enzymes of the phagocyte. In some cases it is suspected that the antigen becomes complexed with ribonucleic acid (RNA) from the macrophage and in this form it is able to activate lymphocytes; in other cases, macrophage RNA alone is thought to be able to stimulate antibody synthesis by lymphocytes. Partial digestion of a protein antigen can reveal hidden antigenic sites of the interior components so that the total number of determinants in the sum of the hydrolytic products of a molecule is often greater than the number of determinants available for reaction with antibodies in the intact molecule. Some low-molecular-weight antigens may be able to stimulate lymphocytes directly without the help of phagocytic cells.

Provided the above criteria of antigenicity are met, the greater the difference between a substance and that of the host animal, the more potent its antigenic qualities are likely to be. Proteins from closely related members of the same species are not as likely to stimulate the immune system as proteins from a completely different species. Serum proteins of the ape or monkey would not be expected to be as immunogenic to humans as would the serum of a nonprimate animal. This principle has been exploited in ascertainment of evolutionary distances between different taxonomic groups of plants and animals.

In summary, antigenicity of a substance is promoted by molecular size, molecular complexity, accessibility of immunodominant groups, digestibility, and degree of foreignness.

Given a substance possessing all of the attributes of a potential antigen, why is it that such a substance is not invariably able to activate lymphocytes in all vertebrate animals possessing a complete immune system? Heredity undoubtedly plays a fundamental role in this regard. The kinds of immune responses that can be made by an individual are ultimately dependent on its genotype. Some species are programmed by their common heredity to be incapable of responding to a substance that is immunogenic in some other species. Even within a species, a wide variation of immunological responsiveness can be demonstrated to a given antigen. Among the potential contributors to the immunological responsiveness of an individual are such factors as the heredity unique to the individual, the number of times the antigen was contacted, preexisting disease states, the dosage of the antigen received at each contact, the route by which it entered the host, the age and sex of the animal, environment or occupation, nutrition, and other aspects of general health. In addition, the patient may be on drugs (therapeutic or otherwise) that could affect the responsiveness of lymphocytes. Other substances may be administered along with an antigen (or may be naturally present) that could prolong its survival in the body or in other ways enhance its immunogenic qualities. So many variables exist that there is no easy answer to questions such as "Why am I allergic to poison oak and my brother is not?"

HAPTENS

Bacterial cells and large, complex molecules such as proteins behave as **complete antigens** in that they are capable of stimulating antibody synthesis in the host and yet can also react with homologous antibodies. The antigenic properties of a bacterial cell are produced by many different antigenic molecules. Any one kind of antigenic molecule may be present thousands of times on a cell. A small chemical group or radical attached to a larger protein or polysaccharide of the cell constitutes each antigenic site. These immunologically and serologically reactive sites are variously referred to as **antigenic determinants, epitopes, antigenic factors,** or **antigenic specificities.** The corresponding antigen-binding sites on an antibody molecule are called **paratopes** or **antibody specificities.** The small molecules that constitute a given antigenic specificity are referred to as incomplete antigens or haptens. They are too small to behave as complete antigens (i.e., they cannot by themselves stimulate an immune response) but they can react specifically with homologous antibodies.

By coupling haptenic groups to much larger "carrier" (**Schlepper**) molecules such as proteins (e.g., bovine serum albumin, BSA), it is possible to confer new antigenic specificities on the hapten-carrier complex. One way this can be done is to attach various chemical groups (e.g., acid radicals, nonionic radicals, aliphatic chains of different lengths, etc.) to an aromatic amine such as analine. The substituted aromatic amine can then be converted to a salt containing a diazo group ($-N^+ \equiv N \cdot$). The diazotized substituted aromatic amine will covalently combine with certain amino acids (lysine, tyrosine, histidine) of a protein Schlepper (Figure 2.1). When the purified diazohapten-conjugated protein is injected into an animal such as a rabbit or goat, three kinds of antibody specificities are commonly produced: (1) hapten-specific, (2) carrier-specific, and (3) those specific for "hybrid" determinants of the hapten-carrier complex.

When antibodies specific for the hapten are combined or conjugated with the hapten-carrier complex, aggregation of antigen-antibody complexes can occur. When cross-linkages (lattice formation) of these complexes become very large, they settle out of solution as visible serological **precipitation** (Figure 2.2). It should be noted at this point that a basic difference between agglutination and precipitation is that the former involves particu-

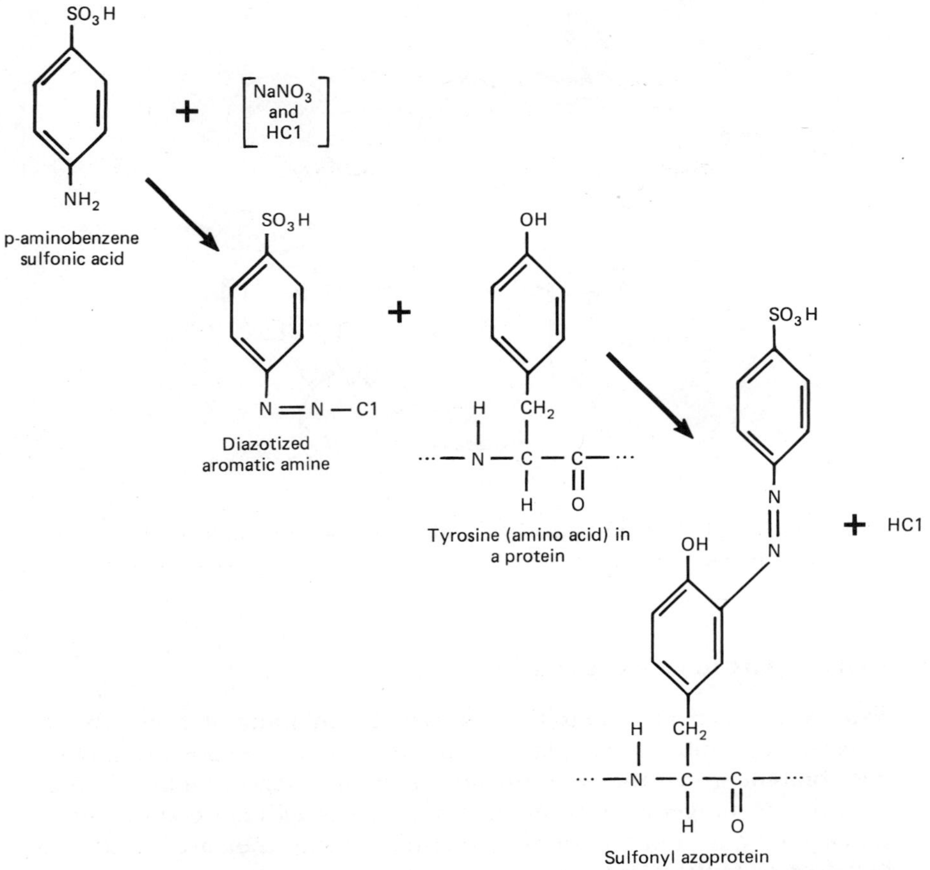

FIGURE 2.1. Formation of a new antigenic determinant on a protein through diazotization of a substituted aromatic amine.

late antigens such as bacterial cells, whereas the latter involves soluble, molecular-size antigens such as proteins or polysaccharides of bacterial capsules.

The ability of an antiserum to cause precipitation of the homologous hapten-carrier complex could be reduced by preincubation with the hapten. Excess hapten would block the combining sites on antibodies with the corresponding specificity so that on subsequent incubation of the treated antiserum with the hapten-carrier complex less precipitation would be observed. This phenomenon, termed the **blocking** or **inhibition reaction,** is widely used in the serological laboratory to demonstrate the presence of **simple** or **nonprecipitating haptens.** They are called simple haptens because, although they can combine with antibody, they cannot produce precipitates. They behave as though they have only a single combining or determinant site. Other haptens are large enough to have two or more combining sites and hence can form precipitates with homologous antibodies. These are called **complex** or **precipitating haptens.** Antibodies can be made to haptens of medical importance by coupling them to large carrier or indicator molecules such as proteins, cells, or latex particles.

Serology and Immunology

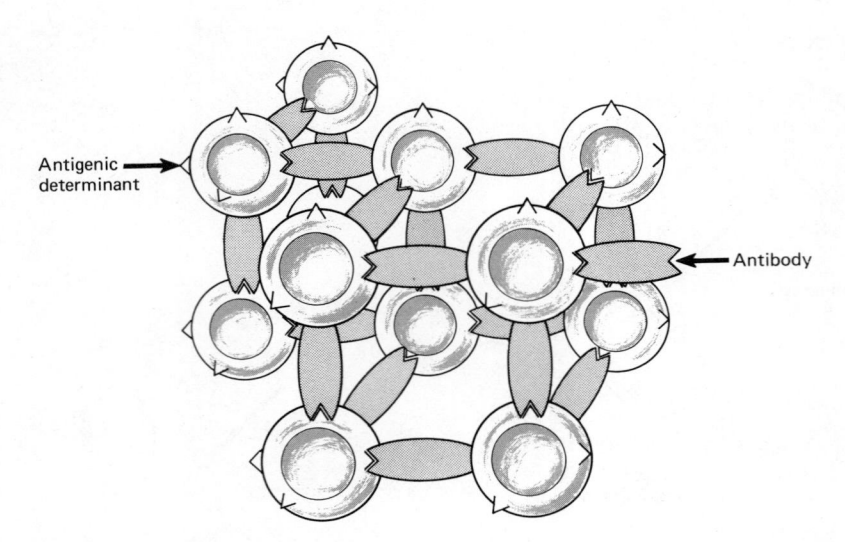

FIGURE 2.2. Lattice formation of antigen-antibody complexes become visible as precipitation (soluble antigen) or agglutination (particulate antigen).

IMMUNOLOGICAL VALENCE

Valence is a term applied to the number of combining sites on either an antigen or an antibody. Simple haptens react as if they possessed only a single combining site; they are functionally **monovalent.** Complex haptens and complete antigens can form large aggregates with antibodies, indicating that they have more than one determinant site; they are functionally **polyvalent** or **multivalent.**

Antibodies of class IgE behave serologically as though they have only a single combining site (monovalent). Unless antibodies have at least two combining sites per immunoglobulin molecule **(bivalent),** they cannot participate in forming aggregates such as those seen in serological agglutination or precipitation reactions. Antibodies of class IgM are known to be polyvalent with up to ten potential combining sites per molecule. All of the combining sites on an antibody molecule are identical regardless of the immunoglobulin class to which it belongs.

Serological valence has no relationship to chemical or ionic valence. As a general rule, most protein antigens have a functional valence of approximately one antibody-binding site per 5,000 to 10,000 molecular weight. The **functional valence** of an antigen is the number of combining sites when in its native state. All of these sites must be on the outer surface of the antigen so that they are accessible to antibodies or lymphocyte receptors. Upon entry into the body, most antigens must become at least partly digested (usually by macrophages), and the "processed" hydrolytic products rather than the intact antigen are the actual immunogenic units. Several antigenic determinants previously hidden internally may be uncovered by partial digestion of an antigenic molecule. Therefore, the **total valence** of an antigen (which includes both the functional valence and the hidden determinants) is usually greater than the functional valence. The portion of the antigenic determinant that fits inside the cavity of a particular antibody-combining site is probably much smaller than the size of a valence unit. When an antibody becomes attached to an antigenic determinant, portions of the antibody may sterically hinder attachment of other antibodies to closely adjacent antigenic sites (Figure 2.3).

ANTIGENIC DETERMINANTS

Much of the early knowledge concerning interactions between antigens and their homologous antibodies resulted from the classical experiments of Karl Landsteiner. The **precipitation inhibition reaction** was used extensively by Landsteiner in his studies on the specificity of serological reactions. The specificity of an antiserum for a hapten was indicated by the degree to which the precipitation reaction was inhibited by related chemical groups.

An alternative method for measuring the specificity of an antiserum for its homologous hapten can be used. A hapten can be coupled to a chicken protein and the azoprotein is then used to produce the homologous antiserum. The same hapten can then be attached to an unrelated carrier molecule such as a horse protein. Reactions of the antiserum with the heterologous azoprotein should involve only the haptenic specificity. If closely related haptens were also attached to the heterologous carrier (horse protein), then the degree of cross-reactivity in precipitation tests with the antiserum would indicate its degree of specificity for the original hapten.

Landsteiner's studies, using artificially conjugated haptens, led to the following general conclusions. Terminal groups in aliphatic chains are commonly the dominant determinants of serological specificity. Strongly ionic groups (either acids or bases) confer high degrees of specificity to the determinant sites. Nonionic groups of nearly equal size and shape can be substituted with little change in serological specificity. The spatial place-

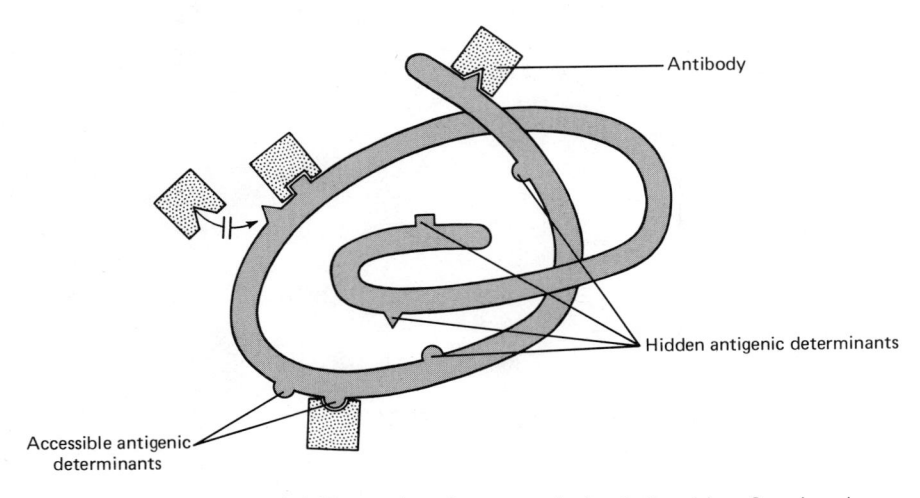

FIGURE 2.3. A model illustrating the numerical relationship of antigenic determinants to immunological valence. The antigen has a valence of three as determined by binding of three antibody molecules. The number of potential antigenic sites is nine; the number of exposed (accessible) antigenic determinants is five. An antibody combining with one antigenic determinant may sterically hinder attachment of another antibody to a closely adjacent determinant.

Serology and Immunology

ment of determinant groups is very important to serological specificity. For example, antisera developed to aniline with a carboxyl group attached at the ortho position on the benzene ring would not cross-react with the same acid radical at the meta or para positions. The same degree of specificity was shown by antisera against the other two substituted anilines (anti-meta-aminobenzoic acid, anti-para-aminobenzoic acid). These observations correlate well with what is now known about the structure of the antibody-combining site and of the forces that are involved in serological binding of antigen and antibody. Serological "bonds" involve relatively weak hydrogen bonds, electrostatic and van der Waals attractions. They only become effective binding forces when the conformation of the antigenic determinant site and the antibody-combining site are of complementary shapes and when the reactive groups are very near one another.

The size of an antigenic determinant varies from one antigen to another, but in general it seems to be quite small compared to the size of the molecule of which it is a part. For example, only 3 to 6 monosaccharide units of dextran may represent the size of the antigenic site (approximately $34 \times 12 \times 7$ Å). Similar estimates of size in terms of amino acid residues have been made in tobacco mosaic virus protein and silk fibroin.

Portions of a determinant on a protein antigen may be contributed by noncontiguous regions of its polypeptide chain (Figure 2.4). In the native state, a globular protein antigen might normally have two components of a determinant site in juxtaposition and in the proper spatial orientation with respect to one another so that serological reaction would occur with the homologous antibody. If the protein becomes denatured (loss of secondary or higher structural levels of organization), then the essential portions of the determinant site might no longer be close together and in the proper spatial relationships for recognition by the antibody-combining site. This is

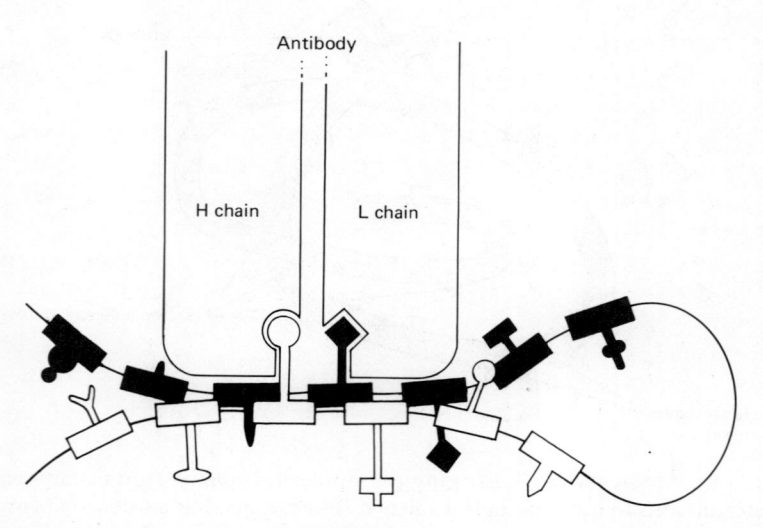

FIGURE 2.4. Portions of an antigenic determinant on a globular protein may be contributed by nonadjacent regions of a polypeptide chain. Denaturation of the protein (loss of native shape) might prevent the antibody from binding effectively. The antibody-combining site consists partly of "heavy" (H) chain and of "light" (L) chain.

an important concept to keep in mind when handling antigens or antibodies in the laboratory. Care must be taken to prevent overheating, repeated freezing and thawing, contamination by chemicals or microorganisms, excessive agitation, or any other condition that might possibly harm the native structures of serological reagents.

Fractionation of Serum

Serum contains an astonishing variety of proteins that function as enzymes, blood-clotting factors, components of the complement system, "transportation proteins," and hormones. A protein can be classified chemically as either an albumin or a globulin. These two groups of proteins are easily separated by chemical treatment of serum with a half-saturated ammonium sulfate solution or a 21.5 percent sodium sulfate solution. Globulins are thereby chemically precipitated, leaving the albumins soluble (in solution). The precipitated globulins can be dissolved in phosphate buffered saline (PBS) solution and then dialyzed against PBS to remove any residual ammonium or sodium sulfate. The dialysate can then be concentrated to any desired degree by pervaporation (evaporation through a membrane). **Immunoglobulins** are proteins that share one or more antigenic sites in common with known antibodies. Therefore, all antibodies are immunoglobulins, but not all immunoglobulins are antibodies. Those immunoglobulins that are not antibodies are usually fragments of antibody molecules. Abnormal plasma polypeptides (usually fragments of functional proteins) excessively produced by neoplastic cells are termed **paraproteins,** and their presence in blood is called **paraproteinemia.**

In addition to chemical fractionation of serum, it is possible to separate additional protein components on the basis of their net electrical charges. If a mixture of proteins differing in net electrical charges in a suitable buffer solution is subjected to an electrical current, the proteins will migrate at different rates. This is the principle of **electrophoresis.** Most biological proteins carry a net negative charge in alkaline buffers, causing them to migrate toward the anode (positive pole). The first successful attempt at electrophoresis was made by Arne Tiselius in a fluid medium. He introduced proteins into the cathodic end of a U-shaped tube filled with buffer and applied an electric current to the solution. The migrating proteins separated according to net charge and were read by a complicated optical scanning system. This technique is called **moving (free) boundary electrophoresis.** It is a complicated technique requiring relatively expensive equipment and is subject to disturbance by convection currents and other problems. Nonetheless, it was possible to separate at least the two major fractions, albumin and globulin, by this technique. The albumins carry the highest net negative charge and hence migrate most rapidly toward the anode. After this discovery various solid or semisolid support media were introduced into electrophoresis. Paper proved to be a useful support for migrating proteins, but higher resolving power (greater number of components separable) has come from the use of cellulose acetate strips or gels made of polyacrylamide, agar, agarose, or starch. The pore size of polyacrylamide gels can be adjusted within a relatively wide range so that separation by net charge can be modified by a sieving effect based on molecular

Serology and Immunology

size/shape. This method improves resolution of proteins that are similar in charge density. Serum can be fractionated into about five bands on agarose but into about twenty by polyacrylamide gel electrophoresis (PAGE). PAGE can be run on horizontal slabs or in vertical rods of gel **(disc electrophoresis).**

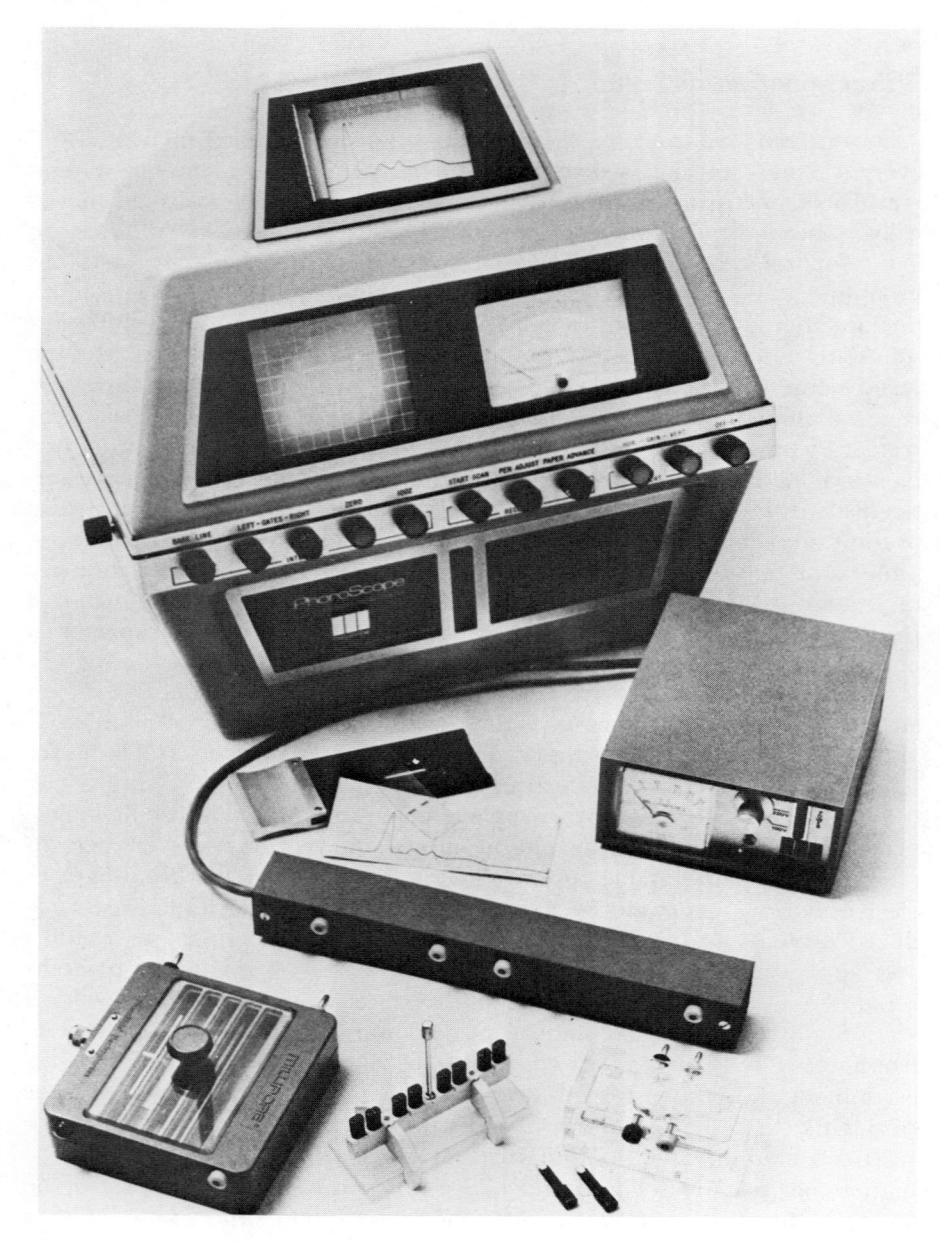

FIGURE 2.5. Equipment used in zone electrophoresis includes buffer chamber, power supply, and densitometer. This technique is used to fractionate serum proteins, LDH isozymes, hemoglobin, lipoproteins, haptoglobin, glycoproteins, cerebrospinal fluid (CSF), and urine. [*Courtesy of Millipore Corp., Bedford, Mass.*]

The term **zone electrophoresis** is applied to all electrophoretic techniques employing support media (Figure 2.5). There are several advantages to use of this method of electrophoretic separation of proteins including simplicity of the technique, relatively inexpensive equipment, less subjectivity to convection currents, permanence of the record, greater resolution, etc. After a serum is zone-electrophoresed, the proteins on the strip or gel may be stained to reveal their relative locations with a protein dye and then the support is destained to remove all the background dye that is not attached to proteins. This leaves a record of stained "bands" or localized regions of protein concentrations called an **electropherogram** (Figure 2.6). Zone electropherograms usually resolve at least four major serum fractions in decreasing order of net negative charge: albumin, alpha (α) globulin, beta (β) globulin, and gamma (γ) globulin. Each purified serum protein typically migrates in one of these four major zones. Almost all antibodies are found in the γ globulin fraction.

Quantitation of the amounts of proteins in various bands of an electropherogram can be obtained by scanning it with a **densitometer.** This requires that the support medium be transparent or relatively so. Cellulose acetate strips are opaque but can be cleared for densitometry after electrophoresis, staining, and destaining by immersion in a glacial acetic acid–methanol solution. The change in optical density (absorbance) can be recorded manually by moving the strips through the light beam by equal increments of length and making plots of the data on graph paper. More

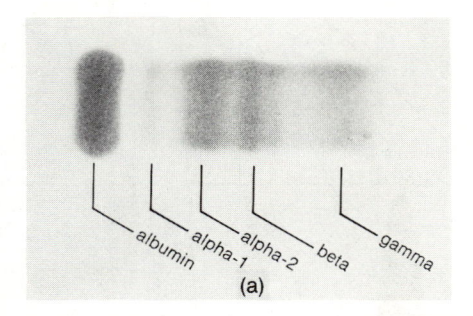

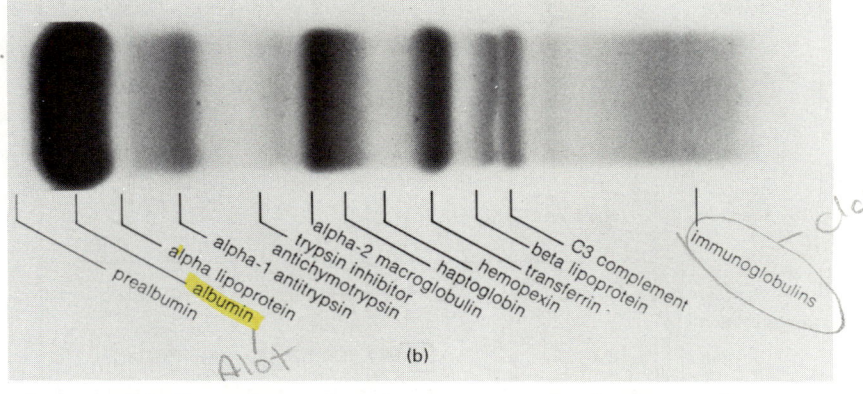

FIGURE 2.6. Zone electrophoresis separates molecules by net charge on conventional support media (*a*) or by a combination of charge and molecular size (shape) on agarose gel (*b*). [*Courtesy of Millipore Corp., Bedford, Mass.*]

Serology and Immunology

commonly, the data are automatically plotted by a mechanical device (integrating densitometer recorder) that also calculates the relative proportions of the total serum profile ascribed to the four major bands of the electropherogram. Typically, albumin proteins plot as a tall narrow peak; the α, β, and γ globulins trail behind as a series of smaller, broader peaks (Figure 2.7). The total area of a peak in such a plot is directly proportional to the concentration of proteins therein. The narrower the peak, the more homogeneous (with regard to net charge) are the corresponding proteins. Therefore, albumins are a relatively homogeneous collection of proteins, but the relatively broad band of the gamma globulins indicates that they are a collection of heterogeneous molecules.

By the technique of **isoelectric focusing,** ampholytes (i.e., electrolytes

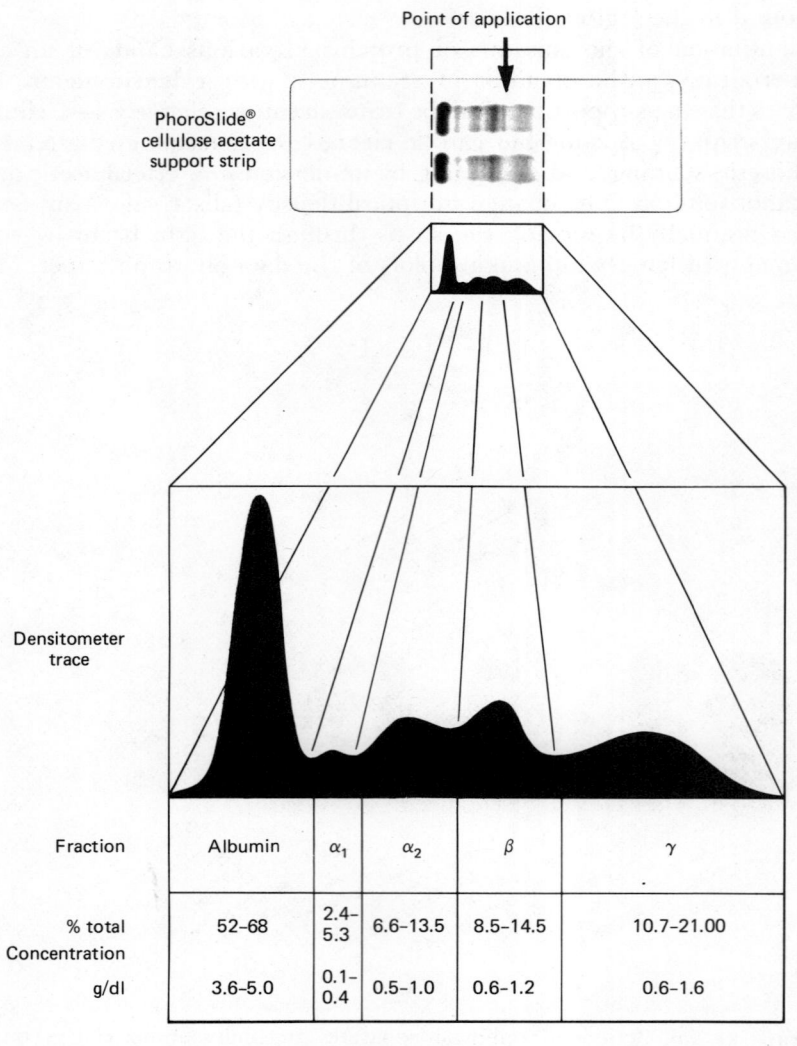

Fraction	Albumin	α_1	α_2	β	γ
% total Concentration	52–68	2.4–5.3	6.6–13.5	8.5–14.5	10.7–21.00
g/dl	3.6–5.0	0.1–0.4	0.5–1.0	0.6–1.2	0.6–1.6

FIGURE 2.7. Zone electrophoresis separation of a normal human serum sample. [*Courtesy of Millipore Corp., Bedford, Mass.*]

such as proteins that contain both acidic and basic groups) can be separated according to their **isoelectric points.** The isoelectric point (pI) of a molecule is that pH at which it has no net charge and hence will not migrate in an electric field. Proteins are least soluble at their isoelectric points. If a mixture of proteins is electrophoresed through a support medium containing a pH gradient increasing from anode to cathode, the various fractions will migrate until they reach their respective isoelectric points. Since different proteins commonly have distinctive isoelectric points, isoelectric focusing can separate (fractionate) a heterogeneous mixture into bands of homogeneous (by pI) proteins.

More recently, techniques have been devised for constructing polyacrylamide gels that have a gradient of pore sizes from one end to the other. When a heterogeneous mixture of proteins is placed at the large pore end and electrophoresed through the gel, molecules are separated by both net charge and size (electrophoretic or molecular sieving). By this method, many more fractions can be resolved than by conventional electrophoresis in gels of uniform pore size (Figure 2.8).

In the technique called **immunoelectrophoresis,** a mixture of protein antigens is first separated by electrophoresis. Antibodies are then added and bands (arcs) of **immunoprecipitates** form where antigens and homologous antibodies have combined. This is another high-resolution system that has revealed over thirty protein fractions in normal human serum. It is discussed more fully in Chapter 5.

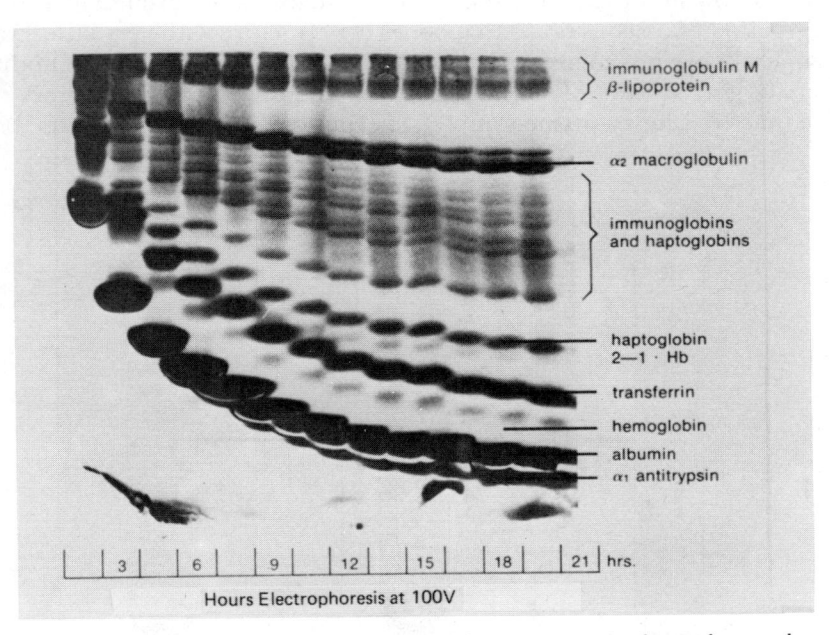

FIGURE 2.8. Electrophoretic sieving of human serum through a polyacrylamide gel containing a gradient of pore sizes. Molecules migrate until they reach a pore size that matches their dimensions and then stop (regardless of the number of hours of continued electrophoresis). Samples were applied at ninety-minute intervals. [*Courtesy of Isolab, Inc., Akron, Ohio.*]

Serology and Immunology

Structure of Immunoglobulin G

Because immunoglobulins are proteins, the antibody molecules of one species behave as foreign antigens when introduced into another species. For example, if human serum (containing numerous chemically diverse immunoglobulins) is injected into a rabbit, the animal should respond with a variety of antibodies to this heterogeneous array of antigens. However, the concentration of structurally identical immunoglobulins with a given specificity in normal serum is too low to allow its detection by immunoelectrophoresis. For a long time, the extreme heterogeneity of antibody molecules and the low concentration of any one kind had precluded isolation and structural analysis of any immunoglobulin. Some "mistakes of nature," although usually quite harmful to individuals with these diseases, have provided immunologists with relatively high concentrations of nearly pure fractions of immunoglobulin molecules. One such mistake was originally discovered in 1847 by the English physician Henry Bence-Jones. He found that patients with the disease called multiple myeloma had a high concentration of an unusual protein in their urine. This substance, called **Bence-Jones protein,** has a peculiar behavior on heating. At room temperature it is soluble, becoming insoluble near 60° to 70°C and again dissolving at about 80°C (Figure 2.9). This behavior is reversed on cooling so that Bence-Jones proteins can be readily isolated from other urine or plasma proteins (few proteins are normally present in urine). Multiple myeloma is a neoplasm (tumor) of plasma cells that **metastasizes** (spreads) from the bone marrow into the soft tissues and into dense bone, eventually causing such erosion of osseous tissue that bones may fracture with very little strain. Plasma cells are not commonly found in bone marrow. Hence, the findings of (1) large numbers of plasma cells and pyroninophilic precursors in a bone marrow **biopsy** (tissue sample), (2) "moth-eaten" holes in dense bone

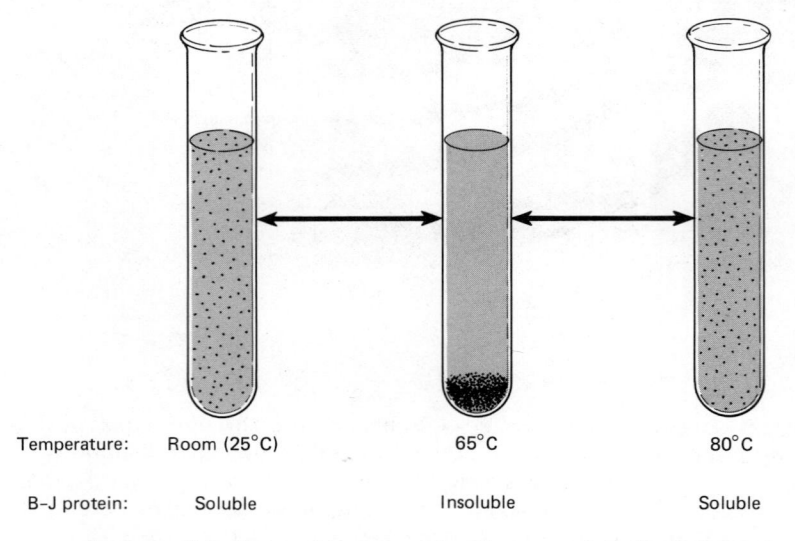

FIGURE 2.9. Bence-Jones proteins (immunoglobulin light chains) are insoluble near 60° to 70°C, but soluble at room temperature or near 80°C.

revealed by X-ray photos, and (3) presence of Bence-Jones proteins in the patient's urine are diagnostic of multiple myeloma. When a plasma cell precursor (lymphoblast) becomes cancerous, it is no longer subject to the normal controls on its cellular proliferation and protein synthesis. A very large clone of cells is thereby produced, all of which have the potential to synthesize and release the same antibody. A high concentration of a single species of immunoglobulin molecule appears as a narrow spike on an electropherogram (Figure 2.10). The proteins in this region are called M (myeloma) proteins and are indicative of a **monoclonal gammopathy** (disease of a single cell type affecting gamma globulin production). If multiple spikes are seen in the γ globulin region of a serum electropherogram, it usually indicates that the patient is suffering from a **polyclonal gammopathy,** involving at least as many different clones as there are protein spikes. These are examples of **immunoproliferative diseases.** When it was discovered that Bence-Jones proteins were polypeptide subunits also found

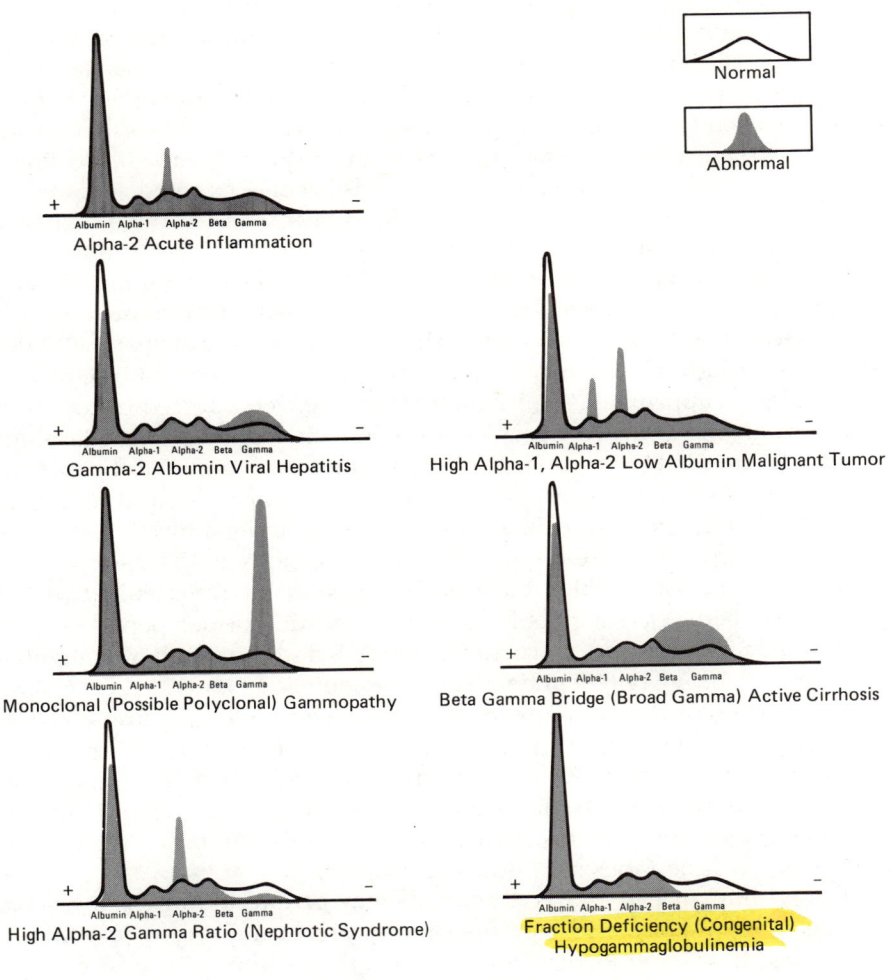

FIGURE 2.10. Major serum protein electrophoretic patterns. [*Courtesy of Gelman Instrument Company, Ann Arbor, Mich.*]

Serology and Immunology

in the abnormal immunoglobulin fraction of the same individual's serum, the way was opened for amino acid sequencing analyses of parts of immunoglobulins. This and other kinds of immunoproliferative diseases have provided immunologists with sufficient quantities of highly purified immunoglobulins so that entire molecules could be structurally analyzed. By using a variety of enzymatic, immunological, and physicochemical techniques, immunochemists have pieced together the gross and fine structures of the immunoglobulin molecule. In 1972, the Nobel Prize in Medicine and Physiology was awarded to Gerald M. Edelman of the Rockefeller University in the United States and Rodney R. Porter of Oxford University in England for their independent work on the structure of immunoglobulin class G (IgG), the predominant form of antibody in most higher vertebrates.

Globular proteins have a complex folded structure that may hide internally covalent disulfide bridges (S—S bonds) between sulfur-containing cystine amino acids (one of the twenty kinds of amino acids found in biological polypeptides). Reducing reagents such as mercaptoethanol can break disulfide bonds and convert them to two free sulfhydryl (–SH) groups through oxidation-reduction reactions. Immunoglobulins are resistant to reducing reagents unless they are first treated with 7 to 8 M (molar) concentrations of urea or guanidine. These latter chemicals disrupt hydrogen bonds that tend to hold globulins in their folded active conformation. As they lose their three-dimensional shape by unfolding into more linear chains, the previously hidden disulfide bonds become exposed and susceptible to cleavage by reducing reagents. The products of such treatment can then be separated in an analytical ultracentrifuge into equal numbers of long and short polypeptide chains. The larger chains (approximately 50,000 MW; MW = molecular weight), called **heavy (H) chains,** are approximately twice the length of the shorter chains (approximately 20,000 MW), called **light (L) chains.** Because an intact immunoglobulin molecule of class IgG is approximately 150,000 MW, it may be inferred to consist of two light chains and two heavy chains connected by interchain disulfide bridges (Figure 2.11). Treatment of the immunoglobulin with the enzyme papain cleaves it into three parts, two of which are identical and bind antigen. Hence, they are called **Fab** (fragment, antigen-binding) components. The third component spontaneously crystallizes at 4°C and is termed **Fc** (fragment, crystallizable). Each of the three major fragments (two Fab and one Fc) behaves as a globular protein, consisting of polypeptide chains tightly folded into compact structures. There is a short stretch of nonglobular ("linear") heavy polypeptide chain between each Fab and the Fc. This flexible portion of the immunoglobulin molecule is called the **hinge region** and permits the bending of the "arms" of intact Ig molecules into Y- or T-shaped configurations. Although proteolytic enzymes such as papain can break many peptide bonds, they cannot hydrolyze globular regions as easily as linear regions of proteins. Papain attacks the linear hinge region and thereby breaks the molecule into three fragments.

Purified human Fab and Fc fragments may be injected into some other animals (goat, rabbit), and they respond by producing the corresponding antibodies. It was found that immunoprecipitates would form when anti-Fab was exposed to either H or L chains, but anti-Fc would combine only

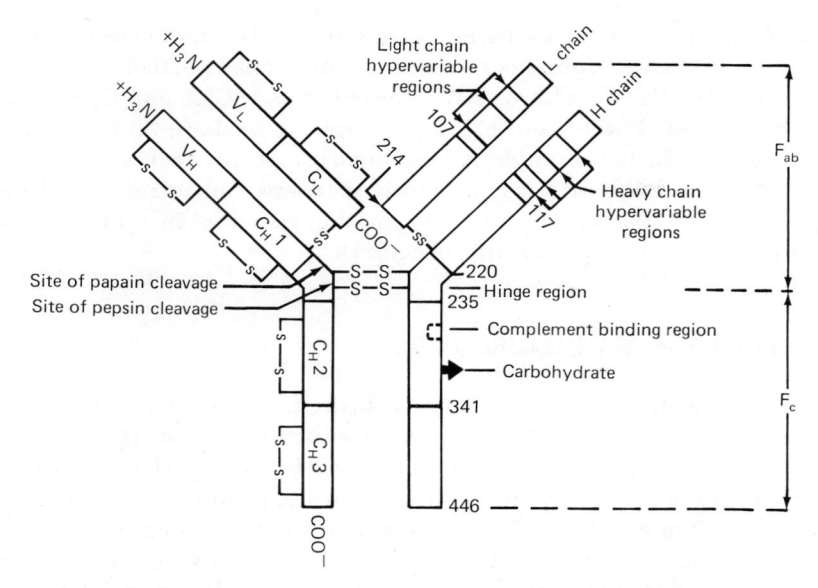

FIGURE 2.11. Diagram of a typical IgG molecule. Within each immunoglobulin molecule, the two L chains are identical and the two H chains are identical. Numbers represent approximate amino acid residues from the N terminus of the respective chain.

with H chains. Therefore, the Fab fragment must be constructed from both H and L chains, whereas the Fc fragment consists entirely of H chains.

Each polypeptide chain (as synthesized from a mRNA) has a free amino group (NH_2) at one end and a free carboxyl group (COOH) at the other end. A Fab unit consists of an entire light chain and the amino-terminal half (approximately) of a heavy chain (**Fd**) joined by an interchain disulfide bridge near their carboxy-terminal ends. A Fc unit consists entirely of the carboxy-terminal half of two heavy chains joined by two disulfide bridges near their amino-terminal ends.

Treatment with the enzyme pepsin produces only two fragments. One of these fragments binds two antigen molecules and consists of two Fab-like units with slightly longer segments of the H chains than occur in Fab fragments from papain treatment. In this component, labeled **F(ab')$_2$**, the two Fab-like fragments are connected by a disulfide bridge between the two H chains near their carboxy-terminal ends. The other product of pepsin digestion, designated **Fc'**, is similar to the Fc component, but slightly shorter. Its two H chains are connected by a single disulfide bridge near their amino-terminal ends.

Bence-Jones proteins are now known to be free dimers or monomers of immunoglobulin light chains. Amino acid sequence analyses of Bence-Jones proteins from different patients have revealed that they are all very similar in composition in the carboxy-terminal half (approximately). This region is labeled C_L (constant-light). The amino-terminal half of a light chain (V_L) is quite variable from one multiple myeloma patient to another. Heavy-chain sequence studies have revealed that approximately one fourth of its length near the amino-terminal end is also quite variable, hence is designated V_H

(variable-heavy). The other three fourths of the H chain consists of three nearly equal (in size) **domains** of relatively invariable, partially homologous amino acid sequences. They are symbolized as C_H1, C_H2, and C_H3 from the N-terminal end. The C_L and C_H regions appear to share 30 to 40 percent homology (similarity of amino acid sequences). It has been suggested that all of these "constant" regions have evolved from an ancestral gene through sequential gene duplications that became differentiated by point mutations and established through natural selection.

Immunoglobulin Classification

When purified human M (myeloma) proteins are injected into a rabbit, antibodies are produced that react with antigenic sites in the constant regions of heavy chains. These antibodies have been used to identify five major **classes** of human immunoglobulins by the technique of immunoelectrophoresis. These classes of immunoglobulins are symbolized IgG, IgM, IgA, IgE, and IgD. The corresponding heavy chains of these immunoglobulins are designated γ (gamma), μ (mu), α (alpha), ϵ (epsilon), and δ (delta), respectively. Similarly, two antigenically defined **types** of light chains are known: κ (kappa) and λ (lambda).

Amino acid sequence differences occurring at a minimum of five different sites in the constant region of lambda light chains serologically differentiate these polypeptides into four **subtypes** found in all normal humans. Each subtype requires a different genetic locus to specify its structure. The Kern marker at position 152 (from the amino end) exemplifies the kind of amino acid substitutions governed by these subtype genes. If glycine is present at this location, the subtype is Kern +; if serene is present, it is Kern −. Similarly, the Oz marker is at position 190. If lysine occupies this site, the subtype is Oz +; substituting arginine makes it Oz − (Figure 2.12). No subtypes have yet been identified in kappa light chains.

Some of the H chain classes have similarly been further defined serologically into **subclasses.** For example, γ chains may be any one of four major subclasses: γ_1, γ_2, γ_3, or γ_4, corresponding to immunoglobulins IgG1, IgG2, IgG3, and IgG4, respectively. At least two major subclasses are known for both μ and α chains. All of the classes, subclasses, types, and subtypes of immunoglobulin H and L chains are **isotypes** and are characterized by being present in all normal people, albeit in different concentrations. For example, IgG is by far the most common class of immunoglobulin and likewise for subclass IgG1.

In addition to the isotypes, several **allotypes** are known. Allotypes are structurally and functionally similar antigenic variants of proteins not common to all members of a species. If only a single form of a gene exists for a given class, subclass, type, or subtype of an immunoglobulin chain, then allotypes are not found. For example, no allotypes have been found in subclasses of lambda light chains, or in heavy chains of classes D, M, or E. However, if two or more alleles exist at any of these isotypic genetic loci, then allotypic antigens are produced. Most of the allotypic variants found to date differ from each other by one or a few amino acid substitutions presumably resulting from a corresponding number of nucleotide substitutions (mutations) in ancestral genes. Three **Km** allotypes are known in

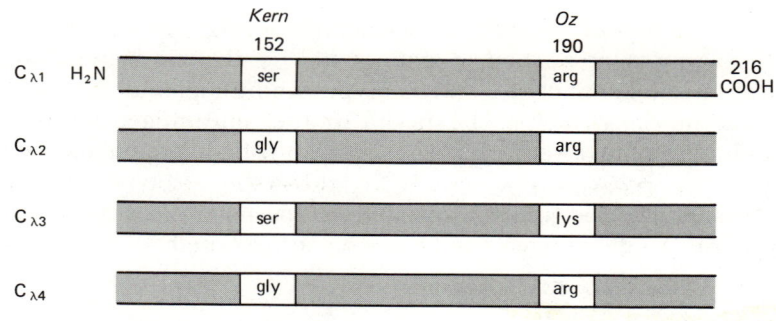

FIGURE 2.12. Four isotypes of lambda light chains are governed by four corresponding genetic loci possessed by all normal people. The Kern antigenic marker is at amino acid position 152 from the amino-terminal end; the Oz marker is at position 190. Glycine at 152 makes the chain Kern+; serine makes it Kern−. Lysine at 190 makes the chain Oz+; arginine makes it Oz−. Other amino acid differences besides those of the Kern and Oz markers are known to characterize each of these four lambda chain subtypes.

kappa light chains corresponding to three allelic forms of the gene for that polypeptide (Figure 2.13). Km allotypes were formerly designated **Inv**. The three constant regions of kappa chains are identical except at positions 153 and 191 from the amino end. Allotype Km (1) has valine and leucine at these two positions respectively; Km (1,2) has alanine and leucine; Km (3) has alanine and valine. More than 24 **Gm** allotypes are known in IgG. Gm (3) has arginine at position 214 in the G1 subclass of heavy chain, whereas Gm (17) has lysine at that same position. Similarly, two **Am** allotypes are known in the A2 subclass of alpha heavy chains. The chemical basis of most allotypic differences is not yet known. The common amino acid sequences shared by all products of an allotypic allelic series are responsible for the isotypic antigenic determinants that all members of the species possess.

The greatest variability in amino acid sequences of both light and heavy chains occurs in the V regions of the Fab fragments. The antigenic differences associated with this kind of variation are called **idiotypes.** It is not known how many idiotypes exist, but the number could very well be in the thousands. A thousand different V regions on both L and H chains potentially could combine in all possible ways to produce 10^6 paratopes. This **combinatorial association** is one source of the vast heterogeneity of antibody-combining sites that typifies the normal immune system.

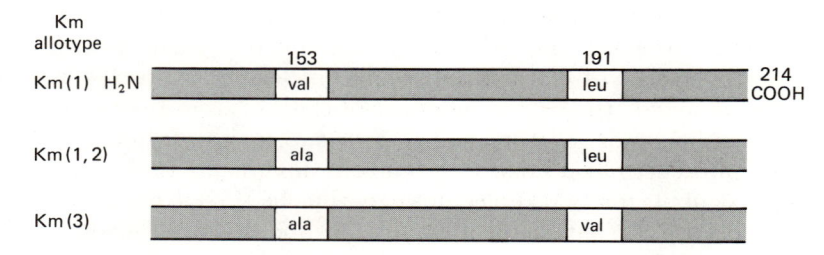

FIGURE 2.13. Three Km (formerly Inv) allotypic variants of the kappa light chain are specified by three alleles of a single structural gene.

Serology and Immunology

For any one immunoglobulin molecule, the two light chains are identical in both isotype, allotype, and idiotype. Likewise, the two heavy chains are identical in isotype, allotype, and idiotype. Immunoglobulins of different classes and subclasses may still be specific for the same antigen. Thus, immunoglobulins capable of reacting with a highly purified antigen may be structurally $(\gamma_1)_2\kappa_2$, $(\gamma_3)_2\lambda_2$, $(\alpha_1)_2\kappa_2$, etc. If we add to these isotype formulas the allotype, subtype, and idiotype differences, the heterogeneity of antibody response to a single antigen can be readily appreciated.

IMMUNOGLOBULIN G

Because most of the preceding discussion of antibody structure has related specifically to immunoglobulin class G, only a few additional comments need be made here. The reason why IgG was first analyzed is indicated by its relatively high concentration in serum. IgG constitutes from 75 to 80 percent of all immunoglobulins in serum. It is highly likely that most myeloma proteins would involve plasma cells making IgG. This was fortunate in that IgG has the smallest molecular weight (150,000) as indicated by its sedimentation constant (6.6S). A molecule of about 7S is likely to be easier to analyze than one of 19S (IgM). IgG has the longest half-life of the immunoglobulins (about thirty days). A long half-life is highly desirable for passive immunity. The only antibodies known to cross the placenta are those of class IgG, and they are of primary importance to immunity of the fetus and newborn baby (neonate). Antibodies of this class are good viral and exotoxin neutralizers. They can participate in precipitation and agglutination with appropriate antigens. IgG antibodies may also be involved in complement-mediated bacteriolysis and opsonization, but they are much inferior in these respects to antibodies of class IgM. The complement system cannot be activated by union of IgG antibody and cognate antigen unless two or more IgG molecules are brought into close apposition on the antigen. The relatively high concentration of IgG in serum makes it a major activator of the complement system, but on a molar basis it is much less effective at this function than multimeric IgM.

IMMUNOGLOBULIN M

All classes of immunoglobulin except IgM have sedmentation rates of approximately 7S. The symbol S is in honor of Theodor Svedberg, inventor of the ultracentrifuge. Generally speaking, higher-molecular-weight substances tend to have larger S values. IgG has a molecular weight of approximately 150,000 (6.6S), whereas IgM has a molecular weight about six times as great (900,000 MW; 19S). The reason for this is that an IgM molecule consists of a complex of five subunits similar in size to IgG molecules (Figure 2.14). Of course, the heavy chains are of class μ rather than γ, and they may have either κ or λ light chains. Two subclasses of IgM (based on antigenic differences in μ chain) are known, designated IgM1 and IgM2. Structural symbols for IgM molecules may thus be $([\mu_2]_2\kappa_2)_5$, $([\mu_1]_2\lambda_2)_5$, etc. Heavy chains γ and α have four domains (1V_H and 3C_H), but μ and ϵ chains consist of five domains (1V_H and 4C_H). The heavy chains of the five individual subunits of an IgM molecule are connected by disulfide bonds near their carboxyl terminal ends to a polypeptide called **J chain**. It is also

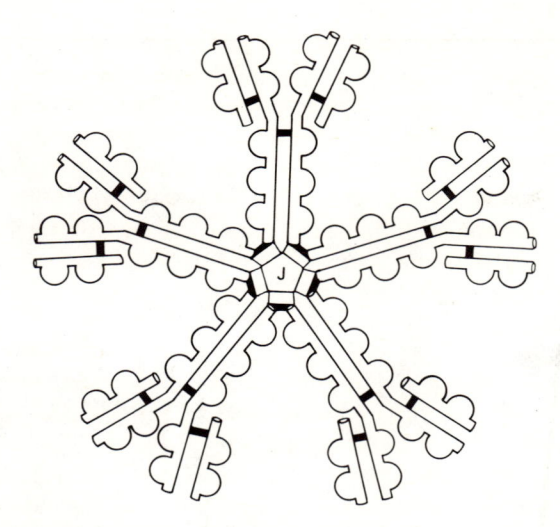

FIGURE 2.14. Structural model of an IgM pentameric molecule. Each of the tetrameric subunits (two H chains plus two L chains) is joined to a polypeptide (called J chain) by disulfide bonds at the ends of the H chains.

assumed that each light chain is linked to a heavy chain by a disulfide bond involving the last or next-to-last residue at the carboxyl end of the light chain and a residue on the heavy chain between the V_H and C_{H1} regions.

Electrophoretically, IgM generally migrates near the beta-gamma globulin boundary (see Figure 2.15). A serum showing a sharp peak in this region may signify a monoclonal gammopathy involving IgM- or IgA-secreting neoplastic cells, whereas a spike further into the γ globulin region is more likely caused by neoplasm of an IgG-secreting cell. It is unfortunate that the symbol γ has been used for both an electrophoretic group of proteins and a class of immunoglobulin heavy chains. The context in which this symbol is used should be carefully noted to avoid confusion.

Although the human IgM pentamer has ten potential antigen-binding regions, it is difficult to demonstrate more than five functional sites. A small protein of molecular weight around 15,000 is bound to each IgM molecule. This protein is called J (joining) chain and constitutes about 1 percent of the immunoglobulin's weight. The function of the J chain is unknown, but it has been suggested that it is required for transport of IgM across the membrane of the plasma cell in the secretion process. It is also theorized that J chains initiate polymerization of the tetrapeptide subunits (2H + 2L chains) into complete pentamers of 19S IgM. Small amounts of IgM have been found in external secretions (colostrum, saliva, mucus of the respiratory and intestinal tracts). In addition to the single J chain of **serum IgM, secretory IgM** also contains another single polypeptide chain now called SC or "secretory component," but formerly called TP (transport piece), T protein, or secretory piece (SP). Despite its name, the biological function of SC is unknown. SC is also found in secretory IgA, but not in IgG or IgE. Plasma cells synthesize L, H, and J chains. Epithelial cells of external mucosal tissue synthesize SC, and it is added to the IgM-J chain complex before being liberated into the exocrine secretion as IgM-J-SC complex.

One might suspect that the large size of IgM would preclude it from

Serology and Immunology

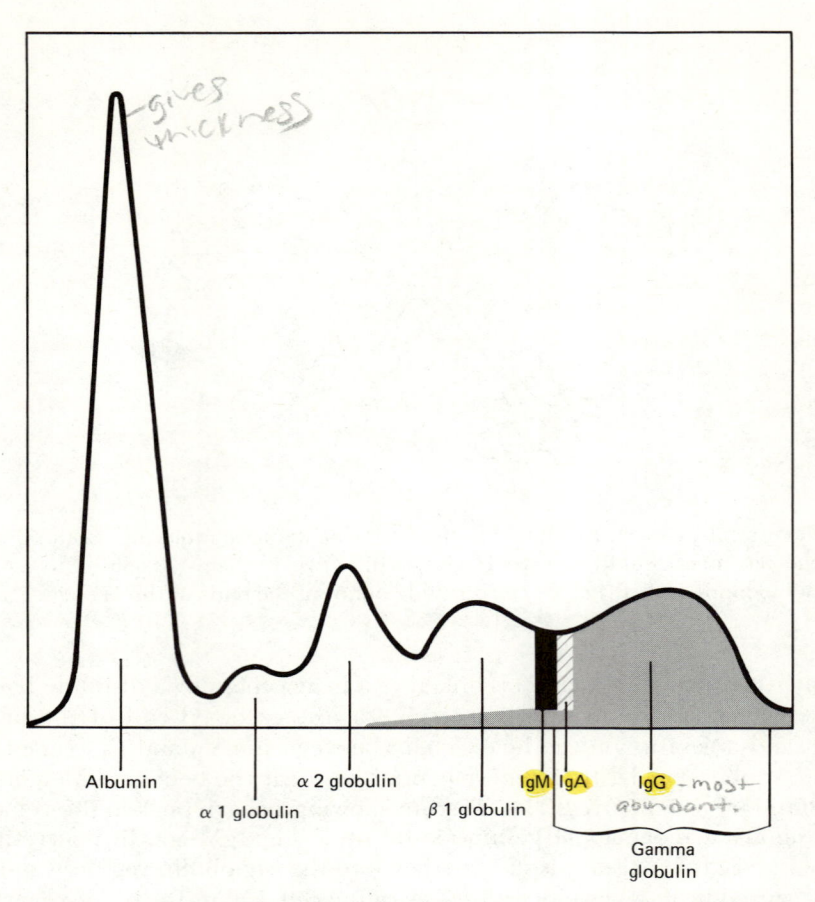

FIGURE 2.15. Typical electrophoretic mobilities of IgA and IgM molecules are near the boundary of the gamma-beta region.

being transported across the placenta from a mother to her child. This is true not only for 19S IgM but also for the much smaller 7S IgA and IgE. However, 7S IgG does pass the placenta. Hence, placental passage of immunoglobulins is not simply a matter of passive diffusion of small molecules. Transplacental passage of IgG in primates is by active transport and requires the Fc region of γ heavy chains. In ruminants (e.g., cattle), IgG antibodies are not transported across the placenta but are secreted in the colostrum and are absorbed from the intestinal tract of the newborn. Because of their large size and multivalence, IgM antibodies are excellent agglutinins but they are unexplicably poor precipitins. They are also excellent complement-fixing antibodies. It is estimated that a single IgM molecule can cause the same degree of red blood cell lysis as 1,000 IgG molecules. It seems that two IgG molecules must attach to neighboring antigenic sites in order to activate complement for initiation of cell lysis. Many more IgG molecules would be required in order to effectively occupy neighboring antigenic sites to the same extent that an IgM molecule could do by its multiple combining sites.

IMMUNOGLOBULIN A

IgA usually migrates electrophoretically between IgM and IgG and is found at the boundary between the β and γ globulin regions (see Figure 2.15). As with IgM, IgA can also be found in serum and in exocrine secretions. Actually, IgA is by far the most predominant immunoglobulin in secretions. It is assumed that IgA is a major immune factor in combating pathogens in the respiratory, urinary, and intestinal tracts. The role of IgA in phagocytosis (opsonic activity) and in protection of infants by its presence in colostrum is equivocal. Heavy chains of IgA molecules are designated α. Two subclasses of IgA are known, IgA1 and IgA2. Both subclasses have disulfide linkages between H chains, but IgA2 is unique in that H and L chains appear to be held together only by noncovalent bonds (no disulfide linkages). Two allotypic variants of the α chain in subclass IgA2 are Am1 and Am2. Serum IgA may be either a 7S monomer of four polypeptide chains resembling IgG in gross structure, a dimer (11S) of two 7S IgA monomers connected to a single J polypeptide by disulfide bonds at the ends of the heavy chains, or possibly even a trimer of three 7S units. Secretory IgA is apparently identical to the dimeric form of serum IgA with the addition of a single SC protein (Figure 2.16). In about 80 percent of secretory IgA molecules, SC is attached by disulfide bonds; in the other 20 percent, it is noncovalently attached. SC appears to contact the hinge region (where oligosaccharide subunits also attach) as well as other places in the Fc portion. The relevance of these structural features to the biological functions of secretory IgA is not yet known. The J chain appears to be essential for polymerization into the dimeric form, for active transport through mucous membranes, and may also be involved in binding SC. The function of SC is unknown. However, salivary and colostral IgA are more resistant to digestion by proteolytic enzymes than other immunoglobulins. The SC portion of secretory IgA may make it resistant to digestion and thereby allow the antibody to remain active longer in the intestinal tract. It has been suggested that secretory IgA can complex with potential pathogens and thereby prevent them from entering mucous membranes and causing infection. Antibodies secreted into the intestinal tract are called **coproantibodies.** It has been suggested that IgA might possibly bind to foods that otherwise would act as allergens and thereby prevent their passage into the intestinal tissues. The monomeric form of IgA (7S) does not appear to activate complement. However, the dimeric form of IgA (11S) does fix

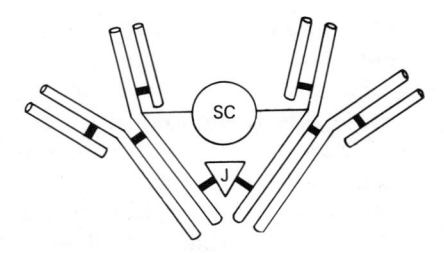

FIGURE 2.16. Dimeric secretory IgA shown attached to J chain and to SC protein. (See text.)

complement. After IgA (11S) binds to the lipopolysaccharide in the wall of gram-negative bacteria, it is postulated that the underlying mucopeptide becomes exposed. This in turn allows the enzyme lysozyme to digest the mucopeptide layer and results in immune-mediated bacteriolysis.

IMMUNOGLOBULIN D

Of all the five classes of human immunoglobulins, IgD is the least understood. It is present in very low concentrations in serum and is produced by less than 3 percent of all myelomas, yet the majority of circulating B cells bear IgD as a cell-surface receptor. Little is known of its biological functions. It has not been detected in exocrine secretions (colostrum, saliva, tears, urine, etc.); it does not fix complement and does not cross the placenta. Approximately 40 percent of patients suffering systemic lupus erythematosus and 20 percent suffering rheumatoid arthritis have antinuclear antibodies of class IgD. Its gross structure seems similar to that of IgG (i.e., a tetramer of two L and two H chains). The H chains are designated δ. The H chains of IgD are longer than those of IgG, and currently this is attributed to an extended hinge region. It contains about 12 percent carbohydrate attached in three regions (in the hinge region and at two other places in the Fc region). Only a single interchain disulfide bridge connects the two H chains. IgD loses its antigen-binding capacity when heated at 56°C for one hour, a feature shared in common only with IgE. Unlike any other immunoglobulin, IgD is denatured at pH 3 and readily aggregates even at physiological pH. These attributes have made study of its ultrastructure very difficult.

IMMUNOGLOBULIN E

The antibody responsible for allergies was formerly called **reagin.** Immunoglobulin E is now known to be equivalent to reagin. The reason why the letter E was chosen for this class of antibody is that it was extensively studied in its reaction with the E antigen of ragweed (a common allergen). Normally, IgE occurs in trace amounts of normal serum (less than 100 ng/ml) but may be elevated up to fifty times the normal level in allergic individuals. Only two IgE-producing myelomas have been found so far. The sedimentation coefficient of 8.2S indicates that it probably consists of four polypeptide chains similar in gross structure to IgG and does not occur in multimeric forms as do IgM and IgA. IgE appears to bind by its Fc fragment to membranes of mast cells, basophils, and perhaps platelets. The cross-linking of homologous polyvalent allergen (antigen of allergy) by IgE then triggers release of pharmacological mediators (e.g., histamine, heparin) of the allergic response. Electrophoretically, IgE migrates as a "fast gamma" or γ_1 globulin. The reason it is 8.2S rather than 7S is because it contains a fourth C_H domain in its heavy ϵ chains. Even more than IgD, IgE is heat-labile, losing its antigen-binding capacity when heated at 56°C for thirty minutes. It behaves as a monovalent antibody, combining with an antigen, but unable to produce precipitates. It does not fix complement and does not pass the placenta. Therefore, children may inherit a genetic predisposition to develop certain kinds of allergies from their parents, but they do not acquire from their parents passive IgE-mediated allergy to any allergens. Not all allergies are IgE-mediated. Allergies triggered by IgG could be passively acquired by babies from their mothers. Table 2.1 summarizes the distinguishing characteristics of all five classes of immunoglobulins.

Antibody Production by Single Cells

According to the clonal selection theory, a plasma cell produces only one kind of antibody. Although some experiments with single lymphoid cells argue to the contrary, most plasma cells seem to produce only antibodies with a single specificity. There are at least three techniques for studying antibody synthesis by single cells. The most popular method is the "plaque-forming cell (PFC) technique" pioneered by Jerne. An individual is first immunized to foreign erythrocytes. Sensitized lymphocytes are then isolated from the spleen or other lymphoid tissues and plated on tissue culture nutrient agar heavily seeded with erythrocytes of the same type used in the primary immunization. Fresh normal guinea pig serum is added as a source of complement. Some lymphocytes programmed to recognize the erythrocyte antigens respond by producing homologous antibodies, forming a radially diminishing antibody concentration gradient around each such cell. The union of IgM and/or IgG antibodies with antigen activates the complement system, resulting in immune lysis of the red cells. This creates a relatively clear area or **plaque** in the light-red, erythrocyte-laden background, with the PFC in the center of each plaque. These plaques are visible to the naked eye. Gram-negative bacterial cells can be substituted for erythrocytes because they also can be lysed by complement and antibodies from suitably sensitized lymphocytes. Even soluble antigens may be used if they can be adsorbed onto erythrocytes or gram-negative bacteria.

The "microdroplet technique" has been used to study antibodies that immobilize certain motile bacteria and antibodies that neutralize the infectivity of certain bacteriophages (bacterial viruses). This method requires the tedious microscopic isolation of individual cells from an immunized individual. Each single lymphocyte is placed in a microdroplet of nutrient medium under a film of oil. After incubation to allow antibody synthesis, the bacteria or phage are added. Each microdroplet must be examined microscopically for immobilization of bacteria (or for inhibition of lysis of added bacterial host cells in the case of antiphage antibodies).

The "immune adherence technique" is a method for identifying antibody-synthesizing and/or antibody-binding cells. Cellular antigens (red cells or bacterial cells) are commonly used, but soluble antigens can also be used if they are coupled to carrier particles such as red cells or acrylic spheres. Following immunization, a suspension of individual lymphoid cells is prepared and incubated with homologous particulate antigen. When the antigen particle contacts a cell bearing homologous membrane-bound antibodies, they adhere to one another. Upon microscopic examination, one often sees **rosettes,** consisting of a central antibody-bearing cell surrounded by several antigen-bearing cells or particles. The central cell may be an antibody-synthesizing plasma cell or it may be a macrophage that has acquired immunoglobulins. Those antibodies that have affinity for mac-

Table 2.1 Distinguishing Characteristics of Immunoglobulin Classes

	Immunoglobulin Class	
	IgG	IgM
Alternate names	—	Macroglobulin
Percent of immunoglobulins in serum	75–85	5–10
Concentration (mg/100 ml serum)	1275 ± 280	125 ± 45
Sedimentation constant	6.6–6.7S	19S
Approx. molecular weight	150,000	900,000
Rate of synthesis (mg/kg body weight/day)	28–33	5–8
Half-life (days)	25–35	9–11
Carbohydrate (percent)	2.5–4	10
Stable at 56° C	Yes	Yes
Pass placenta	Yes	No
Heavy chain class	γ	μ
Heavy chain subclasses	$\gamma_1, \gamma_2, \gamma_3, \gamma_4$ (G1, G2, G3, G4)	μ_1, μ_2 (M1, M2)
Heavy chain constant domains	3	4
Electrophoretic mobility	γ	Slow β (β_2)-Fast γ (γ_1)
Secretory type exists	No	Yes
Polymeric form	None	Pentamer normally
Valency	2	10
J chain present	No	Yes
Complement fixation	Yes (IgG3 > IgG1 > IgG2) IgG4 No	Yes
Relative amount required for serological lysis	High	Low
Serological agglutination	Moderate	Strong
Serological precipitation	Strong	Variable
Serological opsonization	Weak	Strong
Primary immunological functions	Passive immunity for the newborn; viral & exotoxin neutralization; responds best to protein antigens; secondary response to antigens (memory)	Bacterial agglutination; complement-mediated bacteriolysis; opsonization; endotoxin neutralization; responds best to polysaccharide antigens; early (primary) response to antigens

rophages are termed **cytophilic antibodies.** They attach to membrane receptors by their Fc tails, leaving their Fab arms free to bind antigenic determinants.

Genetic Control of Antibody Diversity

The antigen-binding portion of an immunoglobulin is formed by the variable regions of both H and L chains. Since normal animals can immunologically respond to thousands of different antigens, there must be

Table 2.1 (*Continued*)

	Immunoglobulin Class		
	IgA	IgD	IgE
Alternate names	Secretory Ig	—	Reagin
Percent of immunoglobulins in serum	5–15	0.001	0.0003
Concentration (mg/100 ml serum)	225 ± 55 (serum)	0.3–40	16–97 ng/ml
Sedimentation constant	6.8S (serum monomer) 11.4S (secretions)	6.6S	7.9–8.2S
Approx. molecular weight	160,000 (serum) 400,000 (secretions)	180,000	190,000
Rate of synthesis (mg/kg body weight/day)	8–24	0.4	0.02
Half-life (days)	6–8	2–3	2.4
Carbohydrate (percent)	10	12	11.7
Stable at 56° C	Yes	No	No
Pass placenta	No	No	No
Heavy chain class	α	δ	ϵ
Heavy chain subclasses	α_1, α_2 (A1, A2)	None	None
Heavy chain constant domains	3	Possibly 4	Possibly 4
Electrophoretic mobility	$\beta_2 - \gamma_1$	γ_1	γ_1
Secretory type exists	Yes	No	No
Polymeric form	Dimer (secretory) Possibly trimer	None	None
Valency	2, 4, 6	?	1?
J chain present	Yes (secretory form)	No	No
Complement fixation	No	No	No
Relative amount required for serological lysis	—	—	—
Serological agglutination	Weak	?	No
Serological precipitation	Weak	?	No
Serological opsonization	?	?	?
Primary immunological functions	Possibly prevents bacterial and viral invasion of mucous membranes and/or sensitization to food allergies	Unknown; may be involved in certain autoallergic diseases	Allergies; possible respiratory tract defense

some genetic mechanism(s) to generate diversity of polypeptides in the V_L and V_H regions of immunoglobulins. The speculations on this problem are largely centered in either of two theories. According to the **multiple germ line theory,** the variable regions of antibodies with different specificities (capacities for antigen recognition) are determined by a correspondingly large number of genes transmissible from parents to offspring according to the laws of heredity. If there were 100 such genes each for the V_L and V_H regions, then these immunoglobulin chains could be combined in $(100)^2 = 10,000$ different ways. It has been calculated that as little as 10 to 15 percent of vertebrate DNA need be devoted to immunoglobulin production in order to account for the estimated number of antigens to which an individual is responsive.

A different idea is embodied in the **somatic mutation theory.** According to this view, a relatively small number of immunoglobulin genes are carried by the gametes from parents, but they are exceedingly hypermutable in the bodies of offspring. At some relatively early stage of development the progenitor immunoglobulin genes go through a short period of extensive mutations to form a large number of mutant cells each with the ability to synthesize an antibody of different specificity. After this brief period of hypermutability, the genes once again become stable. A slight variation of this idea proposes that one or more genes engage in localized somatic genetic recombinations by crossing over or perhaps by extensive intragenic rearrangements of nucleotide sequences. It appears certain that some germ line genes must exist for immunoglobulins. Further heterogeneity in this regard might be provided by somatic mutation and/or recombination, so that both general theories may be partly correct.

It is now well established that a clone of fully mature plasma cells produces only immunoglobulins with one type of light chain (either λ or κ) and with one class of heavy chain (μ, γ, α, δ, or ϵ). However, it is also known that B cells can switch from production of one class of heavy chain to another during the differentiation process. Recall that the primary immune response is largely IgM and that the secondary immune response is predominantly IgG. This shift is accomplished without changing the type of light chain produced, and the antibody-combining site (containing the heavy and light chain idiotypes) also remains unchanged. For a relatively brief time during this shift (depending on the "life" of the old mRNA), a plasma cell may produce both IgM and IgG molecules with identical idiotypes.

In order to avoid postulating extensive coding redundancy among immunoglobulin genes, it has been suggested that separate genes specify the V and C regions of light and heavy chains and that the products of these genes somehow are combined into single polypeptide chains. If this is true, it represents an exception to the rule that a complete polypeptide chain is the product of a single cistron (functional gene definition).

Recent experiments with embryonic and myeloma DNAs indicate that the V and C regions of κ and λ light chains are coded by nonadjacent genes. The untranslated nucleotide sequence between these V and C genes is referred to as "intervening" or "spacer" DNA (found also in genes for ovalbumin, globin, and tRNAs). After differentiation to plasma cells, the information for the V and C regions of κ chains apparently is carried by a single messenger molecule of about 40S (9,000 nucleotides). This high-molecular-weight transcript is "processed" to remove the intervening nucleotides and produces a 13S (1,200 nucleotides) mRNA. Experimental evidence suggests that these genes become translocated into closer linkage relationships prior to transcription of DNA into mRNA. If translocation of these genes does occur, this may be the event that both commits a plasma cell to the production of a single specific immunoglobulin and activates transcription of the V-C gene complex.

Once the light chain V and C genes have been selected (translocated?) and activated, the plasma cell irrevocably produces only a single kind of light chain. This is not true of heavy chains. During differentiation of a plasma cell, a given V_H region may become associated with more than one of the five C_H regions (classes). At least four models have been proposed for V-C translocations at the DNA level (Figure 2.17). Three of the models (deletion, inversion, and copy insertion) require that the chromosome be broken in two places. The fourth model (excision-insertion) requires four breaks. All four models can be used to explain the juxtaposition of V and C genes for both light and heavy chains. One or more of these rearrangement mechanisms may be operative in any of three gene families: (1) kappa light chains, (2) lambda light chain classes and subclasses, and (3) heavy chain classes and subclasses. Each gene family consists of a tandem array of many structural genes coding for variable regions of heavy and light chains separated from a tandem array of relatively few structural genes for constant regions by spacer DNA. The genes within each family reside on the same chromosome (linked), but each family probably resides on different chromosomes (unlinked).

In humans, the kappa gene family seems to have a single C gene, the lambda C gene family has at least four, and the heavy C gene family (including all classes and subclasses) has at least ten. The number of V genes in each family is unknown, but may run into the hundreds.

Even though each plasma cell may be heterozygous for genetic markers (allotypes) on light and heavy chains, only one of each allele is expressed within a given lymphocyte clone. This phenomenon is called **allelic exclusion,** but the regulatory mechanism by which it operates is unknown. If translocation of V and C regions for both light and heavy chains is required for gene activation, then this event occurs in only one chromosome for each gene family to the exclusion of the homologous chromosome.

Any given antigen-specific V domain can presumably be united with various C domains, thereby permitting each antigen-binding site to acquire a variety of different effector functions, e.g., complement fixation (C_μ or C_γ), transplacental passage (C_γ), secretion across mucous membranes (C_α), or affinity for mast cells (C_ϵ). Any given light chain can associate with any heavy chain, a process called **combinatorial association.** In addition, any given V region of an immunoglobulin chain can associate with any C region of the same gene family, a process termed **combinatorial translocation.** These two mechanisms are responsible for the great heterogeneity of antibody structures that typify the immune response.

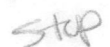

The Antibody-Combining Site

Detailed analyses of the IgG molecule have revealed that there are several positions within the variable regions of both L and H chains that differ much more in amino acid content from one myeloma antibody to another than the rest of the variable region. These positions are termed **hypervariable regions.** There are three hypervariable regions in L chains (near amino acid residues 30, 50, and 95) and four hypervariable regions in H chains (near residues 30, 55, 85, and 105). It was found that the antibody-combining site that binds antigen is composed of the hypervariable regions of both H and L chains. Considerable understanding of the three-dimensional structure of the combining site has recently been obtained from X-ray diffraction studies of Fab fragments and of Bence-Jones dimers (pairs of L chains often found in the urine of myeloma patients). Within the

Serology and Immunology

I. Deletion Model

By looping out and deleting a segment of chromosome, a given V gene could become successively associated with different C genes.

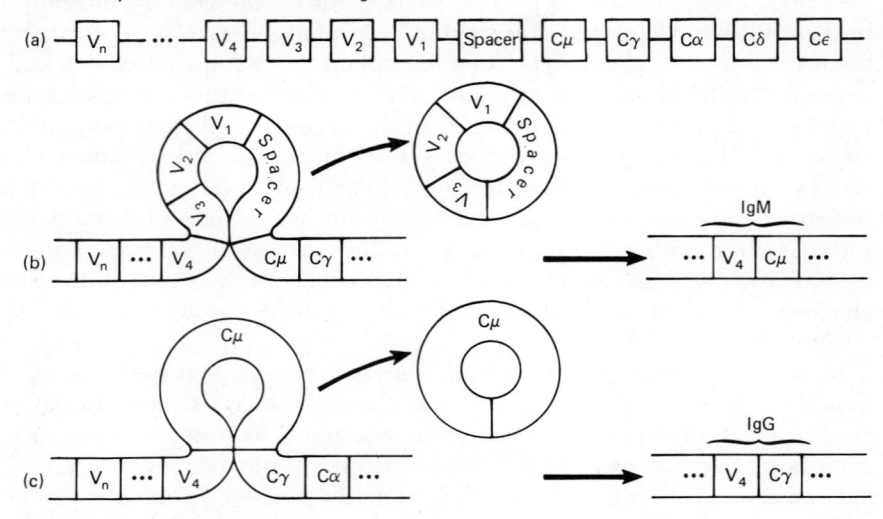

(a) —[V_n]—···—[V_4]—[V_3]—[V_2]—[V_1]—[Spacer]—[Cμ]—[Cγ]—[Cα]—[Cδ]—[Cε]—

(b) [V_n]···[V_4] [Cμ][Cγ]··· → ···[V_4][Cμ]···   IgM

(c) [V_n]···[V_4] [Cγ][Cα]··· → ···[V_4][Cγ]···   IgG

II. Inversion Model

An inversion loop rearranges the V and C genes without loss of any genetic material from the chromosome.

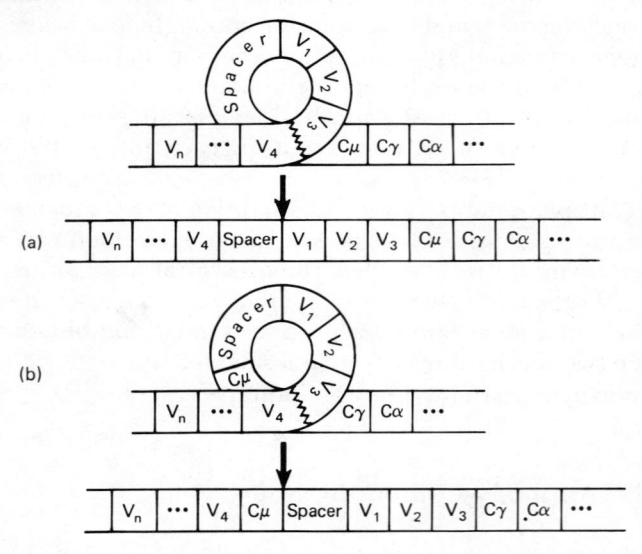

(a) [V_n]···[V_4][Spacer][V_1][V_2][V_3][Cμ][Cγ][Cα]···

(b) [V_n]···[V_4][Cμ][Spacer][V_1][V_2][V_3][Cγ][Cα]···

Fab, the variable (V) and constant (C) domains of an immunoglobulin chain are roughly cylindrical. Within each domain the polypeptide chain is folded back and forth on itself in a sandwich-like configuration.

One layer of the sandwich within the C domain consists of three adjacent (but not contiguous) segments of polypeptides, and the other layer has four. The two layers are covalently connected by a single disulfide bridge. The V domain in both H and L chains has additional loops, but the overall structure is very similar to that of the C domain (Figure 2.18). The two "cylinders" (domains) of a chain are connected by an extended stretch of the polypeptide called the "switch" region. The two domains are rotated

III. Copy-Insertion Model
  (a) A copy of a given V gene is made and inserted next to a given C gene.

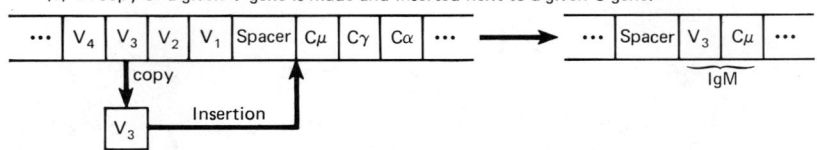

| ... | V_4 | V_3 | V_2 | V_1 | Spacer | $C\mu$ | $C\gamma$ | $C\alpha$ | ... |

→ | ... | Spacer | V_3 | $C\mu$ | ... |
            $\underbrace{\hphantom{V_3 C\mu}}_{\text{IgM}}$

copy → V_3 → Insertion

  (b) Alternatively, several copies of a given V gene are made and inserted adjacent to several C genes. Only one V-C complex would be active at any given time.

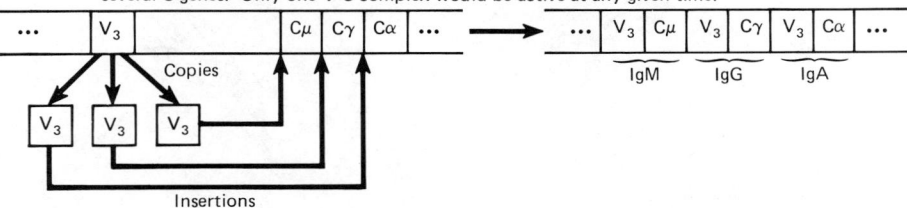

| ... | V_3 | | | $C\mu$ | $C\gamma$ | $C\alpha$ | ... |

→ | ... | V_3 | $C\mu$ | V_3 | $C\gamma$ | V_3 | $C\alpha$ | ... |
         IgM   IgG   IgA

Copies: V_3, V_3, V_3 — Insertions

IV. Excision-Insertion Model
  This model allows a V gene to be snipped out and spliced back into the chromosome adjacent to one of the C genes of the same family.

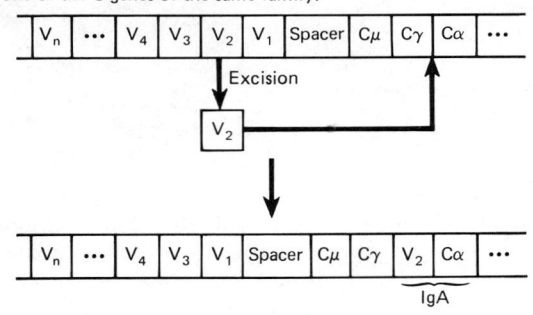

| V_n | ... | V_4 | V_3 | V_2 | V_1 | Spacer | $C\mu$ | $C\gamma$ | $C\alpha$ | ... |

Excision → V_2

↓

| V_n | ... | V_4 | V_3 | V_1 | Spacer | $C\mu$ | $C\gamma$ | V_2 | $C\alpha$ | ... |
                                                                              IgA

FIGURE 2.17. Four models that rearrange the V and C regions within the heavy chain immunoglobulin gene family. The same principles would apply to the kappa and lambda light chain gene families.

with respect to one another on both the horizontal and vertical axes. The three-strand layer of the C domain is on the outside of the molecule and the four-strand layer (containing hydrophobic amino acids) is on the inside. The situation is reversed for the V domain; the four-strand layer is outside and the three-strand layer is inside. The two V domains of H and L chains in a Fab face one another across a water-filled concavity that is the antibody-combining site. There are six hypervariable segments (loops) that line this cavity; none of these segments are more than 17 amino acids long.

Two major factors determine the degree of specificity of the combining site. First, the shape of the site must be complementary to that of the antigen and concave so that a relatively large surface area can interact with the antigen. Second, the side chains of amino acids in the hypervariable regions are positioned in the cavity so that they may fully participate in noncovalent electrostatic bonds (attraction of negatively and positively charged atoms), van der Waals forces (attraction between electrons and

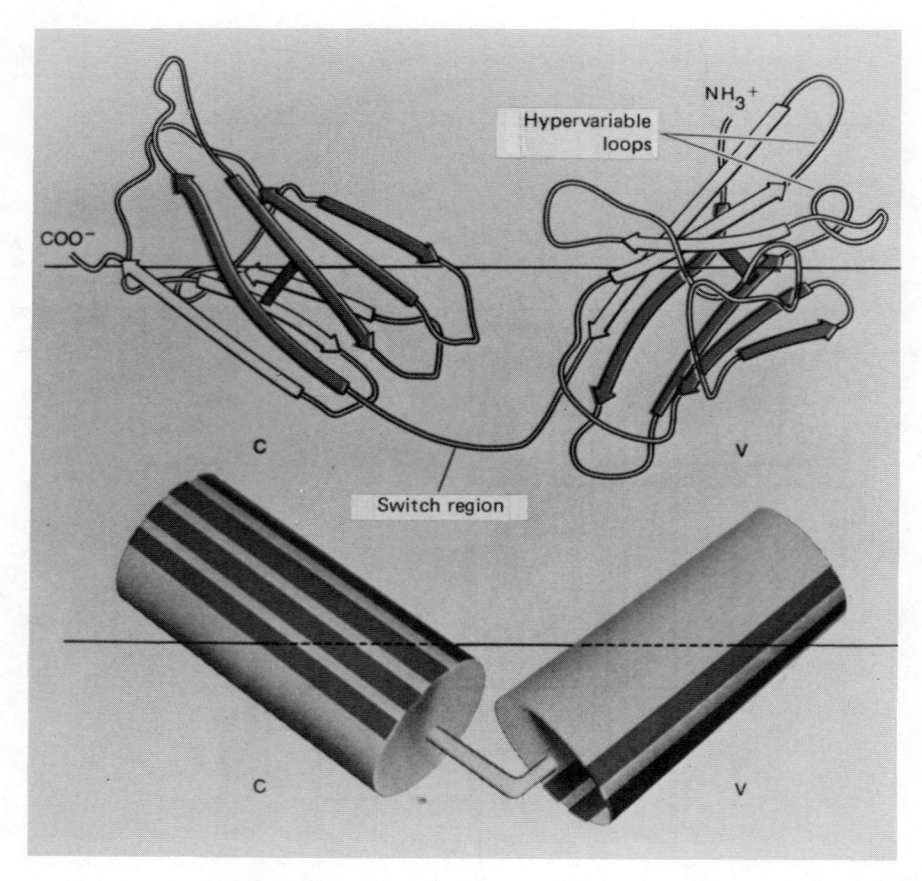

FIGURE 2.18. Light chain of an IgG antibody from a myeloma patient folds into a constant (C) and a variable (V) domain. In the course of evolution the two domains have rotated with respect to each other so that their four-strand layers (*dark arrows*) face in different directions. This rotation has been accompanied by changes in the amino acid composition of the two domains that enable them to perform very different functions when they interact in pairs. For example, the association of two identical light chains in Bence-Jones dimers forms a cavity in which hapten molecules can bind. (Bence-Jones proteins are found in urine of myeloma patients and often exist as pairs, or dimers.) The dimers can thus be considered models for a primitive antibody. In a dimer, the lined areas of the C cylinders are in apposition with one another and the unlined areas of the V cylinders are in apposition with one another. [Source: J. D. Capra and A. B. Edmundson, *The antibody combining site*, Scientific American, *January 1977.*]

atomic nuclei), and hydrogen bonding (attraction of oppositely polarized oxygen and hydrogen atoms) interactions with homologous antigens.

Figure 2.19 presents a model for the binding of a hapten (phosphorylcholine) in the combining site of an immunoglobulin derived from a mouse myeloma. The hapten is bound asymmetrically, closer to the H than to the L chain. The phosphate group of the hapten could form a hydrogen bond with tyrosine residue 33-H and could also form a strong electrostatic interaction with the guanidinium group of arginine 52-H. The choline group of the hapten contains a positively charged nitrogen that could interact with

Antigens and Antibodies

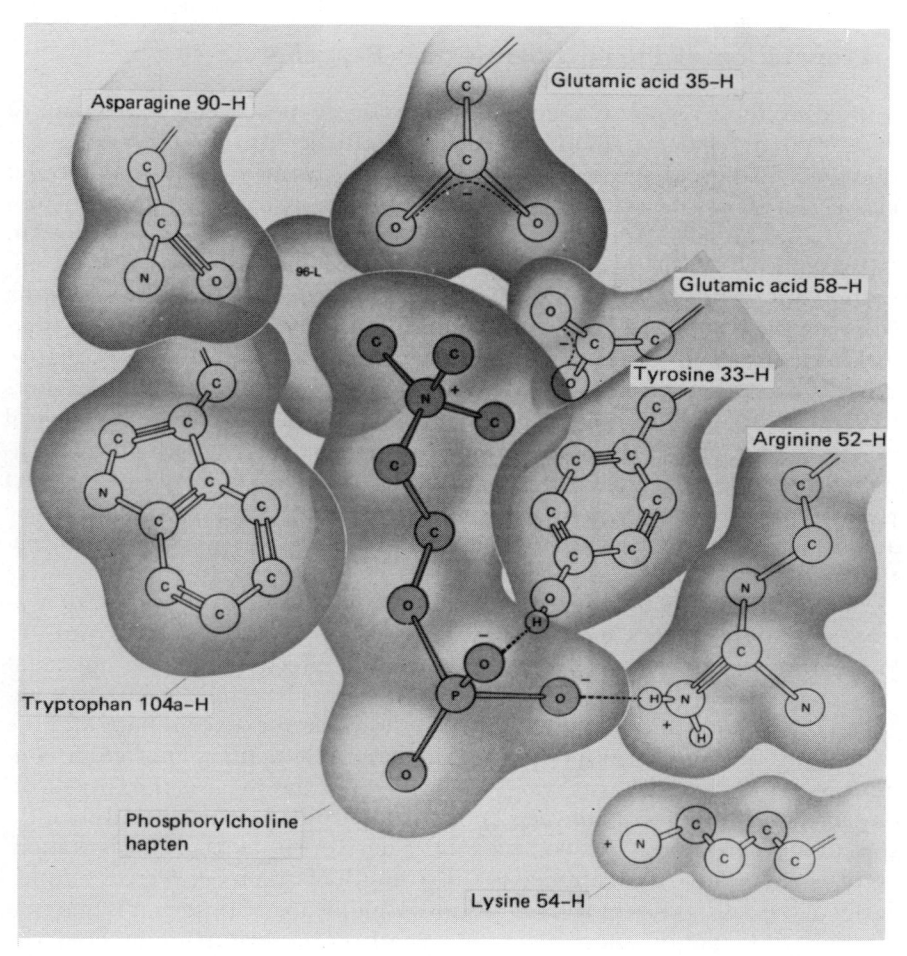

FIGURE 2.19. Model of the binding of the hapten phosphorylcholine (*dark-colored balls*) to combining site of an antibody from a mouse myeloma designated McPC 603 illustrates how the shape of the site is precisely complementary to that of the hapten. In addition, amino acid side chains lining cavity bind to hapten through weak, noncovalent interactions of following types: electrostatic (attraction of positively and negatively charged atoms), hydrogen bonding (attraction of oppositely polarized hydrogen and oxygen atoms), and van der Waals (attraction between electrons and atomic nuclei). This model is based on actual X-ray data. [*Source: J. D. Capra and A. B. Edmundson, The antibody combining site,* Scientific American, *January, 1977.*]

the negatively charged side chain of glutamic acid 58-H. The choline group can also form van der Waals interactions with carbon atoms in both H and L chains. This model was developed from X-ray–diffraction analyses of crystals and may not accurately reflect all of the interactions possible *in vivo.* From the model it is possible to see how antibodies of the same specificity might differ in affinity. For example, if a negatively charged glutamic acid were to be substituted for the positively charged arginine at position 52 in the H chain, the overall topology of the cavity would not change markedly, but the altered immunoglobulin would not be able to bind the hapten as strongly.

Preparation of Purified Serological Reagents

The immune response to a complete antigen (possessing a diversity of determinant sites) usually involves the production of corresponding antibodies of different specificities and belonging to various immunoglobulin classes. Suppose that we have a serum containing two antibody specificities (anti-A and anti-B). If a particulate antigen A is added in large quantity to this serum, all of the anti-A should be absorbed onto the A particles. Centrifugation would bring the A particles and all the absorbed anti-A into a compact mass at the bottom of the tube. Removal of the supernatant fluid yields an **absorbed serum** containing only anti-B immunoglobulins (Figure 2.20). **Absorption** is an immunological term applied to the use of reagents to remove unwanted antigens or antibodies from a mixture by serological reaction. In contrast, the term **adsorption** refers to any nonspecific attachment of soluble substances (such as proteins) to the surfaces of cells or inert particles. Antibodies reacting with the adsorbed substance may cause agglutination of the particles to which they are attached **(passive agglutination).**

The union between antigen and antibody involves only weak, (noncovalent, secondary) forces such as ionic bonds, hydrogen bonds, and van der Waals forces. These weak forces only become effective bonding agents at very close distances. Thus, there must be a very close mirror imagery between the epitope and the paratope; i.e., the antigenic determinant and the combining site on the antibody must be of complementary molecular configurations (lock-and-key analogy). The tighter the fit and the more secondary bonds that form between antigen and antibody, the more difficult it should be to disrupt the complex by such forces as thermal agitation. **Avidity** is a relative term applied to the strength of union between a complex antigen and antibodies of a given serum. A highly avid antiserum is one that binds its homologus antigen tightly. Another antiserum might bind the

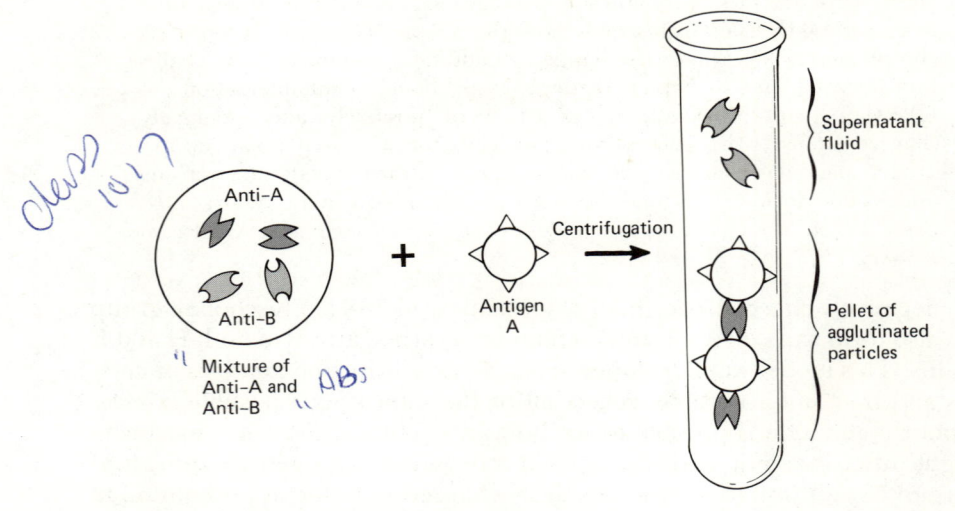

FIGURE 2.20. Absorption procedure for purifying a mixture of antibodies.

same antigen loosely, and in this case the antibodies would appear to be less avid.

As the process of antigenization to a given antigen proceeds, the average affinity of antibodies for that antigen tends to increase. The dosage of antigen can influence the average avidity. For a given antigen, some lymphocytes will have high-affinity receptors and others will have low-affinity receptors. A low dosage of antigen will stand a better chance of being bound by (and stimulating) lymphocytes with high-affinity receptors. Higher dosage of the antigen will also stimulate lymphocytes with lower-affinity receptors. Antigens must bind to lymphocyte receptors before these cells will be stimulated to release antibodies of corresponding specificity. The antigen receptors on certain lymphocytes (B cells) are known to be membrane-bound immunoglobulins. The nature of receptors on other lymphocytes (T cells) is unknown. Thus, a low dosage of antigen tends to generate antibodies of high average affinity, whereas a high dosage of antigen tends to generate antibodies of low average affinity. The selection of lymphocytes in this fashion tends to produce antibodies of higher average affinity as the primary immune response progresses regardless of the initial dosage. As the initial dose of antigen is catabolized and eliminated, progressively lower concentrations of the antigen selectively stimulate lymphocytes with successively higher-affinity receptors. This phenomenon is a logical extension of the clonal selection theory of antibody formation discussed in Chapter 1. Since a more protracted contact with weak antigens is usually required to elicit an immune response, it follows that a broader range of antibody specificities (paratopes) would be expected to appear as antigenization proceeds.

In practice, the terms affinity and avidity are often used synonymously even though they are not exactly the same. **Avidity** refers to the average binding strength exhibited by antibodies of a given serum to a complex antigen (containing a variety of determinants). **Affinity** refers to the strength of binding between antibody and a simple, uniform determinant (hapten). Because of synergisms, the average avidity of a serum may not be equated with a simple summation of affinities for the individual determinants of a complex antigen.

Antibodies bearing similar antigen-combining sites can be purified (as a functional group, not as a chemical group) from a mixture of antibodies by introducing a purified particulate antigen into an antiserum, allowing absorption of the homologous antibodies to occur, removing the antigen-antibody complexes, adding a buffer solution, and heating the complexes to facilitate disunion of antigen and antibody. This process that results in the uncoupling of antigen from antibody is called **elution** and is another method for obtaining a purified antibody reagent. Consider a mixture of bacterial antibodies (anti-A, anti-B, anti-C, anti-D). We introduce pure particulate bacterial antigen C, incubate to allow coupling of antigen and antibody, and centrifuge the particles (and all attached anti-C) to the bottom of the tube. Next, all of the supernatant fluid (containing antibodies anti-A, anti-B, and anti-D) is removed by decantation or aspiration. Isotonic saline or buffer solution is then added to the pellet of particles for a suspending medium, and the tube is heated to 56°C for about fifteen minutes, shaking occasionally to facilitate elution of the antibody. After spinning the tubes in prewarmed centrifuge cups, the purified anti-C may be recovered in the supernatant fluid.

Serological Tests

Serological tests can be performed on a patient's specimen (usually on blood, serum, plasma, urine, or cerbrospinal fluid) for the presence of specific antigens or antibodies. A serological test for a specific antigen ideally is performed using a monospecific antibody reagent, i.e., one containing only antibodies reactive with a single kind of antigenic determinant. It is not always possible, however, to obtain monospecific reagents, especially for typing tissues to be used for grafts. In these cases, polyvalent antisera (containing antibodies of more than one specificity) may have to be used.

Infectious diseases are sometimes diagnosed by finding specific pathogenic microorganisms in the patient. Serology and other departments of the clinical laboratory may aid in diagnosis of cases where no unusual microbe has been found and may serve as confirmation in those cases where a pathogen has been found. Seldom can serological evidence be used exclusively as diagnostic information. Finding serological evidence of an antigen or the **titer** (concentration) of the corresponding antibody serves only as a suggestive indicator of the cause of the disease (**etiology**). As an example, a serologically positive VDRL (Venereal Disease Research Laboratory) test usually indicates present or past exposure to the causative organism of syphilis, *Treponema pallidum*. Malaria, leprosy, and possibly other diseases commonly elicit antibodies that cross-react with the antigen used in the VDRL test. Therefore, syphilis cannot be diagnosed on the qualitative evidence of an antigen-antibody reaction in this test. The quantitative evidence obtained from a serological titration test is likewise subject to suspicion. There is great variability from one individual to another with respect to the titer of antibodies attained by exposure to a specific microorganism and the length of time elapsed since that exposure. As a general rule, antibody titers become apparent shortly after exposure to an antigen and wane with time from that exposure or after recovery from a communicable (microbial) disease. Titration of a single specimen may reveal a certain amount of antibody present in a patient, but one can seldom say that it is indicative of a presently active disease. It is best to obtain **paired sera,** one specimen obtained early in the course of the disease (acute phase) and another sample obtained a week or so later. If the patient is recovered or recovering from the disease, he is in a "convalescent phase." An active or recent disease is indicated if a fourfold or greater antibody titer increase is detected between the acute and "convalescent" samples.

SPECIFICITY-SENSITIVITY

Ideally, the serologist would like to employ tests that are 100 percent specific and 100 percent sensitive. **Specificity** refers to the relative absence of cross-reactivity by antibodies with substances that are chemically related (but not identical) to the inciting antigen. **Sensitivity** refers to the smallest amount of unknown substance (either antigen or antibody) in the patient's specimen that can be detected by the test. If a specimen cross-reacts with natural substances other than the one under test, we say that a **biological false positive** (BFP) result is obtained. Suppose that a laboratory technologist is given 100 samples of sera that do not contain a certain antigen. For example, an antigen such as CRP (C-reactive protein) is routinely present in "heart attack" victims, but is not found in healthy patients. If a test for that same antigen produces three BFP reactions, we say that the test is 97 percent specific. If a serological test fails (for biological reasons) to detect a substance (either antigen or antibody) in a specimen that actually contains the substance, we say that a **biological false negative** (BFN) result is obtained. Given 100 serum samples that all contain a certain antigen, a test that produces five biological false negatives is said to be only 95 percent sensitive. False positive and false negative tests may also be produced by technical errors that are not considered to be of biological origin.

A **screening test** is used for preliminary detection of a specific antigen or antibody in the patient's specimen. A screening test should be 100 percent sensitive if it is to do the job of detecting every individual who has the substance in question. The screening test can afford to be less than 100 percent specific because, if positive, it can be followed by more definitive tests that have a higher specificity rating. The screening test should be relatively quick and cheap. No screening test actually has all of these attributes.

The most sensitive serological tests presently available are radioimmunoassays (RIA) and immunoenzyme tests, some of which can detect picogram (10^{-12} gram) quantities of antigen. Obviously, the use of radioactively labeled materials requires highly skilled technologists, and the cost of the test will be relatively high. Most screening tests cannot boast of either 90 to 95 percent sensitivity or specificity. The VDRL test is a widely used screener for detecting certain antibodies (called **syphilitic reagin**) induced by contact with treponemes. It is a relatively inexpensive test and can be completed in less than ten minutes (following a thirty-minute incubation of serum at 56°C). Because it is known to produce some biological false positives, a positive VDRL test is usually followed by a more specific test (less cross-reactivity) such as the fluorescent treponemal antibody absorption (FTA-ABS) test. The FTA-ABS test requires several hours to complete and is more costly of materials and technologist's time. These are just a few of the realities of serological testing. Discussions of further complications will be deferred to subsequent chapters along with the details of various serological tests.

SELF-EVALUATION

Terms
1. Abnormal plasma polypeptides excessively produced by neoplastic cells.
2. A process used to purify proteins by causing them to migrate differentially in an electric field.
3. The pH at which an amphoteric molecule has no net charge. (2 words)
4. Immunoglobulin light chains that appear in the urine of people with multiple myeloma. (3 words)
5. A nonglobular flexible region in an immunoglobulin molecule between the Fab and Fc fragments.

Serology and Immunology

6. Antigenically distinctive proteins common to all members of a species.
7. Structurally and functionally similar antigenic variants of proteins not common to all members of the species.
8. Antigenic determinants associated with the variable regions of immunoglobulin molecules.
9. The phenomenon in which only one of a pair of genetic markers is expressed by the corresponding region of all immunoglobulins produced by a given plasma cell. (2 words)
10. The phenomenon by which (through one or more of several possible mechanisms) any given V region of an immunoglobulin chain becomes joined to any C region. (2 words)

Multiple Choice

For each question in this section, choose the one best answer from the following:
(a) IgG (b) IgM (c) IgA (d) IgD (e) IgE

1. Which class of immunoglobulin is most common in serum?
2. Which class of immunoglobulin has the longest half-life?
3. Which class of immunoglobulin is predominantly found in secretions?
4. Which class of immunoglobulin is the best at causing serological agglutinations?
5. Which class of immunoglobulin commonly exists as a dimer?
6. Which class of immunoglobulin is responsible for passive immunity of the newborn?
7. Which class of immunoglobulin has a Fc region that exhibits affinity for attachment to mast cells?
8. Which class of immunoglobulin is usually produced earliest in a primary immune response?
9. Which class of immunoglobulin can most efficiently activate the complement system on a molar concentration basis?
10. Which class of immunoglobulin has no well-defined functions?

True-False

1. Albumins remain soluble when serum is treated with half-saturated ammonium sulfate solution.
2. In alkaline buffers, most serum proteins carry a net positive charge and therefore tend to migrate in an electrical field toward the negative electrode (cathode).
3. A protein is least soluble at its isoelectric point.
4. The only covalent force holding light chains to heavy chains within an IgG molecule is disulfide bridging.
5. Amino acids in a polypeptide chain (e.g., L or H chains of immunoglobulins) are conventionally numbered from the carboxyl to the amino ends.
6. The constant region of an IgG heavy chain lies entirely within the Fc fragment.
7. Each immunoglobulin molecule has one kappa and one lambda light chain.
8. Genes for V and C regions of an immunoglobulin chain are thought to be nonadjacent in embryonic lymphocytes, but are moved together during the maturation of plasma cells.
9. The functional valence of an intact antigen is usually less than the sum of the valences in the fragments of the partially digested antigen.
10. Portions of a determinant site on a protein antigen may be contributed by noncontiguous regions of its polypeptide chain.

Immunohematology Part I
The ABO and Rh Blood Group Systems

CHAPTER 3

CHAPTER OUTLINE

The ABO Blood Group System
  Subgroups
  Genetics
  Chemical Structure of Antigens
  Secretion of ABH Substances
  Blood Stains
    Blood Crust Test
    Agglutinin Absorption Test
    Acacia Enhancement Test
The Rh Blood Group System
    The Rosenfield Numerical Code

The Fisher-Race Theory
The Wiener (Multiple Allele) Hypothesis
Antiglobulin
Types of Agglutinins
D^u Antigen
Hemolytic Diseases of the Newborn
  Rh Disease
  ABO Disease
Self-evaluation

Many attempts had been made before 1900 to transfuse blood from one animal to another or from one person to another, often with disastrous consequences. It was only after Karl Landsteiner discovered the ABO blood group system of antigens in 1900 that an immunological understanding of these transfusion incompatibilities began to emerge. It was really not until 1924, when Bernstein showed how these antigens were inherited, that the concept of **systems** of blood group antigens took shape. We now know that antigens on the surface of erythrocytes (blood group antigens) belong to the same blood group system if they are governed by alleles of the same genetic locus (or possibly by alleles of very closely linked loci). Most blood group antigens are not considered to be the direct products of blood group genes. Rather, current theories propose that many blood group gene products are enzymes that attach sugars onto glycoproteins of the erythrocyte membrane, thereby creating new antigenic specificities. Discovery of the ABO system did not prevent all transfusion reactions, however. Slowly it began to dawn on the early immunohematologists (blood group serologists) that there were probably many blood group systems other than the ABO system important for successful transfusions.

The next major discoveries were in 1927 and 1928 when Landsteiner and Levine discovered the M-N types and the P blood group factor, respectively. In 1937, Landsteiner and Wiener discovered the very important Rh blood group system (but delayed reporting this discovery until 1940). The following year (1941) Levine, Burnham, et al. demonstrated that the Rh factor was involved in some cases of maternal-fetal blood group incompatibility responsible for the immunological disease known as **hemolytic disease of the newborn** or **erythroblastosis fetalis.** Since that time, rapid strides have been made in the science of immunohematology. At present, at least fifteen well-defined blood group systems (and more than 100 blood group

Serology and Immunology

factors) are known. The study of blood group antigens is of practical importance from the standpoints of matching bloods for transfusion, providing serological evidence for use in forensic medicine (parentage exclusion, blood stain determinations, etc.), and preventing maternal-fetal incompatability diseases.

Blood group antigens are usually classified as **glycoproteins,** a combination of carbohydrates (sugars) and polypeptides. In many cases (e.g., ABO blood groups) the sugars are the immunodominant groups; in other cases (e.g., MN blood group system) the protein moiety is the immunodominant group. Glycoproteins of cell surfaces serve a variety of "social functions" including regulation of growth and development, intercellular communication, and even malignancy. It is not clear that all glycoproteins of the red cell membrane are blood group antigens. It is also an open question as to what extent any of the known blood group antigens participate in these "social functions."

In addition to their potential roles in numerous normal physiological processes, some blood group antigens may also predispose an individual to specific diseases. Certain blood group antigens may provide the receptor sites by which parasites (from viruses to protozoans) gain entry into susceptible cells. For example, receptor-destroying enzymes (RDE), such as neuraminidase from the cholera bacillus *Vibrio cholerae,* inactivate antigens of the M-N blood group system as well as the influenza virus receptors on the surface of red cells. Thus, these virus receptors and blood group agglutinogens appear to be closely related. About 90 percent of West African Negroes have neither antigens *a* nor *b* of the Duffy blood group system; only about 3 percent of Northern European Caucasians and about 10 percent of Mongoloids of China do not have these antigens. Most West African Negroes are resistant to the endemic protozoan malarial parasite *Plasmodium vivax.* Human blood cells were exposed to a parasite known to cause malaria in monkeys (*P. knowlesi*); similar experiments have not been done with *P. vivax* because it has been difficult to culture it outside the human body. About 80 percent of the cells possessing the Duffy antigens were invaded by this parasite; only about 2 percent of the cells lacking the Duffy antigens were infected. The study of this aspect of immunohematology may ultimately provide more useful knowledge for the conquest of disease than was thought possible a decade ago.

The ABO Blood Group System

There are four major blood groups in the ABO system: A, B, AB, and O. The blood groups are named for the antigens on the surface of the red cells. Thus, group A individuals have the A antigen (factor, specificity, determinant) on their erythrocyte membranes, group B individuals have the B antigen, AB individuals have both A and B determinants, and group O individuals have neither specificity. A unique feature of this blood group system is the fact that antibodies to these A and/or B factors arise naturally in virtually all individuals devoid of these factors, even in the absence of exposure to foreign red blood cells. People with only the A antigen on their cells naturally have anti-B in their serum, people with determinant B on their cells have anti-A in their serum, those of group O have both anti-A

Table 3.1 Serological Reactions in the ABO Blood Group System

Blood Group	Agglutination with Anti-A	Agglutination with Anti-B
A	+	0
B	0	+
AB	+	+
O	0	0

and anti-B, and those of group AB have neither antibody. These facts are known as **Landsteiner's rules.** No other blood group system is known to have this regular, natural, reciprocal antigen-antibody relationship. Thus, the four major blood groups of the ABO system can be identified by the use of two diagnostic antisera, as shown in Table 3.1.

Direct blood grouping can be done on a slide or in a tube at room temperature. The usual procedure (Figure 3.1) is to mix commercial reagent (antiserum of known specificity) with red cells (10 percent saline or serum suspension is used for slide tests; 2 percent is used for tube tests). Ingredients are mixed on the slide with a toothpick. The slide is tilted back and forth and observed over a two-minute period for agglutination. Longer periods of incubation should be avoided because the effects of drying may be interpreted as agglutination **(pseudoagglutination).** Strengths of reactions are graded on a scale from 0 (no reactivity) through +4 (massive agglutination). In the test tube, the ingredients are added, centrifuged, and examined macroscopically for agglutination. Centrifugation brings the cells together rapidly and facilitates the formation of large antigen-antibody complexes. Overcentrifugation should be avoided because unagglutinated cells may become so tightly packed that only severe shaking can dislodge them from the bottom of the tube. Weak agglutinations may miss being detected when tubes are roughly shaken. By gentle rocking of the tube in an almost horizontal position, agglutination can readily be identified if it is present.

One of the most important controls on direct grouping is called **reverse grouping** or **serum grouping.** The patient's serum is tested with suspensions of known group A and B cells. These control cells can be purchased from several commercial sources. They should also be used to test the reactivity of anti-A and anti-B typing reagents. The expected reactions of serum from the four blood groups with these two reagent cell suspensions are given in Table 3.2.

As an example, the serum from an individual of group A contains anti-B; therefore, this serum should agglutinate B reagent cells.

Why are these "natural" anti-A and anti-B antibodies regularly found in reciprocal relationship with B and A blood groups, respectively? In the early days of immunohematology, it was hypothesized that the gene responsible for the blood group antigen also determined the opposite antibody. For example, the gene specifying blood group factor A on the red cells was also responsible for that individual making anti-B in the serum.

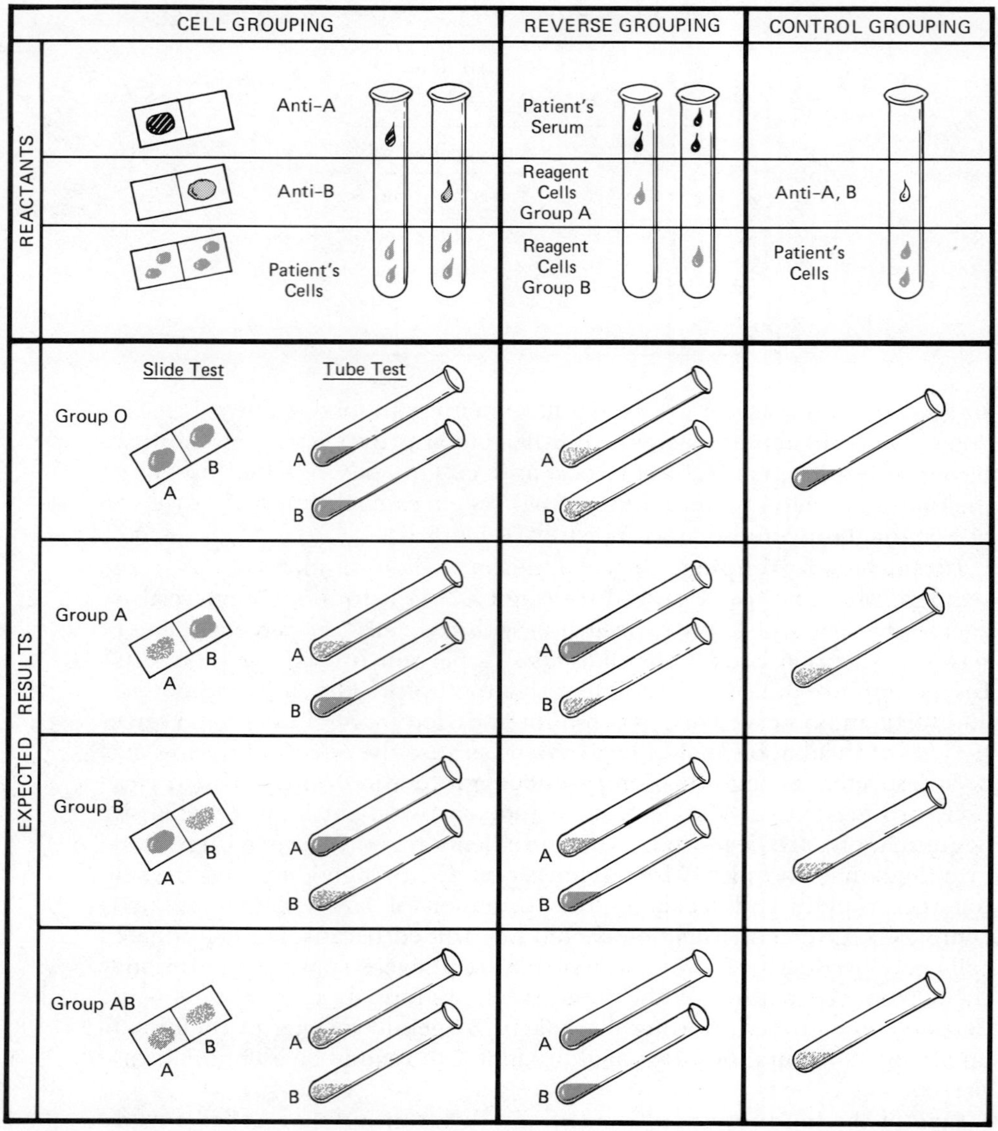

Figure 3.1. ABO blood grouping.

Table 3.2 Reactions of Serum from Different ABO Blood Groups with Reagent Cells

Serum from Blood of Group	Reagent Cells A	B
A	O	+
B	+	O
AB	O	O
O	+	+

Now immunologists are convinced that the production of free antibodies is an acquired characteristic; i.e., the body must by antigenically stimulated before it will release the corresponding antibody from the B lymphocytes. It so happens that the glycoprotein specificities A and B found on red cell membranes are also widely distributed in nature from bacteria to pollens and animal danders. Thus, from birth onward people are literally bombarded with substances carrying the A and/or B determinants, and it is this periodic antigenic exposure that elicits and maintains the titer of the so-called "natural" anti-A and/or anti-B in individuals that lack the corresponding determinants. None of the other human blood group antigens are of such ubiquitous distribution in nature. Hence, no other blood group system has the regular reciprocal antigen-antibody relationship characteristic of the ABO system. For example, the only way an individual can manufacture anti-Rh antibodies is by being exposed to red blood cells carrying this specificity. This may happen artificially as a result of a blood transfusion in either sex, or as a result of a mother becoming naturally sensitized to the red cell antigens of her baby. Any blood group antibodies other than those of the ABO system are therefore called **atypical (irregular) antibodies.**

Because there is neither the A nor the B factor on group O cells, it should be possible to donate group O cells to an individual of any ABO blood group without eliciting a transfusion reaction. Similarly, because group AB individuals have neither anti-A nor anti-B in their sera, it should be possible for them to receive red cells from an individual of any ABO blood group without eliciting an immediate transfusion reaction. This is the rationale for the concept of a **universal donor** (group O) and a **universal recipient** (group AB). Until recently it was common to administer whole blood to all patients. Whole blood may contain antigens on the red cells and antibodies in the serum. Although group O donor cells would not react with anti-A or anti-B in the recipient's serum, both of these antibodies are present in the donor's serum. Hence, when whole blood transfusions are involved, it is imperative that the patient receive blood of identical ABO group. Recently however, many hospitals are beginning to transfuse only cells (packed cells; no serum), especially for treatment of anemia where blood volume is adequate. In this event, the concepts of universal donors and universal recipients are applicable for the ABO blood group system. Another possibility is the use of **blood group–specific substances (Witebsky substances)** to convert a group O donor whole blood into a universal donor. Witebsky substances are soluble haptenic forms of the A and B antigens commercially extracted from the stomachs of domestic animals (horses, hogs). Mixing these Witebsky substances with a unit of group O blood should result in neutralization of the anti-A and anti-B in the serum. That is to say, the antibody-combining sites become occupied by soluble A or B substances so that the antibodies can no longer react with homologous antigens on the red cells. Unfortunately, for reasons as yet unknown, this treatment does not neutralize a cross-reacting antibody known as anti-A,B (anti-C) present in group O serum. Therefore, after treatment of a group O unit with Witebsky substances, it should be subjected to a **titration test.** Treated serum is diluted (usually doubling dilutions $1:2$, $1:4$, $1:8$, etc., out to $1:512$) and mixed in three sets with constant amounts of 5 percent saline cell suspensions of groups A, B, and O cells, respectively (the group

O cells serve as a negative control). The **titer** of the antibodies is the reciprocal of the highest dilution of serum that gives a detectable reaction with the cells. For example, if the greatest dilution of serum that produces a detectable agglutination is 1 : 32, then the titer is 32. If there is no reaction stronger than 1 : 8 with either A or B cells, the titer of the donor antibodies is considered to be sufficiently low as to cause little danger to the prospective recipient.

SUBGROUPS

Approximately 20 to 25 percent of all group A Caucasians have a weak-reacting variant of the A antigen, called A_2. The specificity of the remaining 75 to 80 percent of the A population is termed A_1. Serum from most group B individuals actually contains two kinds of antibodies: anti-A and anti-A_1. Anti-A reacts with both A_1 and A_2 subgroup determinants, but anti-A_1 reacts specifically only with the A_1 subgroup (Figure 3.2). Thus, group B serum can be absorbed with A_2 cells to produce a purified anti-A_1 reagent. Table 3.3 shows the subgroup reactions expected from the use of this purified reagent.

On rare occasions, group A_2 individuals have been known to become sensitized to the A_1 antigen. However, this is considered to be so unlikely that subgrouping is not commonly practiced when selecting donors for blood transfusion.

Extracts from the seeds of certain plants (usually legumes) may cause specific agglutination of red cells; hence they are termed **phytohemagglutinins** or **lectins.** An anti-A_1 lectin can be prepared from seeds of *Dolichos biflorus,* and because it is cheaper than absorbed B serum, it is more commonly used for subgrouping purposes.

Serum from group O individuals actually contains, in addition to anti-A and anti-B, a cross-reacting antibody called anti-A,B or anti-C (the latter term is unfortunate because of possible confusion with anti-C of the Rh system). Weaker and rare subgroups of the A agglutinogen are known (A_3, A_4, A_x, etc.) that are not detected by ordinary anti-A, but that do react with the cross-reacting anti-A,B. Only about 1 in 1,000 group A bloods is A_3 or weaker. Similarly, rare and weak variants of the B agglutinogen are reactive

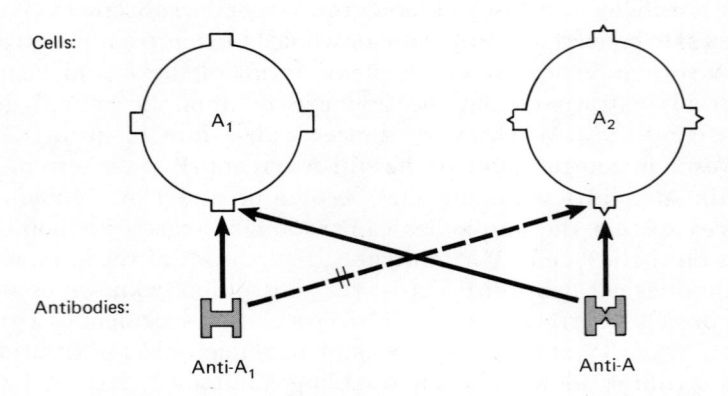

FIGURE 3.2. Models for explaining subgroups of the blood group factor A.

Table 3.3 USE OF ANTI-A_1 FOR SUBGROUPING

Cells	Group B Serum	Anti-A_1
A_1	+	+
A_2	+	0

with the anti-A,B of group O serum. For this reason, it is recommended that direct blood grouping in the ABO system should routinely employ the use of anti-A,B along with anti-A and anti-B reagents. Only blood group O should fail to react with anti-A,B. This single reagent is also used when screening for group O donors (as during disasters when many units of group O blood are needed as "universal donors").

Group A_2 cells react strongly positive with anti-A, whereas group A_3 cells react weakly with anti-A. Other details concerning subgroups of A and B will be deferred to advanced treatises. Subgrouping in newborn infants is unreliable because the receptor is not fully developed until approximately six to twelve months of age. Group A_1 is the most antigenic of the A cells; A_2 is next, then A_3, A_x, etc. However, even weak agglutinogens can cause serious transfusion reactions if the cells are misgrouped. Discrepancies with cell reactions due to weak subgroups of A and B are usually detected by the reverse or serum grouping technique. Some of the most common errors in blood grouping are to classify weak A cells as group O, or to classify AB cells as group B.

The incidence of the ABO blood groups varies from one population or race to another. Table 3.4 lists the approximate incidence of the four major blood groups in three anthropological races. It should be noted that Caucasoids have a relatively low incidence of the B agglutinogen, Negroids are relatively low in the A agglutinogen, and Chinese have a relatively low incidence of the O blood group. This kind of information can be of great value in helping to define racial groups of mankind, a fundamental problem of physical anthropology. Serological information has also been used extensively for studying the population genetics and evolution of various species in both the plant and animal kingdoms.

GENETICS

It is now well established that the four blood groups of the ABO system are determined by three alleles of a single locus. These multiple alleles

Table 3.4 INCIDENCE (%) OF THE ABO BLOOD GROUPS IN VARIOUS POPULATIONS.*

Race	A	B	AB	O
Caucasoid	34–38	12–13	5–6	42–46
Negroid	19–27	21–23	3–6	45–48
Chinese	27–33	25–28	5–9	31–43

* The range of reported values is derived from various studies.

Serology and Immunology

Table 3.5 Inheritance of the ABO Blood Groups

Blood Group (Phenotype)	Genotype(s)
A	$I^A I^A$ or $I^A i$
B	$I^B I^B$ or $I^B i$
AB	$I^A I^B$
O	ii

interact as follows: $(I^A = I^B) > i$. Alleles I^A and I^B are codominant; i.e., each is able to express itself in heterozygous genotypes. Gene i is amorphic and recessive to both I^A and I^B alleles; i.e., i produces no detectable antigenic product, hence it is responsible for blood group O. Table 3.5 displays the genotypes corresponding to the four blood group phenotypes.

There is no serological way to distinguish blood group A individuals as being genetically homozygous or heterozygous. However, this information can sometimes be obtained from pedigree records. For example, if a group A individual has one parent with group O blood, then that person must be heterozygous ($I^A i$). This kind of knowledge can also be used in helping resolve legal cases of disputed parentage. As an illustration, consider a group AB man being sued for paternity of a group O child. A group AB individual cannot transmit i allele to his offspring (barring rare mutation of course) and hence cannot be the parent of a group O (ii) child. This is the **exclusion principle** on which serological tests are admitted in courts of law.

In 1944, the famous comedian Charlie Chaplin was involved in a legal paternity suit with a young starlet named Joan Barry. Miss Barry was group A, her baby was group B, and Chaplin was group O. The mother must have been heterozygous $I^A i$ and transmitted i to her baby; the I^B gene of the baby had to come from its father. Chaplin was genetically ii and therefore could not have transmitted the I^B gene to his baby. Unfortunately, blood group evidence was not admissible in California courts at that time. Chaplin lost his case and was directed to be responsible for the child's support. Parentage cannot be proven serologically, but in certain instances it can be conclusively disproved.

CHEMICAL STRUCTURE OF ANTIGENS

Blood group antigens of the ABO system (and very likely all other blood group systems as well) are glycoproteins. Attached to the proteins of the erythrocyte membrane is a string of five sugars (Figure 3.3) that are considered to be precursor substance of the A and B antigens, called **H substance.** Group O cells have unmodified H substance, but groups A and B have modified most of the H substance by the addition of different sugars. Gene I^A specifies the structure of an enzyme (glycosyltransferase) that recognizes H substance and attaches an N-acetyl-D-galactosamine to the terminal sugar. Gene I^B determines the structure of a different enzyme that attaches D-galactose to the end sugar. A polysaccharide from type XIV pneumococ-

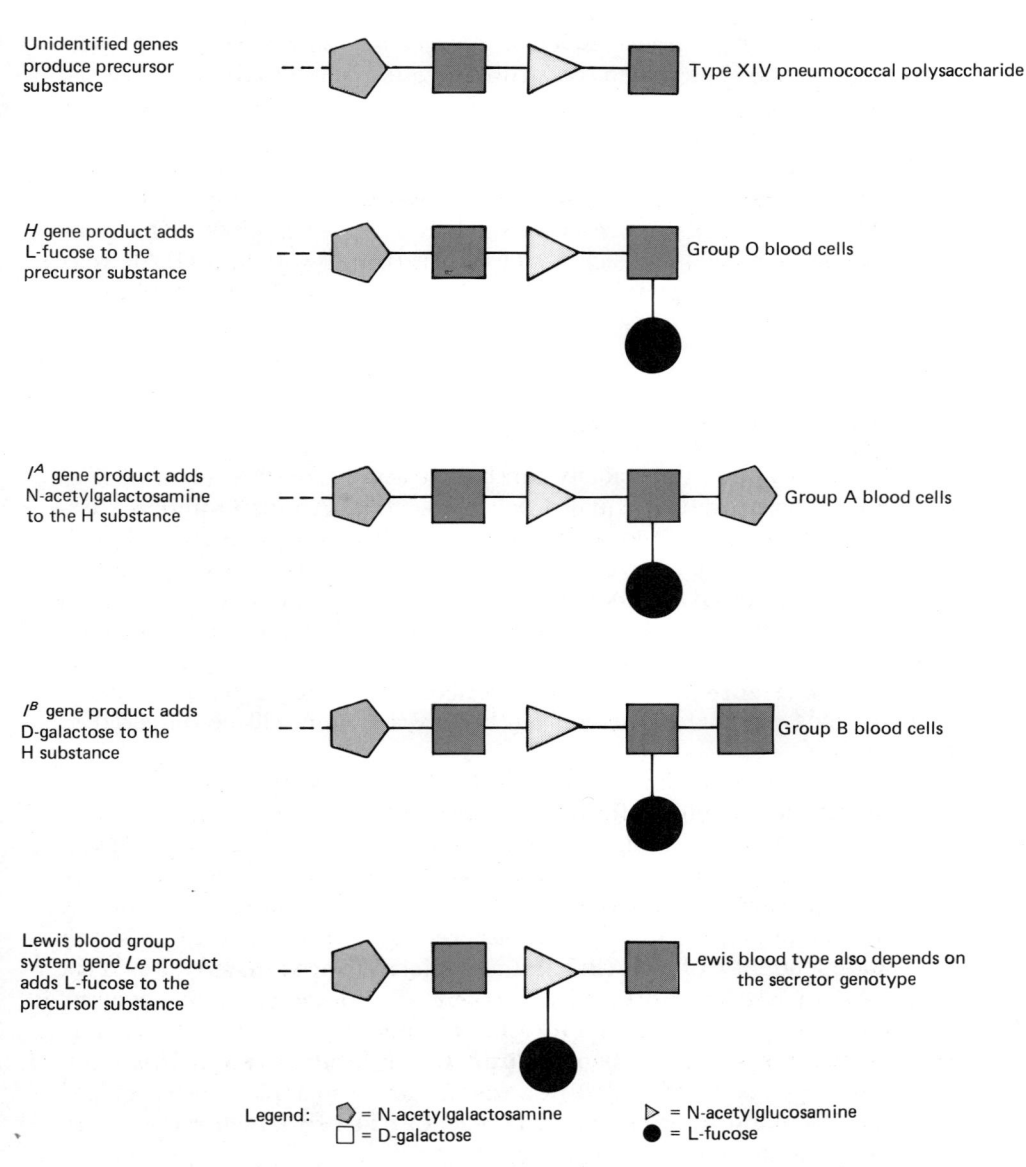

FIGURE 3.3. Diagrammatic representation of the chemical structures of the ABO blood group system antigens.

cus capsule has a structure similar to that of H substance, but it is missing the terminal L-fucose. With rare exceptions, every human, regardless of his ABO blood group, has a dominant gene H (assorting independently of the ABO locus) specifying an enzyme that attaches L-fucose to this precursor, resulting in H substance. Since all the ABO blood groups possess H substance, there is usually no anti-H in the serum. Very few individuals have been found to lack H substance on their red cells, but when it is lacking we find anti-H, anti-A, and anti-B in their sera. Individuals of this kind were first discovered in Bombay, India, and hence their blood was designated as **Bombay blood** (group O_h). These individuals are homozygous for the recessive allele of H (hh). The h allele apparently does not make an active enzyme and hence cannot convert the precursor substance into H substance. Thus, the H locus behaves in an epistatic fashion to the alleles of the ABO locus. That is, none of the ABO genotypes can be expressed unless H is also in the genotype.

Cells of group A_1 seem to have their H substance so well masked that anti-H is sometimes found in the serum of individuals of groups A_1 or A_1B. Most A_1 or A_1B cells do not react with anti-H. Some exceptions, principally in Negroes, are known in which A_1 cells react strongly with anti-H. All weak subgroups of A react strongly with anti-H, presumably because some of the chains of sugars that constitute the A antigen are missing the terminal N-acetylgalactosamine.

SECRETION OF ABH SUBSTANCES

A lectin with anti-H specificity can be extracted from the seeds of *Ulex europeus*. It reacts almost equally well with blood groups O and A_2, less strongly with group B, and weakly or not at all with groups A_1 and A_1B. This lectin is useful in determining the secretor status of certain medicolegal situations, in identifying the ABO group of blood stains, and in classifying genotypes and phenotypes of the Lewis blood group system. Antigens of the Lewis blood group system are closely related to those of the ABO system (Figure 3.3), but are governed by an independently assorting genetic locus. Further discussion of the Lewis system will be deferred to Chapter 4.

People who have the dominant gene *Se* in their genotype have the capacity to secrete water-soluble forms of haptens of the ABO system (A, B, and H substances corresponding to the antigens on the red cells) into various body fluids (saliva, sweat, tears, milk, semen, plasma, gastric juice, etc.). These people are called **secretors.** Others that are homozygous for the recessive allele *(se/se)* are termed **nonsecretors.** The secretor locus segregates independently of the ABO and Lewis loci. Approximately 80 percent of Caucasians are secretors and 20 percent are nonsecretors. Saliva is the most commonly used specimen for determining one's secretor status. The **secretor test** is essentially a **hemagglutination inhibition test.** Saliva is collected in a test tube and boiled in a water bath to inactivate enzymes and bacteria that might interfere with the reaction. The specimen is then spun in a centrifuge to sediment the coagulum, and the opalescent supernatant fluid is used in the test. One drop each of prepared saliva and anti-H lectin are placed in a tube and incubated at room temperature. Then a weak saline suspension of group O red cells is added (group O has the most unmodified H substance). The test is centrifuged and read for agglutination. If no agglutination is seen, we interpret that the saliva specimen contained soluble H substance that bound up all the combining sites on the anti-H lectin so that it could no longer cause agglutination of the red cells. In other words, no agglutination in the test indicates that the person was a secretor of ABH substances. Agglutination in this inhibition test would indicate that the person was a nonsecretor (Figure 3.4). Of course a tube containing saline in place of saliva (or a prepared saliva from a known nonsecretor) should also be run concurrently with the unknown sample as a negative control. The negative control would be expected to show agglutination because it contains no soluble ABH substances to inactivate or neu-

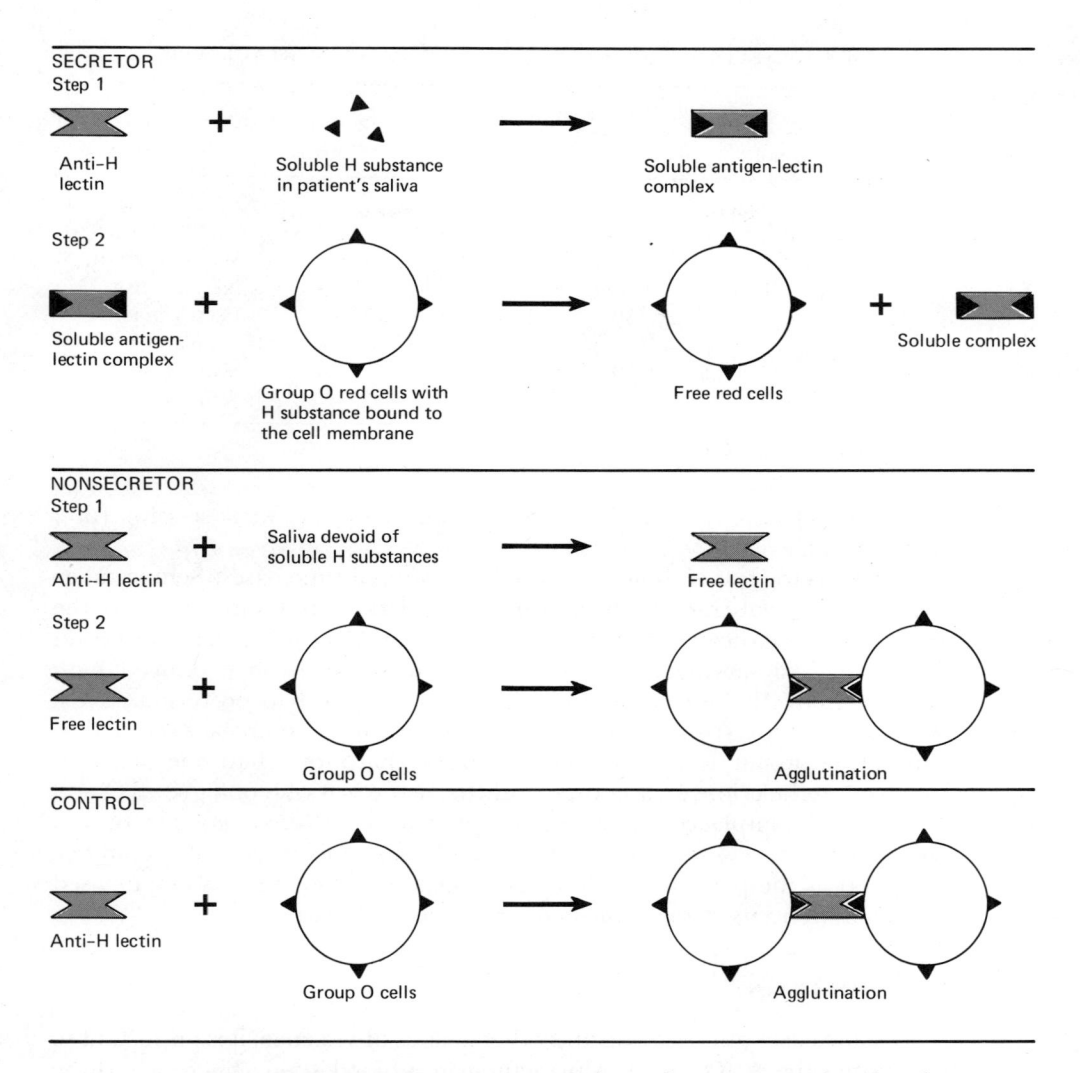

FIGURE 3.4. Diagrammatic representation of secretor testing by the hemagglutination inhibition technique.

tralize the agglutinating activity of the anti-H lectin. People differ considerably in the titer of ABH substances secreted. A titration test (Table 3.6) may be performed, but this is largely of academic interest rather than of practical value. It should be noted that the amount of agglutination tends to increase with increasing dilutions of a secretor's saliva because higher dilutions contain less soluble ABH substances to neutralize the anti-H lectin.

The titer of inhibition tests, including the secretor test, is defined as the reciprocal of the greatest dilution of unknown substance that completely inhibits serological reactivity. For example, in Table 3.6 the first patient's saliva completely inhibited agglutination at one-fourth dilution but not at one-sixteenth. Therefore, the titer is 4. Patient number 2 was unable to completely inhibit agglutination even with undiluted saliva, but since there was less agglutination in the first tube than in the control, we interpret that there was some A, B, or H substance in this individual's saliva inactivating

Table 3.6 EXAMPLES OF SECRETOR TITRATION TEST RESULTS

	Dilutions of Saliva					Control	Interpretation
	Undil.	$1/2$	$1/4$	$1/16$	$1/64$		
Patient							
1	0	0	0	+2	+4	+4	Secretor; titer 4
2	+2	+4	+4	+4	+4	+4	Weak secretor
3	+4	+4	+4	+4	+4	+4	Nonsecretor
4	0	0	0	0	0	0	Lectin inactive; invalid test
5	0	0	0	0	0	+4	Secretor; titer greater than 64

+ = agglutination; 0 = no agglutination

some of the lectin. In other words, the patient was a very weak secretor (titer less than 2).

The secretor test is sometimes used in criminal rape cases. Semen taken from the vaginal tract of the victim is tested for ABH substances. If the victim's saliva indicates she is a nonsecretor and ABH substances are found in the vaginal sample, then the semen must have been produced by a secretor man. If the victim admits in court that she had no recent sexual intercourse aside from the rape, a nonsecretor man could be excluded as the perpetrator unless it was acknowledged that more than one man was involved in the crime ("gang rape"). If the victim was of blood group O and her vaginal sample contained semen with only secreted blood group A substance, then a man of blood group B, whether a secretor or not, could be excluded as the perpetrator. Several other scenarios could also be devised in which an accused innocent man could be excluded.

BLOOD STAINS

In some cases of homocide and other crimes of violence, it is important to determine the ABO group represented in a blood stain. There are three methods in general use for this purpose.

(1) Blood Crust Test. When blood dries, the erythrocytes degenerate, making direct grouping tests impossible. However, the natural blood group antibodies of the ABO system usually can be detected for considerable periods of time after the stain has formed. If the stain has formed a crust on nonabsorbent material (glass, stone, leather, etc.), it can be removed by scraping. Three pieces of comparable size can each be placed on different slides. A drop of a 2 percent saline suspension of groups A, B, and O is added near the three crusts, respectively. A glass cover slip is placed over each preparation so that the cell suspension makes contact with the crust. Antibodies present in the crust may then diffuse out to cause agglutination of cells near this interface. If group A cells are agglutinated, the stain contains anti-A; if group B cells are agglutinated, the stain contains anti-B. Group O cells should not be agglutinated and thereby serve as a negative control. If group O cells are agglutinated, the test is invalid. When the stain is in absorbent material such as cloth, the agglutinins can be extracted by distilled water and evaporated to dryness on a glass slide at room tempera-

ture. The powder residue can then serve as an artificial crust for identification of blood group through the reverse (serum) grouping technique of the blood crust test.

(2) Agglutinin Absorption Test. A, B, and H blood group–specific substances, formerly attached to red cells, can often be detected in stains after the cells have disintegrated. Adding anti-A, anti-B, and anti-H of known titers to blood stain extracts gives these blood group–specific substances opportunity to combine with and neutralize the homologous antibodies. After incubation in the refrigerator overnight, the tubes are centrifuged and the supernatant fluid is transferred to clean tubes for the test. Subsequent addition of saline suspensions of groups A, B, and O cells to the antibody stain preparations may reveal diminished reactivity or nonreactivity, indicating that some or all of the combining sites on the antibodies have become occupied by soluble blood group–specific substances (neutralized). If a stain can neutralize anti-A, then the stain must have possessed the A specificity; if a stain neutralizes anti-B, then it must have had the B determinant. A stain that apparently has failed to neutralize both anti-A and anti-B agglutinins should not be interpreted as group O because there is a possibility that determinants were present but in insufficient amount or they may have become denatured. Conversely, a stain that has absorbed both anti-A and anti-B agglutinins should not be interpreted as group AB because of the possibility of nonspecific absorption by dirt or bacteria in the stain. To account for the latter possibility, an adjacent piece of unstained material should always be included as a negative control. Furthermore, group AB stains should not absorb anti-H lectin, whereas group O stains should absorb it. Additional controls consist of unstained samples of cloth to which are added known group A, B, AB, and O bloods; these are allowed to dry and are tested in parallel with the unknown. These controls should behave as expected if the test results are to be considered valid.

(3) Acacia Enhancement Test. Acacia is a colloid that adsorbs onto the red cell surface, reduces the electrical surface charge, and thereby reduces the repellent force between cells. A 10 percent aqueous solution of gum acacia, when added to a blood stain extract, enhances the sensitivity of a test for blood group agglutinins. Three tubes are set up to receive blood stain extract and a drop of a 1 percent saline suspension of groups A, B, and O cells is added to each tube, respectively. Comparable controls are set up

Table 3.7 POSSIBLE RESULTS OF THE ACACIA ENHANCEMENT TEST FOR DETERMINING THE ABO GROUP OF BLOOD STAINS

Blood Group of Stain	Stain Extract Plus Cells of Group		
	A	*B*	*O*
O	+	+	O
A (or O with anti-A deteriorated)	O	+	O
B (or O with anti-B deteriorated)	+	O	O
Inconclusive	O	O	O
Invalid	+	+	+

Serology and Immunology

using extracts from unstained portions of cloth. The tubes are incubated in the refrigerator, centrifuged, and decanted to remove the dark supernatant fluid. Acacia solution is then added, allowed to incubate at room temperature, and read for agglutination. Interpretation of the results is shown in Table 3.7.

The Rh Blood Group System

Landsteiner and Wiener found an antigenic specificity common to red cells of the rhesus monkey and about 85 percent of Caucasoid humans. It was therefore named the **"rhesus factor"** or **"Rh factor."** Historically, much confusion has surrounded this system because it is the most complicated human blood group system known at present. There are three methods for designating the blood types in this system, two of which are now considered obsolete.

(1) The Rosenfield Numerical Code. R. E. Rosenfield proposed to assign numbers to the blood factors in their order of discovery. This scheme was never widely accepted because it failed to differentiate between genotypes, phenotypes, genes, and agglutinogens. It will not be discussed in this text.

(2) The Fisher-Race Theory. R. A. Fisher and R. R. Race originally championed the theory of three closely linked genetic loci, each with a pair of alleles, to account for the five major blood factors of this system (Figure 3.5). The three contrasting pairs of alleles were designated (D,d), (C,c), and (E,e), respectively. Gene D is dominant to its allele d because gene D is responsible for the antigenic specificity D, whereas gene d produces no detectable antigenic factor. Unfortunately, the other two loci do not consist of dominant and recessive alleles, as expected for upper- and lower-case

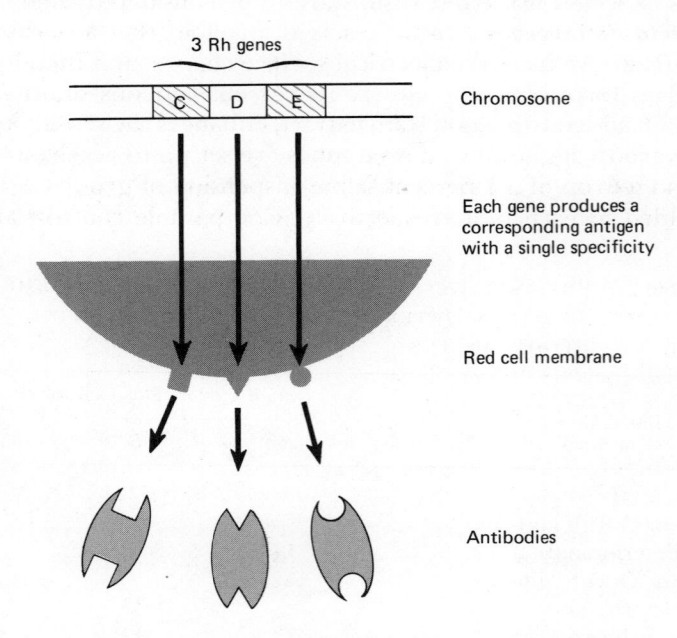

FIGURE 3.5. Model of the Fisher-Race concept of gene control for the Rh blood group system.

symbols. *C* and *c* are actually codominant alleles and thus each specifies an antigenic determinant even when in heterozygous genotypes. The same is true for alleles *E* and *e*. Aside from this source of confusion, the C,D,E system of Fisher and Race was simple to understand and undoubtedly contributed to its preferred use for a time. Fisher and Race envisaged that each blood factor (D,C,c,E,e) stimulated a corresponding antibody in an individual who did not possess the same blood factor. Thus, there was a one-to-one-to-one correspondence for gene–blood factor–antibody. Furthermore, the three genetic loci were considered so tightly linked that crossing over must be extremely rare or nonexistent. Both of these ideas have proven to be erroneous. Many manufacturers of Rh typing reagents still display the DCE nomenclature (in addition to those of the Wiener system) on the labels of their products. Many supervisors of clinical laboratories were trained when the Fisher-Race theory was still considered an accurate representation of the Rh system and may continue to favor its use even though it has been proven to be incorrect. For these reasons, the DCE system will be used liberally in this text.

Since gene *d* is an amorph (making no detectable antigenic product), there is no anti-d. Hence, *DD* and *Dd* genotypes are serologically identical; i.e., both bloods will react with anti-D. Since diploid organisms have a pair of homologous chromosomes bearing the DCE gene complex, a complete genotype for this complex might be *DCe/dCe* (the slash line separates the gene complexes on different chromosomes). One can see from the genotype symbols that blood factors D, C, and e would be present on the red cells and therefore should react with anti-D, anti-C, and anti-e, but not with reagents anti-c or anti-E. Using these five antisera, suppose that a blood specimen is found to agglutinate with anti-D, anti-c, anti-E, and anti-e. We know, therefore, that factors D, c, E, and e are on these cells. There are three possible genotypes that can produce this pattern of blood specificities: *DcE/Dce, DcE/dce,* and *Dce/dcE*. It should be obvious that there are more genotypes possible than serological phenotypes. Actually there are seventeen major phenotypes and thirty-six genotypes. They are shown in Table 3.8 together with their Wiener system counterparts.

So many new serological specificities have been found since the original hypothesis that the number of loci of the DCE system has had to be expanded to more than thirty, and multiple alleles have had to be proposed to account for new "intermediate" factors like C^W, C^V, and C^u. The Fisher-Race scheme has grown to involve such a highly improbable genetic system that it has been discarded for the single-locus multiple-allelic system of Wiener.

(3) The Wiener (Multiple-Allele) Hypothesis. Alexander S. Wiener proposed that a single genetic locus with multiple alleles could account for all of the Rh blood types. Each allele is correlated with the presence of two or three specificities (blood factors) on the red cells. One of the most difficult concepts for the beginner to master in an initial study of immunohematology is the idea that a single gene can be associated with the production of a complex antigen bearing two or more subregions (factors, specificities, determinants), each factor being capable of eliciting an antibody response *in vivo* and a homologous serological reactivity *in vitro*. In other words, it is possible for a gene to produce a blood group antigen that can stimulate the formation of multiple antibody specificities. A complex antigen molecule is

Serology and Immunology

Table 3.8 Rh Genotypes and Their Serological Reactions

| Genotypes | | Reactions with anti- | | | | | Caucasian |
Fisher-Race	Wiener	D	C	E	c	e	Frequency (%)
DCe/dce	R^1/r	+	+	0	+	+	33
DCe/Dce	R^1/R^0	+	+	0	+	+	2
Dce/dCe	R^0/r'	+	+	0	+	+	†
DCe/DCe	R^1/R^1	+	+	0	0	+	18
DCe/dCe	R^1/r'	+	+	0	0	+	*
DcE/dce	R^2/r	+	0	+	+	+	11
Dce/dcE	R^0/r''	+	0	+	+	+	†
DcE/Dce	R^2/R^0	+	0	+	+	+	*
DcE/DcE	R^2/R^2	+	0	+	+	0	2
DcE/dcE	R^2/r''	+	0	+	+	0	*
DCe/DcE	R^1/R^2	+	+	+	+	+	12
DCe/dCE	R^1/r^y	+	+	+	0	+	‡
DCe/dcE	R^1/r''	+	+	+	+	+	1
DcE/dCE	R^2/r^y	+	+	+	+	0	‡
DcE/dCe	R^2/r'	+	+	+	+	+	*
DCE/DCE	R^z/R^z	+	+	+	0	0	‡
DCE/DCe	R^z/R^1	+	+	+	0	+	*
DCE/DcE	R^z/R^2	+	+	+	+	0	†
DCE/dCe	R^z/r'	+	+	+	0	+	‡
DCE/Dce	R^z/R^0	+	+	+	+	+	†
DCE/dcE	R^z/r''	+	+	+	+	0	‡
DCE/dce	R^z/r	+	+	+	+	+	*
DCE/dCE	R^z/r^y	+	+	+	0	0	‡
Dce/dCE	R^0/r^y	+	+	+	+	+	‡
Dce/dce	R^0/r	+	0	0	+	+	2
Dce/Dce	R^0/R^0	+	0	0	+	+	†
dCe/dce	r'/r	0	+	0	+	+	*
dCe/dCe	r'/r'	0	+	0	0	+	‡
dcE/dce	r''/r	0	0	+	+	+	*
dcE/dcE	r''/r''	0	0	+	+	0	†
dCe/dcE	r'/r''	0	+	+	+	+	†
dCE/dce	r^y/r	0	+	+	+	+	‡
dCE/dcE	r^y/r''	0	+	+	+	0	‡
dCE/dCe	r^y/r'	0	+	+	0	+	‡
dCE/dCE	r^y/r^y	0	+	+	0	0	‡
dce/dce	r/r	0	0	0	+	+	15

* = less than 1 percent but greater than 0.1 percent.
† = less than 0.1 percent but greater than 0.01 percent.
‡ = less than 0.01 percent.

therefore viewed as a mosaic of antigenic determinant sites, each of which behaves as a distinctive serological and immunological specificity (Figure 3.6).

The symbols used to represent the alleles are misleading. Despite the upper- and lower-case symbolism, all standard eight Rh blood type alleles are codominant in the sense that they are associated with two or three antigenic factors on the red cells. The capital gene symbol R denotes all alleles that possess the most antigenic factor of the Rh system, Rh_0 (corresponding to D in the Fisher-Race system). The Rh_0 factor is clinically most

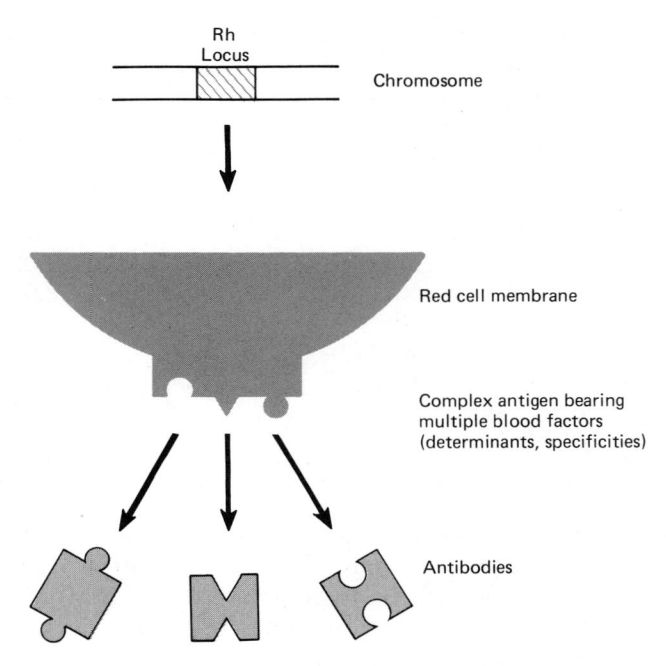

FIGURE 3.6. Model of a complex antigen of the Rh blood group system.

important in blood transfusions and maternal-fetal Rh incompatibilities. The lower-case gene symbol r indicates that the Rh_0 specificity is missing (corresponding to gene d in the Fisher-Race scheme).

There are five standard antibodies in the Wiener concept of the Rh system, corresponding to the blood factors Rh_0, rh′, rh″, hr′, and hr″. There is a reciprocal relationship between the rh factors and the hr factors in that if a gene specifies factor rh′ it fails to specify hr′ (and vice versa); if a gene specifies rh″ it fails to specify hr″ (and vice versa). There is no anti-Hr_0 (hr_0 or hr) to be the antithesis of anti-Rh_0. Comparison is made in Table 3.9 between the blood factors of the Wiener and Fisher-Race schemes. Table 3.10 lists the eight major alleles of the Wiener system and their corresponding antigenic factors in comparison with the Fisher-Race determinants.

It must be remembered that each person has two of these alleles in the genotype. As an example, the genotype R^0/r would be expected to manufac-

Table 3.9 COMPARISON BETWEEN BLOOD FACTORS OF THE WIENER AND FISHER-RACE CONCEPTS OF THE Rh BLOOD GROUP SYSTEM

Wiener	Fisher-Race
Rh_0	D
rh′	C
rh″	E
hr (specificity absent)	d (specificity absent)
hr′	c
hr″	e

Serology and Immunology

Table 3.10 COMPARISON OF WIENER AND FISHER-RACE CONCEPTS OF THE RH BLOOD GROUP SYSTEM

	Wiener Concept		Fisher-Race Concept		Approximate Frequency in Caucasoids of New York City (%)
Gene	Agglutinogen	Blood Factors	Gene Complex	Blood Factors	
R^0	Rh_0	Rh_0, hr′, hr″	Dce	D, c, e	2.5
R^1	Rh_1	Rh_0, rh′, hr″	DCe	D, C, e	51.2
R^2	Rh_2	Rh_0, rh″, hr′	DcE	D, c, E	16.5
R^z	Rh_z	Rh_0, rh′, rh″	DCE	D, C, E	14.9
r	rh	hr′, hr″	dce	c, e	13.4
$r′$	rh′	rh′, hr″	dCe	C, e	1.1
$r″$	rh″	rh″, hr′	dcE	c, E	0.4
r^y	rh_y	rh′, hr″	dCE	C, E	0.02

ture red cells possessing factors Rh_0, hr′, and hr″. On the other hand, a blood that reacts with anti-Rh_0, anti-rh′, anti-hr′, and anti-hr″ could be produced by any of three genotypes: R^0/R^1, R^1/r, and $R^0/r′$. A complete listing of the thirty-six Wiener genotypes and their corresponding serological reactions is presented in Table 3.8.

Most human blood group antigens (with the singular exception of those in the ABO system) are not widely represented in nature. Since the Rh antigens are only present on the red cells of humans (and certain other primates), one must be exposed to foreign erythrocytes in order to develop the corresponding antibodies. Factor Rh_0(D) is by far the most potent antigen for stimulating antibody production in the Rh system. It is the major source of blood transfusion reactions and maternal-fetal incompatibility disease in this system. Hence, blood with the D specificity is said to be **Rh positive;** bloods devoid of the D factor are designated **Rh negative.** Obviously, an Rh-negative person should never be given Rh-positive blood for either of two reasons: (1) to prevent an Rh-negative person from becoming sensitized to the D factor, and (2) to prevent a severe, immediate hemolytic transfusion reaction in an individual already sensitized to the D factor (i.e., one already possessing anti-D).

Other factors of the Rh system are less antigenic than Rh_0. Donor bloods are not routinely typed with any reagent other than anti-D in the Rh system. However, it should be realized that the less antigenic factors of the Rh system may occasionally be involved in incompatibility reactions and that some of these reactions may be life-threatening experiences.

Today there are more than thirty serological specificities known in the Rh system, most of them being extremely rare. It is not within the scope of this text to do more than introduce the student to the major blood group systems. Hence, discussion of other Rh blood factors is deferred to more advanced treatises. However, there is one additional blood factor that deserves attention in an introductory text. This is a weak variant of the Rh_0(D) specificity designated as the D^u factor (by British workers) or as the $\mathfrak{R}h_0$ variant by Wiener. Since the Germanic capital R is foreign to the experience of most people, the symbol D^u will be used in this book. Saline suspensions of red cells bearing the D^u factor fail to agglutinate with even the most potent anti-D antisera. However, these antibodies do combine with D^u cells ("sensitized" red cells), and their presence can be detected by a special reagent known as **antihuman globulin** (AHG), **antiglobulin,** or **Coombs reagent** (Coombs serum). Further discussion of D^u bloods must be preceded by a consideration of the nature of antiglobulin.

ANTIGLOBULIN

To prepare antihuman globulin, whole human serum or purified serum globulin is injected into rabbits or goats. In these animals, human antibodies act as foreign antigens, stimulating the animals to respond immunologically by synthesizing antibodies that react specifically with any globulin (antibody) of human origin. The reason why AHG can react with any human globulin is because within each immunoglobulin class (IgG, IgM, IgA, etc.) the constant regions of heavy chains (C_H) contain identical amino acid sequences and thus are antigenically identical. Within each kappa chain and each subtype of lambda chain, the same is true regarding the constant regions of light chains (C_L). Since normal human serum contains immunoglobulin isotypes, antihuman serum (Coombs reagent) is expected to contain antibodies reactive with all human immunoglobulins. Sera extracted from animals injected with human globulins must be thoroughly absorbed with washed, pooled human cells of groups A, B, and O in order to remove any trace of antibodies against human red cells so that they cannot be a source of agglutination when the Coombs reagent is employed.

It is recommended that the Coombs reagent contain not only antibodies against gamma globulins (the fraction containing most immunoglobulins) but also antibodies against certain beta globulins of the complement system. Such a reagent is called a "broad-spectrum antihuman serum." Following union with blood group antigens, homologous antibodies of classes IgG and IgM can activate the complement system and produce hemolysis. Far fewer antibody molecules are required to detect hemolysis than hemagglutination. Hence, hemolytic reactions greatly increase the sensitivity of the test. Certain antibodies in the Lewis and Kidd blood group systems can best be detected by a broad-spectrum antihuman globulin. This same reagent is also useful in tests for autoimmune hemolytic anemia (AIHA), cold agglutinin disease, paroxysmal cold hemoglobinuria, and certain drug-induced immune hemolytic anemias.

TYPES OF AGGLUTININS

Blood group antibodies may produce hemagglutination in any of three kinds of commonly used media: (1) saline, (2) albumin, and (3) antiglobulin. Blood group antibodies with 19S values are large molecules that behave as **saline agglutinins** or **complete agglutinins;** i.e., they cause agglutination of red cells suspended in saline. They belong to the class of immunoglobulins designated IgM. Agglutinins of class IgG are usually too small to span the gap between antigenic determinants on different cells without the aid of other substances. On the basis of the kind of "helper" substance required for agglutination, 7S agglutinins are classified into two major groups: (1) albumin (high-protein) antibodies, and (2) antihuman globulin antibodies.

Albumin antibodies are so named because of the common clinical practice of adding 22 percent or 30 percent bovine serum albumin (BSA) to enhance their agglutinating capacity. Red cells carry a net negative charge when suspended in a nonelectrolyte medium. Hence they tend to mutually repel one another. This makes it difficult for a small 7S antibody to make contact with different cells simultaneously. Red blood cells also carry a net negative charge in physiological saline solution (0.85 to 0.90 percent NaCl is isotonic with mammalian erythrocytes). Positively charged sodium ions become attracted to the red cell and form around the cell an ionic layer that somewhat reduces the repulsion force between cells. However, the repulsion force may still be too strong to allow 7S antibodies to affect agglutination. Higher salt concentrations would further reduce the repulsion force, but would inhibit antigen-antibody binding. The edge of the cloud of sodium cations surrounding a red cell is known as the "slipping plane" or "shear boundary." The electrostatic potential or voltage (in terms of mV charge per unit of distance) at the shear boundary is called the **zeta potential.**

Amphoteric substances contain positive and negative charges and can therefore react with either acids or bases. Some amphoteric substances, such as albumin molecules, can be used to reduce the zeta potential. Albumin molecules tend to be dipolar; i.e., they have positive and negative regions at opposite ends. The electronegative charges on red cells tend to attract the positive ends of albumin molecules; simultaneously, the negative charges are repelled by the cells, causing the albumin molecules to become nonrandomly oriented in space. Work must be done to orient the albumin molecules in this particular way, and the energy to do this is derived from the electrical field surrounding the red cells. A greater reduction in the zeta potential occurs as a consequence of orienting the dipolar molecules than that added by the fact that the negative portions of these molecules will face outward from the cell. Substances such as albumin or Ficoll that consume electrical energy in this way are said to raise the **dielectric constant** of the medium. By addition of bovine serum albumin or other suitable high-protein colloidal diluents, the zeta potential can be reduced to the point where 7S antibodies can attach to different cells and thereby produce agglutination (Figure 3.7).

It is thought that the negative charge on red cells is mainly attributed to the presence of negatively charged polar groups (such as the carboxyl groups of sialic acid residues) on erythrocyte membranes. Pretreatment of cells with enzymes such as trypsin or neuraminidase may therefore reduce the zeta potential by removing some of these charged residues. Unfortunately, in some cases enzyme treatment can modify blood group antigens so that they no longer can react with their corresponding antibodies.

The sensitivity of hemagglutination tests can be increased by using a low-ionic-strength saline (LISS) solution. LISS contains sodium chloride, glycine, and two phosphate buffers (KH_2PO_4 and Na_2HPO_4). Cells to be tested in LISS should first be washed thoroughly in normal saline and then resuspended to the desired concentration in LISS. Failure to wash cells before adding LISS may cause false positive results. Because it provides a good growth medium for bacteria, LISS should be stored at 4°C and discarded at the first sign of contamination. The addition to LISS of a bacteriostatic agent such as sodium azide is recommended.

The use of a low-ionic-strength BSA reagent also enhances the sensitivity

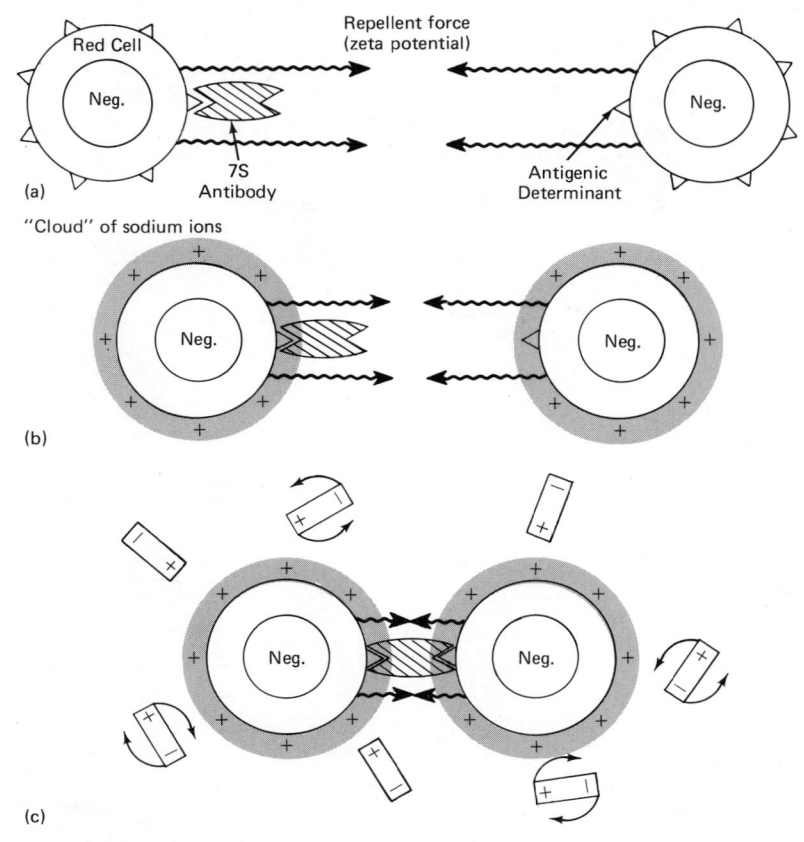

FIGURE 3.7. Models for explaining how the zeta potential between red blood cells is reduced by electrolytes and albumin molecules. (*a*) Red blood cells suspended in a nonelectrolyte medium (e.g., glycerin) have a strong repellent force (zeta potential) because all cells carry the same negative charge. (*b*) The net negative charge on red cells is partially neutralized by positive sodium ions when they are suspended in an electrolyte medium such as physiological saline. (*c*) Addition of a dipolar molecule (e.g., bovine albumin) further reduces the repulsive force by consuming electrical energy in orienting its positive-charged portions toward the cell and its negative-charged portions away from the cell. If the zeta potential is sufficiently reduced, the small 7S antibodies can bridge the gap between cells to affect agglutination.

of hemagglutination tests involving albumin antibodies. It has been shown that greater sensitivity is obtained by using bovine albumin reagents processed to polymerize albumin molecules into dimers, trimers, tetramers, and pentamers.

Those antibodies that can only be detected by antiglobulin reagent behave as though they were **univalent** (having only one combining site; also termed **incomplete antibodies**). This is probably incorrect in an absolute sense. All 7S antibodies probably have two potential combining sites (bivalent) and can behave serologically as **blocking antibodies** (Figure 3.8). A saline suspension of red cells exposed to 7S immunoglobulins may fail to agglutinate because the antibodies are of insufficient size to "bridge the gap" between homologous antigenic sites on different cells. Such cells are

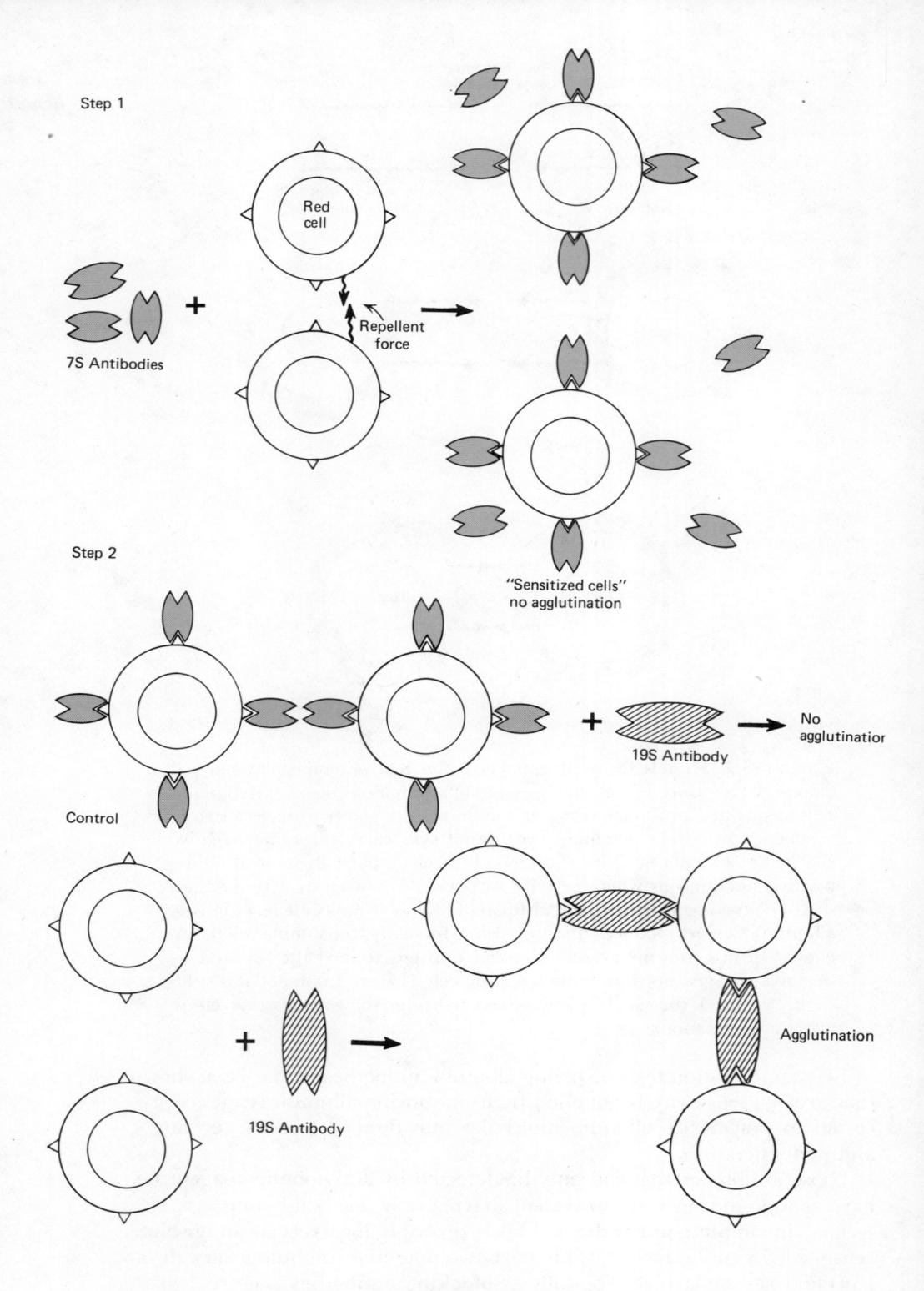

FIGURE 3.8. Model of "blocking" phenomenon that 7S antibodies have on 19S antibody activity.

said to be **coated** or **sensitized** with antibody. Now if we were to add 19S (IgM) saline agglutinins of homologous specificity to these coated cells, they may also fail to cause agglutination because all of the antigenic sites on the red cells are already occupied by 7S (IgG) antibody.

The antiglobulin test is designed to detect coating, blocking, incomplete, or "univalent" antibodies attached to red cells. Coombs serum contains mainly 7S antibodies that combine with immunoglobulins coating red cells, forming an interconnected lattice in three dimensions of sufficient size to settle out as a visible agglutinated mass (Figure 3.9).

D^u ANTIGEN

When a saline suspension of red cells is tested with an anti-D (Rh_0) IgM saline agglutinin, a negative reaction should *not* be interpreted as involving an Rh-negative blood because the possibility exists that a D^u factor is present. By definition, a D^u cell is one that fails to react with complete anti-Rh_0 saline agglutinin, but does react with incomplete anti-D in an albumin-enhanced technique and/or in an indirect antiglobulin D^u test. D^u donor bloods should not be used to transfuse Rh_0-negative recipients. Women who appear Rh negative should be proven to be D^u negative before they are considered eligible to receive treatment for the prevention of sensitization to Rh_0 factor due to an incompatible pregnancy. Because saline anti-D agglutinins fail to detect D^u bloods, they are not recommended for routine Rh typing.

Rh antibodies of class IgG generally have optimal reactivity at 37°C. Direct blood typing in the Rh system can be performed on a slide or in a tube. Slide tests (Figure 3.10) are usually performed on preheated microscope slides using an anti-D reagent of class IgG and whole blood (roughly 50 percent suspension in serum or plasma) or a washed 50 percent suspension of cells in 22 percent BSA. A negative control is run simultaneously and consists of BSA in place of antibody. This control is necessary whether

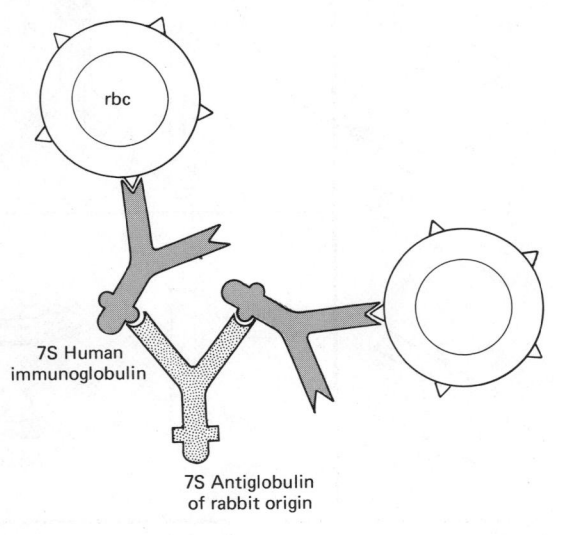

FIGURE 3.9. Model of antiglobulin agglutination of cells coated with 7S (incomplete) antibodies.

Serology and Immunology

washed cells are suspended in BSA or not because BSA is a commonly used diluent in the preparation of commercial blood-typing reagents. The control should not produce agglutination. If the control does agglutinate, the test is considered invalid (nonspecific agglutination) and fresh cells must be washed and retested using a saline agglutinin (devoid of albumin).

A tube test (Figure 3.10) can also be performed using an anti-D reagent of class IgG and a weak suspension of cells in their own serum or plasma. If no agglutination is seen at room temperature, the tube containing antibody is incubated at 37°C to provide optimal thermal conditions for Rh antibody reactivity. If no agglutination is observed at the end of the thermal phase, the tube is filled with saline and centrifuged until the cells are packed at the bottom of the tube. The supernatant wash saline is decanted and the tube refilled. The red blood cells are washed repeatedly (three or four times) in this fashion in order to remove all unreacted antibodies. At the end of the last wash, the fluid is decanted, antiglobulin is added, and the tube is cen-

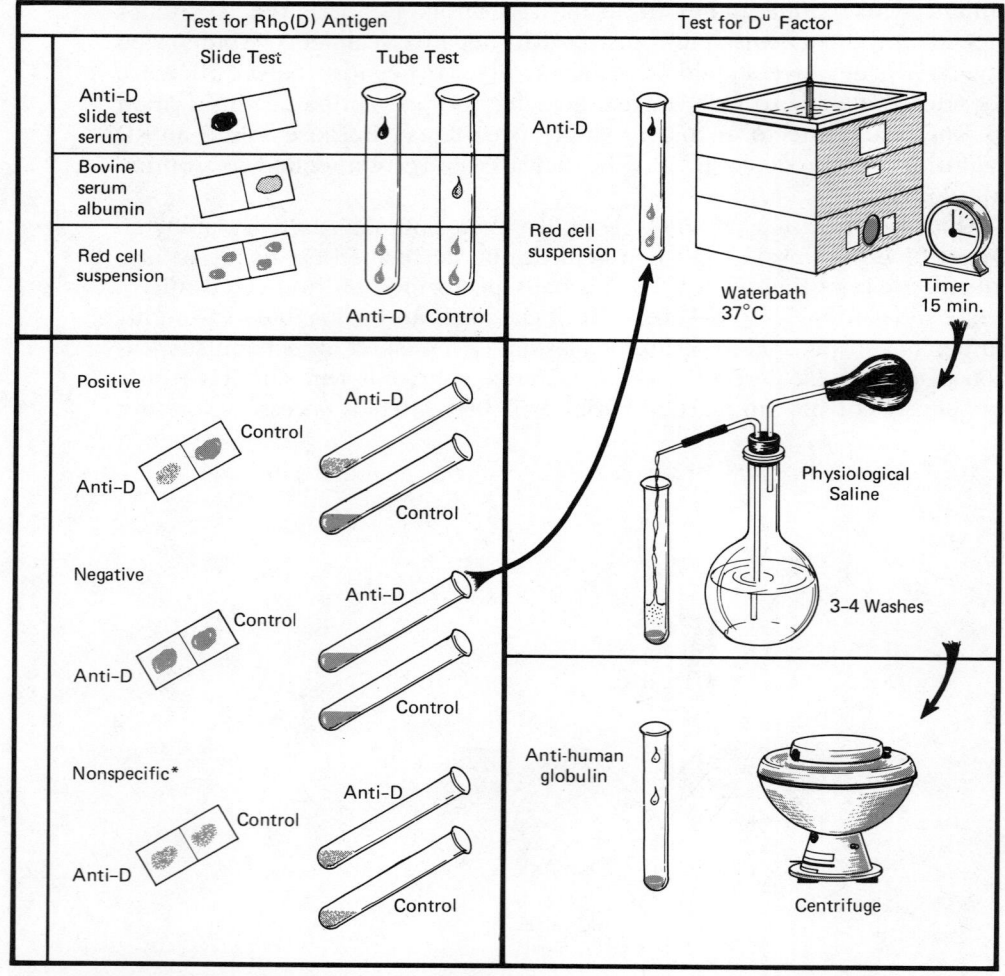

*Cells must be washed and retested with a saline anti-D typing reagent.

FIGURE 3.10. Direct typing for the $Rh_0(D)$ factor.

trifuged and read for agglutination. If no agglutination is seen, then one further test is mandatory. Washed, saline-suspended group O cells already coated with human immunoglobulins (specificity of the antibodies is immaterial) are added directly to the negative Coombs test; the tube is centrifuged and read for agglutination. If no agglutination of these newly added cells (known as **Coombs control cells**) is seen, then either the antihuman globulin was not reactive and/or AHG was not added. If the Coombs control cells do agglutinate, we know that the AHG is reactive, that it was added to the test, and that the cells were washed adequately. The technologist may observe what is called a **mixed-field agglutination** wherein the Coombs control cells agglutinate, but the patient's cells do not. We now infer that the D^u test was indeed negative (i.e., the D factor was not present in any form on the red cells). This confirms that the blood was truly Rh negative.

On the other hand, if agglutination of the patient's cells is observed in the D^u test, one other test must be made. Before it can be concluded that the Coombs reactive antibody attached to red cells is the anti-Rh_0 (anti-D) added in the D^u test, it must be shown that the cells were not previously coated with human immunoglobulins (specificity immaterial). For this purpose, a **direct Coombs test** is performed. A fresh sample of the patient's blood is washed thoroughly and then tested with AHG. If the direct Coombs test is positive (agglutination), it invalidates the D^u test because the cells must have been coated with some kind of antibodies even before exposure to the anti-Rh_0 reagent. If a negative direct Coombs test (no agglutination) is seen (and the subsequently added Coombs control cells agglutinate), then the D^u test results can be considered valid; i.e., the Rh_0 specificity is on these cells as the weak variant D^u. Slide tests cannot detect the D^u factor because cells must be in a tube for the wash process. Any Rh-negative slide test would have to be redone as a tube test. If cell washing is not thorough, some unreacted human globulins may remain in the fluid to neutralize the AHG, giving a false negative reaction. That is to say, free human globulins can occupy the combining sites on AHG so that it becomes unable to bind to the 7S anti-D globulins attached (fixed) to the cells. This is another blocking phenomenon.

Some Rh-negative individuals have been sensitized to manufacture anti-Rh_0 by exposure to D^u blood. Therefore, for purposes of blood donation, any D^u blood should be considered Rh positive. For purposes of receiving blood, many experts recommend that a D^u individual should be considered Rh negative and therefore should receive Rh_0-negative transfusions. If this policy is adopted, then there is no necessity to do a D^u test on recipients, since all transfusion patients who test D negative on direct typing will be given D-negative blood. However, if D-negative donor units are in short supply, some authorities claim that D^u-positive individuals may be given Rh_0-positive blood with little or no risk of either sensitization or transfusion reaction. A few cases have been found in which a D or D^u person appears to have anti-D in his serum. It now seems that both the D and D^u antigens are mosaics of several parts called **cognates.** These cognates are uniform and identical in most people. Occasionally, however, one or more of these parts become altered or deleted (perhaps by mutation) so that the D or D^u antigen takes on a new specificity in a portion of the molecule (Figure 3.11). When such a person receives normal D or D^u blood, he may recognize a

Serology and Immunology

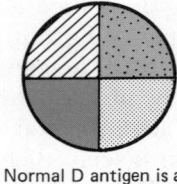

Normal D antigen is a mosaic of several parts (cognates).

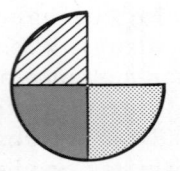

Abnormal D antigen (classified as D^u) is missing one or more cognates.

FIGURE 3.11. Models of D and D^u complex antigens.

portion(s) of that antigen as foreign and produce antibodies against it. Since most Rh-positive people have all of the cognates of the mosaic antigen, this new antibody would appear to react with all Rh-positive cells and would thus appear to be anti-D.

Even when albumin is added to the red cell suspension, some 7S antibodies still behave as blocking (univalent) antibodies and attach to red cells, but fail to produce agglutination. If all 7S antibodies are essentially of the same length and potentially have two combining sites, how can the serological differences between albumin antibodies and Coombs-reactive antibodies be explained? One theory proposes that the difference is in the nature of the homologous antigen rather than in the antibody. As a model system, it is proposed that the Rh_0 factor protrudes from the cell surface on normal Rh-positive cells, but that same factor resides in a depression of the plasma membrane on D^u cells. In the latter instance, only the addition of an antihuman globulin would be instrumental in causing agglutination of the sensitized cells (Figure 3.12). Antibodies of several other blood group systems (e.g., Kell, Duffy, Kidd) react almost exclusively in the Coombs phase. Whereas antigens of the ABO system are found on all tissues of the body, the Rh antigens are located only on the surface of erythrocytes. To date, attempts to extract the Rh antigens in purified form from red cells have not been successful. Hence, very little is known about the chemical structure of the Rh antigens other than hints of interactions between lipids and proteins. Current understanding of the Rh blood group antigens is a long way from providing the kind of information required to verify the validity of current theoretical models concerning the structure of antigens in this system.

Cells that agglutinate weakly with some (but not all) anti-D sera are designated "high-grade" D^u; those that bind anti-D, but agglutinate only with the help of antiglobulin, are called "low-grade" D^u. Thus, D^u cells appear to be a heterogeneous group of intermediates between D positive and D negative. High-grade D^u cells are closer to D, whereas low-grade D^u cells are closer to d (Rh negative). The D^u variants may be inherited in at least two ways. Most of the high-grade D^u cells seem to be produced by gene interaction. When the r' (dCe) gene is on one chromosome and a gene determining the Rh_0 (D) specificity is on the other chromosome, a weakened antigenic product (D^u) is produced. A majority of the low-grade D^u cells (and some of the high-grade variants) are transmitted in classical Mendelian fashion from one generation to the next. This "hereditary" type of D^u is probably governed by a mutant allele. If the patient's cells are found to be D^u posi-

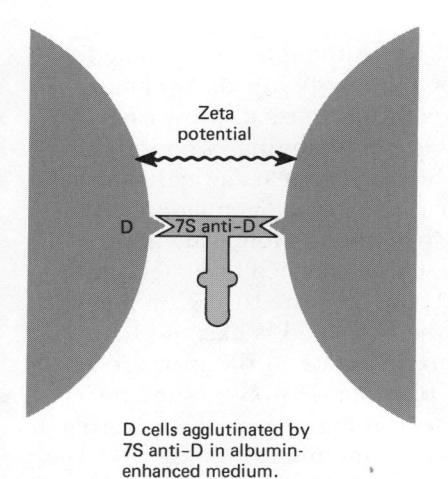

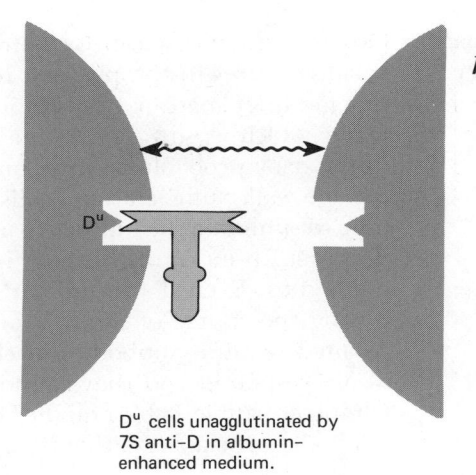

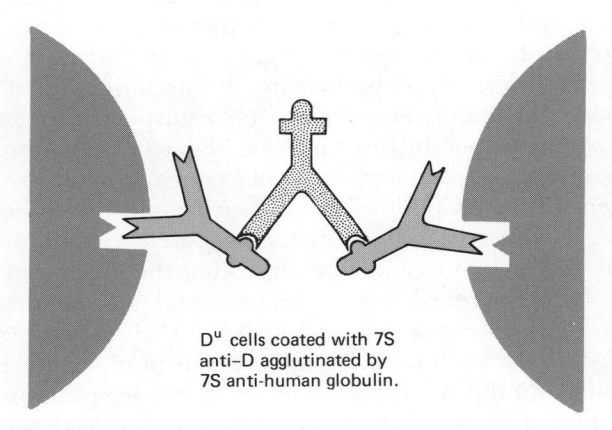

FIGURE 3.12. Models of D and D^u cells.

tive, they should be tested with anti-hr' (anti-c). Those that are positive to anti-c are usually of the low-grade, hereditary variety; those that are negative to anti-c are usually of the high-grade, gene interaction variety (*DCe/dCe*). The hereditary variety should receive only Rh$_0$-negative blood. The gene interaction variety should receive blood that is negative for the c antigen because these patients are more in danger of isoimmunization to c than to D. The hierarchy of antigenic potency is D (Rh$_0$) > c (hr') > C (rh') > E (rh") > e (hr").

Hemolytic Disease of the Newborn

Rh DISEASE

When an Rh-negative mother gives birth to an Rh-positive baby, there is a possibility that some of the baby's red cells will enter the mother's

Serology and Immunology

bloodstream and sensitize her to the Rh factor. Although it is possible for small ruptures in the placenta to occur spontaneously during pregnancy, this mode of maternal sensitization appears to be unusual. Most cases of maternal Rh sensitization by the incompatible Rh determinants on red cells of the baby probably occur at birth when the placenta tears away from the uterine wall. Sufficient fetal cells may enter the maternal circulation at this time to stimulate the mother to make anti-Rh antibodies following delivery. The first Rh-incompatible baby is therefore seldom affected by maternal Rh antibodies. Even if the mother should become sensitized to Rh antigens during the course of the first pregnancy, the first child is likely to be unharmed because antibodies of class IgM predominate in the primary immune response, and they cannot pass the placenta. However, subsequent Rh-incompatible babies might be affected to varying degrees by maternal antibodies of class IgG that typify the secondary immune response (Figure 3.13).

It is common knowledge that mother and fetus do not share a common blood supply. In the placenta, blood vessels of the mother and fetus run very close together but do not fuse (anastomosis). Large molecules and cells cannot pass this placental barrier, but small molecules can often pass freely in either direction. By the process of molecular diffusion across the placenta from areas of higher concentration in the mother's blood to areas of lower concentration in the baby's blood, oxygen, water, and electrolytes are exchanged; by the reverse process, the baby rids itself of metabolic wastes and carbon dioxide. Some nutrients are actively transported to the fetus across the placenta by the expenditure of energy. Maternal antibodies of class IgG are also actively transported across the placenta and enter the fetal circulation. Red cells of an Rh-positive baby in an Rh-sensitized mother become coated with IgG maternal antibodies and become lysed immunologically by complement and/or by macrophages attacking the opsonized cells.

Lysis of baby's cells releases much free hemoglobin. Hemoglobin breaks down into various products, one of which is a toxic yellow pigment called indirect bilirubin. In adult humans, indirect bilirubin is converted to harmless direct bilirubin (bilirubin glucuronide) by the liver enzyme glucuronyl transferase. Free indirect bilirubin normally combines with serum albumin, and this complex circulates until it is absorbed by a liver cell. Inside this

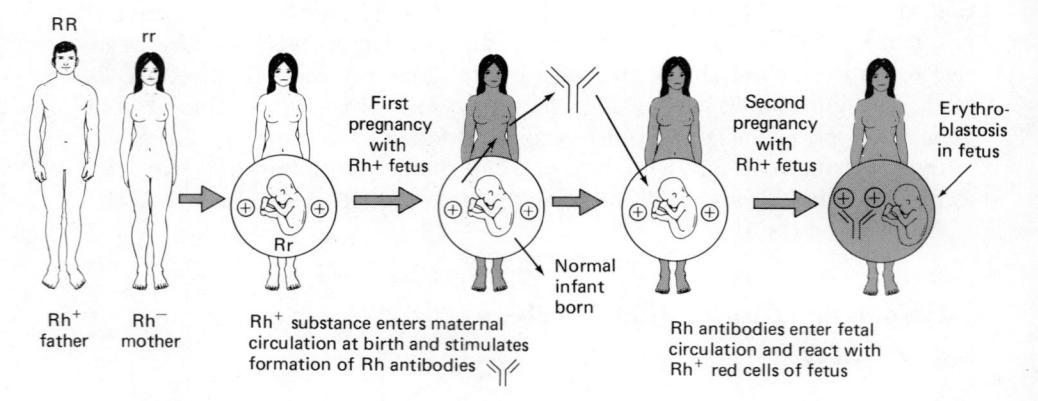

FIGURE 3.13. Steps in the development of Rh disease (erythoblastosis fetalis).

cell, bilirubin is enzymatically cleaved from albumin, conjugated with glucuronic acid, and secreted as bilirubin glucuronide into an adjacent bile canaliculus. Through the secretion of bile pigments into the intestinal tract, hemoglobin breakdown products normally are removed from the body. If albumin fails to complex with free lipid-soluble bilirubin, it can circulate and bind to lipid-rich nerve cell membranes of the central nervous system. As long as indirect bilirubin is bound to albumin, it remains harmless. When all of the binding sites on albumin are saturated with bilirubin, then even small amounts of free bilirubin may be dangerous. There is a clinical test that can determine the degree of saturation of serum albumin; this test is widely used because there is no way at present to measure the amount of free bilirubin in tissues. Competitive binding of other substances with albumin (e.g., heparin, sulfonamides, salicylates, and caffeine) or increased hydrogen ion concentration (acidosis) results in less binding of bilirubin. Fetal livers do not make the enzyme glucuronyl transferase. Hence, the fetus is dependent on the maternal circulation to remove the indirect bilirubin (Figure 3.14). Free indirect bilirubin is extremely toxic. If it is not removed the free bilirubin may cross the blood-brain barrier and deposit in and cause damage to the basal nuclei of the brain, a process termed **kernicterus.** Babies affected by kernicterus can be mentally retarded for life. Anemia is also a common symptom in affected babies, either with or without

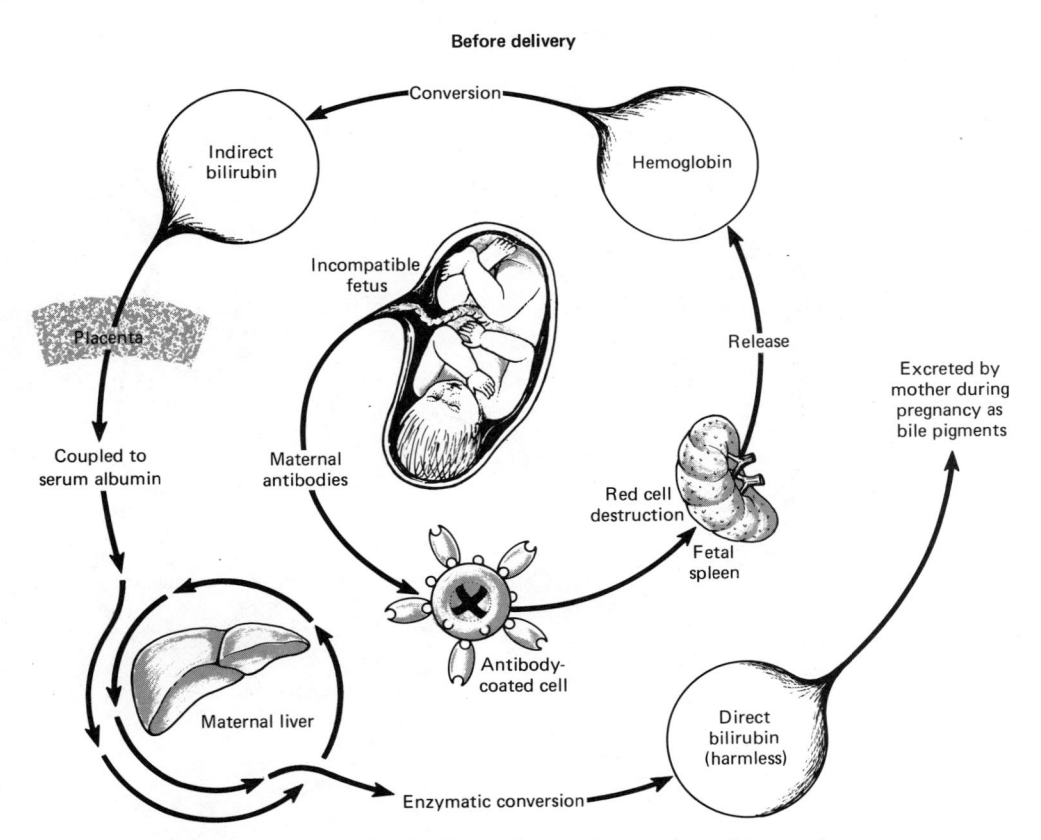

FIGURE 3.14. Prenatal steps in the formation and excretion of hemoglobin derivatives.

Serology and Immunology

kernicterus. These and other sequelae may be so severe as to cause death in the fetal or infant stages (Figure 3.15).

One of the hematological symptoms of this immunological disease is an elevated number of immature (partly nucleated) red blood cells, called **erythroblasts (reticulocytes). Erythroblastosis fetalis** (EBF) or "hemolytic disease of the newborn" is the name given to this disease because it indicates that considerable numbers of nucleated red cells typically occur in the circulation of a fetus so affected. Normally, maturing red cells lose their nuclei before being released from bone marrow (and also from the liver during embryological development) into circulation. When mature erythrocytes are destroyed by this disease, the baby's body attempts to compensate for this loss by allowing immature (nucleated or partly nucleated) erythroblasts to prematurely enter circulation. Unfortunately, these immature red cells do not function as efficiently in oxygen transport as mature erythrocytes; so the baby continues to suffer oxygen deprivation.

In order to simplify the genetics of the Wiener scheme, we can treat all

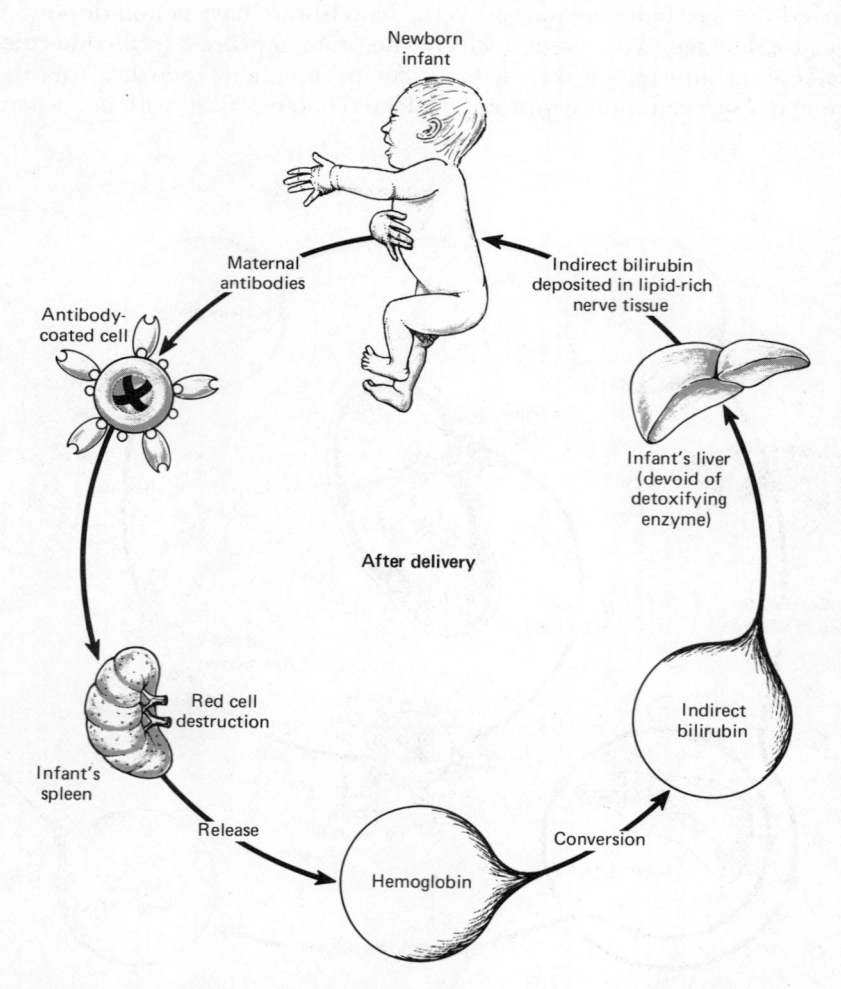

FIGURE 3.15. Postpartum events leading to hemolytic disease of the newborn.

alleles that produce agglutinogens bearing the Rh_0 specificity as though they were one; similarly, all alleles that do not produce this factor can be treated as the alternative allele. Let us designate *D* as the dominant allele responsible for the Rh_0 specificity, and *d* as the recessive allele responsible for the absence of that same factor. If one is testing only for the presence or absence of the Rh_0 factor, blood from individuals of genotype *DD* or *Dd* produces agglutination with anti-D (anti-Rh_0); these individuals are said to be Rh positive. Blood from those of genotype *dd* does not agglutinate; these individuals are said to be Rh negative. Erythroblastosis fetalis (involving the Rh_0 determinant) can develop only when the baby is Rh positive and the mother is Rh negative. If the mother was Rh positive, she should not be stimulated by the Rh_0 factor if it is also present in her baby. An Rh-negative baby, of course, does not have Rh_0 factor and is nonantigenic to the mother in that sense. Babies suffering EBF must be of genotype *Dd*, the mother must be *dd*, and the father must be Rh positive (*DD* or *Dd*). If the father is genetically homozygous *DD*, then all of his children (by a woman of genotype *dd*) should be *Dd* and potentially immunogenic to the mother. If the father is heterozygous *Dd*, then one half of his children (mother *dd*) would be expected to be *Dd*.

Only about one out of every ten marriages involves an Rh-positive man and an Rh-negative woman. Approximately one in twenty-five Rh-negative women bearing an Rh-positive child becomes sensitized to the Rh_0 factor. Why the sensitization rate is so low is incompletely understood. One partial explanation for the low rate of Rh sensitization of mothers by their incompatible babies depends on the ABO blood group system. If the baby's red cells carry the A and/or B antigen(s), and the mother's serum contains the corresponding antibody(s), the baby's cells would come under immediate immune attack when they entered the maternal circulation. For example, cells of a group A, Rh-positive baby would become coated with anti-A in a group B, Rh-negative mother. These antibody-coated cells are very likely to be destroyed before they can cause Rh sensitization of the mother's immune system. Of course, if the mother and baby have the same ABO blood group, or if the baby is group O, then the ABO group of the mother provides no protection against Rh sensitization.

It is a well-known principle of immunology that an optimal dosage exists for each kind of antigen. Too little antigen will not cause the individual to become sensitized; too much of a given antigen apparently "overloads" the immune system, resulting in **immunological paralysis** (unresponsiveness). Perhaps in only a relatively few cases of maternal-fetal Rh incompatibility do sufficient fetal cells escape into the maternal circulation to cause sensitization. Once an individual is sensitized to the Rh factor, he/she may remain so for life. This memory phenomenon is operative (for various lengths of time) for all kinds of antigens, blood group or otherwise. There is no way known at present to purposefully erase immunological memory. Certain drugs and treatments with ionizing radiations can nonspecifically suppress the immune system, but this is certainly not the abolition of a specific immune response.

When specific antibody is passively administered immediately prior to (or simultaneously with) a dose of antigen in a previously unsensitized person, it is generally observed that the individual remains unsensitized. Gorman and Freda (1965) used this principle to prevent sensitization of Rh-negative mothers by their Rh-positive babies. It was found that 7S anti-Rh$_0$ human antibodies, when passively administered intramuscularly to a mother within 72 hours postpartum, would prevent her from becoming sensitized to the Rh-positive cells of her baby (Figure 3.16). The Ortho Pharmaceutical Company of Raritan, New Jersey was the first to make commercially available hyperimmune purified human IgG of Rh$_0$(D) specificity under their trade name RhoGAM. Several other companies have subsequently offered comparable products for sale under their own trade names. The principle underlying the effectiveness of RhoGAM is not completely understood. However, it seems likely that anti-Rh$_0$ antibodies would, upon encountering fetal Rh-positive cells, attach to them, coat them, or sensitize* them. Sensitized cells can be destroyed with the cooperation of complement and/or by phagocytes. Macrophage processing of antigen often precedes lymphocyte stimulation. One theory maintains that if the antigen can be destroyed by the passive immunization before the period of macrophage processing is completed, the antigen becomes neutralized (rendered nonimmunogenic) and the patient remains unsensitized. According to another theory, passively administered antibodies can prevent sensitization by a **feedback inhibition** mechanism. It is well known that many pathways of anabolic biochemical reactions are controlled by feedback inhibition in which an excess end product of a given pathway behaves as an inhibitor of an enzyme for an early step in the pathway. When the end product no longer exists in excess, the early enzyme disassociates from its inhibitor and the whole chain of metabolic reactions resumes. Now when a woman receives RhoGAM, her body seems to recognize that there is ample antibody already available, and by an unknown type of developmental feedback she fails to become sensitized. These two theories of RhoGAM activity are by no means mutually exclusive, nor are they the only theories possible. RhoGAM inhibits sensitization to the Rh$_0$ antigen in better than 99 percent of individuals correctly treated. Because passive immunity wanes rapidly, each time an Rh-negative woman has an incompatible pregnancy (whether it is terminal or ends in miscarriage or induced abortion) she should receive RhoGAM. It is not effective in women already sensitized to the Rh$_0$ factor. Obviously, 7S anti-Rh$_0$ antibodies should not be administered to an Rh-negative pregnant woman because these antibodies can cross the placenta and cause EBF disease if the baby is Rh positive. Likewise, RhoGAM should never be given to an Rh-positive woman because the antibodies would attack her Rh-positive cells and possibly trigger a life-threatening hemolytic episode similar to that of an incompatible blood transfusion.

A sure sign that a baby's cells are under immune attack by maternal antibodies (specificity undetermined) is a positive direct Coombs test. Cells from the baby's umbilicus (cord blood) are normally used because there is some spontaneous blood lost from the cord shortly after birth and therefore it is a convenient source of cells for the test. The cells are washed thoroughly in saline, and then antihuman globulin is added. If agglutination is seen, this is a positive direct Coombs test, indicating that the baby's

---

* The term antibody "sensitization" is synonymous with the attachment or union of antibody to its homologous antigen. When the term "sensitization" is applied to the immune system as a whole, it indicates that the individual has irreversibly recognized a new antigen and has begun to produce a specific lymphocyte response to it.

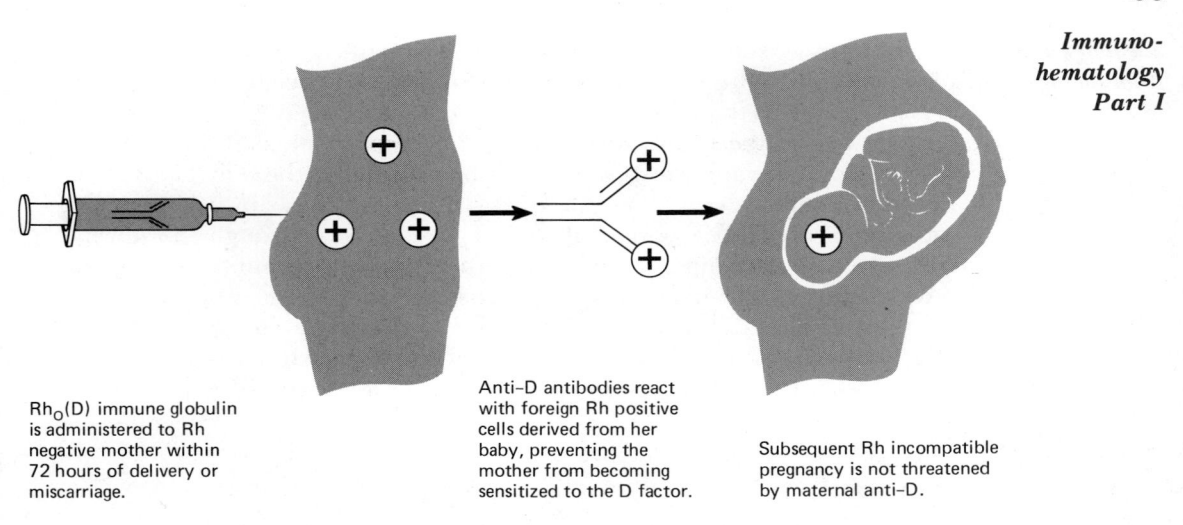

Rh₀(D) immune globulin is administered to Rh negative mother within 72 hours of delivery or miscarriage.

Anti-D antibodies react with foreign Rh positive cells derived from her baby, preventing the mother from becoming sensitized to the D factor.

Subsequent Rh incompatible pregnancy is not threatened by maternal anti-D.

FIGURE 3.16. Prevention of Rh sensitization by Rh₀(D) immune globulin.

cells are coated with maternal antibodies. If the direct Coombs test is negative, a drop of Coombs control cells should be added to the test to confirm that the Coombs reagent is active and that it was added to the test. If a positive direct Coombs test is obtained, an exchange transfusion may be warranted. The attending physician will be watching the bilirubin level of the baby and would probably order an exchange transfusion before the bilirubin concentration reached 5 mg percent (5 mg/100 ml blood). During an exchange transfusion, some of the blood is removed and immediately replaced with fresh Rh-negative blood of the same ABO group. The process is repeated many times in increments of about 5 or 10 ml. Anemia is relieved by the introduction of new functional red cells; bilirubin and maternal antibodies are removed with the baby's serum. If the bilirubin level rises after the first exchange transfusion, subsequent exchange transfusions may be required. Brain damage rarely occurs unless the bilirubin concentration of the blood reaches 20 to 25 mg percent.

Even in normal babies the bilirubin concentration can increase during the first two to four days postpartum, a condition called **physiological icterus.** Icterus (jaundice) is a condition characterized by a yellowish pigmentation of the body due to the accumulation of excessive bile pigment (bilirubin). Treatment of mild cases of physiological icterus or mild EBF may be accomplished by exposing the naked baby to ordinary white light (baby's eyes are protected). Blood coursing near the skin becomes exposed to the light, and a photochemical reaction converts bilirubin to a harmless derivative.

An Rh-negative woman should be regularly monitored during pregnancy for an anti-Rh titer. If her antibody titer increases significantly during pregnancy, the physician might be expected to perform periodic withdrawal of amniotic fluid from her baby, a process termed **amniocentesis.** The level of bilirubin in the amniotic fluid serves as an index of the development and severity of EBF. A bilirubin concentration exceeding 0.27 mg percent in amniotic fluid is considered abnormal; above 0.47 mg percent the fetus is usually distressed, with some degree of circulatory failure present. There are two options open to the physician in severe cases of EBF *in utero.*

Serology and Immunology

If the fetus is sufficiently developed to withstand premature birth, the physician may induce early labor and then perform exchange transfusion. If the fetus is less than 31 weeks of age, premature delivery would probably not be safe for the baby's survival even under optimal conditions. In this case, an intrauterine transfusion might be considered the only alternative. By fluoroscopic examination, the physician locates the baby and inserts a catheter through the abdominal wall of the mother, through the uterine wall, through the amniotic cavity, and through the abdominal wall of the fetus. Group O, Rh-negative cells are introduced into the fetus' abdomen from whence they may be absorbed into its bloodstream to counteract the effects of hemolytic anemia. This procedure is considered dangerous to both mother and fetus and is instituted only as a last resort.

ABO DISEASE

The most common hemolytic disease of the newborn is due to maternal-fetal incompatibility involving the ABO system. Fortunately, most cases of ABO hemolytic anemia are mild or subclinical, and affected babies rarely require exchange transfusions. For reasons not yet understood, anemia is not usually a diagnostic symptom of the disease. Both red cell count and hemoglobin level are usually normal. Some of the more commonly observed symptoms are microspherocytosis, elevated reticulocyte count (greater than 12 percent), elevated indirect bilirubin level (exceeding 12 mg percent) in the first 72 hours postpartum, and jaundice (icterus) appearing in the first 24 hours after birth. A direct antiglobulin test on an affected baby's blood drawn more than 24 hours postpartum usually appears negative. The reason(s) for this is not clear, but some evidence suggests that the antibody resides in vacuoles of the red cell and therefore is not accessible to the antiglobulin. Confirmation of ABO hemolytic disease may be obtained by eluting the antibody from thoroughly washed cells and using the eluate as in a reverse (serum) grouping test against known A and B cells. In contrast to Rh disease, ABO incompatibility may occur in the first-born child and cannot be predicted by any prenatal testing of maternal serum.

Approximately 23 percent of all pregnancies are incompatible in the ABO system, yet only about 1 : 150 of all births actually show clinical signs of ABO disease. There are several possible reasons for this discrepancy. Over 90 percent of all cases of ABO disease involves group O mothers with A or B babies. Only the cross-reacting anti-A,B (anti-C) antibody in group O mothers is 7S IgG immunoglobulin capable of passing across the placenta into the fetal circulation. Anti-A and anti-B are much larger 19S IgM immunoglobulins and cannot usually cross the placenta. A second possible explanation is the fact that A and B antigens are found on virtually all cells of the body, not just the red cells. Maternal anti-A,B that enters the fetus may be absorbed by other tissues and thus is prevented from causing extensive damage to erythrocytes. A third possibility is that the A and B antigens on the red cells of the newborn are not yet well developed, making it more difficult for the homologous antibodies to attack them.

There are many blood group systems other than ABO and Rh that can be involved in hemolytic disease of the newborn, but the involvement of other systems is much less frequent. Whatever the cause, the goal of the treatment is always to repair anemia, eliminate excess bilirubin, and prevent kernicterus.

SELF-EVALUATION

Terms

1. Any group of red cell antigens that are genetically regulated by a single locus (or perhaps a cluster of closely linked genes). (3 words)
2. An immunological disease of the newborn, produced by maternal antibodies to blood group antigens of her baby, resulting in red cell destruction and release of immature red cells into circulation. (2 words)
3. Nonimmune agglutination caused by drying, bacterial contamination, and other non-antibody-mediated phenomena.
4. An ABO blood grouping test involving mixing of patient's serum with cells of known antigenic composition. (1 or 2 words)
5. The strength of the repellent force between red cells of identical negative charge. (2 words)
6. The reciprocal of the highest dilution of serum that gives a detectable (endpoint) reaction with antigen.
7. Extracts from plant seeds that exhibit specific agglutination with red cells.
8. A blood type that possesses anti-H in the serum.
9. Individuals that have soluble A, B, or H substances in their body fluids.
10. An antibody reagent used to detect the union of 7S blood group antibodies with red cells. (2 words)

Multiple Choice. Choose the one best response.

1. A woman of blood group A has a child of blood group B. Which of the following statements is correct? (a) The mother's genotype is incompletely known. (b) The mother's genotype is heterozygous. (c) The father could not be group O. (d) The baby's genotype is incompletely known. (e) More than one of these statements is true.
2. Blood group antigens A and B are classified chemically as (a) glycoproteins (b) lipopolysaccharides (c) nucleoproteins (d) phospholipids (e) amino acids
3. Red cells are classified as A_2 (a) if anti-A_2 is in the serum (b) if the genotype is A_1A_2 (c) if they react only with anti-A_2 (d) if they react with anti-A but not with anti-A_1 (e) if they react with both anti-A and anti-A_1
4. Anti-H (a) reacts best at 37°C (b) is normally found only in the serum of group O individuals (c) does not react with group O cells (d) is commonly involved in hemolytic disease of the newborn (e) is usually inhibited by secretor saliva
5. According to Landsteiner's law, (a) antibodies are present on cells but not in the serum (b) ABO blood groups are inherited by multiple alleles (c) antibodies are present in plasma if the homologous antigen is absent on the red cells (d) all blood groups are inherited according to Mendelian laws (e) more than one of the preceding statements is part of Landsteiner's law
6. The Wiener counterpart of Fisher-Race genotype DCe/dcE is (a) r'/r^y (b) R^0/r (c) R^z/r' (d) R^1/r'' (e) r^y/R^2
7. In the prophylactic treatment of Rh disease (hemolytic disease of the newborn), (a) the erythroblastotic baby is given anti-Rh antibodies soon after birth (b) Rh antibodies are never given to Rh-positive mothers regardless of the condition of their babies (c) the mother is given Rh antibodies soon after she delivers her first erythroblastotic baby (d) all mothers are given anti-Rh antibodies soon after they deliver their first and all subsequent Rh-positive babies (e) none of these statements is correct

Serology and Immunology

8. Which of the following serves as a control for the D^u test? (a) direct blood grouping using anti-D saline agglutinin (b) reverse grouping (c) indirect antiglobulin test using 7S anti-D (d) cord cells washed free of Wharton's jelly (e) direct Coombs test
9. Anti-E should react with cells of genotype (a) R^z/r^y (b) R^1/R^0 (c) r/r' (d) r''/r (e) more than one of these
10. A suspected hemolytic transfusion reaction would be confirmed by (a) elevated levels of serum bilirubin (b) depressed levels of the liver enzyme glucuronyl transferase (c) elevated levels of plasma hemoglobin (d) the appearance of free hemoglobin in the urine (e) elevated levels of serum alkaline phosphatase

True-False

1. Polysaccharide blood group antigens are not the direct products of genes.
2. Blood group antigens themselves are probably not related to resistance against germs.
3. There is no serological way to distinguish blood group A individuals as being genetically homozygous or heterozygous.
4. Blood grouping data can sometimes be used to prove parentage.
5. If agglutination fails to occur in one tube of a hemagglutination inhibition titration test, that tube must be the one with the highest concentration of the substance being diluted.
6. Direct grouping is one commonly used method for establishing the ABO group of blood stains.
7. Albumin enhances serological agglutination by raising the dielectric constant of the reacting medium.
8. It is always safe to administer Rh-negative blood to an Rh-positive person (assuming a match in the other blood group systems).
9. Maternal sensitization to Rh antigens of the baby may be prevented by an incompatibility in the ABO system.
10. Saline (IgM) antibodies are commonly involved in hemolytic disease of the newborn.

Immunohematology Part II
Minor Blood Group Systems, Compatibility Test, Antibody Identification, and Quality Controls

CHAPTER 4

CHAPTER OUTLINE

Minor Blood Group Systems
  Lewis (Le) System
  MNS System
  Kell-Cellano (K-k) System
  Duffy (Fy) System
  Kidd (Jk) System
  P-p System
  Lutheran (Lu) System
  Xg System
  Public and Private Antigens
The Compatibility Test
  Major and Minor Crossmatch
Specific Component Therapy
Alternatives to the Minor Crossmatch
The Auto Control
Patient Screening
Antibody Identification
  Difficulties
Quality Control in Blood Banking
  Equipment
  Procedures
  Reagents
Self-evaluation

Minor Blood Group Systems

For the purpose of blood transfusion, donor and recipient must be a match in the ABO system because "natural antibodies" are a regular feature in the serum of all but AB individuals. The $Rh_0(D)$ specificity is considered highly antigenic, and bloods are also routinely tested for this factor in order to prevent sensitization of Rh-negative individuals. Tests are not commonly made for blood group systems other than ABO and Rh for economic reasons. Some blood factors are so rare that an individual is unlikely to become sensitized to them through a transfusion. Sensitization in itself is not usually harmful, but the second and subsequent contacts with homologous antigen(s) may be traumatic. It is extremely unlikely that an individual would become sensitized to a rare antigen through the first transfusion and then have an incompatibility involving the same rare blood factor on subsequent transfusions (unless the same donor is involved in both cases). Many agglutinogens of these other blood group systems are generally not as antigenic as those of the ABO and Rh systems. Typing reagents are expensive, especially for the rarer antibodies. It would be prohibitively expensive to type each individual for all known blood group factors. In principle, it is desirable to have donor and recipient compatible for all blood group factors, but in reality this is not possible. Therefore, routine grouping in the ABO system and typing in the Rh system, if done correctly, should ensure compatibility in these systems, but makes it possible for a transfusion recip-

Serology and Immunology

ient to become sensitized to antigens of other blood group systems (including those of the Rh system other than D). Once an individual has developed **irregular** or **atypical antibodies** (any blood group antibody other than the "natural" antibodies of the ABO system), a search must be made among potential donors for a blood that lacks the homologous antigen(s). Multiple-transfusion recipients sometimes develop so many antibodies that finding compatible donors becomes a very difficult task. If all the numerous blood factors of an individual were known, it is highly improbable that there would be any other individual (especially if the two are unrelated) possessing exactly the same constellation of red cell antigens. In this sense, the blood factor profile of each individual is virtually unique, analogous to fingerprints. One can thus appreciate the futility of trying to completely match bloods in all blood group systems for transfusions.

LEWIS (Le) SYSTEM

Most blood group systems other than ABO, Rh, MNS, and P-p are named for the family in which a discriminating antibody was first discovered. A. E. Mourant (1946) found an antibody in a patient named Lewis that became known as anti-Le^a; P. H. Andresen (1948) found a related antibody in another patient that became known as anti-Le^b. It was originally believed that the Lewis substances Le^a and Le^b were determined by a corresponding pair of codominant allelic genes *Le*^{a} and *Le*^{b}. According to this genetic hypothesis, only three blood types should exist: Le(a+b+), Le(a+b−), and Le(a−b+). The failure to find Le(a+b+) and the later discovery of Le(a−b−) types caused the original genetic hypothesis to be discarded. Now it is realized that Le^b substance results from the interaction of Lewis and H genes. Recall from Chapter 3 that gene *H* is responsible for H substance, a precursor of A and B antigens of the ABO blood group system. A new genetic theory postulates a dominant gene *Le,* responsible for the Le^a specificity, and its recessive allele *le*, when present in double dose, results in the absence of Le^a substance. Newborn infants do not have Le^a substance on their red cells. Later in life, their red cells may acquire the water-soluble Le^a substance by adsorption from the plasma if they have the appropriate genotype. In other words, the Lewis antigen (Le or Le^a) is not a red cell agglutinogen as such, but must be secondarily acquired by adsorption of the secreted substance in the fluid portion of the blood.

There is a close chemical relationship between the A-B-H substances and the Lewis antigen (Figure 3.3). When both *Le* and *Se* (secretor of ABH substances) genes are in the genotype, their products compete for the same mucopolysaccharide substrate. Hence, secretors of Lewis antigen (*Le*/−) that are nonsecretors of A-B-H substances (*se*/*se*) usually have more Lewis substance in their body fluids than those who are secretors of A-B-H substances (*Se*/−). Red cells from individuals of genotype *Le*/−, *se*/*se* react strongly with anti-Le (anti-Le^a) antibodies and are called blood type Le$_1$; cells from genotype *Le*/−, *Se*/− react very weakly or negatively with anti-Le (Le^a) serum and are called blood type Le$_2$. Red cells of type Le$_2$ are agglutinated by rare sera such as the one originally designated as anti-Le^b. Individuals of homozygous genotype *le*/*le* do not secrete Lewis substances, and therefore their red blood cells do not react with anti-Le serum regardless of the genotype at the *Se* locus (Table 4.1).

Table 4.1 CHARACTERISTICS OF THE LEWIS BLOOD GROUP SYSTEM IN MAN

Possible Genotypes	New Blood Type Symbols	Old Blood Type Symbols	Red Cell Agglutination with Anti-Le (Le^a) Serum	Le Substance Present in Saliva	ABH Substance Present in Saliva
Le/Le se/se Le/le se/se	Le$_1$	Lewis positive Le(a+) Le(a+b−)	+	Yes	No
Le/Le Se/Se Le/le Se/Se Le/Le Se/se Le/le Se/se	Le$_2$	Lewis negative Le(a−) Le(a−b+)	± or 0	Yes	Yes
le/le Se/Se le/le Se/se le/le se/se	le	Lewis negative Le(a−) Le(a−b−)	0	No	Yes Yes No

Typing within the Lewis system is commonly done on both saliva and red cells by using anti-Le (Le^a) antibodies and anti-H lectin. Anti-Le^a is the only blood group antibody other than those of the ABO system that is commonly involved in hemolytic serological reactions. At least one other antibody (Le^d) of the Lewis system has been discovered that distinguishes genotypes *le/le, Se/−* from *le/le, se/se,* but it is not in common clinical use at this time, and further complications of the Lewis system are left to more advanced books on the subject.

MNS SYSTEM

The symbols for this blood group system were derived from the word "iMmuNe" because it was first produced (1927) as an immune response by rabbits to the injection of human blood cells. Two antibodies (anti-M, anti-N) define three blood types: M, N, and MN (Table 4.2). It was originally hypothesized that the agglutinogens M and N were governed by a pair of codominant alleles *M* and *N* (sometimes more correctly designated L^M and L^N, the base symbol L being used in honor of the discoverers Landsteiner and Levine). About twenty years later, two other antibodies (anti-S, anti-s) were discovered to be related to the M-N system. The symbol s was originally used to indicate the presumed absence of S from the red cell. Now we know that s is a blood group specificity, not merely the absence of

Table 4.2 REACTIONS OF THE M-N BLOOD TYPES

Blood Type	Genotype	Agglutination of Red Cells with Anti-M	Agglutination of Red Cells with Anti-N
M	$L^M L^M$	+	0
MN	$L^M L^N$	+	+
N	$L^N L^N$	0	+

Serology and Immunology

factor S. It is therefore currently designated as the MNS system. Since anti-s sera are difficult to obtain and often give inconclusive results, only anti-M, anti-N, and anti-S are commonly used to type in this system. There are two current genetic theories for the MNS system, analogous to those of the Rh system. One theory says that there are two very closely linked loci (L and S). Each gene is responsible for a singular antigenic specificity. The other theory maintains that a multiple allelic series of a single gene locus exists, each allele producing an agglutinogen with multiple specificities. Since the essence of the former theory is easily displayed in tables, it is used for genotypes in Table 4.3, even though the concept of completely linked genes (no crossing-over) is probably erroneous.

Many other blood factors have more recently been found to be genetically related to the MNS system. One factor was named U because of its nearly universal occurrence in Caucasians. U-negative individuals are not uncommon among African Negroes, however. Other factors related to the MNS system, such as Hunter (Hu) and Henshaw (He), were first found in Negroes. Subtypes also exist for the M and N specificities. For example, there is an anti-M_1 that behaves in a manner analogous to that of anti-A_1 of the ABO blood group system.

Antigens of the MNS system are only weakly antigenic for humans and are of little importance in blood transfusions. The presence or absence of the M specificity is a valuable clue in cases of disputed parentage. Agglutinogens M and N are highly antigenic for rabbits, and it is from this source that most typing serum reagents are derived. A potent anti-N lectin can be prepared from seeds of *Vicia graminea*. The M-N substances occur only on erythrocytes and are not found in water-soluble form in body fluids. Treatment of red cells with certain proteolytic enzymes (trypsin, papain, bromelin, ficin) sometimes enhances reactivity of some blood group factors in other systems, but such treatment invariably destroys antigens of the MNS system.

It had long been known that blood of type MN agglutinated less with anti-N reagents than blood of type N. This was formerly attributed to a **gene dosage effect,** wherein two doses of gene L^N in homozygotes ($L^N L^N$) produced more N agglutinogen (and hence stronger reaction with anti-N) than a single dose of L^N in heterozygotes ($L^N L^M$). Some immunohematologists now hypothesize that substance N is a precursor for substance M, analogous to H substance as precursor of A and B. Wiener has proposed a new genetic theory for the M-N types based on this idea. He

Table 4.3 REACTIONS OF THE MNS SYSTEM WITH THREE REAGENTS

Phenotype	Genotype(s)	Anti-M	Anti-N	Anti-S
MS	*MSMS, MSMs*	+	0	+
Ms	*MsMs*	+	0	0
NS	*NSNS, NSNs*	0	+	+
Ns	*NsNs*	0	+	0
MNS	*MSNS, MSNs, MsNS*	+	+	+
MNs	*MsNs*	+	+	0

Agglutination of Red Cells with (column header spanning Anti-M, Anti-N, Anti-S)

proposes that precursor substance N is governed by a gene independent of that for substance M. Virtually everyone is of homozygous genotype $L^N L^N$ and therefore has N substance on their red cells, just as they do H substance. Both M and N specificities are presumed to be on the same molecule just as are H, A, and B. The reason proposed to explain why anti-H lectins react better with O cells than with cells bearing A and/or B specificities is that in the latter case the A and/or B specificities somehow mask or block reactive sites of H substance. This phenomenon is termed **steric interference.** In like manner, M substance is assumed to mask some of the precursor N substance so that anti-N can bind less N agglutinogen in MN than in N blood types. Presumably, N substance is completely masked in $L^M L^M$ homozygotes.

The chemistry of the M and N antigens is just beginning to be unraveled. These are glycoproteins consisting of carbohydrate and protein. Amino acid differences at two positions in the protein moiety (called "glycophoran A") are apparently involved in the M and N specificities. Serine and glycine at positions 1 and 5, respectively, are in the M form of glycophoran A, whereas leucine and glutamic acid occupy these loci in the N form of glycophoran A. However, the carbohydrate moiety must be close to the critical peptide sequence in order for the corresponding antibody to react. If the sugar groups are removed chemically, neither anti-M nor anti-N recognizes the glycophoran A. This is the first case in which antibody recognition has been shown to depend on both carbohydrate and polypeptide.

KELL-CELLANO (K-k) SYSTEM

In 1946, a new antibody (unrelated to other known blood group systems) was found in the serum of a patient named Kelleher. The antibody was named anti-Kell (anti-K) and the homologus blood factor was called Kell (K). Individuals possessing this antigen are said to be Kell positive; those lacking it are Kell negative. This antigen is found in about 10 percent of Caucasians and about 1 percent of Negroes. In 1949, an antibody giving reciprocal reactions to that of anti-K was found in a patient named Cellano. At first, the homologous specificity was designated the Cellano factor; later it was changed to k. Specificities K and k appear to be governed by a single gene locus with codominant alleles K and k, respectively. The use of capital and lower-case letters should be reserved for dominant and recessive allelic relationships. Allen and Rosenfield have proposed the codominant symbols $K1$ (for K) and $K2$ (for k). Unfortunately, K and k became so well established that many modern texts still fail to use proper symbols denoting their codominance. Anti-K1 and anti-K2 can be used to define three genotypes and their corresponding phenotypes (blood groups) in a manner completely analogous to that of the M-N types (Table 4.4). Anti-K2 can only be produced in individuals lacking specificity K2 (genotype $K1K1$). Because gene $K1$ is of relatively low frequency, only about 1 in 500 individuals could become sensitized to factor $K2$ (genotype $K1K1$); hence anti-K2 is rarely encountered as an atypical antibody.

As with most blood group systems, the K-k system has proven to be far more complicated than was originally thought. Two additional antisera (anti-Kp[a] from a person named Penney and anti-Kp[b]) further define the K2 specificity. A very rare antibody called anti-Ku (originally called anti-Peltz)

Serology and Immunology

Table 4.4 REACTIONS OF THE KELL BLOOD GROUP SYSTEM USING TWO ANTISERA

Genotype	Phenotype (Blood Type)	Agglutination Reaction with Anti-K1 (anti-K)	Anti-K2 (anti-k)
$K1K1$ (KK)	K1 (K)	+	0
$K1K2$ (Kk)	K1K2 (Kk)	+	+
$K2K2$ (kk)	K2 (k)	0	+

reacts with a very-high-frequency factor designated Ku (the "u" indicates almost "universal" occurrence of the determinant, analogous to the near universality of factor U of the MNS system). A very rare allele (K^0) of questionable dominance behaves as an **amorphic gene,** associated with the absence of any well-established specificities of the K-k system. In this sense, it is analogous to rare gene $\bar{\bar{r}}$ of the Rh system. In the Rh system, "single-bar" symbols indicate absence of only a single pair of contrasting factors (e.g., rh″ and hr″); "double-bar" symbols indicate absence of two pairs of factors (rh′-hr′ and rh″-hr″). Amorphic genes in serology produce no detectable antigenic product. Deletion or absence of a gene would cause it to behave as an amorph. If the K^0 allele is a deletion, it would behave as a recessive gene and its symbol should be changed to lower case. Table 4.5 lists the reactions of four blood types of the Kell system as defined by these five antisera.

An antibody found in an individual named Sutter (1958) defined a specificity now called Js^a. This blood group factor has so far been found only in Negroes. When a second antibody was found to give reactions antithetical to anti-Js^a, it was named anti-Js^b. All Caucasians are Js^b positive and Js^a negative. The only individuals that have been found to be Js(a−b−) are also of the rare K_0 type. This odd coincidence indicates that the Js^a and Js^b specificities are part of the Kell system, but the exact relationship is still far from clear. Four Js blood types are known: Js(a+b+), Js(a+b−), Js(a−b+), and Js(a+b+).

Antibodies of the Kell system behave as incomplete or blocking antibodies and hence are detected only by the use of antihuman globulin (AHG). When Kell-positive cells that are maximally coated with anti-K1 antibodies are used to titrate an AHG reagent, it is found that the titer is approximately one fourth to one fifth as high as titrations using Rh-positive cells maximally coated with anti-Rh$_0$(D). These results indicate that there

Table 4.5 REACTIONS OF THE KELL BLOOD GROUP SYSTEM USING FIVE ANTISERA

Allelic Gene	Corresponding Antigenic Specificity	K	k	Kp^a	Kp^b	K^u	Gene Frequency in Caucasians
$K1$ (K)	K1 (K)	+	0	0	+	+	0.043
$K2$ (k)	K2 (k) (Kp^b)	0	+	0	+	+	0.947
K^p (k^p)	Kp^a	0	+	+	0	+	0.010
K^0	K$_0$	0	0	0	0	0	Very rare

are probably four to five times more Rh antigenic sites on red cells than there are K1 antigenic sites.

DUFFY (Fy) SYSTEM

When a new antibody was discovered in a patient named Duffy, it defined a new antigen called Duffy factor. Those possessing the antigen were said to be Duffy positive Fy(a+) and those lacking it were Duffy negative Fy(a−). The antibody was designated anti-Fy^a. Later, a second antibody called anti-Fy^b was also found to belong to the Duffy system. The genetics of the Duffy blood group system is remarkably like that of the ABO system. There is a pair of codominant alleles Fy^a and Fy^b corresponding to the specificities Fy(a+) and Fy(b+), respectively, and a recessive amorphic allele fy. Four phenotypes are defined by the use of two typing reagents (Table 4.6). Most Negroes are of blood type Fy(a−b−), a type not found in Caucasians. Anti-Duffy antibodies are usually of class IgG, but AHG is required to detect their union with red cells. It is estimated that there are approximately ten times as many Rh$_0$(D) specificities on erythrocytes as those of the Duffy antigen.

KIDD (Jk) SYSTEM

In 1951, when an antibody belonging to a new blood group system was found in a patient named Kidd, it could not be given the designation anti-K because that symbol had already been assigned to the Kell system. Hence the antibody was designated anti-Jk^a, and its homologous agglutinogen was Jk^a. In 1953, the reciprocal antibody (anti-Jk^b) was discovered. These two antibodies define three Kidd blood types in a manner analogous to the M-N blood types. A pair of codominant alleles determine the two agglutinogens (Table 4.7). Very few people have been found to lack both specificities Jk^a and Jk^b, i.e., blood type Jk(a−b−). These exceptional individuals can make an antibody called anti-Jk that reacts with cells bearing either agglutinogens Jk^a or Jk^b or both. It is hypothesized that individuals of type Jk(a−b−) are homozygous for a rare amorphic allele jk.

Fresh antisera may agglutinate cells suspended in saline, but they quickly lose this ability even when refrigerated. Antihuman globulin may sometimes be used successfully, but is not reliable by itself. Kidd antibodies apparently require complement to effect agglutination even when the AHG technique is used. For best results, it is recommended that the Coombs test

Table 4.6 REACTIONS OF THE DUFFY BLOOD GROUP SYSTEM

		Agglutination Reaction with	
Genotype(s)	Blood Type	Anti-Fy^a	Anti-Fy^b
Fy^aFy^a or Fy^afy	Fy(a+b−)	+	0
Fy^bFy^b or Fy^bfy	Fy(a−b+)	0	+
Fy^aFy^b	Fy(a+b+)	+	+
$fyfy$	Fy(a−b−)	0	0

Serology and Immunology

Table 4.7 REACTIONS OF THE KIDD BLOOD GROUP SYSTEM

Genotype	Blood Type	Anti-Jk^a	Anti-Jk^b
Jk^aJk^a	Jk(a+b−)	+	0
Jk^aJk^b	Jk(a+b+)	+	+
Jk^bJk^b	Jk(a−b+)	0	+
jkjk	Jk(a−b−)	0	0

be used on red cells treated with the enzyme trypsin, and that fresh group AB serum be added as a source of active complement.

P-p SYSTEM

The first antibody of this system was prepared by injecting human cells into rabbits. Later it was found that anti-P occasionally (but not regularly) appears "naturally" (without exposure to foreign red cells) in the blood of P-negative individuals. Apparently a P-like specificity is fairly common in other organisms. P-negative individuals may become sensitized to the P factor through contact with certain parasites (e.g., tapeworms causing hydatid disease). Leaves and flowers of certain mucilaginous plants (e.g., *Tilia* and *Tussilago farfara*) contain a P-like substance and can be used as an immunogen in the production of anti-P. When fed to rabbits, these mucilaginous plants have been reported to produce enteric sensitization. Apparently, fine suspensions of the material can penetrate the intact intestinal mucosa to reach the bloodstream and act as an immunogen.

Originally, anti-P was used to define two blood types. Those with which it reacted were called P positive, and those with which it did not react were called P negative. Subsequently, a rare antibody was found to be related to anti-P in a manner analogous to the way that anti-A is related to anti-A$_1$. Anti-P was then renamed anti-P$_1$. The rare antibody was actually a mixture of anti-P and anti-P$_1$, just as group B (anti-A) serum contains a mixture of anti-A and anti-A$_1$. P-positive individuals are now classified as type P$_1$; P-negative individuals are called type P$_2$. According to Sanger, three blood types can be defined by use of these two antisera. A simple genetic hypothesis proposes that gene P^1 (corresponding to agglutinogen P$_1$) is dominant to allele P^2 (corresponding to agglutinogen P$_2$), and an amorphic allele p is recessive to both P^1 and P^2 (Table 4.8). About 80 percent of Caucasians in the United States are blood type P$_1$, and 20 percent are P$_2$; blood type p is extremely rare. Other rare blood factors (such as P^k) related to the P-p system have been found that will necessitate revision of the "three-allelic

Table 4.8 REACTIONS OF THE P-p BLOOD GROUP SYSTEM

Genotype(s)	Blood Type	Agglutinogen Present	Specificities Present	Anti-P	Anti-P$_1$
P^1P^1, P^1P^2, or P^1p	P$_1$	P$_1$	P$_1$ and P	+	+
P^2P^2 or P^2p	P$_2$	P$_2$	P	+	0
pp	p	None	None	0	0

scheme." At least two other genetic theories have been proposed to account for these rare factors. It is obvious that this system is quite complex and much more work needs to be done to clarify the situation. Antibodies of this system are rarely involved in transfusion reactions. Because these antibodies are usually weak (producing indistinct results), they are of little use in forensic medicine.

LUTHERAN (Lu) SYSTEM

In 1945, an antibody was found in a patient named Lutheran that became known as anti-Lu^a. Eleven years later, a second antibody was found, and it was designated anti-Lu^b. Very few people are Lu^b negative, so that anti-Lu^b is a rare antibody. Almost everyone can be classified into one of three blood types by use of these two antisera: Lu(a+b+), Lu(a+b−), or Lu(a−b+). An individual with the rare blood type Lu(a−b−) has been found, possessing a cross-reacting antibody called anti-Lu. This antibody reacts with both Lu(a+b−) and Lu(a−b+) bloods and cannot be fractionated by absorption with either cell type. Hence it is inferred that anti-Lu cross-reacts with a common specificity (Lu) on both Lu(a+b−) and Lu(a−b+) agglutinogens. In this respect, anti-Lu reacts analogously to anti-C (anti-A,B) of the ABO system, anti-U of the MNS system, and anti-rh^G of the Rh system. In certain families, the rare blood type Lu(a−b−) can be explained by homozygosity for a recessive allele (*lu lu*). In other families, however, it appears to be transmitted as a dominant characteristic. Other factors, such as Auberger (Au), have been found to be related to the Lutheran system, and a comprehensive genetic theory is still awaited. A simplistic view of the Lutheran blood group system (that works well with all but rare bloods) is presented in Table 4.9.

It appears that *Lu* and *Se* (secretor of ABH substances) loci are rather closely linked (recombination frequency estimated at 0.15). Evidence also exists linking the *Lu* and *Le* (Lewis) loci. Therefore, the loci *Lu*, *Se*, and *Le* may all reside on the same autosome, but *Le* may be located so far from *Se* that these two loci may only appear to be assorting independently.

Xg SYSTEM

There is only one blood group antigen known to be governed by a sex-linked genetic locus (i.e., on the X chromosome). This blood factor is called Xg^a and its corresponding dominant allele is *Xg^a*. A single antibody, anti-Xg^a, is used to define two blood types. Those that react with anti-Xg^a are

Table 4.9 REACTIONS OF THE LUTHERAN SYSTEM

Genotype	Blood Type	Agglutination Reaction with Anti-Lu^a	Anti-Lu^b
Lu^{a}Lu^a	Lu(a+b−)	+	0
Lu^{a}Lu^b	Lu(a+b+)	+	+
Lu^{b}Lu^b	Lu(a−b+)	0	+
?	Lu(a−b−)	0	0

Xg(a+); those that do not react are Xg(a−). A recessive "silent" (amorphic) allele *xg* is postulated to be responsible for type Xg(a−). Anti-Xg^a is detected only by the antiglobulin technique. Because it is produced by a sex-linked locus, Xg^a is a very valuable marker for cases of disputed parentage. As for any dominant sex-linked character, this factor must conform to the following rules:

1. Fathers of Xg(a−) girls must also be negative; sons of Xg(a−) women must also be negative.
2. Mothers of Xg(a+) boys must also be positive; daughters of Xg(a+) men must also be positive.
3. If the father is positive and the mother is negative, all sons must be negative and all daughters must be positive.
4. All types of children are possible from negative fathers mated to positive mothers.

PUBLIC AND PRIVATE ANTIGENS

Any blood group antigen found in almost 100 percent of every human population all over the world is called a **public** or **high-frequency antigen.** Examples of such antigens have already been given: H related to the ABO system, U of the MNS system, hr″ of the Rh system, k and Kp^b of the Kell system. Only one other example of a high-frequency antigen will be given here in the I-i blood group system. The reason for discussing this system is the unique way the red cell antigens of an individual change during early childhood. Two antibodies, anti-I and anti-i, detect corresponding specificities I and i, respectively. Virtually all newborn babies are i positive (I negative). However, during the first eighteen months of life, the newly produced red cells become increasingly more reactive with anti-I and each individual then remains I positive throughout the rest of his life. Anti-I is a **cold agglutinin,** reacting at or below room temperature. It is usually a 19S immunoglobulin and therefore is not implicated in hemolytic disease of the newborn, but it can be involved in transfusion reactions. When testing serum for anti-I, it is imperative that cord cells (from the umbilical cord of a baby) be included as an I-negative control. Wharton's jelly, a substance found only in umbilical cords, can be a source of spontaneous clumping of cord cells. All cord cells, therefore, should be thoroughly washed with warm saline before testing to remove any contaminating Wharton's jelly and thus prevent false positive reactions. So few adults are negative for public antigens that these blood factors are seldom involved in transfusion reactions.

To qualify as a **low-frequency** or **private (family) antigen,** its incidence must be less than 1 in 400 among the general population. Furthermore, it must be transmitted as a dominant character and must not belong to any of the previously established blood group systems. Some of the low-frequency specificities of established blood group systems (e.g., Mi of the MNS system, rh^w of the Rh system, and Kp^a of the Kell system) do not really qualify in this respect. Many private antigens have been discovered, but they are often limited to certain families. Because they are so rare, these factors are seldom involved in transfusion reactions.

The Compatibility Test

*Immuno-
hematology
Part II*

MAJOR AND MINOR CROSSMATCH

One of the most critical tests performed in the serological laboratory is the crossmatching of bloods for transfusion. If this test is improperly performed and/or interpreted, there is a risk of harming (or perhaps even killing) the patient by a transfusion incomptability. In this singular instance, the medical laboratory technologist is actually responsible for prescribing "medication" for a patient, as it is the technologist who selects the donor unit that will be transfused into the patient. Blood typing usually begins at the blood bank where agglutination tests are routinely made for antigens of the ABO and Rh blood group systems. The blood bank also normally tests blood for **reagin** (the antibody of syphilis) and for **hepatitis-associated antigen** (HAA; also referred to as **Australia antigen,** AuA, and **hepatitis B antigen,** HBAg). The technologist in the hospital where the blood will be used selects a unit (500 ml) of blood antigenically identical to that of the intended recipient in both the ABO and Rh systems. This requires the hospital technologist to take a sample of blood from the patient and perform direct blood-typing tests using antibody reagents of the ABO and Rh systems. A serological cross-match test is then performed, and if the donor and recipient bloods are found to be compatible, the technician releases the unit to the nurse or physician for transfusion. A compatibility test, when correctly performed and interpreted, should offer confirmation of the ABO groupings and detect the presence of atypical antibodies that could immediately react with cells of either the donor or the recipient. Some serological tests require heating of the serum to inactivate complement. This is never done for compatibility tests, however, because some antibodies may be detected only by their lytic activity in the presence of active complement (complement is destroyed by heating). Complement-mediated immune lysis also requires the presence of calcium and magnesium ions. Most anticoagulants used in blood banking function in the prevention of clotting by binding calcium (also required for coagulation). Therefore, anticoagulated specimens should not be used for crossmatching; serum is preferred.

The most commonly used anticoagulants in blood transfusions are CPD (citrate phosphate dextrose) and ACD (acid citrate dextrose) solutions. Red cells seem to survive better in CPD than in ACD. As the cells age, they progressively lose more potassium. Blood cannot be used for transfusion if stored more than twenty-one days. The fresher the blood, the better it is likely to be for the patient. Technologists should not be surprised if electrolytes such as potassium are greatly elevated in a posttransfusion patient given relatively old blood. The amount of 2,3-diphosphoglycerate (2,3-DPG) in blood is an indication of the affinity of hemoglobin for oxygen. Bloods preserved in CPD have higher levels of 2,3-DPG than those of comparable age in ACD. Rapid or massive transfusions can cause citrate to reach toxic levels in the recipient. This can be prevented by the simultaneous administration of calcium gluconate solution. Ethylenediamine tetra-acetic acid (EDTA) is a chelating agent that also binds calcium. It is commonly used for hematological tests such as hemoglobin estimations. EDTA damages platelets and greatly inhibits complement activity and therefore is not recommended for use in blood transfusion work.

Serology and Immunology

Artificial blood made from fluorochemicals has recently been used successfully in at least eight cases. In one of these, it replaced about 25 percent of the blood of a surgery patient whose religion forbade blood transfusions. Artificial blood remains in the body for a relatively short time; it is excreted in about a week. Its future use, therefore, will probably be limited to emergency situations in which suitable replacement blood cannot be immediately obtained.

A compatibility test actually consists of two parts. The **major crossmatch** involves mixing donor's cells with recipient's serum. It is designed to detect antibodies in the recipient's serum that could react with red cell antigens of the prospective donor. The **minor crossmatch** involves mixing recipient's cells with donor's serum for the reciprocal purpose. The major test is considered more important because of the possible destruction of the donor cells by complement-mediated immune lysis. Furthermore, globulin-coated (opsonized) cells are usually recognized as foreign material by the reticuloendothelial system and may also be destroyed by this mechanism. Ruptured red blood cells release hemoglobin. Free hemoglobin is converted enzymatically into bilirubin and other products normally excreted as bile pigments. However, when massive red cell destruction occurs (as in an incompatible transfusion) excessive bile pigments may accumulate in the blood and produce a yellowish tinge in the skin known as **jaundice.** Bile pigments may be toxic in high concentration and result in lower nephron nephritis and, in severe cases, death. These phenomena are important parts of the **hemolytic transfusion reaction.** Agglutination is rarely a problem *in vivo* because of the rapid destruction of incompatible donor cells. The major compatibility test is critical for the welfare of the patient. The minor test is usually considered less important because of the large dilution of donor antibodies that occurs when a unit of blood is transfused into an adult (approximately 5 liters of total blood is in a normal adult). However, if the donor antibodies are in high titer, even this large dilution factor may be insufficient to prevent widespread erythrocyte destruction. Thus, the minor test should not be considered trivial for the well-being of the patient.

There is considerable variation in the optimal conditions for reactivity of different blood group antibodies (Table 4.10). In order to detect any of three major types of antibodies (saline, albumin, and AHG-reacting), the compatibility test should be performed in three phases (Figure 4.1).

1. The **room temperature phase** requires two tubes labeled I and II. Both tubes receive two drops of serum* and two drops of an approximate 5 percent red blood cell suspension in their own serum or saline. In addition, tube I receives 22 percent bovine serum albumin (BSA) to enhance the reactivity of certain 7S antibodies. The tubes are spun immediately in a centrifuge and examined macroscopically (by naked eye) for agglutination and/or hemolysis. Saline agglutinins may be detected in either tube; albumin antibodies may be detected in tube I. If no reaction is seen in either tube, they should be shaken and tested in phase 2.
2. The **warm (thermo) phase** is designed to detect antibodies that react optimally at 37°C (normal human body temperature). Both tubes

---

* Two drops of serum are recommended to assure reactivity of antibodies in low titer.

FIGURE 4.1. Three-phase compatibility test.

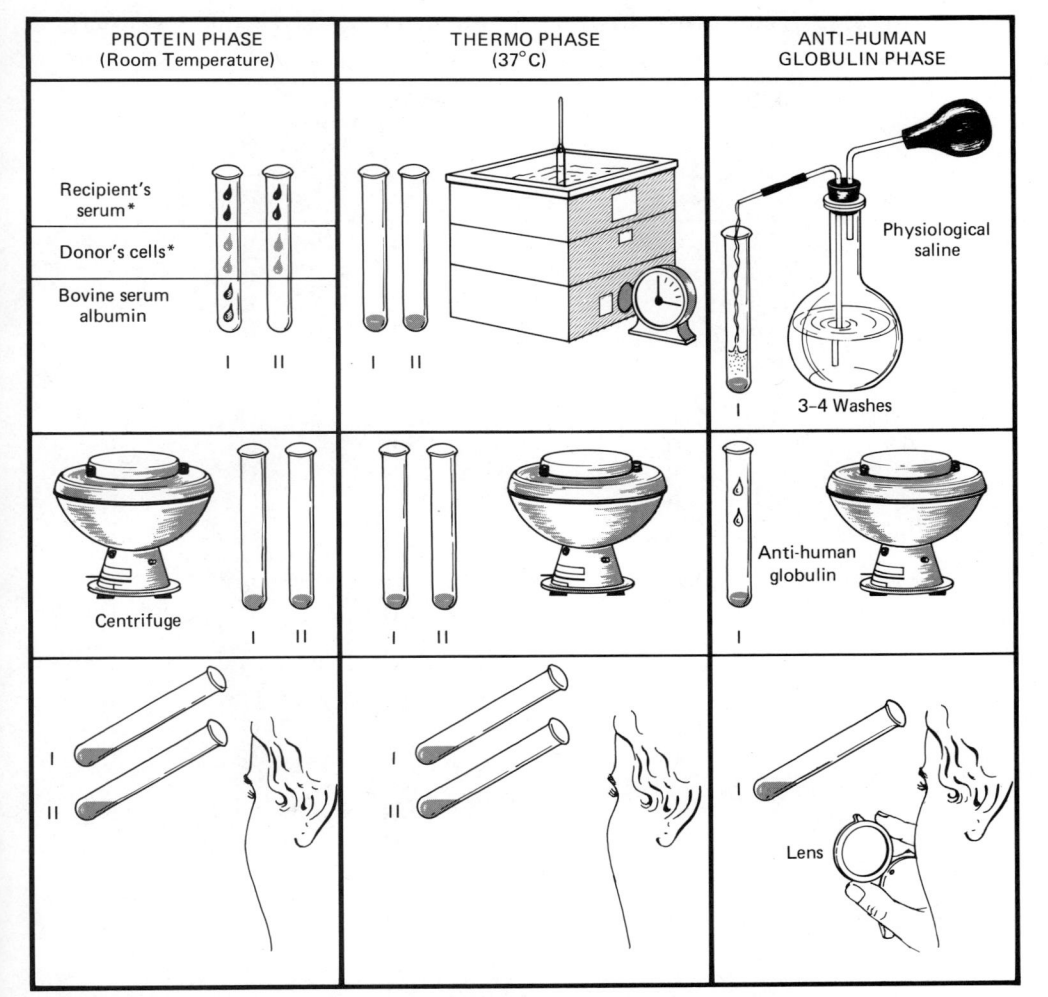

*A minor compatibility test can be performed by the method illustrated, substituting donor's serum and recipient's cells.

from phase 1 are incubated (either in a dry heating block or in a water bath) at 37°C for at least fifteen minutes, centrifuged, and examined macroscopically for agglutination and/or hemolysis. If there is still no reactivity, tube I should be tested in phase 3.

3. The **Coombs phase** (or **antihuman globulin phase**) should detect almost any blood group antibody that failed to react in phases 1 or 2. Tube I (containing BSA† from the thermo phase) should be shaken and then thoroughly washed by filling with physiological saline solution, mixing thoroughly, and centrifuging until all cells are at the bottom of the tube. Decant the wash saline, disperse the cells by shaking, refill with fresh saline, and repeat the wash cycle at least two more times (total washes three or four). Washing the cells thoroughly is

† The sensitivity of the test is increased when BSA-treated cells are carried through the antiglobulin technique.

Table 4.10 REACTIVITY OF SELECTED MAJOR BLOOD GROUP ANTIBODIES UNDER VARIOUS TEST CONDITIONS

Blood Group System	Antibody	RT Saline	37°C Saline	High Protein RT	High Protein 37°C	AHG
ABO	A	U	R	U	R	R
	B	U	R	U	R	R
	O/H	U	R	U	R	R
	A_1	U	R	U	R	R
Rh	D (Rh_0)	R	O	U	U	U
	C (rh')	R	O	U	U	U
	E (rh'')	R	O	U	U	U
	c (hr')	R	R	U	U	U
	e (hr'')	R	R	U	U	U
Kell-Cellano	K1 (Kell)	O	R	O	R	U
	K2 (Cellano)	R	R	U	R	U
MNS	M	U	R	U	O	R
	N	U	R	U	O	R
	S	R	O	R	O	O
	s	R	R	V	V	U
Lewis	Le^a	U	O	U	O	R
	Le^b	U	R	U	O	R
Duffy	Fy^a	R	R	R	R	U
	Fy^b	R	R	R	R	U
Kidd	Jk^a	R	R	R	R	U
	Jk^b	R	R	R	R	U
Lutheran	Lu^a	U	R	U	R	R
	Lu^b	R	R	R	R	U
P	P_1	U	R	U	R	R

RT = room temperature; AHG = antihuman globulin.
O = occasionally reactive, but undependable.
R = rarely reactive or nonoccurring.
U = usually reactive.
V = variable reactivity.

extremely important to remove all unreacted globulins (antibodies). If any free globulins remain after the wash cycles, they may inactivate the Coombs reagent and result in a false negative reading. This inactivation involves a blocking antibody phenomenon. Soluble globulins can occupy the combining sites on the AHG reagent so that it fails to

Enzyme Treatment	Optimum Temperature	Approx. % of Donors Antigenically Negative (Compatible with Antibody)		Comments
		White	Negro	
U	4–20	54	68	All antibodies of this
U	4–20	87	79	system are naturally
V	4–20	V	V	acquired
V	4–20	11	9	{May appear in groups A_2, A_2B, or weaker subgroups of A
U	37	15	7	Most common atypical antibody
U	37	34	69	{Rarely occurs alone; often
U	37	73	84	in combination with anti-D
U	37	20	5	{Often with anti-E; most
U	37	2	2	common in D-positive people
U	37	92	99	Potent antibody
O	37	8	1	Easily produced by K 1K 1 people
V	4–20	21	25	Antibodies of this system
V	4–20	28	23	may be inhibited by enzymes
V	20–37	45	45	
V	37	10	3	Extremely rare
O	4–20	78	80	May be lytic with complement
O	4–20	28	44	{Reacts stronger with group O and A_2 cells
R	37	34	90	May be inhibited by enzymes
R	37	17	68	
O	37	25	9	Highly labile; use fresh
O	37	25	57	samples; may require complement
U	20–37	92	96	Both antibodies are very
	37	<1		rare
U	4–20	21	6	Natural antibody; often appearing with "cold autoagglutinins"

combine with globulins attached to the red blood cells. After the last wash solution is decanted, the remaining drop of cells is shaken, AHG is added, and the tube is centrifuged and read both macroscopically and microscopically. If there is still no reactivity observed, one final control must be made. Coombs control cells (also called Coombs check cells and a variety of other names) should be added to the tube, mixed, centrifuged, and read macroscopically. A truly negative compatibility test should leave the AHG reagent free to react with the globulin-coated 5 percent saline suspension of washed Coombs control cells. Thus, agglutination of the control cells confirms the fact that AHG was added to the test and that the washing of the cells was adequate.

In the performance of a compatibility test, four tubes will actually be needed—two for the major test and two for the minor test. No unit of blood should be transfused into a patient unless it has passed the compatibility test, i.e., without reacting in any of the three phases on either the major or minor sides. A negative-reacting pair of donor-recipient bloods in a compatibility test verifies that the ABO grouping was done correctly and ensures that the patient will not suffer an immediate transfusion reaction. The transfused blood should survive for several weeks in the recipient. However, it should be realized that even though a donor and recipient have been determined to be compatible by this test the donor's blood may stimulate the patient to make antibodies against any foreign blood group antigens other than $Rh_0(D)$ factor and those of the ABO system.* Tests for antigens of other blood group systems are not routinely performed in crossmatching unless the patient is known to possess an **irregular** or **atypical antibody** (any blood group antibody other than those of the ABO system). As an example, suppose that the recipient is of rare genotype $K1K1$ (possessing only the K1 antigen) and the donor is $K1K2$ or $K2K2$ (having K2 antigen of the Kell-Cellano system). The patient may recognize K2 as foreign and eventually make anti-K2 antibodies (become sensitized to the K2 factor). This sensitization reaction may take several weeks before detectable titers of anti-K2 can be developed. By that time, the transfused cells have probably survived long enough to benefit the patient. The next time this patient needs a transfusion, he will already have anti-K2 as an atypical antibody in his serum. This may make it more difficult to find a compatible donor because more than 90 percent of the donor population possesses the K2 factor. The most expedient way to find a compatible blood for a patient sensitized to K2 is to do direct typing on prospective donor units using anti-K2 reagent. A blood that fails to react with anti-K2 is probably $K1K1$, and a compatibility test should be run only on donors that are K2 negative and also a match for the $Rh_0(D)$ factor and for the ABO antigens.

There are four possible kinds of reactions in a complete compatibility test. Examples of each are as follows.

1. Major side incompatible—compatible on the minor side.
   In this case, the recipient has one or more antibodies that react with antigens on the donor's cells.
   Example: If the recipient's serum contains anti-K1, and the donor's cells are K1 positive, and no atypical antibodies are in the donor's serum, then we would see a reaction (indicating incompatibility) on the major side, but no reaction on the minor side.
2. Major side compatible—minor side incompatible.
   This pattern of reaction indicates that the donor's serum contains one

---

* All bloods to be crossmatched are first determined to be identical in ABO group and for the $Rh_0(D)$ factor by direct typing.

or more antibodies that are attached to antigens on the recipient's cells.

Example: Suppose that the donor was actually group O, but was mistyped as group A. When the group O serum of this potential donor is mixed with group A recipient cells, the natural anti-A in the serum would react on the minor side, indicating incompatibility. There would be no reaction on the major side because although the group A serum of the recipient contains anti-B, it will not react with group O cells of the donor.

3. Incompatibility on both sides.

Here we have detected antibodies in both recipient and donor bloods that are reacting reciprocally with homologous antigens on red cells.

Example: A male recipient is group O, Rh positive (genotype R^0/r'), Lu(a−) with anti-Lu^a in his serum as a result of a previous transfusion of Lu(a+) cells. Blood from a prospective female donor is group O, Rh positive (genotype r''/r), Lu(a+) with anti-rh' (anti-C) in her serum as a result of sensitization by an incompatible pregnancy. A major side incompatibility occurs when the recipient's anti-Lu^a reacts with Lu(a+) donor's cells. A minor side incompatibility occurs when donor's anti-rh' (anti-C) reacts with recipient's rh'(C) factor.

4. No reaction on either side of the test.

This result indicates that the donor and recipient bloods are compatible. There are no antibodies of the recipient that will react with antigens of the donor, and vice versa. However, there may be one or more antibodies in either donor's or recipient's sera for which there are no corresponding antigens on the other's cells.

Example: If the recipient's serum contained anti-Rh$_0$(D) and the donor's cells were Rh$_0$ negative, there would be no incompatibility detected.

SPECIFIC COMPONENT THERAPY

It is becoming standard procedure in many hospitals to transfuse only specific blood components, where possible, rather than whole blood. **Packed cells** (plasma components removed by sedimentation or cetrifugation) can be used for patients whose oxygen transport capacity is subnormal. Units of blood to be used as packed cells are usually collected into "twin" packs. After the cells have settled at 4°C for 24 hours (or by centrifugation), the plasma is transferred into the second (twin) pack without opening the unit (sterile transfer). Some of the plasma-citrate is also transferred so that the cells will flow through the tubing during a transfusion (packed cell volume approximately 70 percent). Packed cells are used in cases where it is desired to increase the patient's **hematocrit** (proportion of red blood cells in whole blood) with the least disturbance of blood volume, as in severe anemia and intrauterine transfusion. The use of packed cells also reduces the risk of overloading the circulatory system, eliminates the possibility of toxic effects of anticoagulants, and minimizes the chances of allergic reactions to foreign plasma proteins of the donor.

It is usually wise to avoid transfusion of white blood cells if possible. Leukocytes carry histocompatibility antigens (Chapter 10) that could sensitize the patient and make it more difficult to find a compatible donor

Serology and Immunology

should he ever need a tissue or organ transplant. Platelets alone can be transfused if the patient's platelet count is low (thrombocytopenia). If the patient has hemophilia A (deficient in blood coagulation factor VIII), the deficiency can be replaced by transfusion of antihemophilic globulin. Plasma is seldom administered merely to replace a blood fluid deficiency. A plasma expander, such as a dextran solution, can do this. By a technique called **plasmapheresis,** blood can be withdrawn from a donor, the plasma separated from the cells, and the cells returned to the donor. The plasma extracted from packed cells of healthy donors can then be used as a source of blood-clotting factors or antibodies for use as typing reagents.

ALTERNATIVES TO THE MINOR CROSSMATCH

When only packed cells are transfused, a minor crossmatch test need not be made, but a major crossmatch would still be mandatory. If whole blood is needed, some laboratories prefer to substitute an **atypical antibody screening test** on donor serum in lieu of a minor crossmatch. Several companies offer these screening cells for sale, usually as a two-reagent kit. A typical kit contains two bottles of approximately 5 percent saline suspension of washed group O red cells. These two reagents are selected cells that contain between them virtually all of the clinically important blood group antigens (Table 4.11). Therefore, any donor's serum that fails to react with either of these **reagent cells** (as they are sometimes called) may be considered devoid of atypical blood group antibodies and hence should be compatible on the minor side (provided there is a match in the ABO system). Since reagent cells are always group O, any reactions in which they participate must involve atypical antibodies (blood group antibodies other than those of the ABO system). A screening test for atypical antibodies is performed in three phases analogous to those of the compatibility test (Figure 4.2). Two drops of the patient's serum are delivered into each of four tubes labeled I, IA, II, and IIA, respectively. Two drops of BSA go into tubes IA and IIA. A drop of reagent cell I goes into tubes I and IA; a drop of reagent cell II goes into tubes II and IIA. The tubes are mixed, centrifuged, and examined for agglutination and/or hemolysis. Saline agglutinins may be detected in any of the four tubes; albumin agglutinins may be detected in tubes IA and/or IIA. If no reaction is seen in the room temperature phase, all four tubes are incubated at 37°C for a minimum of fifteen minutes, centrifuged, and read. If still no reactivity is observed, then an **indirect antiglobulin (Coombs) test** is performed on tubes IA and IIA. The cells are thoroughly washed to remove all unreacted globulins and then exposed to AHG reagent. All negative antiglobulin tests are confirmed by the addition of Coombs control cells. It should be emphasized that a **direct** Coombs test is performed on fresh cells of the patient to determine if they have been coated *in vivo* with any kind of blood group antibodies. The **indirect** Coombs test is performed on the patient's serum to determine if any atypical blood group antibodies are present. This requires that the patient's serum be first mixed *in vitro* with reagent cells of known antigenic composition. After this exposure, the reagent cells are treated as they would be in a direct antiglobulin test.

Donor screening (i.e., testing donor's serum for atypical antibodies) does not provide a check on ABO grouping because reagent cells are always group O. Therefore, some laboratories prefer to use a minor crossmatch

Table 4.11 A Two-Cell Atypical Antibody Screening Kit

Antigens	Cells I	II
D	+	+
C	+	O
E	O	+
c	O	+
e	+	+
C^w	O	O
K	+	O
k	+	+
Kp^a	O	O
Kp^b	+	+
Js^a	O	O
Js^b	+	+
Fy^a	+	O
Fy^b	+	O
Jk^a	+	+
Jk^b	+	O
Le^a	+	O
Le^b	O	+
M	+	+
N	+	+
S	+	O
s	+	+
P_1	+	+
Lu^a	O	O
Lu^b	±	+
Xg^a	+	O
Vel	+	+

+ = antigen present on the cell; O = antigen absent.

because it should confirm direct ABO grouping. However, there are several advantages in using donor screening rather than a minor crossmatch.

1. Donor screening need be done only once on a unit of blood in order to detect any atypical antibodies. If atypical antibodies do exist in the donor's serum, it may require several to many minor crossmatches before a recipient is found whose red cells lack the homologus blood factor(s).
2. Units of blood may be checked for atypical antibodies as they are received. This can save time in crossmatching. Crossmatching must sometimes be done under "stat" conditions. (*Statim* is a Latin word meaning "immediately." Its abbreviation "stat" on an order for a laboratory test indicates that it should be done as quickly as possible.) Stat crossmatching is often required for accident victims who have hemorrhaged (massive loss of blood). In this case, the technologist's job is to find a compatible unit of blood for the patient as quickly as possible. Obviously, if several donor units have been previously

Serology and Immunology

Phase 1: Room Temperature Phase ("Immediate Spin")

Phase 2: 37°C (warm) Phase

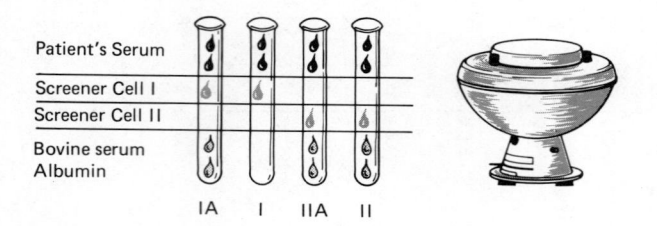

37°–30 min.

Phase 3: AHG Phase

3–4 Washes

FIGURE 4.2. Detection of atypical antibodies.

screened and found to contain no atypical antibodies, the technologist need not perform the minor crossmatch.

3. If donor screening is performed shortly after a serum sample is drawn, complement should still be reactive. Lytic antibodies can be detected only if active complement is present. The lytic activity of complement tends to wane as the unit of blood ages. Donor blood is commonly drawn into a plastic bag containing an anticoagulant (e.g., sodium citrate) that prevents clotting. Minor crossmatches or donor screening on stored units of blood must use plasma instead of serum. Most of the anticoagulants in common use for blood transfusions* prevent clotting by binding calcium. This cation is essential for binding at least one of the complement components in immune lysis. Minor crossmatching or donor screening on plasma is therefore un-

---

* Commonly used anticoagulants for transfusion are CPD (citrate phosphate dextrose) and ACD (acid citrate dextrose).

likely to detect lytic antibodies. A segmented pilot tube attached to each unit of blood allows the technologist to obtain repeated samples without danger of contaminating the unit as a whole. Blood is freshly drawn from a hospitalized patient (recipient) into a dry tube and allowed to clot. Serum containing active complement is thereby always used in the major crossmatch. Actually two tubes must be drawn from every patient if both a major and a minor crossmatch are to be performed. A "dry" tube is used for obtaining serum for the major crossmatch; a "wet" tube, containing anticoagulant fluid (or powder), is used to obtain red cells for the minor crossmatch. If donor screening is done in lieu of a minor crossmatch, only a dry tube sample need be taken from the patient. All cells used in crossmatching should be washed free of anticoagulant and suspended in saline or serum, but never in plasma.

4. Donor screening can detect the presence of virtually all clinically important blood group antibodies, even those for which no homologous antigens exist in the recipient. If atypical antibodies are found in a donor's serum, it is possible to record this information for the future safety of the donor. Many hospitals receive most of their blood from local or regional blood banks. It is possible for information concerning donors to flow from hospital laboratories to blood banks to the family physician of the donor. Unfortunately, this flow of information is seldom (if ever) routinely transmitted. However, if the donor and recipient are members of the same family, and the transfusion is to be performed directly from one family member to another by the family physician, there is a good chance that information on atypical antibodies of family members screened as possible donors will come to the attention of the family physician. Blood found to possess a rare atypical antibody (or antigen) is often much more valuable as a source of commercial blood-typing reagent (or reagent cells) than as a donor unit of whole blood.

5. During an emergency, when group O blood is used as a universal donor for a recipient of another group, the minor crossmatch will be incompatible because of the natural anti-A and anti-B in group O serum. In this case, donor screening should be done to detect atypical antibodies that would otherwise be missed.

THE AUTO CONTROL

Many people have **cold agglutinins** that react nonspecifically at 5°C. These antibodies are usually not considered to be clinically significant, and crossmatching at this temperature is not recommended. An **auto control** should be run simultaneously in the cross-match test, using patient's cells and patient's serum. If the auto control is negative, a corresponding incompatible crossmatch is probably caused by a specific antibody. On the other hand, if the auto control is positive and the corresponding crossmatch is incompatible, the patient has a nonspecific agglutinin that may be masking the presence of one or more specific antibodies. In this case, the patient's blood should be absorbed by allowing a sample to clot at refrigerator temperature. Cold agglutinins attach to the clot, leaving the serum free of cold antibodies. A second sample, collected in anticoagulant, provides cells for

Serology and Immunology

the auto control. These cells should be washed thoroughly with warm (37°C) saline to remove (elute) any cold autoantibodies. If a 5 to 6 percent saline suspension of the washed cells is tested with the absorbed serum and gives no reactivity, then the serum is considered fully absorbed and ready for use in crossmatching or in tests with screener cells.

PATIENT SCREENING

The use of group O screener cells (reagent red blood cells) to detect the presence of atypical blood group antibodies in the patient's serum should be tempered by knowledge of the following facts.

1. Patient screening should never be used as a substitute for a major crossmatch. It is recommended that patient screening be done prior to the crossmatch. If an atypical antibody is found in the patient's serum, then the most expedient procedure is to identify the atypical antibody(s) by the methods outlined in the final section of this chapter. Once these antibodies are known, direct typing should be performed on donor units for the *absence* of the corresponding blood factor(s). A donor unit found not to possess the corresponding blood factor(s) should then be subjected to a complete compatibility test with the patient.
2. If patient screening reveals the presence of an atypical antibody, then the hospital laboratory or blood bank is in a better position to anticipate problems in finding a donor match. This becomes increasingly important for transfusions involving multiple units.
3. Even if only low titers of atypical antibodies have been detected and identified in the patient prior to transfusion, a donor unit of blood should be selected that is devoid of the homologus antigen. In this way, the patient will not be restimulated (as a booster immunization) to rapidly produce the corresponding antibody (anamnestic reaction) that could trigger a delayed transfusion reaction.
4. Most of the companies that sell screener cell kits attempt to provide cells that are not influenced by dosage effects. Some antibodies react weakly with a single dose of antigen, but react strongly with a double

Table 4.12 CELL PANEL FOR ANTIBODY IDENTIFICATION

Cell No.	\multicolumn{6}{c} Rh-hr						Kell				Duffy
	D	C	c	E	e	C^w	K	k	Kp^a	Kp^b	Fy^a
1	+	+	0	0	+	+	0	+	0	+	0
2	+	0	+	+	0	0	0	+	0	+	0
3	+	0	+	0	+	0	0	+	0	+	0
4	0	+	0	0	+	0	+	+	0	+	+
5	0	0	+	+	+	0	0	+	0	+	+
6	0	0	+	0	+	0	+	0	0	+	+
7	0	0	+	0	+	0	0	+	0	+	+
8	+	+	0	+	+	0	0	+	+	+	0

* Vell is a high-frequency antigen lacking in about 1 in 4,000 individuals.

dose. Anti-N often reacts weakly with MN cells, but strongly with N cells. If a patient's serum contains anti-N and the donor's cells used in the crossmatch are MN, then the presence of anti-N may go undetected. On the other hand, if one of the screener cells was M and the other was N, then anti-N should be detected. Anti-rh' (c) is another antibody showing dosage effects. Red cells with only a single dose of c factor (as in genotype *DCe/dce*) react weakly with anti-c. A stronger reaction is commonly seen with cells of genotypes *DcE/DcE* or *DcE/dce*. Again, commercial screener cell kits attempt to provide at least one vial of reagent cells with a double dose of factor c. If a patient's serum contains anti-c, then potential donor cells can be directly tested with high-titered antiserum; only those testing c negative would be selected for the compatibility test.

5. If the reactivity of the reagent screener cells is better than that of donor cells in the pilot tube, then a weak atypical antibody in the patient's serum might best be detected by testing it with the screener cells.

Antibody Identification

Once an atypical antibody has been discovered in a patient's serum by use of screener red cells, the next logical step is to determine its specificity. For this purpose, a commercial 5 percent saline suspension panel of washed reagent red cells (usually eight to ten vials) is employed. These cells are all group O so that natural antibodies of the ABO system will not be reactive with them. They are a selected group, the antigenic pattern of which offers a good chance for antibody discrimination (Table 4.12). All reagent cells have a limited lifetime and should not be used past the expiration date printed by the supplier on the labels. Toward the end of the dating period some of the antigens lose some reactivity and may not react as strongly with weak antibodies as they did when they were fresh.

An antibody identification test is performed in a manner analogous to a major crossmatch (Figure 4.3). The number of tubes needed corresponds to the number of vials in the panel, plus one additional tube for an auto

	Kidd	Lewis		P	MNS				Lutheran		Sex-linked	
Jk^a	Jk^b	Le^a	Le^b	P_1	M	N	S	s	Lu^a	Lu^b	Xg^a	Vel*
+	0	0	3+	3+	+	+	0	+	0	+	+	2+
0	+	0	0	1+	+	0	+	0	0	+	+	4+
+	0	0	1+	4+	0	+	0	0	0	+	+	3+
+	+	0	0	0	+	+	+	+	+	+	+	2+
0	+	3+	0	2+	+	+	0	+	0	+	+	1+
0	+	0	2+	3+	+	+	0	+	0	+	0	2+
+	+	0	1+	0	+	+	+	+	+	0	+	3+
+	0	2+	0	0	+	0	0	+	0	+	0	3+

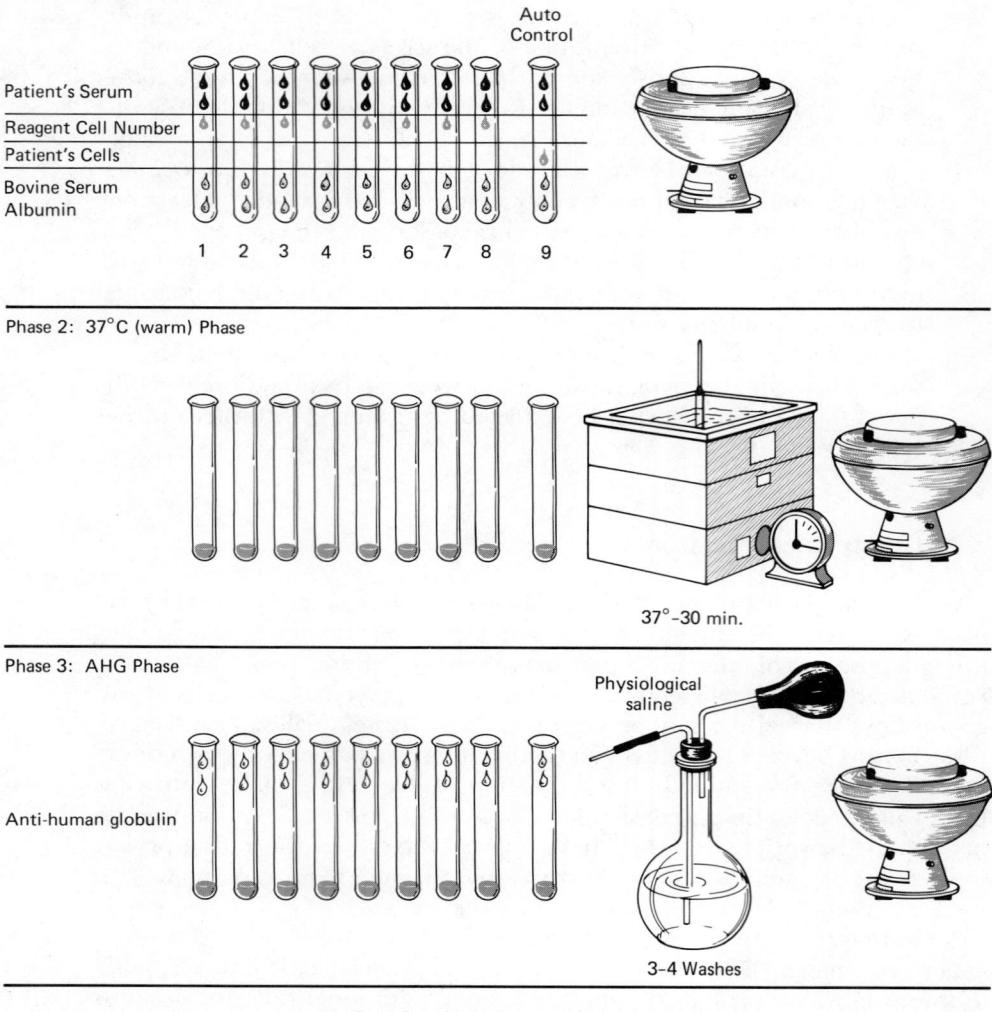

FIGURE 4.3. Identification of atypical antibodies.

control (testing the patient's cells against his own serum). Each tube is carried through the three phases of the compatibility test: (1) room temperature, (2) 37°C, and (3) antiglobulin. Any negative antiglobulin tests are confirmed by the use of Coombs control cells.

It may not be discerned from the screener test whether only a single atypical antibody or multiple antibodies are present in a patient's serum. Recipients of multiple transfusions may have produced two or more atypical antibodies, making it increasingly more difficult to find compatible donors for them.

Suppose that a patient's serum reacts with a cell panel as shown in Table 4.13. The best way to proceed is to note all reagent cells of the panel that failed to react with the patient's serum in any phase of the test. We can infer that our atypical antibody(s) is not directed against any of the antigens present on these nonreactive cells. We may cross off all antigens on the nonreactive cells of the protocol that failed to react with the serum. For

Table 4.13 Hypothetical Example of Results Obtained on a Patient's Serum with the Panel of Reagent Cells Shown in Table 4.12

Patient's name _____ Tom Jones _____

ABO group _____ 0 _____

Rh type _____ Pos _____

Direct antiglobulin test _____ Neg _____

Screener test for atypical antibodies _____ Pos _____

Results of test with cell panel:

Cell No.:	1	2	3	4	5	6	7	8	Auto Control
Room temp. saline	0	0	0	0	0	0	0	0	0
Room temp. albumin	0	0	0	0	0	0	0	0	0
37°C saline	0	0	0	0	0	0	0	0	0
37°C albumin	0	0	0	0	0	0	0	0	0
Antiglobulin	0	0	0	4+	4+	4+	4+	0	0
Coombs control	4+	4+	4+					4+	4+

example, in Table 4.13 cell 1 failed to react; hence we infer that the atypical antibody(s) is not directed against factors D, C, e, C^w, k, Kp^b, Fy^b, Jk^a, Le^b, P_1, M, N, s, Lu^b, Xg^a, and Vel. Similarly we can infer from nonreactive cell 2 that, in addition to those antibodies already eliminated by cell 1, we can also eliminate antibodies against factors c, E, Jk^b, and S. Cell 3 fails to eliminate any additional antibodies. Cell 8 eliminates antibodies against Kp^a and Le^a. This leaves antibodies against factors K, Fy^a, and Lu^a. Notice that the pattern of reactivity, involving cells 4, 5, 6, and 7 could be accounted for solely by anti-Fy^a because the corresponding Fy^a factor is present on each of these cells. However, anti-K and/or anti-Lu^a could also be present in addition to anti-Fy^a because they react with some of the same cells (but not all) as anti-Fy^a. It is clear that anti-Fy^a must be present because of reactivity of the serum with cell 5 (possessing factor Fy^a, missing factors K and Lu^a). Anti-Lu^a can be eliminated because it typically is reactive at low temperatures in saline, and no such antibody was detected in this test. Anti-K typically reacts only in the antiglobulin phase (as does anti-Fy^a) and therefore cannot be eliminated on the basis of its "phase reactivity." There are at least two additional clues that may help to resolve the question of anti-K. If direct typing is performed on the patient's cells with reagent anti-K and they are found to be K positive, then anti-K should not be present in this person's serum. If the patient's cells are K negative however, anti-K *could* be present in the patient's serum. In the latter case, absorption of the serum with appropriate cells may reveal the presence or absence of anti-K. If we have an available source of cells that are Fy^a positive and K negative (such as panel cell 5), we could absorb anti-Fy^a from the serum and see what reactivity remains. If we retest the absorbed serum against the eight-cell panel and find reactivity with cells 4 and 6, then the presence of anti-K is confirmed.

On the other hand, if retesting the absorbed serum gives no reactivity with any cells of the panel, then anti-K was not present. To adequately absorb any serum usually requires a packed cell volume at least equal to that of the serum sample. Obviously, the 5 percent red cell suspensions in the small vials of the commercial panel cells would probably not provide enough cells for absorption purposes; this is not the purpose of panel cells. Before embarking on a search for cells that are Fy^a positive and K negative, it might be wise to calculate the chance of finding such a cell in a random sample of Caucasians. The Fy^a factor is present in approximately two thirds and the K factor is absent in approximately nine tenths of such a population. The combined probability is $((2/3)(9/10) = {}^{18}/_{30} = 0.6$. Thus, 6 out of 10 units of blood selected at random from this population would be expected to be suitable for this absorption, a high enough probability to warrant the search. Alternatively, if cells can be found that are K positive and Fy^a negative, their use in an indirect antiglobulin test with the patient's serum may reveal whether or not anti-K is present. However, the probability of finding such a blood from a random sample of Caucasian donors is very low. K-positive individuals constitute only about one tenth and Fy^a-negative individuals constitute about one third of such a population. The combined chance of finding such a blood is $(^1/_{10})(^1/_3) = {}^1/_{30}$ or about 3 percent, hardly worth making the search. These calculations also reveal why no cells of the panel were K positive and Fy^a negative—they are just too "rare."

It should be noted that the two cells of the screener cell kit may also provide information that may help to identify atypical antibodies by following the same "elimination procedure" as described for the panel cells.

Very few atypical antibodies (e.g., anti-Le^a) commonly are involved in hemolysis; so this type of reaction may also aid in antibody identification. Treatment of red cells with proteolytic enzymes (e.g., trypsin, bromelin, papain, ficin) may be used to enhance the reactivity of certain blood group factors (e.g., P_1, Lewis, Kidd) and thereby aid in identification of the corresponding antibodies. These enzymes remove from red cells certain membrane components such as sialic acid (with their negatively charged carboxyl groups), thereby reducing the zeta potential and enhancing reactivity of cells with antibodies. However, some blood group factors (e.g., Fy^a, M, N, S) are destroyed by enzyme treatment, and this can also provide a valuable clue in identifying an atypical antibody.

Occasionally the racial origin of the patient is helpful in antibody identification. Some blood group factors are rare in one race and common in another. For example, in the Sutter-Kell blood group system, factor Js^a appears to be found only in Negroes; virtually all Caucasians are Js^b positive and Js^a negative. Therefore, anti-Js^b would not be expected in the serum of Caucasians.

If the patient has never had a blood transfusion or has never been pregnant, then an atypical antibody in that person's serum must be of "natural" origin. A few atypical blood group antibodies are known to be produced "naturally" (i.e., without exposure to foreign red cells in this case). Among the "naturally occurring" atypical antibodies are anti-Lewis, anti-M (most), anti-N (rare), anti-S (some), anti-Kp^a, anti-P_1, anti-Lu^a, and anti-I. Hence, if a patient has never had the opportunity to be sensitized by foreign cells, then an atypical agglutinin in his serum probably is one of these "naturally occurring" antibodies.

DIFFICULTIES

Not all antibody identification tests are as easily solved as the foregoing example. Some of the possible sources of difficulty are as follows.

1. Dosage effects. If a patient's serum contains anti-N, it probably would react more strongly with cell 3 (homozygous for factor N) than it would with cells 1, 4, 5, 6, or 7 (heterozygous for factor N). If the antibody is weak, its reactivity with heterozygous cells may appear to be negative. This can be a profound source of confusion in the analysis of such tests.
2. Variable strengths of antigens. In Table 4.12, a variation in reactivity (4+, 3+, 2+, 1+) is apparent with some of the panel cells, even in the presence of high-titered antibody (e.g., Le^a, Le^b, P_1, and Vel).
3. Weak antibodies. The specificity of an antibody is very difficult to detect unless it reacts 1+ or stronger. Some blood group antibodies may increase in strength with time due to continued stimulation (e.g., by an incompatible pregnancy). The strength of an antibody in a given patient may therefore change significantly from one sampling to another.
4. Antigen not present on the panel cells. Some rare antibodies may have no antigenic counterpart on the reagent cells of the panel. Perhaps the antibody is a new one belonging to an as-yet-unidentified blood group system. Both these possibilities are quite remote. If the problem cannot be resolved at the local level, it may be referred to a consultation laboratory.
5. Contamination. Various nonspecific reactions may be observed as a result of microbial and/or chemical contamination of the serum and/or the reagent cells. When contamination is suspected, a new sample of serum should be drawn and retested against a fresh cell panel, paying particular attention to cleanliness of all glassware and purity of reagents such as saline.

Quality Control in Blood Banking

In order to ensure that serological test results are valid, quality control measures must be in daily operation within the laboratory. A comprehensive quality control program must include at least three major areas: (1) equipment, (2) procedures, and (3) reagents.

EQUIPMENT

The blood bank refrigerator must be monitored daily for a temperature variation no greater than $\pm 1°C$ within the range of 1 to 6°C. A permanent record of these daily checks must be maintained by each laboratory issuing blood for transfusions. The refrigerator must be equipped with an alarm so that variations outside the prescribed storage range will be immediately known by personnel in the building. Centrifuges should be calibrated periodically to ascertain if the rotor speeds attained agree with the dial settings. Timers on centrifuges also need periodic checks as do all timing devices, whether or not they are integrated with other pieces of equipment. Constant temperature devices (dry blocks or water baths) should be checked daily for uniformity of prescribed temperatures. The entire laboratory should be maintained at a uniform comfortable temperature. Automated pipetes should be monitored regularly for accuracy in delivery of prescribed quantities of fluids. If the laboratory has an automated cell washer, it must be constantly monitored because incomplete cell washings may produce false negative antiglobulin (Coombs) tests. The efficiency of washing can be checked by the addition of known sensitized cells (Coombs control cells) to all negative antiglobulin tests.

PROCEDURES

Laboratory technologists should read the directions supplied with each shipment of immunological reagents (antisera, reagent cells, etc.) because manufacturers may change procedures from time to time. The serum-to-cell ratio should be standardized for all red cell tests according to directions provided by the reagent manufacturer. Standardization of red cell concentrations can be accomplished by matching the patient's cell suspension to that of commercial sources of reagent red cells of specified concentration. At regular intervals, an exact standard cell suspension should be prepared by hematocrit (blood cell volume) as a control against which other suspensions are adjusted by visual comparison. Groups of related tests (e.g., tests with anti-A, anti-B, and anti-A,B) should be read together in order to detect variations in the strength of agglutination. Grading of positive reactions and comparison with pictures of graded agglutinations are highly recommended. Most errors in the clinical laboratory are not made in the performance of tests, but rather in the recording and transcribing of results onto the proper forms and reports. The strengths of positive results, as well as unusual reactions (e.g., hemolysis, mixed-field agglutination, etc.) and interpretations of the results, should be carefully recorded in the correct places. The lot number of each reagent used should be recorded.

There are two ways to control ABO grouping tests: (1) testing the cells with anti-A,B and (2) reverse grouping (which is controlled reciprocally by direct red cell grouping). For control of Rh typing, some laboratories have the tests performed in duplicate by different technologists or by one technologist using different lot numbers of antisera. Both slide and modified tube tests should also be controlled by exposing the test cells to bovine serum albumin since this substance is used as a diluent in the preparation of the reagent. The ideal negative control for Rh antisera is not 22 percent or 30 percent BSA, but rather one that contains all of the constituents in similar concentrations to that of the antisera (minus the Rh antibodies) and is manufactured by the same process. Such Rh control reagents are now commercially available. All negative Rh tests must be confirmed by the D^u test. A positive D^u test must be confirmed by a negative direct antiglobulin (Coombs) test. If not used as alternatives for compatibility tests, antibody screening tests on the recipient and donor sera serve as controls of the major and minor cross-match tests, respectively. An auto control, consisting of the patient's or donor's serum and his own red cells, should be run in parallel with an antibody identification test. If an antibody has been identified in the intended recipient and a donor has been selected that lacks the corresponding antigen, then a nonreactive major crossmatch also served as confirmation of correct atypical antibody identification. If the selected donor is incompatible, then identification of atypical antibodies was either incomplete or erroneous. Coombs control cells are used on all negative Coombs tests to control the efficiency of red cell washings and to confirm that antihuman globulin was added to the test.

REAGENTS

Each time a reagent is used the technologist should inspect the label to ensure that it is the correct reagent and that it is still "in date" (i.e., it has not exceeded the date specified on the label by the manufacturer). Daily controls on reagents are required to prove that they are reacting as specified and that they have not deteriorated in storage or become contaminated. Positive controls are designed to demonstrate that the reagents have not lost sensitivity and are still able to detect weak antigens or weak antibodies. Negative controls demonstrate that reagents have not lost specificity (perhaps by contamination). Both positive and negative controls should be run under the same conditions (temperatures, centrifuge speed times, incubation times, volumes, etc.) as the reagents would encounter in tests where they would normally be employed. A daily blood bank reagent control program should include (1) antihuman serum controls, (2) reagent red cell controls, and (3) antiserum controls.

A "broad-spectrum antihuman (Coombs) serum" is one prepared against whole human serum and contains antibodies reactive with immunoglobulins (electrophoretic gamma globulin fraction of serum) as well as nongamma globulins (including most of the components of the complement system). Purified antihuman IgG is also commercially available to assist in the characterization of proteins bound to red blood cells that have reacted with a broad-spectrum antihuman serum. Anti-IgG is useful as an aid in diagnosis of warm antibody autoimmune hemolytic anemias, cold agglutination disease, drug-induced hemolytic anemias, drug-induced positive antiglobulin tests, and hemolytic disease of the newborn. Antihuman serum should agglutinate Coombs control cells as a positive control of the antigamma activity of the reagent. A positive control on the antinongamma activity (mainly beta globulin complement components) of antihuman serum is a test with red cells sensitized with complement. Fresh human serum contains complement. Exposing group O cells to fresh normal serum (containing no atypical antibodies) and a 10 percent sucrose solution apparently allows complement to become attached nonspecifically (without the aid of antibodies) to red cells. Complement can be destroyed by heating serum at 56°C for thirty minutes. Saline suspensions (5 percent) of such complement-sensitized cells (CSC), unsensitized cells (USC), and immunoglobulin-sensitized Coombs control cells (CCC) are employed in the antihuman serum control tests. Antihuman serum is added to three tubes, each containing one of the three kinds of cells (CCC, CSC, and USC). A comparable set of three saline control tubes substitutes saline for antihuman serum. If the broad-spectrum Coombs reagent is satisfactory, it should produce results as shown in Table 4.14.

In the reagent red cell controls, the cells are tested with diluted antiserum to demonstrate that they are capable of detecting even low titers of an-

Table 4.14 EXPECTED RESULTS FOR REAGENT CONTROL TESTS (SEE TEXT)

ANTIHUMAN SERUM CONTROLS

	Coombs Control Cells (CCC)	Complement-Sensitized Cells (CSC)	Unsensitized Cells (USC)
Antihuman Serum	RT +	RT +	RT Neg
Saline	Neg	Neg	Neg

REAGENT RED CELL CONTROLS

	Reagent Red Blood Cells (Human)									
	Screener Cells for Atypical Antibodies								Reverse Grouping Cells		
	1				2				A_1	B	A_2
Dilute anti-D	Sal RT Neg	Alb RT Neg	Alb 37°C Neg	AHS +	Sal RT Neg	Alb RT Neg	Alb 37°C Neg	AHS +			
Dilute anti-A,B									RT +	RT +	

ANTISERUM CONTROLS

	Screener Cells for Atypical Antibodies							
	1				2			
Bovine albumin	RT Neg	37°C Neg	AHS Neg	CCC +	RT Neg	37°C Neg	AHS Neg	CCC +
Anti-D	RT +				RT +			
Anti-A	Neg				Neg			
Anti-B	Neg				Neg			
Anti-A,B	Neg				Neg			

	Reverse Grouping Cells											
	A_1				B				A_2			
Bovine albumin	RT Neg	37°C Neg	AHS Neg	CCC +	RT Neg	37°C Neg	AHS Neg	CCC +	RT Neg	37°C Neg	AHS Neg	CCC +
Anti-D	Neg	Neg	Neg	+	Neg	Neg	Neg	+	Neg	Neg	Neg	+
Anti-A					RT Neg				RT +			
Anti-B	RT Neg				+							
Anti-A,B					+				RT +			

tibodies in serum samples. Anti-D (anti-Rh₀) serum for slide and modified tube tests is diluted 1:50 and exposed to screener cells for detection of atypical antibodies. Most commercial screening reagent cells consist of two vials of different cells that, as a set, contain most of the clinically important blood group antigens. These two screener cells are both usually D-positive and are simply labeled 1 and 2 in Table 4.14. The sensitized cells are tested in both saline and albumin suspensions at room temperature, in albumin at 37°C, and (following washing) with antihuman serum (AHS). Because the concentration of the antibody is so weak, agglutination is expected to occur only in the tubes with antihuman serum. Reagent cells used for reverse grouping (groups A_1 and B) are tested with a 1:50 dilution of anti-A,B at room temperature.

The antiserum controls in Table 4.14 consist of testing bovine serum albumin, anti-D, anti-A, anti-B, and anti-A,B with appropriate reagent human red cells. In addition to showing that the antisera have lost neither sensitivity nor specificity, these controls will also demonstrate that reagent cells for reverse grouping (groups A_1, A_2, and B) are $Rh_o(D)$ negative and D^u negative. In addition, these tests will prove (by a negative direct antiglobulin test) that the various reagent cells have no attached globulins. Reverse grouping cells therefore are tested the same way as screener cells for atypical antibodies in these controls. Anti-A and anti-A,B are tested with B cells for specificity, and with A_2 cells for ability to detect weak subgroups of A. Anti-B is tested with A_1 cells for specificity and with B cells for adequate sensitivity. The expected results for all of these reagent tests are given in Table 4.14.

SELF-EVALUATION

Terms

1. A theory that homozygotes produce twice as much of the corresponding blood group antigen as heterozygotes. (2 words)
2. A phenomenon in which the presence of one antigen blocks antibody access to another antigen. (2 words)
3. An adjective descriptive of genes that produce no detectable product (e.g., no blood group antigen).
4. Any blood group antigen found in almost 100 percent of every human population.
5. The antibody of syphilis.
6. A yellowish staining of the integument, sclerae, deeper tissues, and body excretions with bile pigments.
7. Abbreviation of a Latin word meaning "at once; immediately."
8. A general name for blood group antibodies other than those of the ABO system.
9. Antibodies that cause clumping of red cells at about 5°C. (2 words)
10. A test designed to determine if a pair of bloods can be mixed without any serological reactivity.

Multiple Choice. Choose the one best response.

1. Which of the following blood group systems is most closely antigenically related to the ABO system? (a) Lewis (b) MNS (c) Kell (d) Duffy (e) Kidd
2. The Cellano blood group factor is also designated (a) P (b) Lu^a (c) Xg^a (d) s (e) none of these

Serology and Immunology

3. In the performance of an antiglobulin test, the presence of free serum proteins (a) usually facilitates agglutination (b) may cause lysis (c) may produce a false negative reaction (d) enhances the sensitivity of the test (e) may produce a false positive reaction
4. Suppose that a pair of bloods is determined compatible by a correctly performed compatibility test. Which of the following statements is incorrect? (a) An immediate transfusion reaction should not occur. (b) The Rh typing is confirmed. (c) The ABO grouping is confirmed. (d) The recipient could become sensitized to a foreign blood group antigen. (e) Blood group antibodies may be undetected in either donor or recipient.
5. The auto control in a compatibility test contains (a) patient's serum and reagent red cells (b) patient's cells and donor's serum (c) patient's cells and BSA (d) patient's serum and patient's cells (e) none of these
6. Which of the following does not help resolve problems arising from a test for atypical antibody identification? (a) differential absorption (b) direct typing (c) enzyme-treated cells (d) parental ABO group and Rh type (e) phase reactivity
7. Which of the following is not an advantage of donor screening? (a) donor units need be screened only once (b) provides a check on the ABO grouping (c) screening can be done before the crossmatch test (d) eliminates the need for a minor crossmatch (e) more than one of these
8. If a cross-match test is incompatible on both the major and minor sides and no error has been made in ABO grouping, then (a) both bloods have different atypical antibodies (b) both bloods have the same antibody (c) the donor has an antigen that is not present in the recipient (d) the recipient has an antigen not present in the donor (e) more than one of these is correct
9. In crossmatching, the test that is most likely to detect the greatest variety of clinically important blood group antibodies is the (a) saline agglutination test (b) complement (fresh serum) hemolysis test (c) cold agglutination test (d) antiglobulin test (e) albumin-enhanced test at 37°C
10. If 80 percent of Caucasians in the United States are blood type P_1, 20 percent are P_2, and 90 percent are K negative, then the probability that a blood chosen at random from this population would be P_1 and K positive is approximately (a) 2 percent (b) 8 percent (c) 16 percent (d) 18 percent (e) none of these

True-False

1. Patient screening (testing patient's serum with reagent red blood cells) may be substituted for a major crossmatch.
2. In a test for atypical antibody identification, if a patient's serum reacts with a reagent red cell that does not possess a certain antigen, then the corresponding antibody must not be present.
3. Low-frequency blood group antigens are so named because they rarely stimulate antibody formation when introduced into an individual lacking them.
4. Some human blood group antigens have been found in only certain races.
5. Lewis blood types are postulated to be jointly determined by the Le and S loci.
6. Antigens of the MNS system are only weakly antigenic for humans and are usually of little importance in blood transfusions.
7. Antibodies of the Kell system usually are reactive only in the antiglobulin phase.
8. No blood group antibodies other than those of the ABO system are known to be produced by stimulation of substances other than red cells.
9. The gene responsible for the Xg^a antigen cannot be transmitted from a father to his son.
10. The compatibility test is the most critical test (in terms of patient welfare) performed in the serological laboratory.

Precipitation

CHAPTER 5

CHAPTER OUTLINE

Precipitation in Liquid Medium
  Quantitative Procedure
  Ring Test
  Practical Applications of Fluid Precipitin Tests
Precipitation in Gel Medium
  Immunodiffusion Tests
    Single Diffusion–Single Dimension
    Single Diffusion–Double Dimension
    Double Diffusion–Single Dimension
    Double Diffusion–Double Dimension
  Immunoelectrophoresis Tests
    Single Reactant Moving in One Dimension
    Single Reactant Moving in Two Dimensions
    Double Reactants Moving in One Dimension
    Double Reactants Moving in Two Dimensions
  Capsular Precipitation
Self-evaluation

Precipitation in Liquid Medium

Immunological **precipitates** are insoluble complexes formed by the union of antibodies **(precipitins)** and soluble antigens **(precipitinogens).** Lattice formation requires that both the precipitin and the precipitinogen be at least bivalent. As an example of an *in vitro* precipitation test, let us consider the case of egg albumin (ovalbumin, OA) and rabbit anti-OA. One way to set up the test is to serially dilute the antigen with saline and mix it with a constant amount of antibody. IgG is a much better precipitating antibody than IgM, whereas the reverse is true of agglutination. IgA is a poorer precipitin than IgM, and IgE is nonprecipitating. The tubes are incubated and then macroscopically scored for the degree of precipitation. Precipitates tend to form more rapidly as the temperature increases to about 40 or 45°C. More complete precipitation is usually obtained between 0 and 4°C. A convenient (although arbitrary) scale of recording relative reactions is to assign +4 to the tube containing the greatest amount of precipitate; +2 would indicate half of the greatest amount seen in the test. Table 5.1 displays the hypothetical results of an idealized precipitation test. Precipitation in either of the controls invalidates the test. It should be noted that at lower dilutions (higher concentrations) of antigen there is little or no precipitate formed. As the antigen is diluted further, more precipitate is formed, until a maximal amount is reached. If the antigen is diluted still further, the amount of precipitate declines until it disappears. The ratio of antigen dilution to antibody dilution at which maximum precipitation occurs is the **equivalence point.** Little or no difference in the amount of precipitation may be observed in one or more tubes on either side of the equivalence point of some titrations, thereby establishing an **equivalence zone.** The ratio of dilutions of antigen and antibody producing a visible serological reaction most rapidly constitutes the **optimal proportion** (OP). The OP is usually at or near the middle of the equivalence zone so OP and equivalence zone are often used interchangeably. At equivalence, all of the reactants (both antigen and antibody) are involved in formation of the precipitation lattice. Neither free antigen nor free antibody can be detected in the supernatant fluid. Concentrations of antigen higher than at equivalence may result in either a weak precipitation reaction or no precipitate being formed. This region is called a **prozone** (prezone, zone of inhibition). If the supernatant fluids ("supernates") of tubes in the prozone are separately diluted and tested with antiserum, they can be shown to contain free antigen. In other words, the prozone is a region of antigen excess. Similarly, antigen dilutions greater than the equivalence point will result in a weak reaction or no precipitate being formed. This is called the **postzone** (Figure 5.1). If antigen is added to supernatant fluids from the postzone, precipitates will form because this is a region of antibody excess. The **zoning phenomenon** (prozones, postzones) is a major deterrent to the use of fluid precipitation tests in the clinical laboratory. *In vivo* precipitation reactions are probably rare because of zoning phenomena. Agglutinating systems are less susceptible to prozones, but they can occur (e.g., see VDRL test, Chapter 6).

Each antigen-antiserum system has its own characteristic OP zone. Unless one knows *a priori* approximately the dilutions of antigen and/or antibody where equivalence exists, a precipitation test may be falsely negative because prozoning or postzoning has occurred. Of course, if one has the time, dilutions of reactants over much greater ranges can detect the region within which the OP zone occurs. With much finer dilutions in that region the OP zone can then be accurately located. This is a time-consuming process, however, and does not lend itself readily to a clinical situation. Nonetheless, it has been used extensively in research and has yielded much information concerning the nature of antigens and antibodies and details of their interactions.

Performance of a precipitation test according to the methodology just described is the **Dean and Webb** or **alpha (α) procedure.** It is not the only way that a precipitation test can be performed. In the **Ramon** or **beta (β) procedure,** the antibody is diluted and added to constant amounts of anti-

Table 5.1 Hypothetical Results of an Idealized Precipitation Test in Which Antigen Is Serially Diluted (Antigen Is Egg Albumin; Antibody Is Undiluted Rabbit Anti-Egg Albumin)

	Dilutions of Egg Albumin (Antigen)					Controls*	
	1:500	1:1,000	1:2,000	1:4,000	1:8,000	Antigen	Antibody
Antigen (ml)	0.5	0.5	0.5	0.5	0.5	0.5 (1:500)	0.5 S
Antibody (ml)	0.5	0.5	0.5	0.5	0.5	0.5 S	0.5
Precipitation	±	+2	+4	+1	0	0	0
Supernate contains uncombined							
Antigen	Yes	Yes	No	No	No	Yes	No
Antibody	No	No	No	Yes	Yes	No	Yes

* S = saline.

gen (Table 5.2). Precipitation occurs in a much narrower range of reactant dilutions in the Ramon than in the Dean and Webb procedure. In contrast to the Dean and Webb procedure, the prozone seen in the Ramon titration is due to antibody excess, and the postzone is due to antigen excess. Much less antibody is needed for a Ramon test than for a Dean and Webb test. The smallest amount of antibody that will cause precipitation with a given amount of antigen is detected by the Ramon method. The Dean and Webb method detects the smallest amount of antigen that can give a visible reaction with a given amount of antibody. The precipitin titer of an antiserum determined by these two methods seldom agrees. In a Dean and Webb test, the antigen can produce precipitates over a broader range of dilutions because it is multivalent. On the other hand, precipitation occurs within a much narrower spread of dilutions in the Ramon procedure because the major precipitating antibody is bivalent and therefore more easily diluted beyond its functional concentration. The Dean and Webb procedure is more extensively used because different antisera will precipitate over a rela-

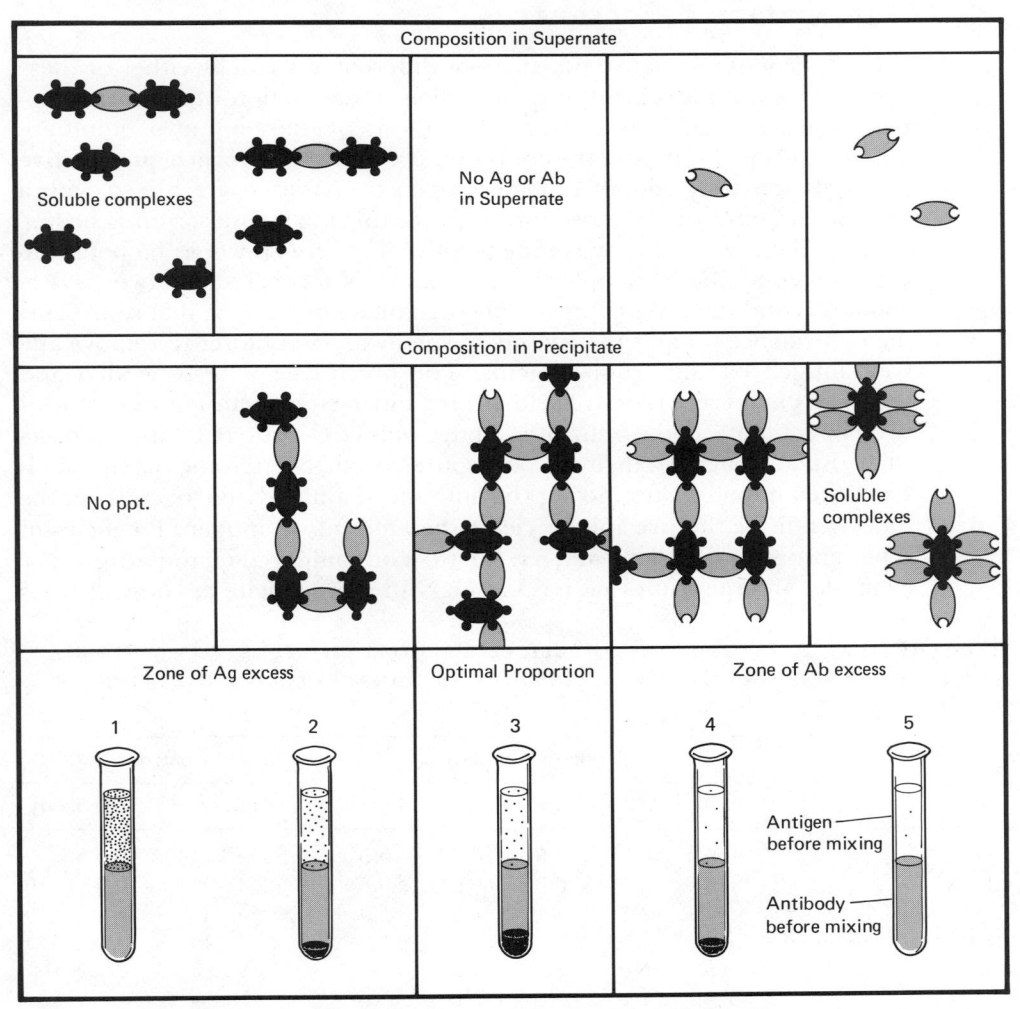

FIGURE 5.1. Major zones of a fluid precipitation test using a constant amount of antibody and diminishing amounts of antigen.

Serology and Immunology

tively wide range of antigen dilutions and thereby allow comparison of potencies under essentially identical conditions.

The optimal ratio is a constant characteristic for any given antigen-antiserum system. For example, if a one-tenth dilution of an anti-OA preparation precipitates most rapidy with 1 : 400 egg albumin, the optimal ratio of the antigen preparation to the antiserum is $(1/10) \div (1/400) = 40 : 1$. If this same antiserum is diluted one fifth, it would be expected to give maximal precipitation with an antigen dilution that makes the OP = 40 : 1; i.e., the antigen dilution should be $1/200$. It should be emphasized that the OP is constant for a given combination of antigen preparation and a particular antiserum. It will vary from one antigen preparation to another and from one antiserum to another even for the same antigen (e.g., OA) and the same antibody "specificity" (e.g., anti-OA). For reasons explained previously, the OP values derived from Dean and Webb (constant antiserum) and from Ramon (constant antigen) methods seldom agree.

QUANTITATIVE PROCEDURE

Comparisons of relative potencies of different antisera by either of these procedures do not constitute quantitation. Quantitation of precipitin potency must ultimately be expressed in terms of the amount of immunoglobulin in a precipitate at the equivalence point. To perform a **quantitative precipitation test,** dilutions of an antigen preparation are mixed with a constant amount of an antiserum (α procedure). The antiserum is heated prior to the test to destroy complement that otherwise would be bound to the antigen-antibody complex. The mixture is incubated for two days at about 4°C and then centrifuged. The precipitate in the tube that represents the equivalence point is thoroughly washed with cold buffer to remove any free antigen or antiserum proteins. The precipitate is resuspended and analyzed chemically (micro-Kjeldahl) for nitrogen content (an indicator of protein content). If the antigen is a pure polysaccharide (e.g., pneumococcal capsular material), then the only source of nitrogen in the precipitate is from the antibody. Subtracting the amount of antibody nitrogen from the total weight of the precipitate yields the amount of antigen. Potencies of other antisera to the same antigen can then be compared quantitatively. For example, an antiserum that has 0.8 mgN in a precipitate at equivalence is

Table 5.2 Hypothetical Results of an Idealized Precipitation Test in which Antibody Is Serially Diluted. Antigen Is Constant at a Dilution of 1:1,000

	Dilution of Antibody					Controls*	
	1:10	1:20	1:40	1:80	1:160	Antigen	Antibody
Antigen (ml)	0.5	0.5	0.5	0.5	0.5	0.5 (1:1,000)	0.5 S
Antibody (ml)	0.5	0.5	0.5	0.5	0.5	0.5 S	0.5 (1:10)
Precipitation	0	+1	+4	0	0	0	0
Supernate contains uncombined							
Antigen	No	No	Yes	Yes	Yes	Yes	No
Antibody	Yes	Yes	No	No	No	No	Yes

* S = saline.

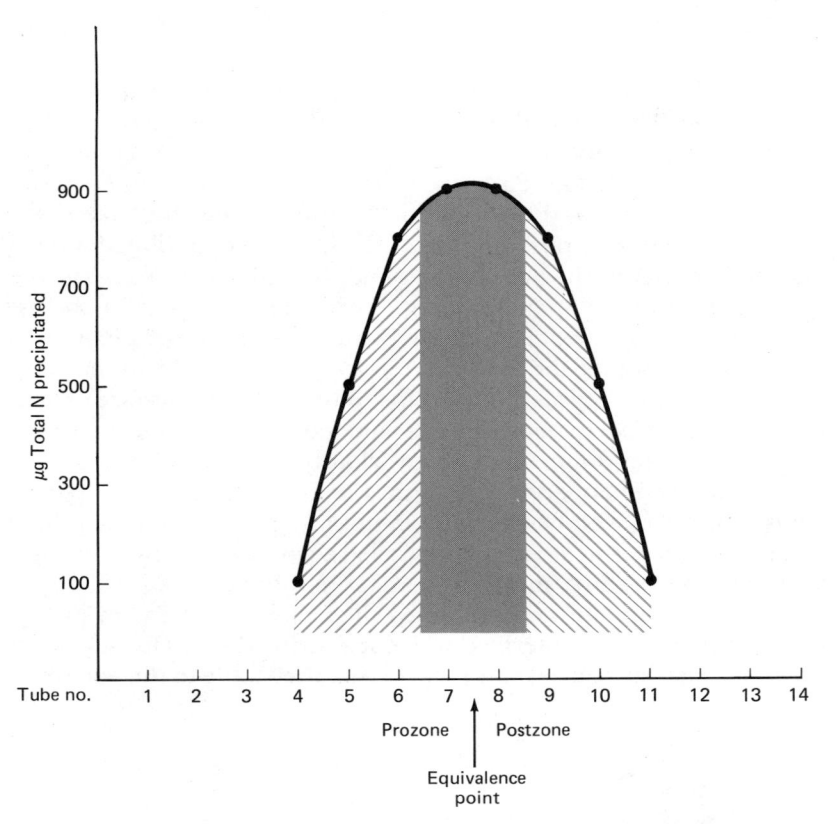

FIGURE 5.2. Idealized quantitative precipitation curve for an R-type antiserum. The shaded area represents the zone of flocculation for an H-type antiserum.

twice as potent as one with 0.4 mgN. If a purified protein antigen is used, the amount of antigen nitrogen added to the tube would need to be determined. Subtracting this amount from the total weight of the precipitate gives the amount of antibody nitrogen. Figure 5.2 is a diagram of an idealized quantitative precipitation curve representative of the antisera from most species. Since the rabbit is a widely used source of precipitating antisera, the curve is typical of **R** (rabbit) **type** antisera. Antiserum from the horse may behave much differently; it usually precipitates in a narrow zone around the equivalence point and precipitation is completely inhibited outside this zone. An explanation for **H** (horse) **type** (or **flocculating***) antisera is elusive. Not all horse antisera display the flocculating property. The antitoxins against diphtheria and tetanus toxins that are sometimes used for passive immunity of humans are commonly produced by hyperimmunization of horses with toxoids. Precipitation tests can be used to determine the precipitating potency of these horse antitoxins (see Chapter 7). A serological titer indicates only the ability of the antibody to combine with its antigen; it does not necessarily indicate its potential for neutralizing toxins (biological potency).

* The term "flocculation" has also been loosely used for any type of serological precipitation as well as for certain agglutinations (especially those involving the colloidal particles of syphilis tests and the flagellar antigens of *Salmonella* species).

Serology and Immunology

RING TEST

A simple qualitative precipitation test that avoids the zoning phenomenon is the **ring** or **interfacial test.** It is usually performed in small-diameter glass tubing (approximately 5 mm inside diameter) in order to conserve antiserum. A long, slender Pasteur pipet is used to deposit about 10 mm of undiluted antiserum on the bottom of the tube, care being taken to avoid depositing any on the upper portion of the tube. The undiluted antibody is usually the heavier of the two reagents and therefore must form the bottom layer to prevent gravitational mixing. Then the antigen solution (usually diluted 1 : 100 or greater) is delivered with a clean Pasteur pipet so that it forms a layer on top of the antiserum. Care must be taken so that virtually no mixing of antigen or antibody occurs initially at the interface. The tubes are incubated at room temperature and observed at about five-minute intervals for the development of a hazy, cloudy, or milky layer at or near the interface. Someone apparently thought this precipitate looked like a ring, but it is actually a layer, best seen by shining a light through the side of the tube and observing it against a black background. Precipitation is commonly seen within thirty minutes. If not, the tubes can be incubated overnight in the refrigerator and examined the next day. A band of precipitate initially formed at the interface will not remain there. During overnight incubation, such large precipitates form that they settle to the bottom of the

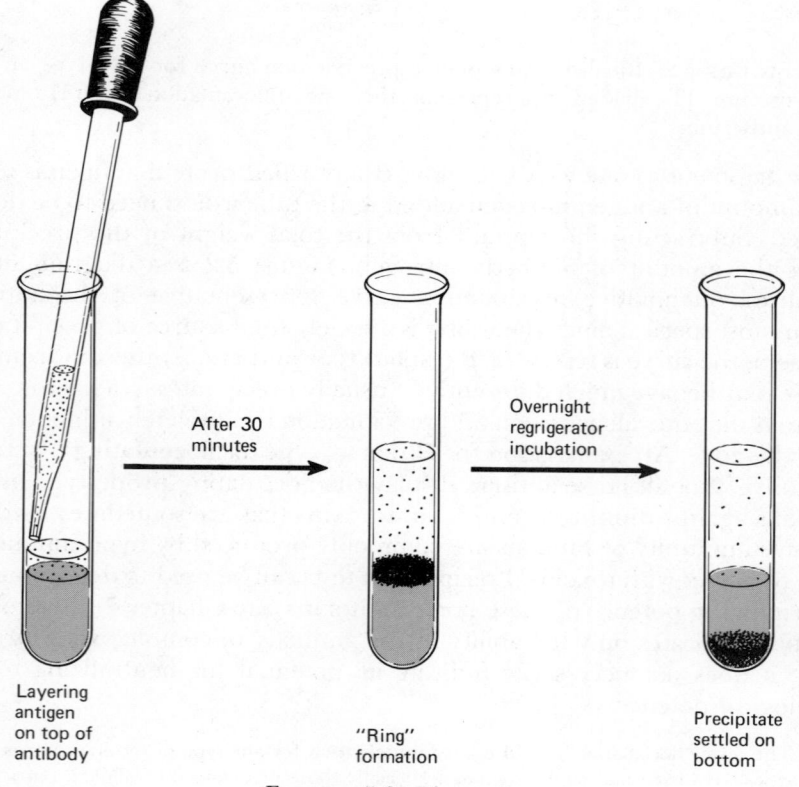

FIGURE 5.3. Ring test.

tube (Figure 5.3). Measurement of the height of such precipitates is a crude way of assaying the results.

The reason why no zoning occurs is because both reactants diffuse into one another until sufficiently diluted to allow precipitation to occur. In other words, the reactants eventually reach their own optimum proportions. The ring test can be used for relative titration of antisera by making serial dilutions of antigen (e.g., $1/100$, $1/1{,}000$, $1/10{,}000$, $1/100{,}000$). The titer of an undiluted antiserum is expressed as the reciprocal of the greatest dilution of antigen giving a detectable precipitate. It is not uncommon for rabbits injected with foreign proteins (e.g., horse serum) to yield antisera with titers of $1/100{,}000$ or more. The sensitivities of precipitation tests are compared with those of other serological and immunological tests in Table 5.3.

PRACTICAL APPLICATIONS OF FLUID PRECIPITIN TESTS

Ascoli developed the ring test in 1902 to detect the thermostable capsular antigens of anthrax bacilli in extracts from tissues or hides of animals suspected to be infected. Boiling does not destroy the antigenicity of these antigens. The tissue is finely divided in a Waring blendor, extracted with boiling water, and filtered. This fluid is then used as the antigen in a "thermoprecipitin" (heat-extracted antigen) ring test with high-titer antianthrax serum. The same principle can be applied to animals suspected to have died of the plague.

Table 5.3 SENSITIVITIES OF SOME SEROLOGICAL AND IMMUNOLOGICAL TESTS

Test	Lower Limit of Antibody Nitrogen Detectable (μg/ml)
Fluid precipitation	
Interfacial (ring) test	20–30
Quantitative, colorimetric	3–10
Quantitative, nephelometric	0.05–3
Gel precipitation	
Ouchterlony	3–15
Oudin	12–110
RID	3–10
IEP	50–200
Agglutination	
Bacterial	0.01
Hemagglutination	
Direct	0.5–1
Passive (indirect)	0.001–0.003
"Flocculation" test (VDRL)	0.2–0.5
Passive cutaneous anaphylaxis in guinea pigs	0.01–0.03*
Prausnitz-Küstner skin test in man	0.01*
Toxin neutralization	0.003–0.01
Complement-mediated hemolysis	0.001–0.03
Radioimmunoassay	0.0001–0.001
Virus neutralization	0.00001–0.0001
Bactericidal test	0.00001–0.0001

* = μg N total

Another clinical use of the fluid-phase precipitation technique is in the serological typing of bacteria. R. C. Lancefield originally used the ring test to serologically classify various strains of streptococci into what came to be known as "Lancefield groups." Currently, eleven groups of hemolytic streptococci are recognized. Most of the streptococci involved in human disease are in group A. Group-specific polysaccharides can be extracted from a pure culture of a *Streptococcus* by autoclaving, by dilute hydrochloric acid, by formamide, or by an enzyme (called the "Maxted antigen") from *Streptomyces albus*. The precipitinogen extract (called "Rantz antigen") is layered onto group-specific antisera for a ring test.

The high sensitivity of a precipitation test lends itself to the detection of even very small amounts of contaminating substances in otherwise pure preparations. The name "coctoantisera" (cocto = heat modified) is given to the high-titered precipitins used to detect adulterated foods (e.g., horsemeat contaminants in so-called "pure beef" hamburgers, the presence of rye or other grains in "pure wheat flour"). These antisera are commonly produced by injecting rabbits with heated (70°C for one hour) sera of the animals in question or with heated tissue extracts.

Another forensic application of the precipitin test is the identification of species origin for a blood stain. For example, a blood-stained piece of cloth may be an important piece of evidence in a murder trial only if it can be proved that the blood is of human origin. The blood stain is extracted from the cloth by soaking it in saline. As with all precipitation reactions, the reagents should be transparent. If not transparent, they must first be clarified by filtration or centrifugation prior to use in precipitation tests. A ring test, employing high-potency antiserum, can detect whether or not the proteins extracted from a blood stain are of human origin. To have validity in court, the results of the test must be substantiated by suitable controls run simultaneously with the unknown stain: (1) The antiserum used must be shown to be reactive with bloods of other humans; (2) the antiserum must not be reactive with bloods of other vertebrate species likely to be present at the scene of the crime (e.g., dogs, cats, meats of domesticated animals); (3) the antiserum must not precipitate with the saline used to extract the stain; (4) if the source of the antiserum is from hyperimmunized rabbits, normal rabbit serum must not react with the antigen extract; (5) an extract from an unstained portion of the cloth must not react with the antiserum; (6) an extract from an unstained portion of the cloth should not inhibit reactivity of the antiserum with homologous blood.

One of the most widely used fluid-phase precipitation tests performed in the clinical laboratory is for detecting a substance called CRP. Serum from patients with pneumococcal pneumonia possesses a protein that reacts with the C-polysaccharide of the pneumococcus. This substance, called **C-reactive protein** (CRP), is not an antibody. It behaves as a precipitinogen when mixed with anti-CRP. This antibody is usually obtained from rabbits injected with purified CRP. During many necrotic, inflammatory, or infectious diseases, CRP is manufactured by the liver and released into the plasma. CRP binds to bacterial cell wall phosphorylcholine residues and thereby activates complement-mediated opsonization and cytolysis of the foreign cells. CRP is consistently present in sera of patients with acute myocardial infarction (MI, necrosis of heart muscle due to blockage of the local blood supply by a clot) and active rheumatic fever. It is not present in serum from healthy people, and it disappears rapidly from the blood after recovery from disease. The presence of CRP in a patient with MI or rheumatic fever is considered to be the most sensitive indicator of necrosis and inflammation. The level of CRP in the serum indicates the intensity of the disease and the response of the patient to treatment. The test is not diagnostic, however, because CRP may also be produced in patients with malignancies, pregnancies, active tuberculosis, viral infections, pneumococcal pneumonia, bronchial asthma, vascular occlusions, and certain other bacterial infections.

Lipids tend to make serum cloudy. Therefore, the patient should be fasted for at least four hours prior to drawing the specimen for the precipitation test or any other test using serum. The CRP precipitation test can be performed in small-diameter capillary tubes. A small amount of clear anti-CRP is drawn into the tube, the outside of the tube is wiped clean, and an equivalent amount of patient's serum is drawn in (Figure 5.4). Care must be taken to avoid an air bubble between the two fluids. The contents are mixed well and the tube is allowed to stand in a plasticine block for two

Step 1: Draw up the C-reactive protein antiserum into the 0.8 mm I.D. capillary tube. Using the fingertip for control, fill about one-third of the tube. Wipe the outside of the tube clean.

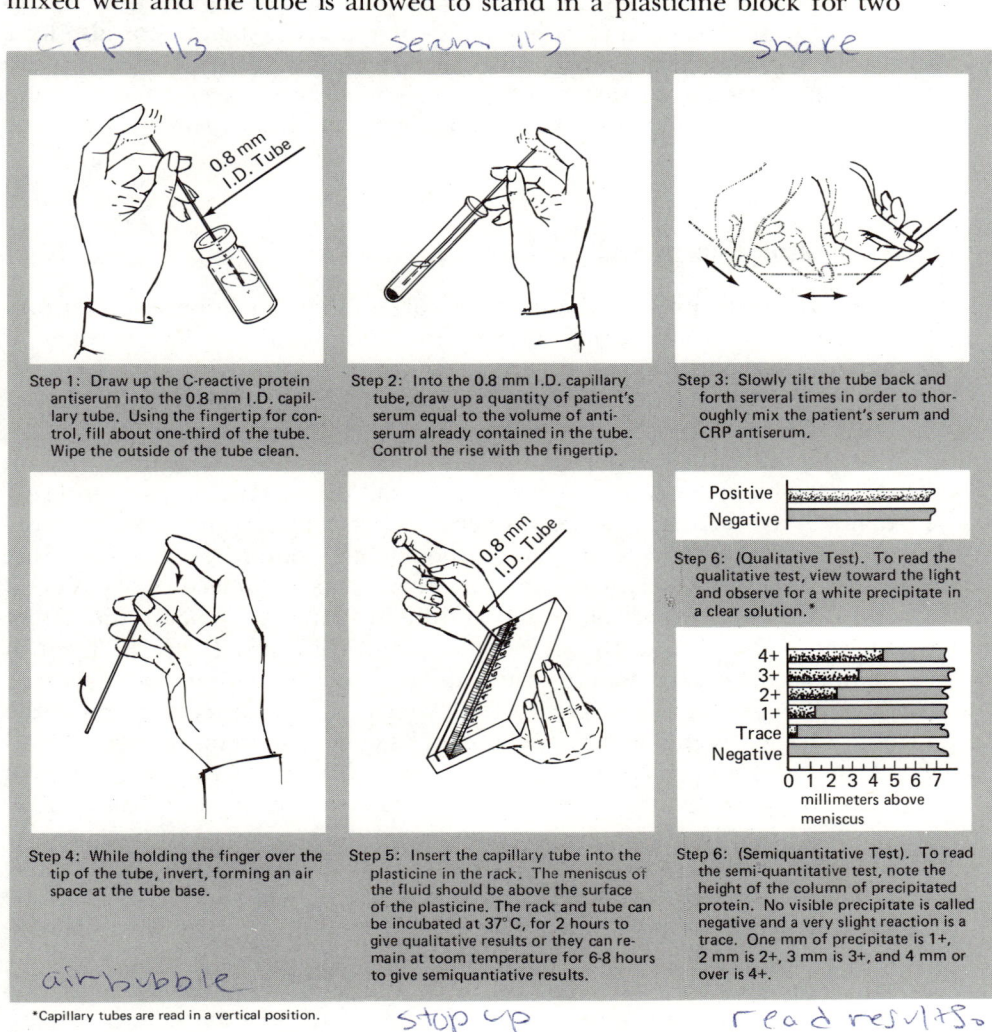

Step 2: Into the 0.8 mm I.D. capillary tube, draw up a quantity of patient's serum equal to the volume of antiserum already contained in the tube. Control the rise with the fingertip.

Step 3: Slowly tilt the tube back and forth serveral times in order to thoroughly mix the patient's serum and CRP antiserum.

Step 6: (Qualitative Test). To read the qualitative test, view toward the light and observe for a white precipitate in a clear solution.*

Step 4: While holding the finger over the tip of the tube, invert, forming an air space at the tube base.

Step 5: Insert the capillary tube into the plasticine in the rack. The meniscus of the fluid should be above the surface of the plasticine. The rack and tube can be incubated at 37°C. for 2 hours to give qualitative results or they can remain at room temperature for 6-8 hours to give semiquantiative results.

Step 6: (Semiquantitative Test). To read the semi-quantitative test, note the height of the column of precipitated protein. No visible precipitate is called negative and a very slight reaction is a trace. One mm of precipitate is 1+, 2 mm is 2+, 3 mm is 3+, and 4 mm or over is 4+.

*Capillary tubes are read in a vertical position.

FIGURE 5.4. Capillary tube precipitation test for C-reactive protein.

hours at 37°C (or six to eight hours at room temperature). The two-hour result is read as either positive (precipitation) or negative (no precipitation). A "semiquantitative" result is obtained from the six-to-eight-hour test. The height of the precipitate is measured and scored as shown in Figure 5.5. A +4 reaction is indicative of a very severe inflammatory process. The capillary tubes should be sterilized with dry heat prior to use because bacterial growth during the six-to-eight-hour incubation period could be a serious source of error in reading the test. A known positive serum (containing CRP) should be run as a control simultaneously with the patient's serum.

Fluid precipitation tests have also been widely used for nonclinical research purposes. Landsteiner used precipitation tests in his studies of the nature of antigenic determinant sites and haptens. Precipitation tests can be used to determine the hosts on which blood-sucking insects have fed. The degree of cross-reactivity of an antiserum with antigens from species in other taxonomic orders or classes can yield estimates of "serological distances" that reflect approximate degrees of genetic relationship. Phylogenies constructed from serological data agree very well with "evolutionary trees" based on morphological criteria. Precipitation tests also have a role in checking the purity of pharmaceutical proteins. For example, a protein fraction may appear to be homogeneous by ultracentrifugation and electrophoresis and yet prove to be antigenically heterogeneous by a precipitation test.

Precipitation in Gel Medium

There are two major disadvantages of fluid precipitation tests: (1) prozoning or postzoning phenomena and (2) ambiguity in the number of antigen-antibody systems in heterogeneous mixtures. Allowing precipitating antigens and antibodies to react in semisolid media (gels) has neither of these disadvantages. Soluble antigen and/or antibody can diffuse through the pores of the gel until their concentrations reach the optimum ratio and there form a stable immunoprecipitate. In other words, the reactants eventually arrive at their own equivalence concentrations and thereby avoid prozones or postzones of soluble (nonvisible) complexes that otherwise might be falsely interpreted as a negative reaction. Molecules of different sizes tend to diffuse through gels at different rates. In general, the higher the molecular weight, the slower the rate of diffusion. If two antigens of identical molecular weight (but different concentrations) are moving through a gel, they are likely to form precipitates in different parts of the gel with their homologous antibodies. The combination of different molecular weights and concentrations of reactants makes it highly probable that each antigen-antibody system will form its own precipitation band. However, since it is possible for two antigen-antibody systems to have similar diffusion rates and concentrations that allow them to precipitate in the same region of the gel, the number of precipitation bands observed must be interpreted as the minimal number of antigen-antibody systems in the mixture.

Gel precipitation tests are said to be **single-diffusion** tests if only one reactant (usually antigen) is moving, and **double-diffusion** tests if both antigen and antibody are moving through the medium. Reactions in tubes

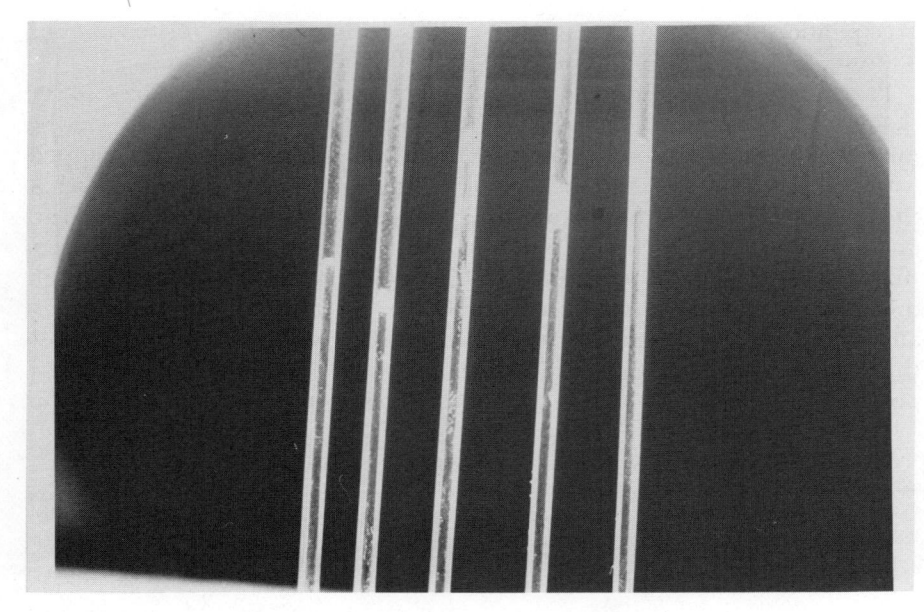

FIGURE 5.5. Photograph of C-reactive protein capillary tube tests. Reactions range from negative on the left to 4+ on the right. [*Courtesy of Elliot Scientific Corp., New York City.*]

essentially have only one effective dimension (single dimension) for antigen and antibody migration, *viz.*, up and down. If circular holes (wells) are cut in a gel on a flat surface (e.g., in a Petri dish), antigen or antibody diffuses from the wells radially (double dimension). Therefore, there are four combinations of reactions in gels by these two criteria: (1) single diffusion–single dimension, (2) single diffusion–double dimension, (3) double diffusion–single dimension, and (4) double diffusion–double dimension. In addition to immunodiffusion tests, one or both reactants may be caused to migrate through the gel by electrophoresis. An immunoelectrophoretic test exploits both the electrophoretic and the serological properties of antigens and thereby can yield high resolving power in identifying the number of antigen-antibody systems in a mixture.

Each of the four immunodiffusion techniques has an immunoelectrophoretic counterpart. All eight of these methods are summarized in Table 5.4. Some of these tests are named after those who first developed them or made significant improvements on the original techniques. Some of the tests are known by more than one name. Many types of gelling substances have been used as the support medium (e.g., agar, agarose, polyacrylamide, cellulose acetate, gelatin, starch, etc.) with varying degrees of success. The most widely used medium is agarose (approximately 0.7 percent); all other substances have one or more disadvantages that seriously limit their use.

IMMUNODIFFUSION TESTS

Single Diffusion–Single Dimension. Precipitation as a serological phenomenon was discovered by Kraus in 1897. It seems incredible that it took immunologists almost fifty years to discover the advantages of gel

Serology and Immunology

precipitation over fluid precipitation. The earliest of the gel techniques (Oudin, 1946) was a single diffusion–single dimension method.

Protein solutions seldom coagulate (denature) at temperatures lower than 65°C. Fortunately, agarose congeals at about 45°C. Antibody can be mixed with liquid agarose at about 60°C and when cooled becomes trapped within the gel matrix. Antibody mixed with liquid agarose is deposited at the bottom of a tube. After allowing the mixture to gel, it is overlaid with an antigen dilution. The concentration of the antigen must always be greater than the equivalence concentration. The mobile antigen diffuses through the gel containing immobilized antibody, forming insoluble antigen-antibody complexes until the size of the complex becomes too large to pass through the pores of the gel. A band (disc) of precipitate forms at that position, but does not stay there. Soon the concentration of antigen on top

Table 5.4 Techniques of Immunological Precipitation in Gels

Number of reactants moving	1	1	2	2
Number of effective dimensions	1	2	1	2
Diffusion	Oudin (1946)*	Radial immuno-diffusion (RID)† Feinberg (1957) Mancini (1963)	Oakley and Fulthrope (1953)*	Ouchterlony and Elek (1948)*
Electrophoresis	Rocket immuno-electrophoresis† Laurell technique Single electro-immunodiffusion (single EID)	Crossed immuno-electrophoresis* Double-crossed immunoelectro-phoresis Two-dimensional immunoelectro-phoresis Ressler (1960) Laurell (1965)	Double electro-immunodiffusion (double EID)* Crossed antigen-antibody electro-phoresis Counter electro-phoresis Crossing over electro-phoresis Counter immunoelec-trophoresis (CIE) Counter current immunoelectro-phoresis Immuno-osmo-phoresis (IOP) Electrosyneresis Immunoelectro-osmophoresis (IEOP) Counter migration electrophoresis	Immuno-electrophoresis (IEP) (IE)* Grabar and Williams (1953)

* = qualitative results.
† = quantitative results.

of the band causes the precipitate to solubilize because of antigen excess. But at the same time, antigen at the bottom of the band is forming new precipitate. The band thus migrates down the gel with time. Several factors influence the rate of this migration including the concentrations of antigen and antibody, the temperature, and the pore size of the gel. At its equivalence concentration, the antigen stops moving and a stabilized band of precipitate forms. R-type antisera tend to form precipitate bands with "fuzzy" edges because smaller amounts of precipitate exist on either side of equivalence. H-type antisera typically form bands with clean margins because "flocculation" is complete within the equivalence zone and it is completely inhibited outside that zone (Figure 5.6). If two bands of precipitate are seen, it is inferred that at least two antigens (e.g., specificities A and B) are present, but the specificity of each band would be unknown. It might be possible, for example with purified antigen A, to absorb the antiserum, repeat the test, and observe which band is missing. The remaining band in this case would belong to antigen B. Alternatively purified antigen A could be added to the test, causing band A to migrate further down the gel column and leaving band B at its equivalence position (Figure 5.7).

The Oudin technique can also be adapted for rough estimation of antigen concentration by comparing the position of a precipitate band of an unknown specimen with one formed by a reference sample (of known concentration) in a replicate tube. For example, if a reference band of CRP stabilized at 10 mm into the gel whereas an unknown sample in a separate tube stabilized at 7 mm, then the test specimen has approximately 70 percent of the CRP concentration of the reference. If the patient's specimen stabilizes more than 10 mm below the gel surface, the only valid conclusion is that the test specimen contains more CRP than the reference specimen.

Single Diffusion–Double Dimension. This technique is commonly called radial immunodiffusion (RID) or the Mancini test. It is a very popular method for quantitating a variety of proteins normally found in serum including immunoglobulin classes, components of the complement system, transferrin, alpha-1 antitrypsin, alpha-2 macroglobulin, and lysozyme.

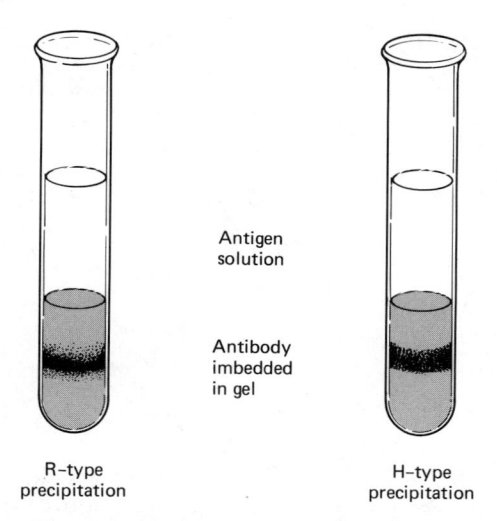

FIGURE 5.6. Single diffusion–single dimension gel precipitation tests with R- and H-type antisera.

Serology and Immunology

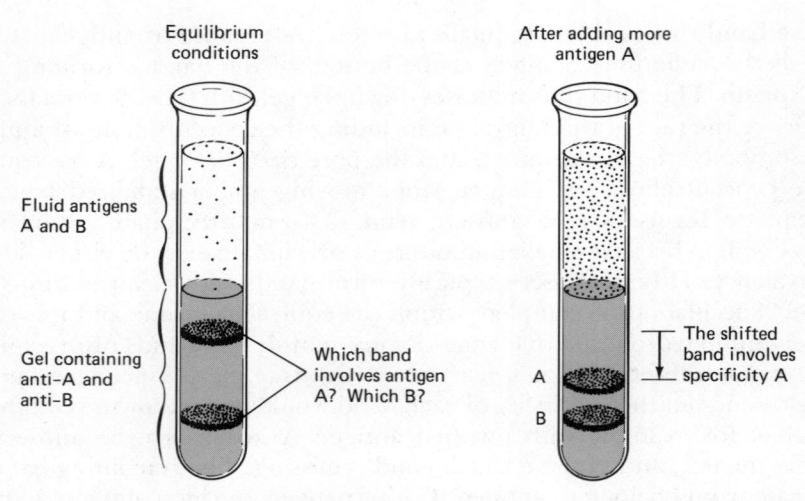

FIGURE 5.7. Method for determining the specificity of a precipitate band in an Oudin test.

Antibody is mixed with hot liquid agar, poured onto a flat surface such as a slide or Petri dish, and allowed to solidify. Circular wells are cut in the gel and loaded with a specific amount of antigen. Care must be taken to avoid damaging the gel. Any irregularity, such as a nick, in the gel surrounding the well will produce an abnormally shaped precipitation ring that yields invalid data. Wells must not be overfilled; antigen should not be allowed to touch the flat surface of the gel. Except when being loaded, RID plates must be kept covered to prevent evaporation of fluids and hardening of the gel. A ring of precipitate expands from the well as the antigen diffuses toward its equilibrium concentration. RID plates are commercially available in a size resembling a microscope slide. Antibody embedded in the gel is an expensive reagent and hence these tests must be performed as micro techniques if the cost is to be kept as low as possible. The surface area of the

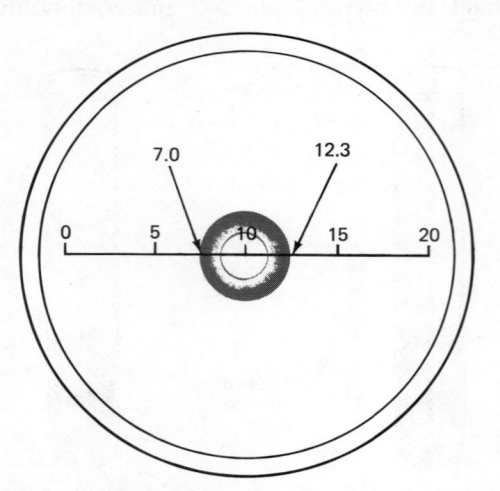

FIGURE 5.8. Reading the diameter of a RID precipitation ring by means of a magnifying glass containing a 20 mm scale with 0.1 mm divisions. More accurate readings are obtained in the central region of the scale. In this example, the ring diameter is 12.3 − 7.0 = 5.3 mm.

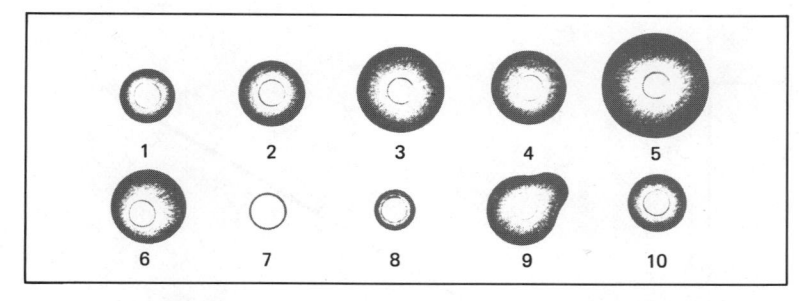

FIGURE 5.9. RID plate for quantitating IgG. Wells 1 to 3 contain IgG reference standards (1 = 725, 2 = 1,450, 3 = 2,900 mg percent). Unknowns in wells 4 and 10 fall within the range of the standards and therefore can be quantitated. Samples in wells 5 and 8 are too high and too low, respectively, to be measured against these standards (high-range and low-range standards sometimes are available). Sample 6 was spilled on the surface of the gel; the well for sample 9 was nicked (both invalid). Sample in well 7 was agammaglobulinemic.

precipitate disc is directly proportional to the original antigen concentration. The diameter of the disc is proportional to the logarithm of the concentration. Diameters of precipitation discs are commonly read with a magnifying glass containing a calibrated scale (Figure 5.8). Commercial RID kits provide antigen standards (i.e., antigens of known concentration), which should be run simultaneously with the unknowns. For example, Figure 5.9 shows an RID plate for quantitating the concentration of immunoglobulins of class IgG in patients' sera. Three of the ten wells in the gel plate are loaded with 2 lambda (microliters) of reference standards. The other wells can then be used to test the same amount of seven patients' sera. All of the standard reference sera should be represented on each RID plate in order to avoid between-plate variability. The three reference standards should plot as a straight line on semilog paper (antigen concentration on the log scale; diameter of the precipitation disc on the linear scale). If the three points do not fall on a straight line (they usually do not), the line of best fit should be drawn such that the distance from the line to each of the plot points is minimized (Figure 5.10). The concentration of antigen (in this case IgG) in a patient's serum can now be determined by drawing a vertical line from the measured diameter of the precipitation disc up to the standard line, and thence by a horizontal line that intersects the concentration scale. Manufacturers of RID kits choose their reference standards with such a wide range of values that it is unlikely to be exceeded by that of the patient. If, however, a patient's serum does plot outside the values of the standards, its concentration cannot be accurately calculated. It is not appropriate to simply extend the standard line beyond the levels measured. Extrapolation beyond the available data is always pseudoscientific. There are two methods for reading RID tests: (1) the kinetic (Fahey) method, and (2) the end-point (Mancini) method. Kinetic methods measure the disc while it is still expanding (e.g., after 18 hours or as specified by the manufacturer). The end-point method measures it when it essentially has stopped expanding. The obvious advantage of the kinetic method is that results can be obtained in a shorter period of time. The Mancini method uses a higher antibody concentration and is considered to produce more reliable results than the Fahey method.

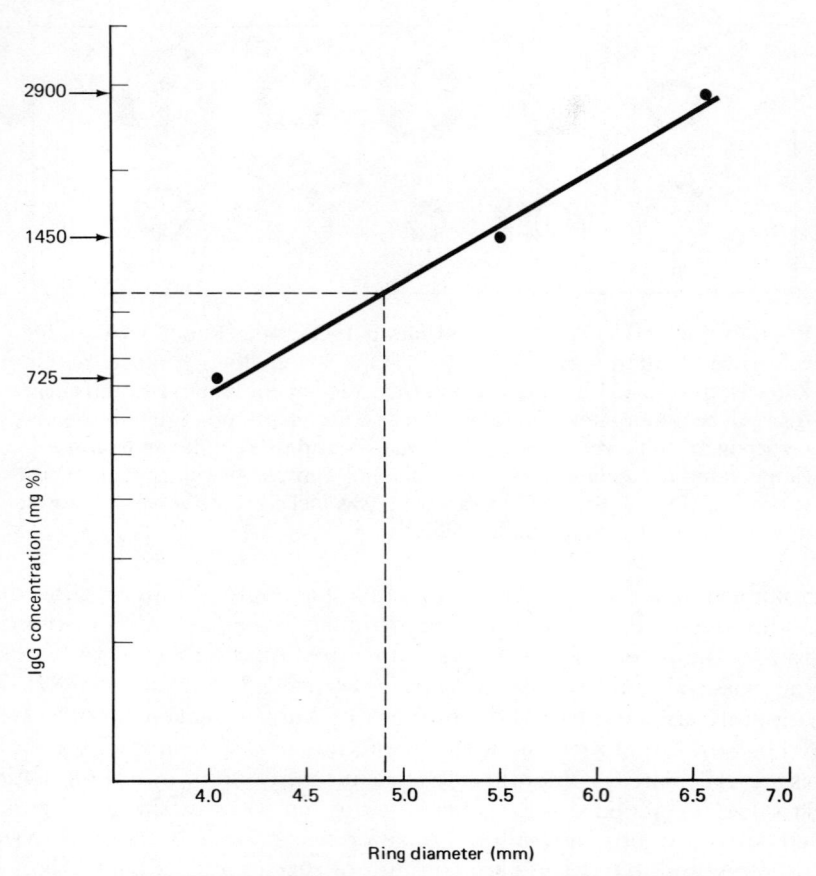

FIGURE 5.10. Standard curve plotted on two-cycle semilog paper for the reference standards shown in Figure 5.9. A patient's sample with a ring diameter of 4.9 mm is estimated to contain 1,100 mg percent IgG (dashed line).

The precipitate ring continues to grow to the edge of a Fahey plate because of its lower antibody content. It therefore cannot be used for an end-point determination. Mancini plates, however, can be used for a timed assay if desired. The end-point method usually produces an almost linear plot on semilog paper. The standard curve for the kinetic (timed-assay) method is constructed by connecting adjacent plot points with straight lines ("curvilinear").

RID can also be adapted to detect and quantitate antibody titers. For example, anti-influenza virus antibody can be placed in a well of a gel containing a uniformly distributed, immobilized influenca virus antigen. This test has the major disadvantage of the large amount of costly purified viral antigen required for incorporation in the gel. Commercial sources for an influenza RID test are not yet available.

Double Diffusion–Single Dimension. Oakley and Fulthrope (1953) modified the Oudin technique by overlayering antibody with neutral agar, allowing it to gel, and then overlayering the gel with antigen. Both antigen and antibody diffuse through the gel and form bands (layers) of precipitates near their zones of equivalence concentrations. In the Oudin technique, antigen must initially be in greater concentration than its equivalence point with reference to the uniform concentration of immobilized antibody in the gel. In the Oakley-Fulthrope technique both reactants can be diluted by diffusion so that the initial concentration of antigen does not need to be greater than the equivalence point with reference to the original concentration of antibody. Otherwise, there are no essential differences (advantages, disadvantages) in the application of these two methods.

Double Diffusion–Double Dimension. The chief advantage of the Ouchterlony technique over other immunodiffusion tests is its ability to detect serological identity (or lack thereof) in two or more antigen-antibody systems. A suitable pattern of wells is cut in an agarose plate (Petri dish or

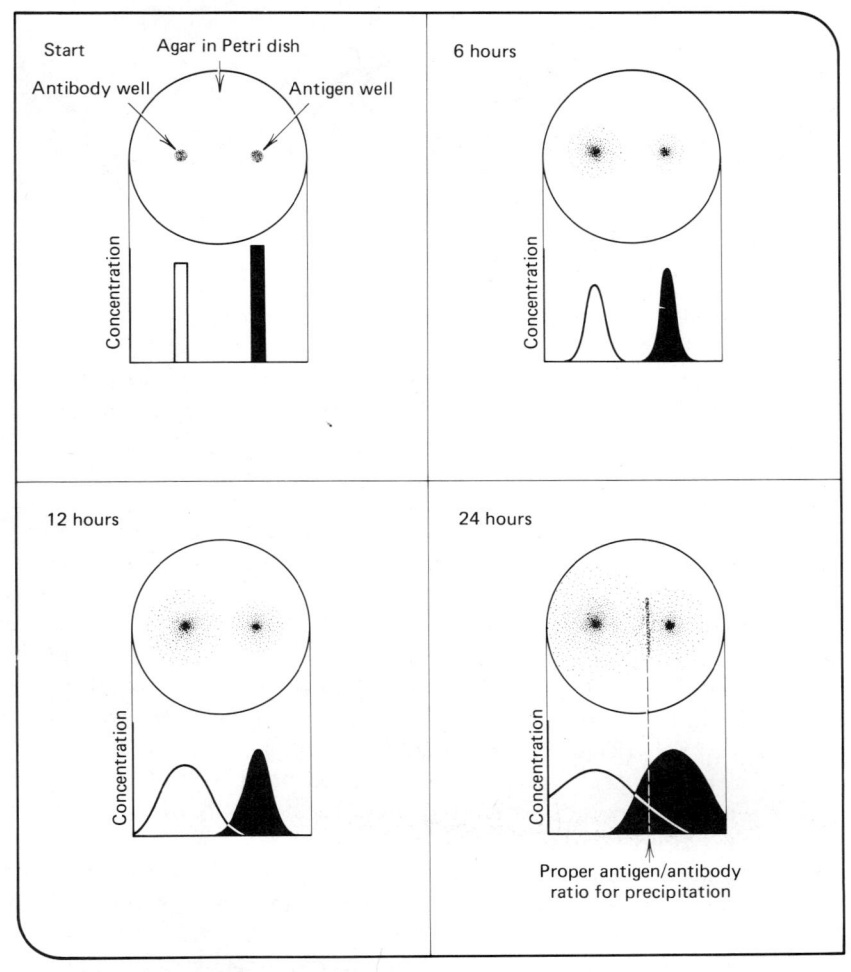

FIGURE 5.11. Ouchterlony gel "double diffusion in two dimensions" method of visualizing antigen-antibody reactions. An antigen solution is placed in one well cut in a layer of agar, and an antibody solution is placed in another well. These materials diffuse radially from their respective wells toward one another. When the optimal precipitation ratio of the counter-diffusing materials is reached, at a point in the gel volume lying between the two wells, a line of precipitation is formed in the gel. [*Courtesy of Millipore Biomedica, Bedford, Mass.*]

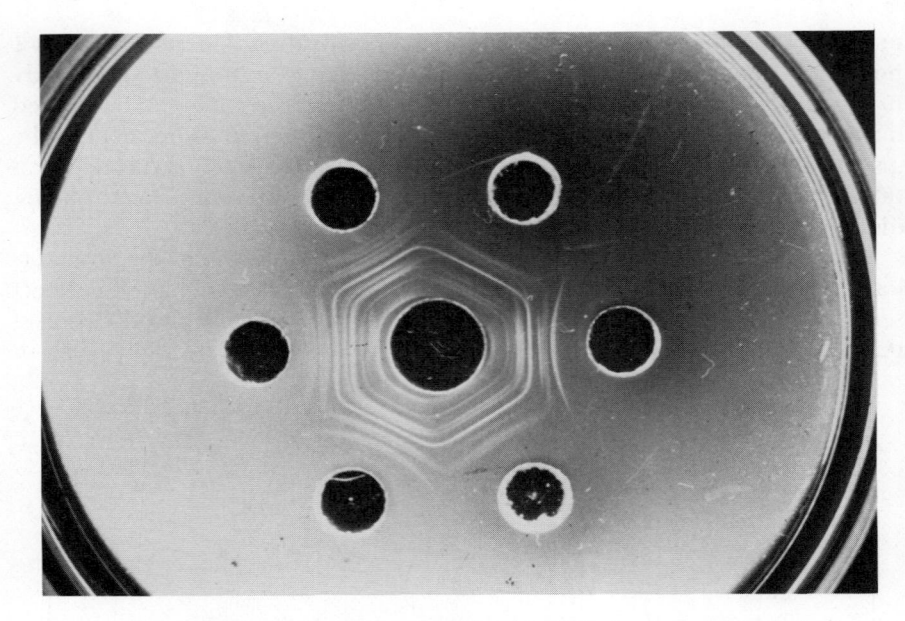

FIGURE 5.12. Ouchterlony plate agar double diffusion in two dimensions. Formation of opaque, visible bands between polyvalent antiserum in central well and homologous components of various antigens in peripheral wells. [*Courtesy of Elliot Scientific Corp., New York City.*]

microscope slide), loaded with the reactants, covered to prevent evaporation, and incubated (at room temperature or under refrigeration) until lines of precipitate have fully developed (Figures 5.11 and 5.12). Sodium azide or some other bacteriostatic agent may be added to the gel to inhibit bacterial growth on the plate.

There are four possible patterns of reaction with two antigen wells and one antibody well (Figure 5.13). A fused band of precipitate around the antibody well is a reaction of serological identity (Figure 5.13a). Antigens that are serologically identical need not be chemically identical molecules. For example, an antibody made against human IgG molecules could produce precipitation with whole IgG molecules, with Fab or Fc fragments, or with heavy or light chains. An anti-L chain antibody, however, could react with L chains, Fab fragments, or whole IgG molecules, but not with H chains or Fc fragments. If the lines of precipitation cross one another (Figure 5.13b), it indicates that the antigens are serologically distinct (reaction of nonidentity). Spur formation is seen in a reaction of single partial identity (Figure 5.13c). In this case, the line of precipitate involving antigen B is superimposed over the right side of the band of identity involving antigen A. The spur points in the direction of the well of lower antigenic complexity. Double spurring is seen in the reaction of double partial identity (Figure 5.13d). It is easily confused with a band of nonidentity. Fortunately double spurring reactions are rare.

If one side of a band of identity is closer to the antibody well than is the other side of the band (Figure 5.14), it could indicate that either the concentrations and/or the molecular weights of the two antigens are different. In general, the antigen of higher molecular weight will exhibit a slower diffusion rate. The precipitation line tends to be concave around the well with

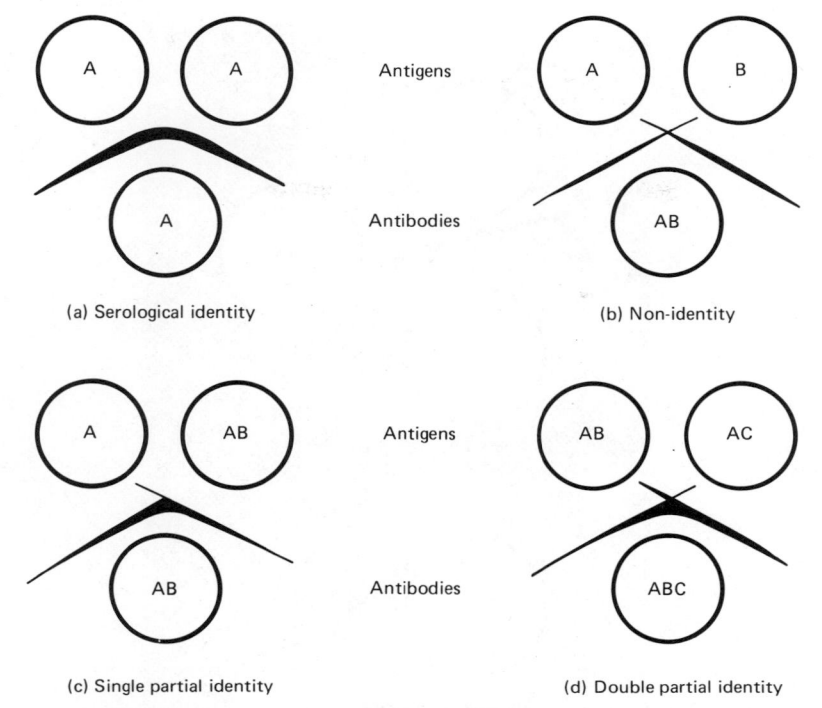

FIGURE 5.13. Ouchterlony immunodiffusion test patterns. Antigens are in the top wells; antibodies are in the lower well.

the slowest-diffusing molecules, If antigen and antibody are approximately of equal molecular weights, a straight line of precipitation is usually produced. Two bands of identity are shown in Figure 5.14. The antibody recognizes a common specificity (e.g., A) in both antigens 1 and 2. It also recognizes another common specificity (e.g., B) in both antigens 1 and 2. If the specificity and titer of the antibody for the two antigens are identical, then the cause of the crossed bands of identity is probably a reflection of differential antigen titers. The antigenic determinant in lower concentration of well 1 (indicated by the closest band to well 1) is in higher concentration in well 2 (indicated by the nearest band to the antibody well). The

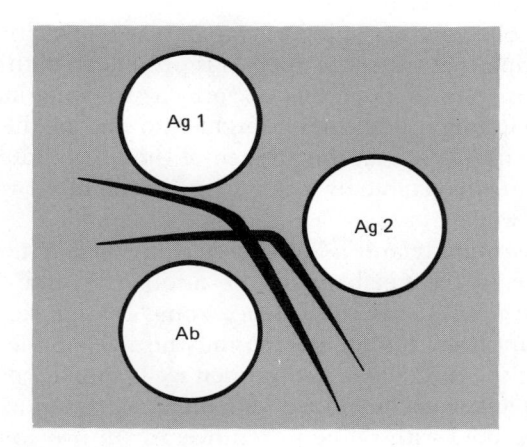

FIGURE 5.14. Asymmetrical reactions in two bands of identity.

Serology and Immunology

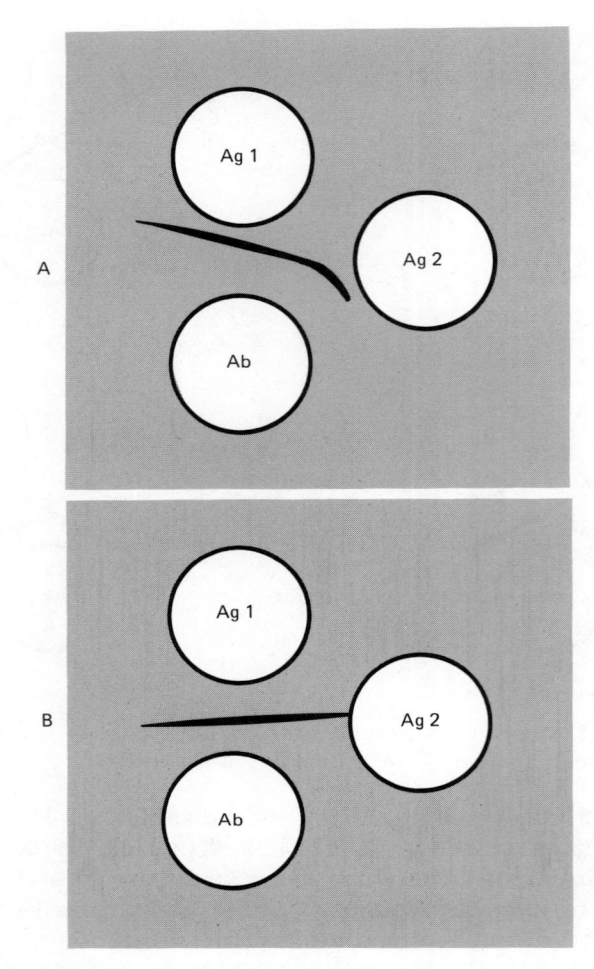

FIGURE 5.15. Ouchterlony patterns indicating that the corresponding antigen in the precipitate is present in well 2 (A) and absent in well 2 (B).

reverse is true of the other antigenic determinant, being of higher concentration in well 1 and lower in well 2.

On occasion, a blunting or slight curving of a precipitation band may be observed, indicating that the same antigen is present in both wells, but is of insufficient titer in one of the wells to form a precipitation line (Figure 5.15A). If a precipitation line goes straight into one of the antigen wells (Figure 5.15B), it indicates that the antigen of the precipitate is not present (at least in amounts detectable by this system) in the other well (a negative reaction for that well).

A high-titered antibody and a low-titered antigen may not produce any visible precipitate in the gel because the antibody could not diffuse far enough to dilute itself to its equivalence zone. In this case, preliminary dilution of the antibody and/or decreasing the size of the antibody well and/or increasing the distance to the antigen wells should correct the problem. Weak precipitates can be visually enhanced by staining. Prior to staining, the plate is soaked with saline to remove any unprecipitated proteins, covered with a saline-moistened piece of filter paper, and allowed to dry.

The filter paper cover prevents unequal drying on the plate or slide and thereby inhibits cracking of the agarose. The dried specimen should be carefully rinsed with water to remove any filter paper fibers before staining. After exposure to a protein stain such as acid fuchsin, the residual stain is removed (destained) with acetic acid–methanol solution and the plate is air-dried. In this form, the laboratory has a permanent record of the test. RID plates can also be preserved in this fashion, the only requirement being that the gel be thin and flat.

IMMUNOELECTROPHORESIS TESTS

Single Reactant Moving in One Dimension. The "rocket" technique of Laurell may be considered the electrophoretic counterpart of the Oudin test in that a single reagent (antigen) is migrating electrophoretically in essentially a single dimension through a gel containing immobilized antibody. It differs from the Oudin technique in that it is performed on plates rather than in tubes, it is a quantitative rather than a qualitative method, and it employs electrophoresis rather than diffusion to move the antigen. The pH of the agarose-antibody medium must be 8.6, the isoelectric point for immunoglobulins. Under these conditions, antibody molecules have no net electrical charge and therefore will not tend to migrate when current is passed through the gel. Filter paper wicks are applied to each end of the gel slab and the other ends are immersed in trays of buffer solution. Circular wells are cut at one end of the gel and loaded with a measured amount of antigen. Electrodes are applied to the buffer trays in such a way as to cause migration of the antigen toward the center of the gel (e.g., antigens that are electronegative at pH 8.6 would tend to migrate toward the anode during electrophoresis). The current is turned on and the antigen is pulled into the gel forming a cone- or rocket-shaped band of precipitate (Figure 5.16). Reference standards of known antigen concentration must be run simultaneously with the unknowns on the same gel plate (analogous to the standards of an RID plate). The length of the rocket is proportional to the log of the antigen concentration. The concentration of antigen in any sample can be determined from the line of reference standards plotted on semilog paper, just as in RID. Electrophoresis must continue until the rocket stabilizes at equilibrium, otherwise a rounded or blunted apex can be seen. If sharp rockets fail to develop within four hours, the antigen should be diluted and run again. There are two advantages of the rocket technique over the RID technique: (1) it requires less time, and (2) rocket lengths (being longer than the discs of RID) may be read with less error. Some disadvantages of rocket tests are the requirements for special electrophoresis equipment and relatively large slabs of gel requiring more antibody.

Single Reactant Moving in Two Dimensions. Ressler's method of two-dimensional immunoelectrophoresis is a research technique for fractionating serologically active components of a complex mixture of proteins such as whole serum. Antigen is first electrophoresed in neutral agarose to separate components by net charge. At the end of the run, the strip of agarose is transferred to a larger glass plate or plastic sheet. Liquid antibody-agarose (pH 8.6) is poured on the plate, making contact at one end with the neutral agarose segment containing the antigen (Figure 5.17). After the gel has

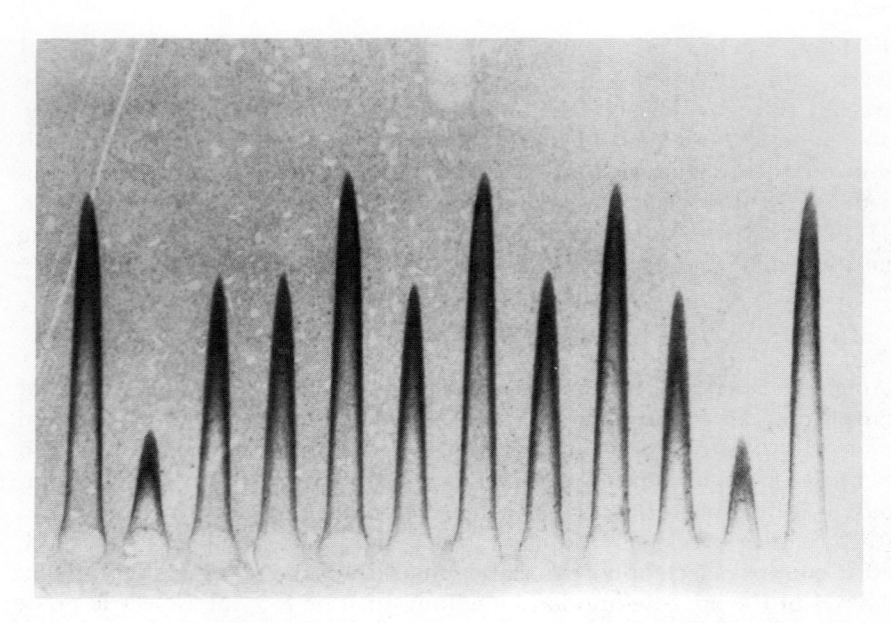

FIGURE 5.16. Electroimmunoassay method ("rocket" immunoelectrophoresis) for serum protein quantitation. The length of a peak is proportional to the concentration of the antigen applied. [*Courtesy of Millipore Biomedica, Bedford, Mass.*]

congealed, filter paper wicks are placed at each end, and current is applied in such a way that the antigenic components now migrate into the antibody gel (i.e., at right angles to the direction of the first electrophoresis). Electrophoresis may require up to twenty hours. Electrophoresing for long times or at high voltages generates heat, and heat tends to distort precipi-

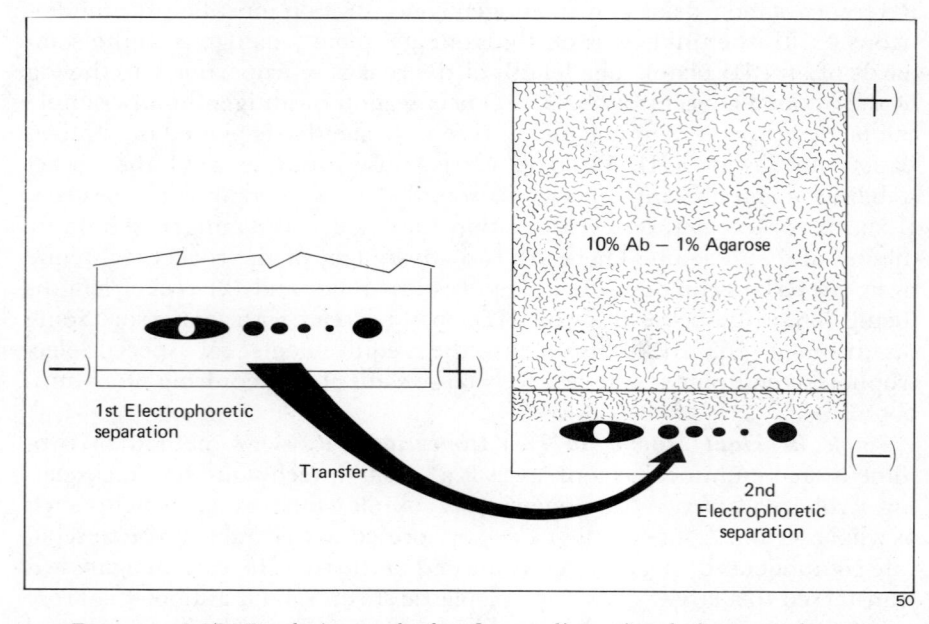

FIGURE 5.17. Ressler's method of two-dimensional immunoelectrophoresis. (See text.) [*Courtesy of Lab-Ed, Inc., Wichita, Kans.*]

tate bands. Consequently, anything that can be done to prevent overheating during any kind of electrophoresis is likely to give better results (e.g., periodic replacement of tray buffer with refrigerated stock, ice packs under and/or on top of the chamber, etc.). After turning off the current, the plate is removed from the electrophoresis chamber, excess proteins are removed by several saline washes, and the plate is covered with filter paper and dried in preparation for staining as previously described. The resulting immunoelectropherogram resembles a landscape of mountain-shaped precipitate peaks (Figure 5.18). The heights of the peaks cannot be compared with one another as an indicator of relative concentrations of the various antigenic components because variable titers of the corresponding antibodies are unknown. Quantification of antigenic concentrations is possible by simultaneously running reference standards, but this is not commonly done. At pH 8.6, gamma globulins are at their isoelectric point and should not migrate during the second run. Ressler's technique therefore cannot be used to analyze the heterogeneity of antigens in the gamma globulin fraction of serum unless these proteins are modified so as to make them electronegative at this pH. This is a time-consuming, costly, and difficult technique. It is not likely to be of much use in clinical laboratories. This technique has mainly been used in the research laboratory for identification of the heterogeneity of certain proteins such as alpha-1 antitrypsin.

Double Reactants Moving in One Dimension. Double electroimmunodiffusion (double EID) is also called counter immunoelectrophoresis (CIE) and several other names (Tables 5.4). Both antigen and antibody move essentially linearly toward one another through neutral agar under the influence of an electric current. Since both reactants are moving, EID usually requires a relatively short run time (thirty to sixty minutes). It is a qualitative technique widely used in the clinical laboratory for identifying the presence

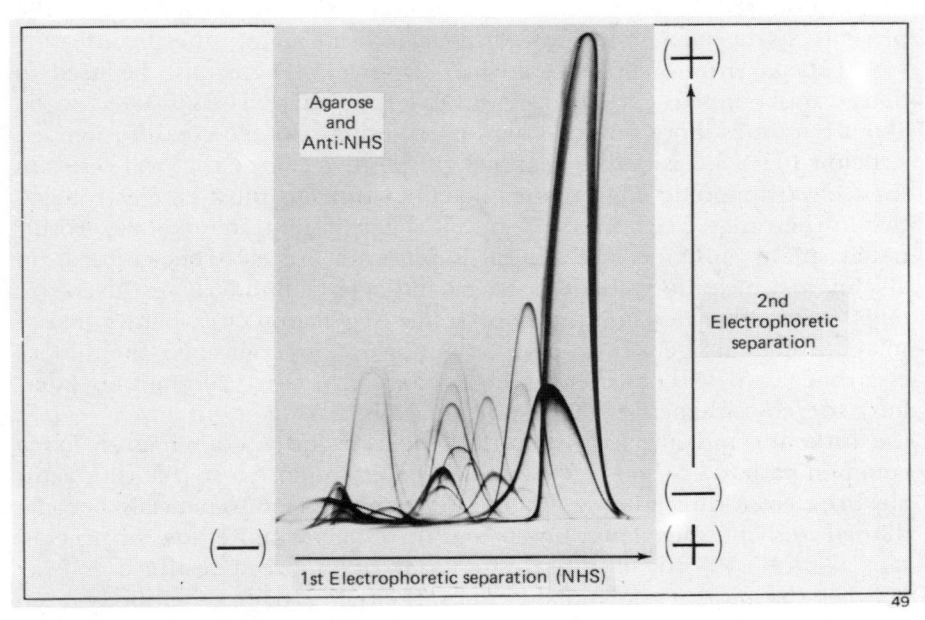

FIGURE 5.18. Photograph of immunoelectropherogram by Ressler's technique using whole human serum antigen and antinormal human serum (anti-NHS). [*Courtesy of Lab-Ed, Inc., Wichita, Kans.*]

Serology and Immunology

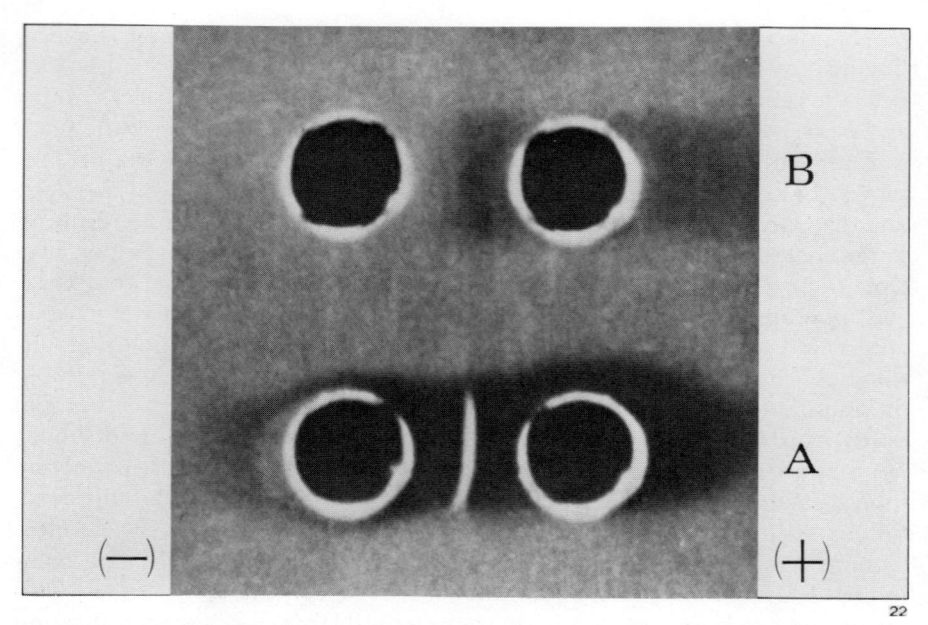

FIGURE 5.19. Photograph of CIE as used in screening donor bloods for HAA. Antigens in wells at left (cathodic end) are migrating toward the anode (+). Antibodies in wells at right are migrating toward the cathode (−). B = negative reaction; A = positive reaction. [*Courtesy of Lab-Ed, Inc., Wichita, Kans.*]

of an unusual protein in serum (e.g., Australia antigen and/or antibody, IgM screening of newborns, alpha fetoprotein, detection of circulating fibrinogen or fibrin split products in patients with disseminated intravascular coagulation [DIC], etc.). Since IgM is too large to normally pass the placenta, its detection in the newborn may indicate an intrauterine infection with rubella virus or cytomegalovirus. Double EID can also be used to detect antibodies to certain bacteria and fungi. CIE is considered to be about ten times more sensitive than Ouchterlony double gel diffusion.

Below pH 8.3, antibodies bear a slight positive charge that will result in their electrophoretic migration cathodally. Antigens must be electronegative in the range pH 8.2 to 8.3 so that they will migrate anodally. Fortunately, many substances of clinical importance are electronegative at an alkaline pH including albumins, alpha and beta globulins, many glycoproteins, polysaccharides, and nucleoproteins. Acetylation or carbamylation of many protein antigens (including immunoglobulins) can make them more electronegative (without altering the serological reactivity of immunoglobulins), thereby enhancing their anodic migration. Antigen (in a well nearest the cathode) and antibody (in a well nearest the anode) migrate on a common path toward one another during electrophoresis so that they actually are driven through one another. The reactants automatically become diluted to their equivalence points and form one or more lines of precipitate (Figure 5.19). Ideally, it is desired to have the precipites form midway between the antigen and antibody wells. If either antigen or antibody is too highly concentrated, equivalence may not be attained and precipitates will not be observed. This problem can be corrected by preparing dilutions of antibody and/or antigen and determining the optimum dilutions for each system. Commercially prepared kits for use in clinical laboratories contain pretitrated antibody in a concentration designed to produce precipitates with homologous antigen in the range of antigen concentrations likely to exist in clinical situations. Nevertheless, a negative CIE test on an undiluted sample should not be considered as proof of the absence of the antigen. Known positive and negative controls should be run on the same plate with the unknowns.

In addition to the slight positive charge on the antibody molecules at pH 8.2 to 8.3, another force called **electroendosmosis** aids in their cathodic migration. Electroendosmosis (endosmosis) is the flow of hydronium ions (H_3O^+) in the buffer that can carry with it electrically neutral or other positively charged molecules. The antigen must be sufficiently electronegative to move anodally against the "buffer flow" in the opposite direction.

Double EID can also be modified to detect serological identity (or nonidentity) of a known antigen with an unknown antigen if the antibody is not monospecific (polyvalent). A single antibody well is cut to overlap two antigen wells in a triangular pattern (Figure 5.20A). Patterns of identity, partial identity, or nonidentity may be obtained, as in double gel diffusion. If one antigen is in much lower titer than the other, this triangular technique can be modified by increasing the diameter of the well in which the weaker antigen is placed (Figure 5.20B).

Double Reactants Moving in Two Dimensions. The first of the immunoelectrophoretic techniques to be developed is still called immunoelectrophoresis (IEP). It, like the Ressler technique, is mainly a qualitative method for fractionating complex mixtures of antigens. It was by this technique that immunoglobulins of classes G, M, and A were initially differentiated. In the clinical laboratory it can be used for typing and identification of abnormal proteins. It is widely used in the pharmaceutical industry to monitor the purity of products sold for human consumption. Antigen is usually placed in a well near the center (or sometimes near one end depending on the pH) of a gel plate and then electrophoresed through neutral agarose to separate components by net charge. This may require one to four hours. The gel plate is then removed from the electrophoresis

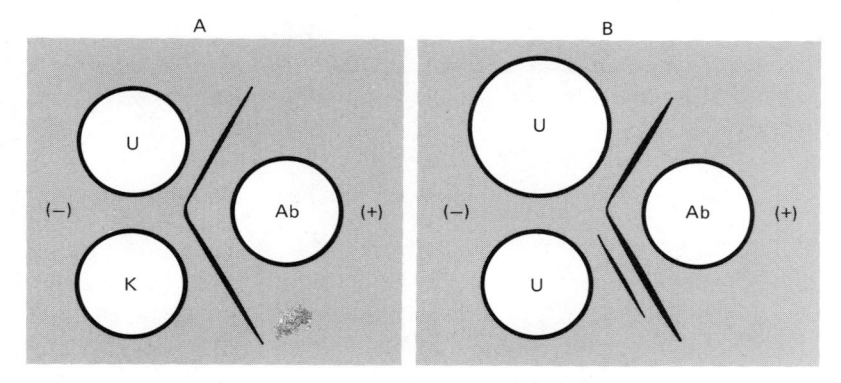

FIGURE 5.20. Detecting serological identity of two antigens (U = unknown, K = known) by triangulation modification of CIE (A). If one antigen is much less concentrated than the other, the weaker antigen can be placed in a larger well (B). The smaller well contains at least one antigen not present in the larger well.

chamber and a narrow trough is cut in the gel on one or both sides and parallel to the path of antigen migration. The trough is loaded with antiserum, and both antibody and antigen are allowed to diffuse overnight (sixteen to eighteen hours). Each antigen component will diffuse radially from its locus of highest concentration in a geometry corresponding to the shape that existed at the end of the electrophoretic run. Antibody molecules will diffuse in a geometry reflective of the trough, but the only effective direction for producing precipitates is the perpendicular distance between the antibody trough and the electrophoretic direction of antigen migration. Stable arcs of precipitates will occur in the gel where antigen and antibody reach their equivalence concentrations. The plate or slide can be dried and stained for ease in visualization of the bands or for retention as a permanent record of the test (Figure 5.21).

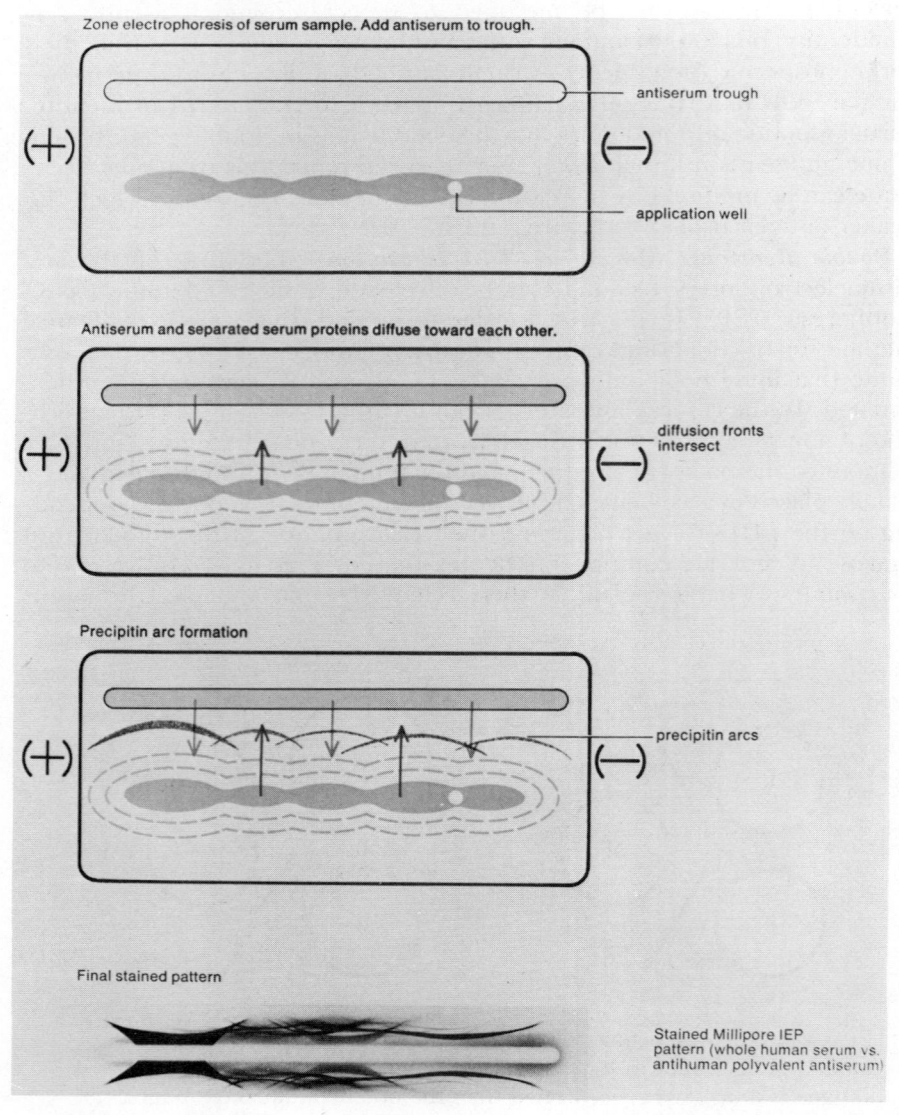

FIGURE 5.21. Steps in immunoelectrophoresis. [*Courtesy of Millipore Corp., Bedford, Mass.*]

Several methods are available for identifying the antigenic composition of a given immunoprecipitin arc among the several bands produced by a heterogeneous antigenic mixture immunoelectrophoresed against a polyvalent antiserum. By IEP of the antigenic mixture against a monospecific antiserum, the position and shape of the resulting arc should correspond to one of the arcs in the immunoelectropherogram produced by an identical procedure using the polyvalent antiserum (Figure 5.22).

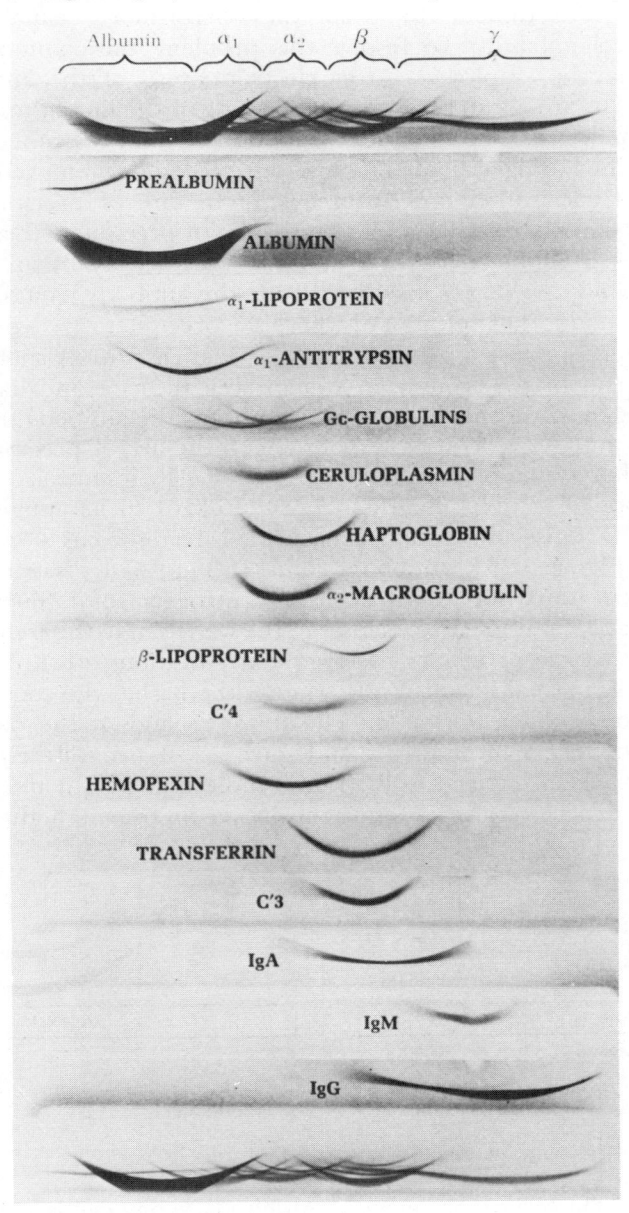

FIGURE 5.22. Composite photograph from IEP patterns obtained using the Millipore Immunoelectrophoresis System. Normal human serum (NHS) was used as the sample. Antisera challenges included polyvalent anti-NHS (top and bottom patterns) and various monospecific antisera. [*Courtesy of Millipore Biomedica, Bedford, Mass.*]

Alternatively, a purified antigen can be electrophoresed simultaneously with an antigen mixture on the same gel. A trough is then cut midway between and parallel to the path of antigen electroporesis. Polyvalent antiserum is loaded into the trench, and immunodiffusion produces a single immunoprecipitin arc with the purified antigen that has its mirror image among the several arcs of the antigenic mixture on the opposite side of the trough.

Sometimes it is difficult to locate the mirror-image band among a "jungle" of other bands. To resolve this problem, the common antigen technique may be employed. After electrophoresis of the antigen, two parallel troughs are cut in the gel on either side of the line of migration of the antigen mixture. One is loaded with antibody and the other is loaded with the purified antigen. Antibody and pure antigen will move in a linear front toward each other and form a straight line of precipitate. This straight line should be continuous with the arc of precipitate formed by its electrophoresed counterpart. Alternatively, the identity of an unknown precipitate band may be resolved by cutting the antibody trough so that it terminates at about the midpoint of where the precipitate arc is expected to develop (determined by a previous conventional IE run). A short distance beyond the end of the trough, a circular well is made and loaded with purified antigen. If the line of precipitate between the antibody trough and the purified antigen well fuses smoothly with the arc of precipitate from the electrophored component, they are serologically identical.

The position of a precipitate band, with regard to its antigen well of origin and the antiserum trough (trench), is referred to as a "well-trench position." In Figure 5.23A, antibody against IgG molecules is reacted with a patient's serum (top) and a normal serum control (bottom). Since the precipitate at the top of the figure is closer to the well than to the trench, it may be inferred that the patient has a lower concentration (titer) of IgG than that present in normal serum. Furthermore, the higher the concentration, the thicker or broader the band. The thinner band of the patient also reflects the subnormal level of IgG. In Figure 5.23B, two different antigens (X and Y) have been subject to IEP. Lower molecular weight antigens (Y in this case) are expected to be closest to the antiserum trench; higher molecu-

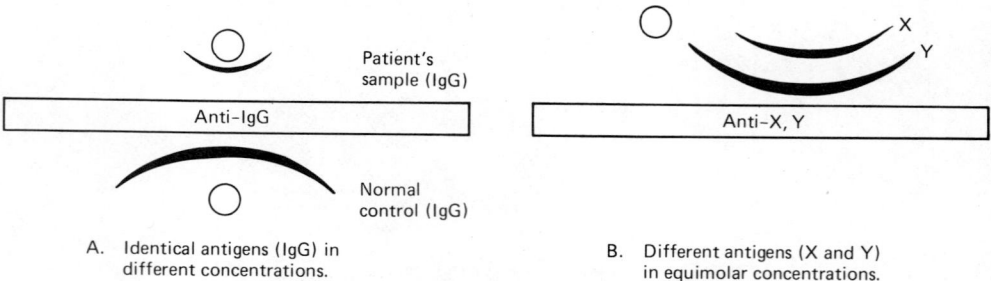

FIGURE 5.23. Well-trench positions. At left (*A*), subnormal level of IgG antigen in patient's sample is indicated by its precipitation arc being thinner and closer to the well than to the trench (as compared to the normal control on the bottom). At right (*B*), with equimolar concentrations of two different antigens (X and Y) the precipitate arc nearest the antigen well is expected to involve the antigen of higher molecular weight.

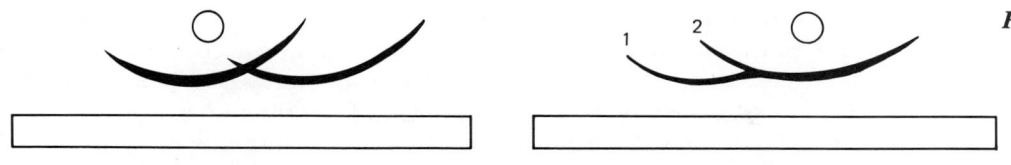

A. Serological nonidentity

B. Serological partial identity

FIGURE 5.24. Serological nonidentity (*A*) vs. partial identity (*B*) in immunoelectrophoresis.

lar weight antigens (X in this case) are expected to diffuse slower from their electrophoresed position and hence be closer to the antigen well.

Serological nonidentity is illustrated in Figure 5.24A by crossing of the arcs. Figure 5.24B is an example of partial identity of two antigens differing in electrophoretic mobilities and antigenicities, yet sharing some antigenic determinants. In this instance, line 1 could represent the kappa L chain specificity and line 2 could represent the lambda L chain specificity as detected by an antiserum made to whole IgG molecules. These spurs share a common antigenicity in the constant region of the gamma heavy chain, but the constant regions of the kappa and lambda light chains are antigenically distinct.

Figure 5.25A represents two electrophoretically different proteins that share a common antigenic specificity. This might occur if anti-Fc was allowed to react with a mixture of Fc fragments and whole IgG molecules. Partial enzymatic digestion of a protein could leave the undigested residue with a different net charge than that of the intact native protein. In this case, the abnormal protein would be displaced electrophoretically with respect to the normal protein (Figure 5.25B).

A variation of IEP, called *direct immunoelectrophoresis,* was developed by E. Alfonso and A. T. Wilson in 1964. After the sample has been electrophoresed in agar, a polyvalent antiserum is spread over the gel rather than being placed in a trough as in routine IEP. This procedure enhanced the precipitation pattern but resulted in some loss of resolution.

In 1969, C. A. Alper and A. M. Johnson used a similar approach with monospecific antiserum and called it *immunofixation electrophoresis.* This is a high resolution technique for (1) identification of monoclonal proteins, (2) phenotyping of plasma proteins such as α_1-antitrypsin and ceruloplasmin,

A. Crossreactivity of electrophoretically different antigens

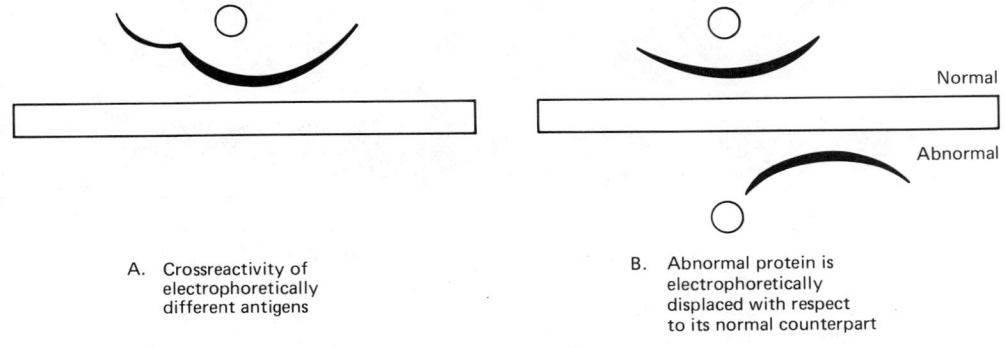

B. Abnormal protein is electrophoretically displaced with respect to its normal counterpart

FIGURE 5.25. Serological cross-reactivity of electrophoretically different antigens (*A*), and electrophoretic displacement of an abnormal protein (*B*).

Serology and Immunology

(3) study of protein polymorphism, (4) identification of components causing abnormal electrophoretic patterns such as antitrypsin, macroglobulin, C3 component, etc., and (5) demonstration of specific antibodies. Following electrophoresis or isoelectric focusing, monospecific antibodies are applied to the gel surface. They diffuse into the gel and form immune complexes

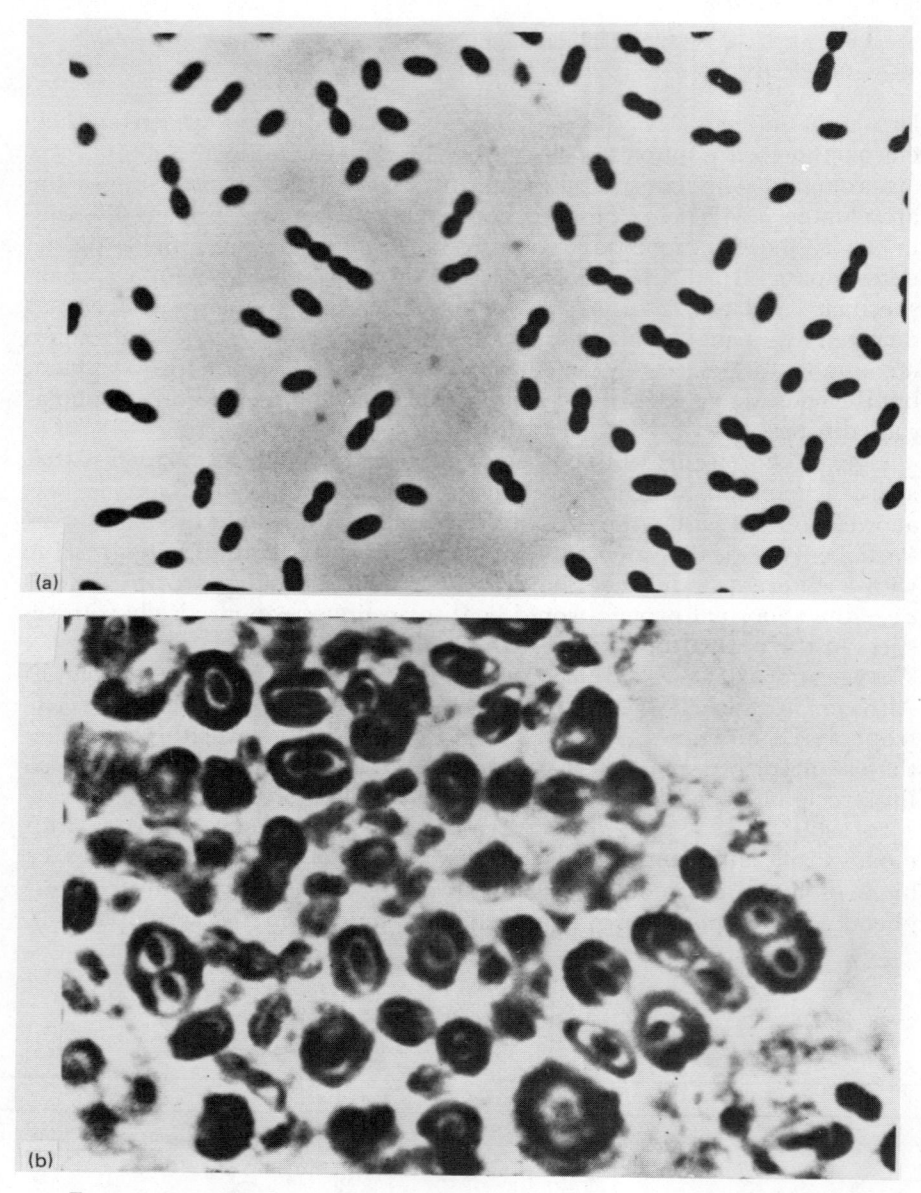

FIGURE 5.26. Encapsulated type III pneumococci: (a) in normal serum, and (b) in serum containing antibody against the capsular polysaccharide. Note the aggregation and apparent swelling caused by the antibody, which increases the optical density of the capsules (Neufeld's "Quellung" phenomenon). (Phase contrast ×2,000). [*From* Immunology for Students of Medicine *(3rd ed.), 1970, by J. H. Humphrey and R. G. White, Blackwell Scientific Publications Limited, Oxford, England.*]

with their homologous antigens at the sites to which they have migrated. These complexes are too large to wash out of the gel's pore structure provided that slight antibody excess is present; all unprecipitated proteins are washed out. Sensitivity can be enhanced by applying a protein stain or by reacting the immunoprecipitates with a second antibody labeled with either a fluor, an enzyme, or a radioisotope (see Chapter 8). Much less antiserum and time is required if cellulose acetate support strips are used instead of agarose or starch gels. Electrophoresis is accomplished on a large strip. About 25 μl of a monospecific antiserum is applied to smaller strips (1 × 2 cm); these small strips are applied to the large strip at the sites where the electrophoresed components are expected to be located (determined by staining an adjoining electropherogram track from the same source). After 60 seconds, the small antibody strips can be removed and the large strip is washed and stained.

Capsular Precipitation

Neufeld (1902) observed through the microscope that encapsulated bacteria seem to swell when exposed to homologous antisera. Methylene blue is commonly used to render the capsules more visually distinctive. Agglutination may also occur in addition to the swelling phenomenon. The German term for "swelling reaction" is "Quellung reaktion." It is doubtful that the capsule actually swells as a result of immunoprecipitate complexes (Figure 5.26). The deposition of a protein (antibody) on the nearly transparent polysaccharide layer of the bacterial capsule enhances visualization of the capsule. The capsular antigens of *Streptococcus pneumonia* are haptenic polysaccharides known as **soluble specific substances** (SSS). A Quellung reaction occurs in a matter of minutes. It is the easiest and most rapid technique for identifying the more than eighty serological types of capsule in *Streptococcus pneumoniae*. It is also used for typing and identifying serotypes of *Hemophilus influenzae, Klebsiella pneumoniae,* and *Neisseria meningitidis.*

SELF-EVALUATION

Terms

1. Soluble antigens involved in serological aggregation.
2. The ratio of dilutions of antigen and antibody producing a visible serological reaction most rapidly. (2 words)
3. In a Ramon titration test, the absence of precipitation in tubes containing high concentrations of antibody.
4. A qualitative fluid precipitation test in which antibody is carefully overlaid with antigen in small-diameter tubes.
5. A protein that usually rapidly appears in the serum following myocardial infarction or rheumatic fever. Its titer is indicative of the severity of the disease and it disappears rapidly following recovery. (2 words)
6. A single diffusion–single dimension gel precipitation test in a tube, named for the man who first developed it in 1946.
7. A double diffusion–double dimension precipitation test in a flat gel, named for its discoverer.

Serology and Immunology

8. Common name given to the precipitates of an immunoelectrophoresis test involving a single reactant moving in a single dimension.
9. The cathodic flow of hydronium ions of a buffer in a double EID test.
10. A precipitation reaction in gel produced by allowing antibody to diffuse outward from a trough cut in the gel parallel to the line along which antigens were previously separated by net charge.

Multiple Choice. Choose the one best answer.

1. Precipitation requires that (a) antigen be monovalent and antibody be multivalent (b) antigen be polyvalent and antibody be univalent (c) both antigen and antibody have ten or more reactive sites (d) both antigen and antibody be at least bivalent (e) none of the above is correct
2. Tubes in the prozone of a Dean and Webb titration (a) contain antibody excess (b) contain antigen excess (c) contain both antigen and antibody excess (d) are unlikely to have either antigen or antibody excess (e) possess none of the above properties
3. Antisera that cause almost total flocculation within a relatively narrow zone around the equivalence point and do not precipitate outside this zone are typically derived from (a) horses (b) chickens (c) rabbits (d) guinea pigs (e) sheep
4. The most widely used support material for immunodiffusion tests is (a) starch (b) agar (c) agarose (d) gelatin (e) polyacrylamide
5. Which of the following is a quantitative precipitation technique? (a) double electroimmunodiffusion (b) immunoelectrophoresis (c) Ouchterlony (d) radial immunodiffusion (e) more than one of these
6. The precipitation technique that is able to distinguish serological identity from nonidentity in two or more unknowns is (a) double diffusion from wells in a flat gel (b) single diffusion from wells in a flat gel (c) single electroimmunodiffusion (d) all of these (e) none of these
7. A Quellung reaction is most likely to occur with (a) rickettsiae (b) acid-fast bacteria (c) viruses (d) spirochetes (e) encapsulated bacteria
8. The precipitation technique in which antigen and antibody move essentially linearly in opposite directions is (a) Oakley and Fulthrope (b) immunoelectrophoresis (c) double electroimmunodiffusion (d) Ouchterlony (e) more than one of these
9. Which of the following is not a practical application of a fluid precipitation test? (a) Lancefield grouping of streptococci (b) detecting serological identity of two or more antigens (c) distinguishing human from animal blood stains (d) detecting adulterated foods (e) more than one of these
10. Which of the following is not an advantage of the rocket technique over RID? (a) requires less time (b) less expensive (c) easier to read with less error (d) all of these are advantages (e) none of these are advantages

True-False

1. Precipitation occurs over a broader range of dilutions in a Ramon than in a Dean and Webb titration.
2. At the equivalence point of a precipitation test, neither free antigen nor free antibody is found in the supernate.
3. The presence of IgM in newborn infants may indicate intrauterine viral infection.
4. Zone phenomena are more likely to be a problem in gel than in fluid precipitation reactions.
5. A test for CRP is routinely performed on patient's suspected of having suffered a myocardial infarction.

Precipitation

6. The diameter of a precipitation ring in a RID test is linearly related to the concentration of the antigen.
7. A precipitation test in a tube can be used to detect serological identity of two or more unknowns in that same tube.
8. In general, precipitation tests are more sensitive than agglutination tests.
9. Detection of IgM in newborn infants is suggestive of an intrauterine infection with rubella virus or cytomegalovirus.
10. A "spur" of precipitate in the Ouchterlony gel diffusion test points to the well containing the lower antigenic complexity.

CHAPTER 6

Agglutination

CHAPTER OUTLINE

Direct Immune Agglutination
  Hemagglutination
    Cold Agglutinin Test
    Heterophile Agglutinin Test
  Bacterial Agglutination
    Tests for Febrile Agglutinins
    Streptococcus MG Agglutination Test
  Serological Tests for Syphilis
    VDRL Test
    RPR Test
Direct Nonimmune Agglutination
  Viral Hemagglutination
  Hemagglutination Inhibition
Indirect (Passive) Agglutination
  Passive Hemagglutination Tests
    Rubella Test
    Serum Hepatitis Test
  RF Test
  Inhibition Tests
    Pregnancy Tests for HCG
    Drugs of Abuse
  Reversed Passive Agglutination Tests
Self-evaluation

The immunological aggregation or clumping of insoluble particles is termed **agglutination.** The participating antigen is called an **agglutinogen,** and the antibody is called an **agglutinin.** There are three major categories of agglutination reactions: (1) direct immune agglutination, (2) direct nonimmune agglutination, and (3) indirect (passive) agglutination. This chapter is divided into three major divisions corresponding to these three major categories of agglutination reactions.

Direct, immune agglutination involves antibodies reactive with antigens of the native particle. For example, in ABO blood grouping, anti-A and anti-B react with native antigenic determinants of the red cell and directly cause hemagglutination. Lectins (phytohemagglutinins) are not antibodies; hence the direct hemagglutination of blood group O cells by anti-H lectin is considered to be a nonimmune reaction. Red blood cells coated with nonagglutinating antibody can be passively agglutinated by reacting the washed complex with antihuman serum (Coombs reagent). Since antiglobulin antibodies are causing the agglutination, it is an immune reaction. However, the Coombs antibody is not combining with an antigen of the erythrocyte, but rather with an antigen (immunoglobulin in this case) attached to the cell. Therefore, the cells are only indirectly (passively) agglutinated. Hemagglutination reactions pertaining to blood banking have been discussed in Chapters 3 and 4 and will not be considered further in this chapter.

Direct Immune Agglutination

HEMAGGLUTINATION

Cold Hemagglutinin Test. Nonspecific cold hemagglutinins are commonly found in sera of patients with primary atypical pneumonia, a respiratory disease caused by *Mycoplasma pneumoniae*. These antibodies cause hemagglutination at about 4°C but not at normal body temperature (37°C). They are capable of agglutinating the patient's own red cells (autohemagglutinins) as well as those of other people or other species. Not all cases of primary atypical pneumonia have autoagglutinins, but as the severity of the disease increases, there tends to be a greater incidence of positive tests and the titers also tend to be correspondingly elevated. Detectable titers of these cold agglutinins generally are found toward the end of the first week or during the second week of the disease. Titers increase to a maximum during the second to fourth week and are greatly decreased or absent in four to six weeks. A single convalescent serum titer of 1:32 to 1:64 is suggestive of primary atypical pneumonia, but as is true of almost all serological tests, a fourfold or greater rise in titer from paired sera (one taken early and another taken several days or a week later) is much more meaningful. Cold agglutinins may also be produced by other diseases including liver disorders (e.g., cirrhosis), chronic sepsis, acquired hemolytic anemia, leishmaniasis, and black water fever. Most of these diseases have symptoms that easily distinguish them from those of primary atypical pneumonia (fever, headache, malaise, productive cough, and chills characterize pneumonia).

Blood for a cold agglutinin test must be taken with a warm syringe, placed in a warm tube, and kept warm in transit to the laboratory. The sample is allowed to clot in an incubator or water bath at 37°C. The serum is separated from the clot by centrifugation in prewarmed cups. These precautions are necessary to avoid adsorption of the cold agglutinins to the clot and a subsequent low titer or false negative test. Prepared serum can be stored in a refrigerator or freezer until tested. Doubling serial dilutions of the serum are made (1:4 to 1:1024) and added to a 1 percent washed saline suspension of group O red cells. The patient's cells may be used instead of group O cells if kept warm through the washing procedure to prevent adsorption of cold agglutinins. A negative control (with saline substituted for serum) is always run simultaneously with the test. It is advisable to also run a known positive control serum as a check on the suitability of the blood cells employed in the test. The rack of tubes is shaken and kept overnight in the refrigerator at 0° to 5°C. Each tube is immediately read for hemagglutination as it comes from the refrigerator; tubes must not be allowed to warm up because the cold antibodies will be eluted and agglutination may fail to occur. The end-point titer of the serum is the reciprocal of the highest dilution that gives +1 or better agglutination (Figure 6.1). As a final control, all tubes should be incubated at 37°C and reread after two hours. Failure to observe any hemagglutination would confirm that only cold agglutinins are present.

Heterophile Agglutinin Test. Infectious mononucleosis (IM) is probably caused by the Epstein-Barr virus (EBV) of the herpes group. It is primarily a disease of young adults (16 to 25 years of age) and thought to be transmitted with difficulty, and then usually by intimate oral contact. This "kissing

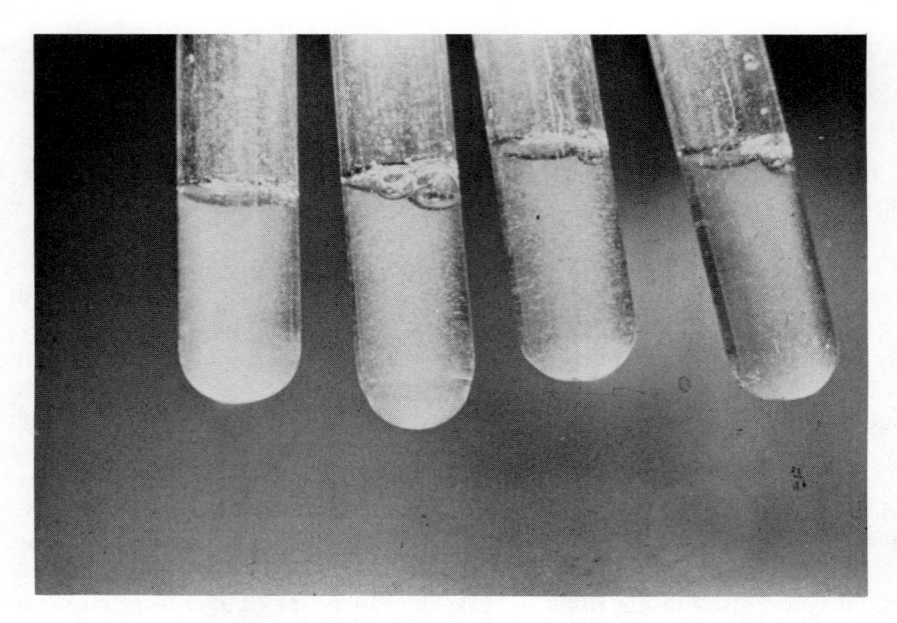

FIGURE 6.1. Cold agglutination titration. Left to right: tubes 1 through 3 exhibit decreasing amounts of type O red cell agglutination by the patient's serum at refrigerator temperature. Tube 4 has no agglutination. The titer is the reciprocal of the dilution of the patient's serum contained in tube 3. [*Courtesy of Elliot Scientific Corp., New York City.*]

disease" is common in populations of college or university students and on military installations. Symptoms of the disease include enlargement of lymph nodes, lymphocytosis, atypical lymphocytes, and fever. **Heterophile (heterophil, heterogenetic) antibodies** are commonly present in serum of patients suffering with IM. In general terms, a heterophile antibody is one that cross-reacts with antigens from a source different from the one that stimulated primary immunization. As far as clinical serology is concerned, the term "heterophile antibody" refers to any human serum that will agglutinate sheep red cells. Heterophile antibodies can be present in normal sera, but are usually elevated in titer in sera from IM patients. Here again, single titers are not of much diagnostic value, but a fourfold or greater difference in titer of paired sera is considered to be indicative of a pathological condition. It is not considered to be specifically indicative of infectious mononucleosis because patients with **serum sickness** are known to have elevated titers of heterophile antibodies. This disease occurs several days to weeks after exposure to a large dose of horse serum (or other foreign sera) and is a common sequela of passive immunization. Even normal healthy people can have titers of heterophile agglutinins up to 320 as a consequence of contact with the ubiquitous Forssman antigen. In 1911, Forssman found that rabbits injected with guinea pig kidney emulsions produced an antibody that could agglutinate sheep erythrocytes (Figure 6.2). The Forssman "antigen" is actually a polysaccharide hapten, but its chemical structure is presently unknown. Its distribution follows no phylogenetic system, being present or absent almost at random without regard to the degree of genetic relatedness of the species. For example, it is present in the mouse (Forssman positive), but not in the rat (Forssman

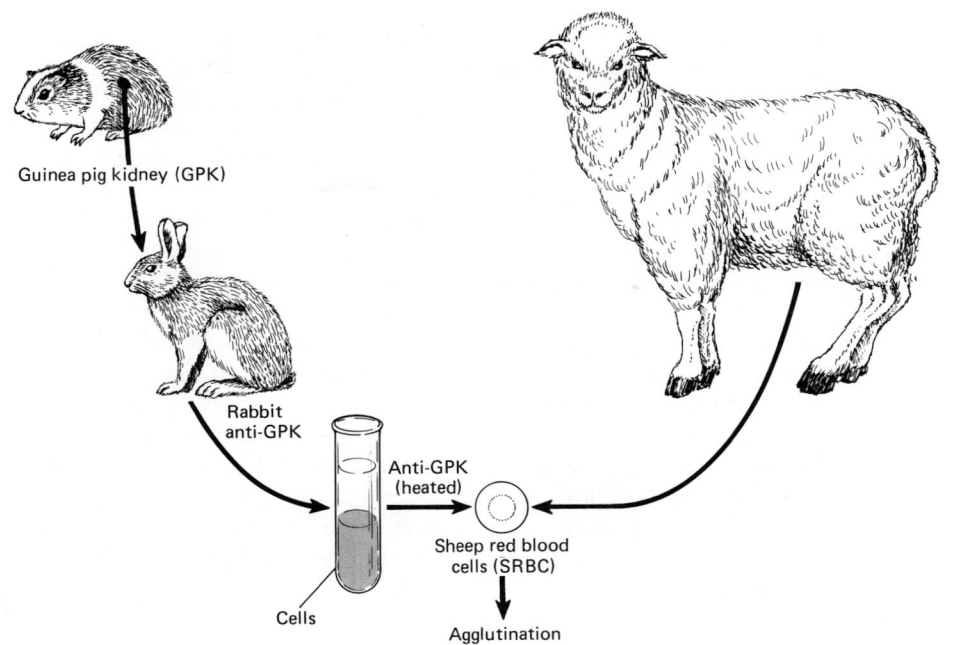

FIGURE 6.2. Production of the classical Forssman-type heterophile antibody.

negative); the horse is positive, but cattle are negative; etc. Even within a species its presence or absence is not constant. For example, in humans it is present in individuals of blood groups A and AB, but not B or O. Furthermore, it has variable distribution in tissues of a Forssman-positive individual. Most guinea pig tissues are positive, but their erythrocytes are negative. The situation is just reversed in the sheep, being present only on the red cells. Some strains of *Salmonella* and *Pasteurella* are Forssman positive, as is *Shigella dysenteriae, Streptococcus pneumoniae,* and *Bacillus anthracis.* It is undoubtedly through contact with Forssman-positive microorganisms that some people develop anti-Forssman titers of heterophile agglutinins. There are many heterophile systems other than the Forssman system, but it is the best known. It has become common practice to equate any heterophile antibody as belonging to the Forssman system, but this is incorrect. For example, horse serum probably contains other heterophile antigens in addition to the Forssman antigen.

A rapid plate screening test would normally be performed on a serum from a patient suspected of having infectious mononucleosis. A drop of patient's serum is added to a drop of 5 percent saline suspension of washed sheep erythrocytes on a glass slide. The slide is mechanically rotated and then read immediately for agglutination. A known positive control serum should be run simultaneously. Agglutination of the sheep red cells indicates that a heterophile antibody is present. The next step is to determine if the titer of the heterophile antibody is sufficiently elevated to be of clinical importance. The titration test for heterophile antibodies is called the "presumptive test of Paul-Bunnell." It requires heat inactivation of the patient's serum at 56°C for thirty minutes to destroy native complement. Doubling dilutions of the serum are made (1 : 7 through 1 : 7168). A constant amount

Serology and Immunology

of 2 percent saline suspension of washed sheep erythrocytes is added to each tube. The rack of tubes is shaken and incubated either at room temperature for two hours or in a water bath at 37°C for one hour. Brief centrifugation of the tubes after incubation accelerates the clumping. A negative control is run concurrently with the test, substituting physiological saline for serum. The reciprocal of the highest dilution that shows agglutination is the titer. A titer of 1 : 224 or greater is considered to be presumptive evidence of IM provided the patient has not recently been exposed to horse serum and shows clinical and hematological evidence of infectious mononucleosis. For example, several kinds of abnormal lymphocytes may be present in a patient with mononucleosis, but the most common is one with an eccentrically placed nucleus containing coarse stranded chromatin and a basophilic cytoplasm with a "moth-eaten" (vacuolated) appearance.

A differential heterophile test (Davidsohn's) is used to confirm the results of the presumptive test and to differentiate between the three major types of heterophile antibodies. First, two aliquots of the patient's serum are separately absorbed with guinea pig kidney tissue (GPK) and with beef (cattle, ox) erythrocyte antigen (BE). Then the absorbed sera are titrated for their residual contents of sheep agglutinins. Forssman antibodies are absorbed by GPK but not by BE. Hence the presumptive test titer should be markedly reduced or disappear in GPK-absorbed sera but not in BE-absorbed sera (Table 6.1). A heterophile antibody produced by serum sickness is absorbed by both GPK and beef cells. Heterophile titers should be low or absent in the absorbed serum. Finally, the heterophile antibody of infectious mononucleosis is absorbed by beef cells but not by GPK. Sheep cell agglutinins will remain in the GPK-absorbed serum but not in the serum absorbed with BE. The differential test is considered to be positive for IM if the heterophile titer of the guinea pig–absorbed serum is not more than three tubes (doubling dilutions) lower than the titer of the unabsorbed serum (presumptive test) and the BE-absorbed serum is devoid of heterophile antibodies.

Lyophilized boiled guinea pig kidney antigen and boiled beef erythrocyte antigen are commercially available. The patient's serum is heat inactivated at 56°C for thirty minutes. An aliquot of the serum is placed in a tube with the reconstituted boiled guinea pig kidney antigen; another aliquot is mixed with reconstituted boiled beef erythrocyte antigen. The tubes are incubated at room temperature for one hour, and shaken at fifteen-minute intervals to enhance absorption. They are then centrifuged and the clear supernatant fluid is used for the titration test (dilutions begin with 1 : 7 as in

Table 6.1 DIFFERENTIAL ABSORPTION OF HETEROPHILE ANTIBODIES

Type of Heterophile Antibody	Absorption by Guinea Pig Kidney Antigen	Absorption by Beef Erythrocyte Antigen
Forssman	Yes	No
Serum sickness	Yes	Yes
Infectious mononucleosis	No	Yes

the presumptive test). A negative saline control is also included with the titration test. Sheep red cells should be fresh or less than one week old. A weakly reactive result may be observed in the first few tubes that becomes stronger with greater dilutions. This prozone phenomenon occurs only with high-titer heterophile sera. Zoning is seldom a problem with agglutination reactions and is one of the major reasons why agglutination tests are preferred over precipitation tests.

Davidsohn's differential test for IM has been modified into a rapid plate test that can be performed in less than five minutes. These newer plate tests are a great saving in technologist's time (and cost to the patient) and have largely replaced the Davidsohn test. A typical commercial test kit contains a bottle each of GPK, BE, and indicator cells. It is now known that horse erythrocytes preserved in sodium citrate solution remain useful for at least three months. Horse cells are three to four times more sensitive than sheep cells and sixteen times more sensitive than formalinized horse cells (treating red cells with formalin is a common preservative technique). A drop of patient's serum is placed on the left and right sides of a glass slide. A drop of GPK reagent is added to the serum at the left, and a drop of BE is added to the serum on the right. A drop of indicator cells is placed near each serum. Using a toothpick, each absorbing reagent is mixed thoroughly with its drop of serum (about ten revolutions) and then the indicator cells are stirred into the mixture with another ten revolutions. The slide is observed for agglutination no longer than one minute after mixing. If agglutination is stronger on the right side than on the left side of the slide (Figure 6.3), the test is considered negative (the patient does not have heterophile antibodies generated by IM). No agglutination on either side or equal amounts of agglutination on both sides is also considered to be a negative test. A posi-

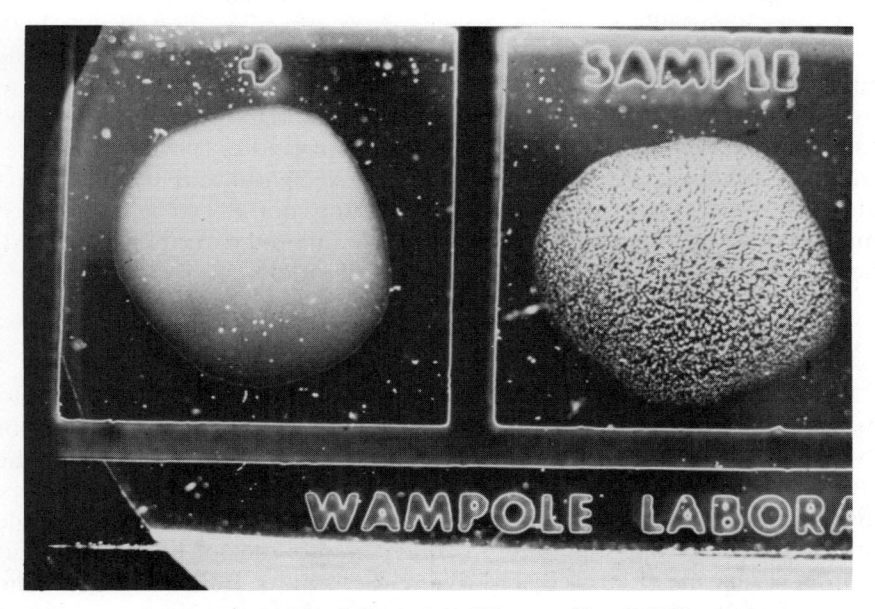

FIGURE 6.3. A negative differential slide test for infectious mononucleosis. Negative agglutination is at the left with GPK-absorbed serum; positive agglutination is at the right with BE-absorbed serum. The indicator particles are horse cells. [*Courtesy of Elliot Scientific Corp., New York City.*]

tive test is indicated by a stronger agglutination on the left than on the right side. The rapid slide test can also be made semiquantitative by making doubling dilutions and testing a drop of each dilution as is done in the qualitative test (using undiluted serum). End-point titers determined by a rapid differential slide test cannot be equated with those from slide tests by other manufacturers nor with the titers from a presumptive (tube) test with sheep cells. There is no correlation of IM heterophile titer with severity of the disease. As with most serological tests, a significant (fourfold) elevation in titer between sera taken a week or so apart usually is indicative of active disease or recent contact with the causative agent. These kits should also provide a known positive control serum that should be run in parallel (on another slide) with the test. Serum or plasma mixed with anticoagulants (EDTA, sodium oxalate, potassium oxalate, sodium citrate, ACD solution, or heparin) may be used. Heat inactivation of the serum is not required, but heated serum may be used if desired. The heterophile antibody of IM can usually be detected by the sixth to the tenth day after onset of illness. Highest titers tend to occur during the second or third week. Detectable titers may persist for at least six weeks.

More recently, a rapid card test kit has become available that does not require differential absorptions to identify the antibody of infectious mononucleosis. This test uses an IM antigen reagent prepared from horse erythrocyte IM receptor glycoprotein. This antigen does not agglutinate in the presence of Forssman antibodies. It consists of lipid particles into which an antigen isolated from horse erythrocyte membranes has been incorporated. Charcoal particles are added to enhance visualization of the agglutination reaction. After mixing under a humidifying cover on a mechanical rotator, the coagglutination of the charcoal particles appears as black clumps against the white background of the plastic-coated card. The test is read macroscopically as either reactive or nonreactive. The kit has both positive and negative control sera that should be run concurrently with the patients' samples. Plasma should be diluted 1:4 because of the tendency to produce atypical reactions when unheated plasma is tested in the undiluted state. Serum may be used instead of plasma, but neither specimen requires heat inactivation. Plasma samples should be tested within twenty-four hours after collection and should not be frozen. Serum samples can be kept frozen until needed for the test. The test can be quantitated directly on the card, thereby eliminating the need for test tube dilutions.

BACTERIAL AGGLUTINATION

Most bacteria have a cell wall adjacent to and surrounding the cytoplasmic membrane. Gram-positive cell walls consist of a thick inner layer of glycopeptide and a thinner outer layer of teichoic acid (Figure 6.4), the latter containing the major surface antigens consisting of various proteins, glycoproteins, and polysaccharides. Gram-negative cell walls have a single inner layer of glycopeptide and an "outer membrane" of lipoprotein and lipopolysaccharide (LPS) referred to as **endotoxin** or **Boivin antigen.** The polysaccharide side chains of the LPS project above the outer membrane and are the major sites for antibody or complement attachment. A few bacteria do not have cell walls. Cells without walls are called **protoplasts.** A group of bacteria called "mycoplasmas" (Family = *Mycoplasmatales*) contain

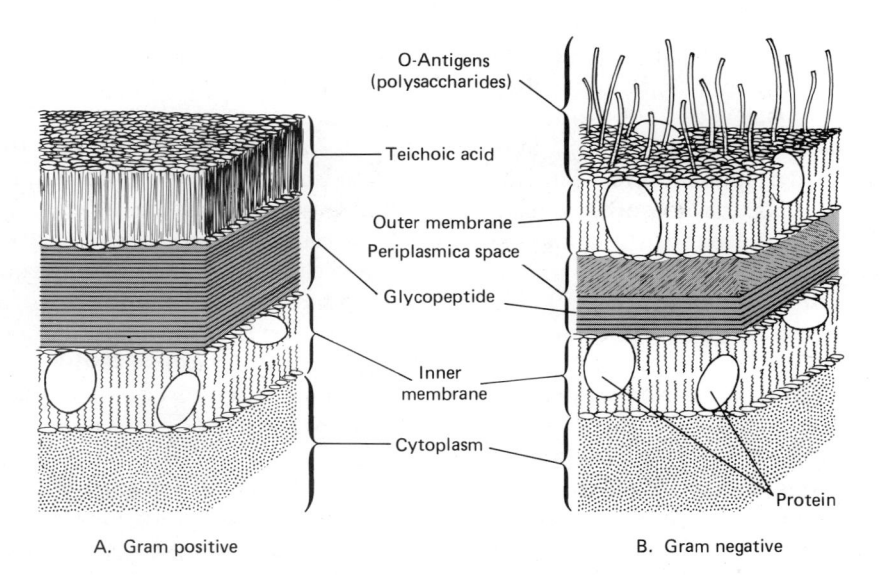

FIGURE 6.4. Composition of bacterial cell walls.

natural wall-deficient forms. Some bacteria of other genera (either gram-negative or gram-positive) may spontaneously lose part or all of their cell walls and fail to react with antisera against antigens of the cell wall. These are called **L forms.** The proteins of the cytoplasmic membrane are the major antigenic determinants of protoplasts.

Many bacteria have a gelatinous slime layer external to the cell wall. If this layer has some tendency to adhere to the outer wall surface, it is termed a **capsule.** Capsules may consist of polysaccharides (as in several strains of streptococci) or complexes of polysaccharides and proteins or polypeptides (e.g., *Bacillus anthracis*). Encapsulated cells tend to resist phagocytosis and thereby become virulent. Most capsular materials are usually complete haptens when separated from the rest of the cell. The union of antibodies with capsules often renders the organism susceptible to phagocytosis (opsonization phenomenon). Killed encapsulated (phase I) *Bordetella pertussis* is utilized in the production of a vaccine against whooping cough; no immunity to this organism results from exposure to unencapsulated (phase IV) *B. pertussis*.

Some bacteria (e.g., genus *Salmonella*) are motile because they possess long, whiplike structures called flagella. They are composed of proteins called flagellins and are usually strongly antigenic. Some gram-negative bacteria possess shorter, hollow-cored protein appendages called **pili** or **fimbriae** that should not be confused with flagella. Pili may function in conjugation to transfer DNA from a donor to a recipient cell. Some pili furnish receptor sites by which certain RNA viruses can attach and introduce their genetic material into the host cell. Some bacteria may use pili to attach to human mucosal cells. Neither flagellar antigens nor pili antigens seem to contribute to virulence of bacteria or their ability to induce immunity. However, flagellar antigens are diagnostically important in serological classification of bacteria such as *Salmonella*.

Flagellated bacteria of the genus *Proteus* swarm across the surface of a solid medium, forming a thin film of growth. The Germans Weil and Felix

Serology and Immunology

likened this to the mist produced by breathing on glass and referred to this type of bacteria as "hauch" (breath, film, emanation). Nonmotile (nonflagellated) bacteria did not produce a breath mist and were referred to as "ohne hauch" (without a breath). Subsequently, all flagellated bacteria and the flagellar antigens have been called **H** type; all nonflagellated bacteria and the **somatic** (body) **antigens** have been called **O** type. Antibodies against cell wall determinants (O antigens) cause bacteria to clump into compact, granular or hailstone-like masses that are not easily disrupted by vigorous shaking (O-type agglutination). Antibodies against flagellar antigens produce a loose, filmy, "flocculent" type of agglutination (H-type agglutination) that is easily disrupted by vigorous shaking. Antisera made in response to flagellated bacteria are expected to contain antibodies against both H and O antigens. However, the flagella seem to take precedence in the clumping process, resulting in H-type agglutination.

Antigens associated with bacterial capsules are called **K antigens.** The presence of a capsule may block the underlying cell wall antigens (O antigens) from immune attack. One of the best-known K antigens, designated Vi, is found in typhoid bacilli and certain other *Enterobacteriaceae*. It was originally thought that the Vi antigen contributed to virulence, but this may not always be true. The Vi antigen can interfere with bacterial agglutination by antibodies directed against O antigens of the cell wall. Fortunately, this inhibitory activity of Vi and related K antigens of other enteric bacilli can be abolished by heating the bacterial suspension prior to testing. Complement is also destroyed by heating, thereby preventing lysis of some gram-negative bacteria in the presence of homologous antibodies. This is why bacterial suspensions are routinely heated before antisera directed against O antigens are added to them in agglutination tests. Colonies of encapsulated strains of *Streptococcus pneumoniae* growing on nutrient agar plates appear to have smooth borders and are called S strains. Mutant strains that have lost the capsule produce colonies with rough borders and are called R strains. Virulence in *S. pneumoniae* is lost with the capsule.

The terms **antigenic variation** or **dissociation** may be used for any change in a cell or organism (usually genetically controlled) that results in the appearance of new or altered antigens or that results in loss of antigens. Bacterial dissociation may involve loss of flagella (H-O variation), partial or total loss of polysaccharides from the LPS layer in gram-negative rods **(S-R variation),** loss of capsular antigens such as Vi, appearance of new antigens as a consequence of bacteriophage infection **(phage conversion, lysogenic conversion),** or alternating changes in flagellar antigens **(phase variation).** In viruses, the term **immunological drift (antigenic drift, antigenic shift)** refers to the appearance of new viral antigens (new strains of a virus) and the rapid spread of the new strain among the nonimmune host population. Naturally, K antigens are not present in R strains that have lost their capsules. In cell walls of *Salmonella* species there is a common core polysaccharide that has been modified in the evolution of these species by the addition of other monosaccharides to create specific O antigens. R mutants of *Salmonella* lose the repeating side-chain oligosaccharides that determine "S-phase" O-antigenic specificities and are left with the common core polysaccharide (the R antigen).

There is so much antigenic diversity in some of the gram-negative species that infection by (or vaccination with) one serotype may provide little or no protection to a different serotype. For example, there are well over 1,000 serotypes known in the genus *Salmonella*. Each serotype is defined by its constellation of O and H antigens. Many of these antigens are shared by different serotypes. Certain shared O antigens are used to define **serogroups,** the latter given designations A to I and over 60 Arabic numerals. Figure 6.5 illustrates a slide agglutination test with one of these group specific antisera. For example, all members of serogroup B contain the somatic antigen 4; all members of serogroup C_1 possess O antigens 6 and 7, etc. About forty serogroups have been established for *Salmonella*. The Vi antigen is not used to define either serogroups or serotypes, but is usually included in the **antigenic formula** of the serogroup if it is present. As an illustration, the antigenic formula of *S. typhi* is 9, 12: Vi: d. Determinants 9 and 12 are somatic (O) antigens, and d is a flagellar (H) antigen. *S. enteritidis* has the antigenic formula 1, 9, 12: g, m. Determinants 1, 9, and 12 are O antigens; g and m are H antigens.

To complicate matters further, the flagellar (H) antigens of *Salmonella* species experience antigenic changes called **phase variations** at relatively high frequencies (1×10^3 to 1×10^5 cell divisions). H antigens characteristic of the serotype are called **specific antigens** or **phase 1 antigens;** those common to several serotypes are called **group antigens** or **phase 2 antigens.** Phase 1 antigens are designated by lower-case letters, phase 2 antigens by numbers. Some species have antigens of only one phase (either phase 1 or phase 2) and are called **monophasic.** In the above example, *S. typhi* has, in addition to its O antigens, only the phase 1 antigen d; it has no phase 2 antigens. Other species have both phase 1 and phase 2 antigens and are said to be **diphasic,** as exemplified by *S. typhimurium* with the antigenic formula

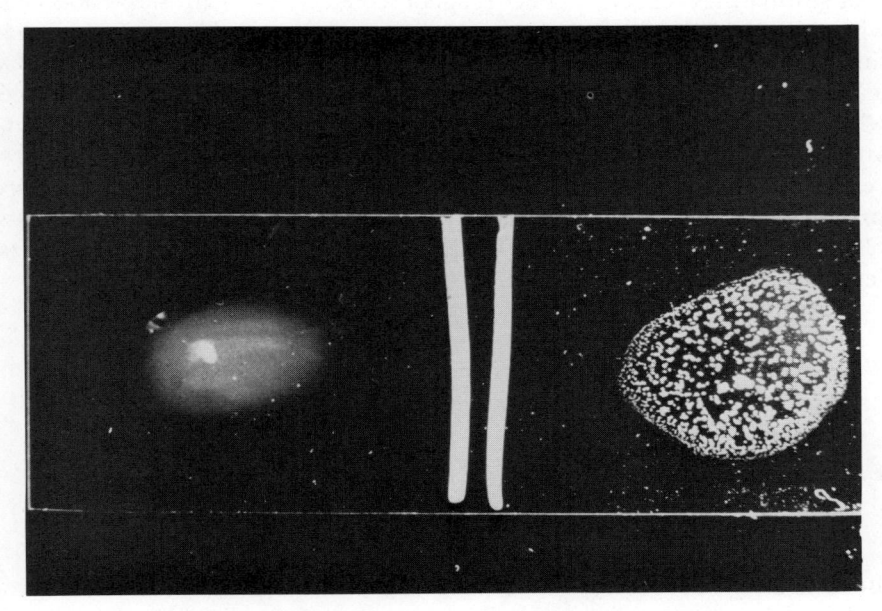

FIGURE 6.5. Slide agglutination with *Salmonella* group antiserum. Left: Negative agglutination with *Escherichia coli* culture. Right: Positive agglutination with *Salmonella* group-specific antiserum, thereby establishing identity of strain as a *Salmonella* as well as its membership in the same group as that of the antiserum. [*Courtesy of Elliot Scientific Corp., New York City.*]

1, 4, 5, 12 : i : 1, 2. The somatic antigens (1, 4, 5, 12) are listed first followed by a colon; then the phase 1 antigen(s) (in this case i) is given followed by another colon, and finally the phase 2 antigen(s) is designated (1, 2).

Monophasic variants can be easily isolated from a diphasic culture by inoculating the latter on soft "motility agar" containing antibodies against one or more of the group phase antigens. For example, the motility of an inoculum of *S. typhimurium* in group phase (1, 4, 5, 12 : 1, 2) will be inhibited by flagellar agglutination with the antigroup serum antibodies 1, 2. However, a specific phase 1 variant (1, 4, 5, 12 : b) is able to migrate through the agar and can be isolated at a distance from the original inoculum.

Bacterial agglutination tests serve two major functions in the clinical laboratory. Serological identification of microorganisms can be obtained in minutes as opposed to the days required for many biochemical tests. Even when no organism can be isolated from a patient, serological diagnosis of the causative agent is considered proven (in the absence of a recently administered vaccine) when there is a fourfold or greater increase in antibody titers between paired sera (acute vs. convalescent samples). Regardless of the antibacterial titer, a single specimen is of little diagnostic value because antibodies may be present as a result of a previous infection, purposeful immunization, or serological cross-reactions with other organisms. This is why each patient's past history of infection or immunization must be taken into consideration by the physician in order to make a valid interpretation of the test results.

The sensitivity of bacterial agglutination tests can be enhanced by a **coagglutination** technique. At least one commercial source is available for serotyping streptococcus groups A, B, C, and D and gonococcus by coagglutinating reagents. The reagent consists of dead staphylococcus whole cells coated with specific antibodies of class IgG. The immunoglobulins readily attach to protein A of the staph cells by their Fc portions, leaving the Fab regions free to bind the homologous antigens. For example, when a suspension of group B streptococci is exposed to a reagent bearing anti-group B IgG, an agglutination lattice forms that is a mosaic of staph reagent cells and strep B test cells (coagglutination). Larger clumps are produced with the coagglutination reagent than without it, making it possible to detect agglutination in weaker bacterial suspensions (greater test sensitivity).

Table 6.2 SOME FEBRILE DISEASES AND THEIR ETIOLOGICAL AGENTS

Disease	Etiological Agent
Enteric fever	
Typhoid fever	*Salmonella typhi**
Paratyphoid fevers	*Salmonella cholerasuis**
	Salmonella enteritidis†
Brucellosis (undulant fever)	*Brucella melitensis*
Tularemia	*Franciscella tularensis* (formerly *Pasteurella tularensis*)
Rickettsial diseases (e.g., typhus)	See Table 6.3

* Monotypic species.
† Common serotypes in U.S. include *paratyphi A, paratyphi B,* and *typhimurium.*

Tests for Febrile Agglutinins. **Febrile agglutinins** are agglutinating antibodies produced in response to various fever-producing bacteria. These microorganisms cause typhoid fever, paratyphoid, brucellosis, tularemia, and typhus (Table 6.2). When *Salmonella* species serve as the antigens, it is called a **Widal test.** Both O and H antigens are commercially available (or easily prepared) for agglutination in a Widal test. Because rickettsiae are obligate intracellular parasites, the cost of producing specific rickettsial antigens is relatively high. In 1916, E. Weil and A. Felix found that some rickettsial antibodies would agglutinate certain bacterial strains of *Proteus* (OX-19 and OX-2 of *P. vulgaris,* and OX-K of *P. mirabilis*). *Proteus* antigens were much less costly and became routinely used in the **Weil-Felix** test to detect cross-reactive (heterophile) antibodies induced by some of the rickettsiae (Table 6.3).

The various antigens described above can be employed in a slide agglutination test to screen for febrile agglutinins. If a febrile agglutinin is found it can be titrated. Doubling dilutions of the patient's serum (1:20 through 1:320) are mixed with a constant amount of an appropriate dilution of bacterial antigen (killed with heat, phenol, or formalin) on ceramic or glass ringed slides. Three controls should be run simultaneously: (1) antigen control (no serum), (2) known positive serum control, and (3) known negative serum control. The slide is rotated and tilted on an illuminated frosted glass surface for no longer than three minutes and scored for agglutination. Prozoning may occur in the lowest dilutions, but this is easily detected and corrected in the titration. The reciprocal of the highest dilution of serum producing agglutination is the end-point titer (some workers prefer to use the greatest dilution giving +2 or 50 percent agglutination as the end point). The tube test is considered preferable to the slide test, but requires a much longer time to perform. Dilution of the patient's serum is made as before, the bacterial antigen is added, and the tubes are shaken and incubated at 52°C for eighteen hours (*Brucella* species are incubated at 37°C for eighteen hours) or at 37°C for twenty-four to forty-eight hours. Controls are run as with the slide test. The test is scored for agglutination and interpreted in accordance with the criteria of Table 6.3. Negative results do

Table 6.3 TYPICAL WEIL-FELIX REACTIONS

Diseases	Agglutination with Proteus Strain			Causative Organism
	OX-19	OX-2	OX-K	
Epidemic typhus	+4	+	0	*Rickettsia prowazeki*
Murine typhus	+4	+	0	*R. mooseri*
Brill-Zinsser disease	0	0	0	*R. prowazeki*
Rocky Mountain spotted fever	*	*	0	*R. rickettsii*
Scrub typhus (Tsutsugamushi fever)	0	0	+2	*R. tsutsugamushi*
Rickettsial pox	0	0	0	*R. akari*
Trench fever	0	0	0	*Rochalimaea quintana*
Q fever	0	0	0	*Coxiella burnetii*

* Reactivity is exceedingly variable from one case to another.

Serology and Immunology

not rule out infection. Narcotics addicts tend to have higher-than-average titers to *S. typhi* O and H antigens. These enteric fevers respond well to broad-spectrum antibiotics. Effective treatment in early stages of the disease tends to inhibit further rise in antibody titers. Serological cross-reactions are common among members of this group of organisms; so it is important that a full battery of antigens representing all relevant serogroups be included in the test.

Results of the Weil-Felix test can at best give only a presumptive diagnosis. Some rickettsial diseases cannot be detected at all with *Proteus* antigens. Regardless of the outcome of this test, the sera should be sent to the state public health department laboratory for confirmation by agglutination tests using specific rickettsial antigens.

***Streptococcus* MG Agglutination Test.** An alternative to the cold hemagglutinin test for primary atypical pneumonia involves the agglutination of a nonhemolytic strain (MG) of "streptococcus" by unheated patient's serum. Although this organism is not involved in the etiology of the disease, heterophile antibodies are often produced by patients with the disease that specifically cross-react with a capsular polysaccharide of this strain of the "streptococcus." No special techniques are required for collecting the specimen. Clot formation may be allowed at any suitable temperature (even refrigeration is acceptable), but the serum should not be heat-inactivated. Doubling serial dilutions of the patient's serum are made as in the cold agglutinin test. To each of these dilutions is added a constant amount of bacterial suspension. Positive and negative controls are run simultaneously. The rack of tubes is shaken and allowed to incubate overnight at room temperature. The tubes are read for the degree of bacterial agglutination on a scale like that of hemagglutination. The end-point titer is the reciprocal of the highest dilution of serum producing clumps that do not dis-

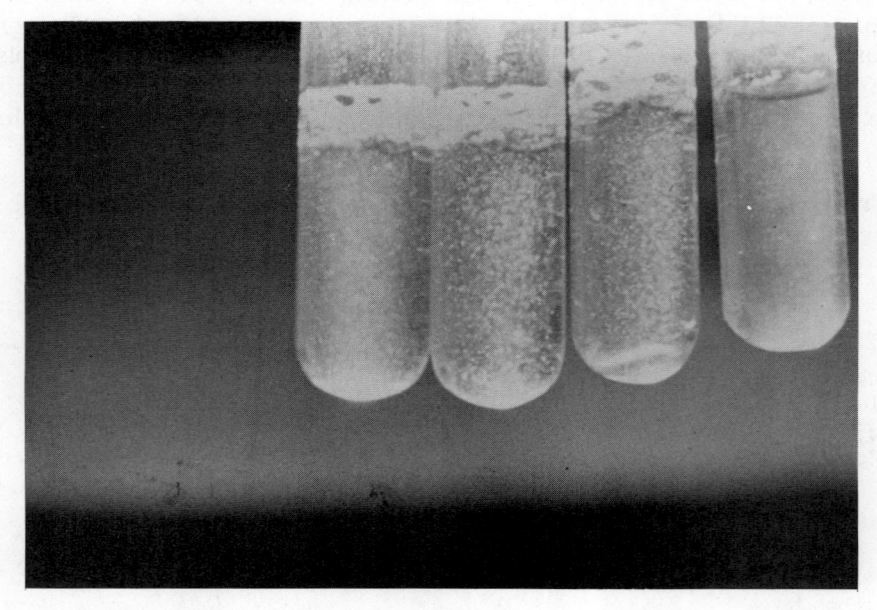

FIGURE 6.6. Serum *Streptococcus* MG agglutination titration. Left to right: Tubes 1 to 3 positive; tube 4 negative. Titer is reciprocal of serum dilution in tube 3. [*Courtesy of Elliot Scientific Corp., New York City.*]

solve on shaking (Figure 6.6). End-point dilutions of 1 : 20 or greater are suggestive of disease, but again a fourfold or greater titer increase on paired sera is of more diagnostic value.

Some patients with primary atypical pneumonia develop only cold hemagglutinins and others develop MG bacterial agglutinins. Therefore, it may be desirable to run both tests when this disease is suspected. Not all patients with the disease produce either or both of these agglutinins; so a negative test(s) does not rule out the possibility that the patient has primary atypical pneumonia.

SEROLOGICAL TESTS FOR SYPHILIS

Syphilis is a contagious venereal disease caused by the spirochete *Treponema pallidum*. This organism apparently cannot penetrate the skin unless a break occurs in the epithelial layer. After a ten to sixty-day incubation period, a painless, inflammatory reaction produces a characteristic ulcerated lesion of primary syphilis called a **chancre,** usually at the site of entry of the treponeme. The lesions usually heal spontaneously but the infection persists. Syphilis is easily cured by penicillin if treated early, but the spontaneous remission of the chancre may lull the affected individual into a false sense of security so that he/she fails to seek medical treatment. In untreated individuals, six weeks to six months after the chancre disappears a generalized skin rash and other abnormalities signal that syphilis has reached the secondary stage. Clinical symptoms then usually disappear (latent syphilis) for various periods. Latent syphilis may continue throughout life, it may terminate with spontaneous cure, or it may advance to tertiary syphilis. In its advanced stages, syphilis can cause blindness, insanity, paralysis, vascular disease, bone and joint lesions, and ulcers of skin and mucous membranes. Pregnant women with active syphilis (even primary syphilis) can transmit the organism to their babies. As of 1979, only eight states did not require some kind of premarital blood test for syphilis in order to determine if medical treatment is required.

Serological tests for syphilis (STS) are of two major kinds: (1) tests for specific treponemal antibodies of class IgG and (2) nonspecific reagin tests. *Treponema pallidum* hemagglutination (TPHA) test kits are commercially available. The antigen is *T. pallidum* adsorbed onto red cells. Antitreponemal antibodies can react with the specific antigen and cause passive agglutination of the red cells. Other nonagglutinating tests for specific treponemal antibodies include the *Treponema pallidum* complement fixation (TPCF) test, the Reiter protein complement fixation (RPCF) test, and the fluorescent treponemal antibody absorption (FTA-ABS) test. The principles of these kinds of tests are presented in the next two chapters.

Syphilitic reagin is an IgM antibody produced by people who have been infected with treponemes. It nonspecifically reacts with a variety of tissue phospholipids presumed to be released as a consequence of microbial damage during infections. Antigenicity of these lipid haptens perhaps is enhanced by spontaneous complexing with some "Schleppering" agent (carrier or adjuvant) present in the serum and thereby induces the production of reagins. An alcoholic extract of normal beef hearts, called **cardiolipin,** is the conventional source of antigen for detecting the presence of reagin in serum. Sensitivity of the reaction is enhanced by the addition of lecithin and cholesterol. Lecithin also helps neutralize the anticomplementary properties of cardiolipin; cholesterol increases the effective reacting surface and the complement-fixing capacity of cardiolipin with reagin.

VDRL Test. A test developed by the **V**enereal **D**isease **R**esearch **L**aboratory, called the **VDRL test,** is one of the most commonly used screening tests for reagin. It employs an alcoholic solution of the cardiolipin-lecithin-cholesterol antigen (VDRL antigen) and a special buffered saline containing sodium chloride, formaldehyde, secondary sodium phosphate, and primary potassium phosphate. Detailed directions for performing the test (in U.S. Public Health Service or state Departments of Public Health publications) must be followed exactly. Only the broad outline of the test will be presented here. When the VDRL antigen is mixed with buffered saline, it forms short rod particles of uniform size that can easily be seen at 100× magnification. When reagin combines with these antigen particles, they agglutinate and the clumps can be seen with the naked eye or a hand lens. This reaction has historically been called a "flocculation" and is commonly discussed along with precipitation phenomena in many serology texts. It is clearly not a precipitation reaction, however, because the antigen is not soluble; it is a particle easily seen in the light microscope, and hence the VDRL reaction is technically an agglutination. Perhaps it was thought to be more like a precipitation reaction because small clumps on a slide can be detected only by observation under the microscope, and zoning reactions are sometimes a problem. Blocking antibodies (7S) may be responsible for some prozone agglutination reactions.

The VDRL test is a slide test performed as either a qualitative or quantitative procedure. All sera for use in VDRL tests must be heated at 56°C for thirty minutes within four hours of testing in order to inactivate heat-labile nonspecific inhibitors of the VDRL test reaction. After cooling to room temperature, 0.05 ml of undiluted serum is pipetted into a ring of a paraffin-ringed or ceramic-ringed slide for the **qualitative test.** One drop of antigen is added from a syringe specially calibrated to deliver 1/60 ml per drop. The slide can be mechanically rotated at 180 rpm for four minutes and read at 100× for agglutination according to Figure 6.7. In scoring agglutination, attention should be paid not only to the size of the aggregates, but also to the amount of free antigen in the background. This is why it is so important that exactly 1/60 ml of antigen be used. More than this amount of antigen could give smaller clumps and be interpreted as weaker reactions. Three serum controls of known reactivity (R, WR, N) should be run simultaneously with the patient's serum. The nonreactive serum control should show only free antigen particles, uniformly distributed in the field of vision. Any roughness or nonrandom distribution in the nonreactive serum control may indicate that (1) the antigen has been rendered unusable (possibly by failure to store it in the dark or because it is outdated), (2) the antigen was improperly prepared, or (3) other technical errors have been made. High-titered sera may produce a weakly reactive zonal agglutination. If this is suspected, a **quantitative test** is performed by serially diluting the patient's serum and retesting. If agglutination becomes stronger at early dilutions, a zonal reaction is confirmed. The end point is the greatest dilution of serum that produces a +2 or stronger reaction.

There is no correlation between the amount of reagin in a patient's serum and the severity of the disease. Reagin is not usually detected by the VDRL

Agglutination

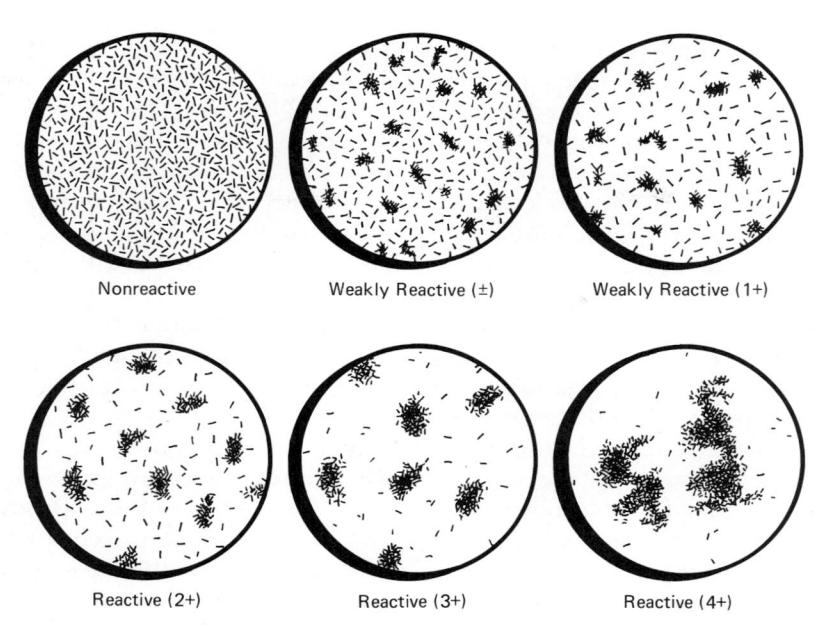

FIGURE 6.7. Degrees of reactivity as microscopically observed in the cardiolipin microflocculation test. [*From U.S. Army Technical Manual TM 8-227-1. Laboratory Procedures in Clinical Serology, October 1960.*]

test until about four to five weeks after infection. Therefore, a negative VDRL test is no proof that an individual has not been infected. Once stimulated, reagin levels tend to climb to a maximum titer during the secondary stage of the disease. After that, the reagin titer tends to decrease to a fairly stable level during late syphilis. A fourfold or greater increase in reagin titers when paired sera are tested is suggestive evidence of syphilis. Of course, if chancres and other lesions of syphilis are present, reagin tests only offer confirmation of the diagnosis. There are many diseases, however, that stimulate reagin production. For example, 100 percent of malaria cases have reagin titers; 60 percent of leprosy; 20 percent of typhus fever, vaccinia, atypical pneumonia, infectious mononucleosis, lupus erythematosus; 10 percent of trypanosomiasis and infectious hepatitis; 5 percent of rheumatoid arthritis; etc. Needless to say, there are many opportunities for BFP (biological false positive) reactions to occur in VDRL tests. One of the advantages of reagin tests is that reagin disappears relatively soon after the patient is cured. Specific antitreponemal antibodies, on the other hand, may persist long after the patient is cured. Antigens for the specific tests are the treponemes or their extracts. They must be cultured in rabbit testes because *in vitro* culture has not been possible; therefore, the cost of these antigens is relatively high.

Other "flocculation tests" for syphilis (e.g., Kahn, Kline, Mazini) also employ a cardiolipin antigen. They differ from the VDRL test and from one another in such factors as the composition of the antigen, the amount of antigen used, the magnification at which the test is read, flat vs. concave slides, etc.

RPR Test. Other tests for detecting reagin are also available. One of the most popular alternatives to the VDRL test is the **rapid plasma reagin** (RPR) test. This test uses the VDRL cardiolipin antigen modified by the incorporation of choline chloride and inclusion of charcoal indicator particles. The choline chloride inactivates inhibitors so that the serum or plasma does not have to be heated prior to the test. The coagglutination of the charcoal particles renders the serological reaction easily visible to the naked eye and therefore does not have to be read under the microscope. The RPR test is performed on plastic-coated cards within 14- or 18-mm circles or teardrop-shaped reaction areas. The patient's serum (or plasma) is mixed with the RPR antigen on the card, and it is mechanically rotated at 100 rpm for eight minutes under a humidifying cover to prevent evaporation. Then it is read macroscopically in the wet state for agglutination (Figure 6.8). Only two reactions are recognized: (1) reactive—showing any type of clumping, and (2) nonreactive—showing slight roughness or no clumping. The test can be quantitated on the card if desired.

The antigen supplied with the RPR kit requires no preparation. This is a distinct advantage over the VDRL test where improper preparation of the antigen can lead to spurious results. The RPR test has not been approved for testing spinal fluids, whereas the VDRL has been so approved. Biological false positive reactions occur in both types of tests. BFP reactions in RPR tests have been reported to be associated with many of the same diseases that produce BFP reactions in VDRL tests. Other related treponemal diseases such as pinta, yaws, and bejel produce positive reactions in RPR tests, but they should not be considered false. The concentrations of anticoagulants EDTA and heparin are not critical, but an excess of potassium oxalate or sodium fluoride may cause improper RPR results. Even low concentrations of positively charged chemicals (e.g., quarternary ammonium compounds) may produce false positive reactions in RPR tests.

Direct Nonimmune Agglutination

VIRAL HEMAGGLUTINATION

In 1941 J. C. Hirst discovered that influenza virus (myxovirus) agglutinates chicken red blood cells. Since then, many other viruses have been found to have nonserological hemagglutinating properties including vaccinia, variola, dengue, ECHO group, Coxsackie group, mumps, some members of the encephalitides group, parainfluenza viruses, rabies, and many more. The type of erythrocytes agglutinated varies from one virus to another. For example, influenza viruses seem to react best with red cells of the chicken, guinea pig, or human group O. Viruses are noncellular, obligate intracellular parasites. In their mature infectious stage, viruses consist of a core of nucleic acid (either RNA or DNA) that carriers the genetic information, surrounded by a protein coat called a **capsid** (Figure 6.9). The capsid possesses binding sites for specific attachment to receptor sites on host cells. A complete, potentially virulent virus particle is called a **virion**. The capsid usually consists of many identical subunits called **capsomeres**. The capsid of some viruses may also be surrounded by remnants of a highly modified host cell membrane acquired when the virus was released by a "budding" process. This lipoprotein layer is called a **peplos** or **envelope**. Many of the proteins detected in the peplos are synthesized by the host cell according to viral genetic instructions and become incorporated into its plasma membrane prior to virion release by budding. These proteins are

Agglutination

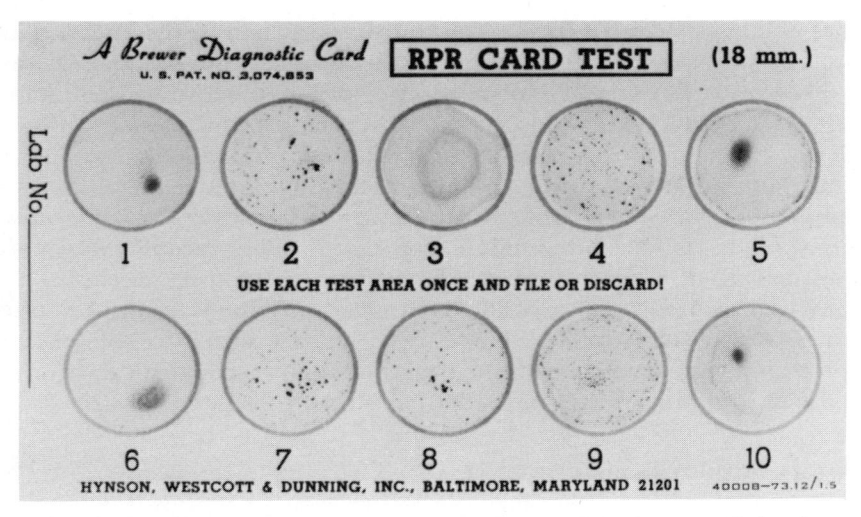

FIGURE 6.8. RPR card test for syphilitic reagin. This photograph is of a file card containing dried specimens. Positive reactions are in circles 2, 4, 7, 8, and 9. Swirling of the card during the test tends to cause unagglutinated charcoal particles (circles 1, 3, 5, 6, and 10) to congregate in one area.

organized within the peplos into discrete structural subunits called **peplomeres,** which may be visualized by electron microscopy. The peplomeres serve as specific binding sites by which the virion can attach to susceptible host cells in the initial stage of the infection process. Antibodies produced in response to proteins of the capsomeres or peplomeres play an important role in specifically neutralizing the infectivity of virions before they can attach to target tissues. A few viruses such as those of the herpes group pass directly by membrane fusion from an infected cell into an adjacent healthy cell. Antibodies produced in response to a virus that spreads in this fashion do not produce immunity because the antibodies cannot enter the cells and the virus is rarely exposed extracellularly. If the host cell membrane's molecular structure is sufficiently modified by viral infection to represent a "foreign" antigenic determinant, it may be attacked by T lymphocytes.

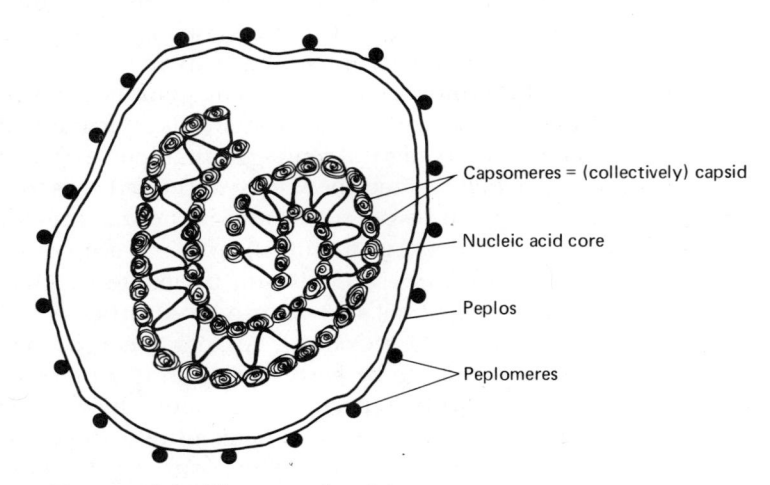

FIGURE 6.9. Diagram of a virion.

Serology and Immunology

Since children with defective B cell functions (agammaglobulinemics) can recover from most viral diseases of childhood, T cell immunity to viruses is inferred to be an extremely potent source of defense against these pathogens.

Two kinds of viral peplomeres are found on influenza virions: (1) hemagglutinin, and (2) neuraminidase. Hemagglutinins are glycoprotein complexes and are responsible for attachment of viruses to specific receptors on red blood cells. Neuraminidase (sometimes called **receptor destroying enzyme** or RDE) is an enzyme that hydrolyzes neuraminic acid linkages of many mucoproteins and probably is involved in some way with the infection process. This enzyme can destroy receptor sites on host cells and thereby interfere with the viral hemagglutination reaction or can reverse a viral hemagglutination reaction that has already occurred.

HEMAGGLUTINATION INHIBITION

Some viruses cause hemagglutination (HA) of certain red blood cells. This knowledge is used by state and federal virology laboratories as an aid in the identification of certain kinds of viruses. Specific antiviral antibodies can combine with these HA viruses and "neutralize" their ability to cause hemagglutination. The **hemagglutination inhibition** (HI) test is widely used in hospital laboratories as an aid in detecting exposure of patients to specific viruses. In the HI test, the patient's serum is incubated with known hemagglutinating viral antigen (inactivated virus) and then the mixture is exposed to red cells. The absence of agglutination of the red cells is indicative of a positive test (specific antiviral antibody is present). The HI test can also be used with an antibody of known antiviral specificity to identify and titrate an unknown virus isolated from a patient. Many problems are involved in isolation of a virus, and only a few research or reference laboratories are equipped and staffed to do this kind of work. Hence, in hospital laboratories, the HI test is almost invariably performed to determine the titer of a specific antiviral hemagglutinin in a patient's serum. The major disadvantage of the HI test is that the patient's serum may contain substances (usually sialic acid–containing mucoproteins) that nonspecifically inhibit agglutination. In addition, the patient's serum may also contain native agglutinins for the erythrocytes used as indicator cells. Therefore, a serum to be titrated for its antiviral activity must first be treated to remove the nonspecific inhibitors of viral hemagglutination and to remove any native hemagglutinins for the indicator cells. The methods used to remove nonspecific inhibitors of viral hemagglutination vary considerably depending on the viral antigen and the source of the red cells to be used in the test. For example, sera to be tested for anti-influenza antibodies can be treated with heat (56°C for thirty minutes), trypsin, receptor-destroying enzyme (RDE) of *Vibrio cholerae,* or potassium periodate (KIO_4). In a case of suspected rubella, the patient's serum can be adsorbed with kaolin. Studies by CDC (Center for Disease Control, Atlanta, Georgia) have shown that HI rubella test titers tend to be higher (indicating a more sensitive test) if the serum is treated with heparin–manganous chloride or dextran sulfate rather than kaolin. Nonspecific hemagglutinins can be adsorbed from the patient's serum prior to the test by exposure to the same type of erythrocytes as will be used in the test. Because the pure viral antigen is so expensive, the HI test is usually performed in Microtiter plates (wells in a plastic block) using less than 0.1 ml of the antigen preparation per well.

As an example of how an HI test is performed, let us consider a test for antirubella virus antibodies. Before the HI test can be performed, a hemagglutination (HA) test must be done to standardize the antigen. Inactivated rubella virus is commercially available. Serial doubling dilutions of the antigen are made with a buffer solution from 1:4 through 1:512. A constant amount of chicken erythrocytes is added to each well including a cell control containing only buffer and cells. The plate is shaken and incubated at 4°C for up to one and one-half hours or until a compact button of cells forms in the control well (a negative reaction). The virus can elute from the cells at higher temperatures or after prolonged incubation; so these conditions must be avoided in the test. Agglutination is indicated by adherence of the red cells to the bottom of the well as a film of cells that does not flow when the plate is tilted (Figure 6.10). The last well (greatest dilution of antigen) that shows complete agglutination contains 1 hemagglutination unit (1 HA unit).

Three serums are used in an HI test: (1) patient's serum, (2) known positive control serum, and (3) known negative control serum. All three sera are adsorbed with kaolin for twenty minutes at room temperature with frequent shaking. Alternatively and preferentially, the sera can be treated with a 1:1 mixture of heparin–manganous chloride for fifteen minutes at 4°C. The treated sera are centrifuged and then adsorbed with chicken erythrocytes at 4°C for one hour. After another centrifugation, the kaolin-adsorbed supernatant fluids are pipetted into clean tubes and heated at 56°C for thirty minutes (sera treated with heparin–manganous chloride should not be heat inactivated). The sera are now ready for the HI test.

Doubling dilutions of the treated sera are made (1:10 through 1:160). Four units of virus antigen are added to each well. If the end-point dilution of the antigen titration was 1:32 (containing 1 HA unit), then 4 HA units would be in 32/4 = 1:8 dilution. The plate is shaken and incubated at 4°C for one hour. Indicator cells are added, the plate is shaken, and it is again incubated at 4°C up to one and one-half hours or until the cell control well (containing only buffer and cells) develops a compact button. A kaolin-treated serum control well is also run simultaneously, containing treated patient's serum, buffer, and indicator cells (no virus antigen). The wells are read for agglutination. The end-point HI titer is the reciprocal of the high-

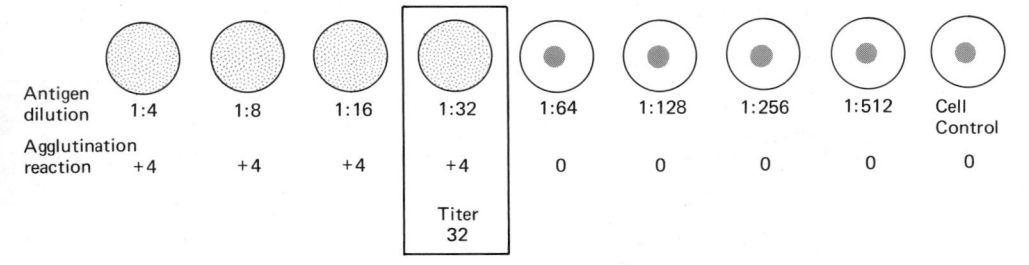

Antigen dilution	1:4	1:8	1:16	1:32	1:64	1:128	1:256	1:512	Cell Control
Agglutination reaction	+4	+4	+4	+4	0	0	0	0	0
				Titer 32					

FIGURE 6.10. Hemagglutination (HA) test for standardizing rubella antigen. In this example, the titer of the viral antigen is in the well with the highest dilution of antigen showing complete agglutination (as indicated by a lacy pattern of indicator cells coating the bottom of the well).

Serology and Immunology

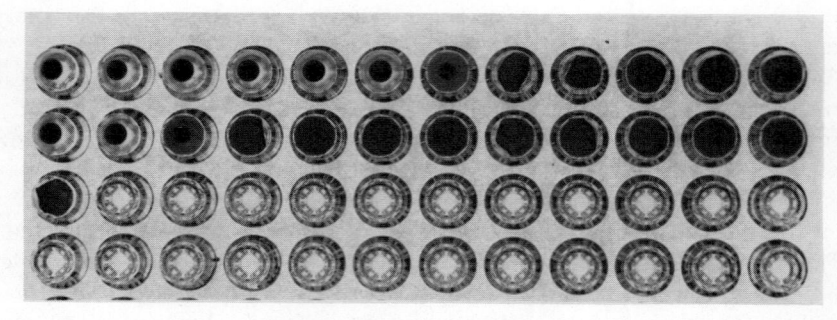

FIGURE 6.11. Titration of specimens for rubella virus hemagglutination inhibition antibodies in Microtiter plate. The HI end point of the convalescent specimen (top row) is in well 6 from the left. Viral hemagglutination is completely inhibited in wells 1 to 6. Well 7 is partly agglutinated and wells 8 to 12 are completely agglutinated. The end point of an acute specimen (second row) is in well 2. A virus hemagglutination control is in the third row. The bottom row contains empty wells. All serum specimens are serially diluted left to right. Microtiter plates are viewed from beneath by reflection in a mirror.

est serum dilution that completely inhibits hemagglutination (Figure 6.11). The positive serum control should inhibit hemagglutination within one dilution of the titer specified by the manufacturer of the kit. Agglutination should be observed in all dilutions of the negative control serum; no agglutination should be seen in either the treated patient's serum control or the red cell control (no antigen added).

One more control should be run concurrently with the HI test. This control is called the **antigen dilution confirmation test.** This is a **backtitration** of the virus antigen to confirm that 4 HA units were added to each well of the HI test. If it was determined from the antigen standardization test that a 1 : 8 dilution of virus contained 4 HA units, then five wells would be set up containing serial doubling dilutions with buffer from 1 : 8 through 1 : 256. A constant amount of indicator cells is added, the plate is shaken, and it is incubated at 4°C for up to one and one-half hours, or until the cell control well forms a compact button. If there were four HA units in the 1 : 8 dilution of virus, then there should be complete agglutination only in the first three wells of the antigen dilution confirmation test (Fig. 6.12). If more than three wells show agglutination, the antigen used in the HI test needs to be diluted further. If less than three wells have agglutination, more virus needs to be used in the HI test.

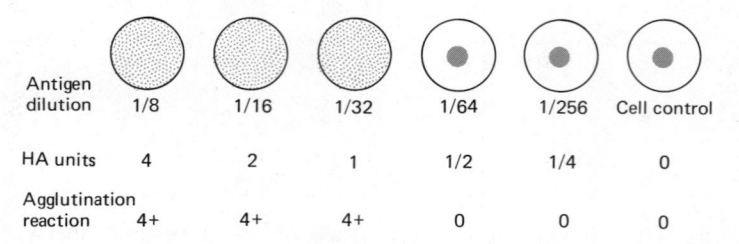

Antigen dilution	1/8	1/16	1/32	1/64	1/256	Cell control
HA units	4	2	1	1/2	1/4	0
Agglutination reaction	4+	4+	4+	0	0	0

FIGURE 6.12. Example of an antigen dilution confirmation test for rubella virus. If 4 HA units are in one-eighth dilution of the virus, then 1 HA unit should be in one fourth of this amount ($1/4 \times 1/8 = 1/32$).

A rash usually develops within two to three weeks after exposure to rubella virus, but subclinical cases are not uncommon. HI antibodies can usually be detected about two weeks after initial infection. Therefore, some patients may have an HI titer when the rash first appears. Maximum titers usually develop within five weeks and remain elevated for a relatively long time. If the HI test is being used as a screener to establish the immune status of an individual (e.g., premarital examination, potential candidate for rubella vaccine), then only one sample is taken. An HI titer of 1 : 10 or greater in the screening test may be considered indicative of current infection or immunity. If rubella disease is suspected to be active in a patient, a blood specimen should be obtained within three days of the appearance of the rash, and a second specimen obtained about three weeks later. A fourfold or greater rise in HI titer between these paired sera may be considered as confirmation of a rubella infection. If no rise in titer is noted, the patient probably did not have a rubella infection in that time interval. If the titers in both specimens are less than 1 : 10, the patient is probably not immune. Rubella (German measles) is a relatively benign, self-limiting illness in all postnatal infections. However, if a nonimmune pregnant woman becomes infected during the first trimester, the consequences to her baby may be very severe. If the baby is not stillborn, it may have one or more congenital defects including cataracts, deafness, heart defects, enlarged liver and spleen (hepatomegaly, splenomegaly), encephalitis, meningitis, mental retardation, abnormally small head size (microencephaly), anemia, and many other abnormalities. If a pregnant woman shows clinical signs of rubella during early gestation, attempts at passive immunization can be made. However, administration of immune gamma globulin to pregnant mothers has not been conclusively demonstrated to be effective in preventing damage to their babies. Some women choose to undergo therapeutic abortion to prevent the birth of a rubella-damaged child. Whatever the decision, the consequences are often unpleasant, especially today when rubella could have been prevented by prior immunization. All preschoolers (both boys and girls) should be immunized against rubella. If this were done, within one generation most women of childbearing age would be immune and surrounded by other people most of whom also were immune and incapable of passing on the disease. Premarital blood testing of women for HI titers can reveal those who are not immune to rubella and in need of immunization. The decision to immunize women of childbearing age (married or otherwise) must be based on (1) establishment that the woman is not already pregnant (pregnancy testing) and (2) thorough understanding by the woman of the dire consequences that could ensue if she were to become pregnant soon after exposure to the live virus vaccine. The attending physician would probably ask the woman to sign a legal document releasing the physician from liability if she were to become pregnant soon after the vaccination. Inactivated ("killed") virus vaccines have not proven effective; so for now, attenuated live virus vaccines are the only ones available.

Although differing somewhat in details and ramifications, HI tests for other antiviral hemagglutinins follow procedures essentially similar to those of the rubella test. For example, there are three serotypes of the influenza virus that affect humans. Serotype A is responsible for epidemics or pandemics; type B is seen in local outbreaks of the disease; type C is rare and of localized incidence. Type A virus causes influenza in swine, horses, and ducks as well as humans; types B and C infect only humans. The type A virus can mutate to new antigenic forms and thereby can spread rapidly into an epidemic in the nonimmune population. This phenomenon is called **immunological (antigenic) drift** or **shift,** and the ensuing success of the virus in spreading throughout the population is a classical example of how natural selection functions in the evolutionary process. An antigenic shift may involve the hemagglutinin protein determinant (H_x) and/or the neuraminidase protein determinant (N_x). Influenza type A_0 (H_0N_1) was the cause of the 1918 pandemic. It experienced an antigenic shift about 1947 and became type A_1 (H_1N_1). Another shift to type A_2 (H_2N_2) was responsible for the Asian flue of 1957. This shift was interesting in that both the H and N determinants mutated at about the same time. The Hong Kong flu epidemic of 1968–1969 was caused by type A_3 (H_3N_2). In 1977, it appeared as though an antigenic shift had occurred in Russia reverting back to the A_0 (H_0N_1) type. Reversion to this older type of virus could again cause an epidemic because most people are too young to have contacted it before and consequently are nonimmune. Fortunately, an influenza vaccine can be prepared quickly after a new serotype appears. However, there is no way to predict in what direction it will shift in the future. So while "flu shots" can offer some short-lived protection to the currently prevalent forms of influenza virus, they may confer little or no long-term protection because of the antigenic differences that arise with antigenic shifts. Diagnosis of a recent influenza infection requires at least a fourfold rise in HI titers between paired sera collected two to three weeks apart. Consequently, results of the HI test provide little or no guidance for the management of the patient with acute influenza. Diagnosis of the antigenic type of virus responsible for an outbreak of flu in a community can aid in management of clinically similar cases and dictate the type of vaccine most likely to be effective.

Indirect (Passive) Agglutination

In this class of agglutinating phenomena, the antigen with which the antibody reacts is soluble. Fluid precipitation tests require relatively large aggregates of antigen-antibody complexes to appear as a visible reaction to the naked eye. Therefore, the sensitivity of fluid precipitation tests is relatively low. Zonal reactions can occur outside the region of optimal proportions, making false negative reactions a common problem. By attachment of soluble antigens to inert carrier particles, the antigens become serologically detectable by the indirect or passive agglutination of the large particles. In other words, the agglutinins are not reacting with native determinants of the carrier particle, but rather with antigens or haptens attached to the particle. Among the kinds of particles employed for passive agglutination are red cells, latex particles, colloidal charcoal, bentonite, and collodion. One of the problems in using cells as carrier particles is the possibility of "natural" antibodies or cross-reactive antibodies in the patient's serum against cellular (carrier) antigens, thereby producing false positive passive agglutination reactions. This problem may be eliminated by pretreatment of the serum with uncoated cells to absorb the antibodies directed against cellular antigens. Erythrocytes are good carrier particles because they readily adsorb polysaccharides and lipopolysaccharides. However, erythrocytes have a short shelf life and soon begin to autolyse. Red cells treated with formaldehyde or glutaraldehyde turn dark brown, but become resistant to lysis and can even be frozen or lyophilized. Polysaccharides adsorbed onto red cells can spontaneously elute and become haptenic inhibitors of passive agglutination by homologous antibodies. It is therefore important to wash such reagent cells immediately prior to use in a serological test. Treatment of red cells with tannic acid tends to stabilize the adsorbed polysaccharides. In addition, tanned red cells adsorb proteins readily, making them very useful indicator particles for antibodies directed against soluble protein antigens. The addition of normal rabbit serum (NRS) or other colloids to diluting saline inhibits the tendency toward spontaneous agglutination by tanned red cells. Tanned cells tend to be easily lysed; so they are usually formalinized prior to being tanned. Chemicals such as dinitrofluorobenzene (DNFB), bisdiazotized benzidine, and toluene diisocyanate can be used to covalently couple the soluble antigen to the red cell. A tanned, formalinized red cell to which the soluble antigen is covalently bound becomes a long-lived, stable indicator particle of great utility in passive hemagglutination reactions. Passive agglutination tests are usually very sensitive, able to detect as little as 0.03 μg of antibody nitrogen, and serum titers of over 1:1,000,000 are not uncommon.

PASSIVE HEMAGGLUTINATION TESTS

Rubella Test. Antibodies to rubella virus can be detected by a passive hemagglutination (PHA) test. A commercial kit typically contains (1) lyophilized, stabilized erythrocytes, sensitized with a soluble rubella virus antigen, (2) a positive control serum, and (3) a dilution buffer. If a negative control serum is not included in the kit, one should be provided by the user. The test is performed in disposable V-bottom Microtiter® plates. Microtiter is the registered trademark of Cooke Laboratory Products (Division of Dynatech Laboratories, Inc.), Alexandria, Virginia. The Microtiter system is commonly used for titrations by serial doubling dilutions or for tests that use only microliter (lambda) quantities of costly reagents. The specimen (or control sera) are added to the buffer, followed by the reconstituted erythrocyte reagent. After about two hours of incubation at room temperature, the plate is examined for agglutination by looking at the bottom of the plate reflected in a mirror. A positive result is indicated by a dispersed settling pattern of agglutinated cells in a well. A negative result is indicated by a sharp, compact button of unagglutinated cells in the V bottom of a well.

Anti-rubella antibody titers, as determined by the PHA test, exhibit a delayed rise relative to hemagglutination inhibition (HAI) titers, but continue to rise for three or four months. Once the PHA antibody concentration reaches a plateau, the titers of antibody as determined by both methods are comparable. According to the Center for Disease Control (CDC), "The presence of any level of HAI antibody equal to or greater than 1:8 indicates past rubella infection at some undetermined time, and thus immunity to primary infection." Under this condition, there is no need for the patient to be vaccinated. The PHA test is recommended for testing specimens from individuals with clinical symptoms of rubella or suspected exposure to rubella virus. However, for determining recent rubella infection in a pregnant woman, the PHA test should not be used. In this special case, a HAI test is recommended.

Serum Hepatitis Test. Hepatitis is another viral disease for which a passive hemagglutination test is commercially available. Serum hepatitis is considered to be one of the major hazards to both patients and technologists in transfusion of blood and blood products or working with these substances in the clinical laboratory. Hepatitis B surface antigen (HB_sAg) is thought to be a component of the hepatitis B virus (HBV). It was formerly described as Australia antigen (AuA). This antigen is shed into the blood by hepatitis patients and by chronically infected carriers of HBV. Several tests are available for detecting HB_sAg in serum or plasma. The least sensitive ("first-generation") test is agar gel diffusion. "Second-generation" tests for HB_sAg are five to ten times as sensitive as first-generation tests; they include counterelectrophoresis, complement fixation, and reversed passive latex agglutination. "Third-generation" tests, such as radioimmunoassay and reversed passive hemagglutination, are about 100 times as sensitive as first-generation tests.

Diagnosis of serum hepatitis can be confirmed by detecting either HB_sAg or anti-HB_s in the patient's serum. Following recovery, HB_sAg disappears from the serum, but anti-HB_s tends to persist. The reagent used for detecting anti-HB_s in the passive hemagglutination test kit consists of highly purified HB_sAg conjugated to human group O red blood cells. The test is performed in wells of a Microtiter® plate. The serum sample is mixed with the viral reagent cells, incubated, and centrifuged. The plate is placed at a 60° angle and read. A specimen containing anti-HB_s will passively agglutinate the reagent cells and produce a distinct button of cells at the bottom of the well. If the specimen is negative (no antibody present), the unagglutinated cells will flow down the vertex of the well. The test can be performed as a screen for detecting the presence of anti-HB_s or as a titration test for determining the end point of antibody present.

The kit should be supplied with at least three controls: (1) a cell control consisting of human group O red blood cells from the same source as that used to prepare the reagent cells, (2) a positive control serum containing anti-HB_s, and (3) a negative control serum. The cell control may agglutinate if atypical blood group antibodies in the sample are homologus with blood group antigens on the reagent cells. Natural and acquired agglutinins to human red cells are usually in low titers. As an indication of anti-HB_s, a sample should therefore have a titer with reagent cells at least fourfold greater than that found with control red cells. Microorganisms can produce metabolites that cause nonspecific agglutination of red cells. The manufacturer should specify the expected end-point titer for the positive control serum. The end point of titration is the greatest dilution that gives a complete button of reagent cells. The positive control serum should show a reaction pattern within two dilutions of the specified titer; lower titers indicate a loss of sensitivity; higher titers may indicate nonspecific agglutination of cells.

It is possible to determine if a positive reaction is a true or false positive. The test serum is mixed with several dilutions of a serum known to contain HB_sAg. A control titration with untreated serum is performed simultaneously. Reagent cells are then added. If the end-point titer of the serum mixed with HB_sAg is reduced, the sample is a true positive. If the end point is not diminished, it is a false positive.

The incidence of serum hepatitis among volunteer blood donors may vary from 4 percent to 20 percent; among commercial donors, rates are often higher. The greatest incidence of HB_sAg and highest titers of anti-HB_s are found in patients who have been multiply exposed to blood or blood products, such as those who have received multiple blood transfusions or hemophilic patients who have received specific clotting factors. In general, the incidence of anti-HB_s tends to increase with age, leveling off at age fifty. It is higher among those of lower socioeconomic status. Those especially at risk include institutionalized children, hospital and lab personnel, and dialysis unit patients and personnel.

RF TEST

Rheumatoid arthritis is a chronic systemic disease of unknown etiology characterized mainly by recurrent inflammatory episodes involving the synovium (lining of the joint cavity). About three times as many women suffer from this form of arthritis as men. Farm workers seem to be twice as susceptible as urban workers. It is hypothesized that rheumatoid arthritis is an autoimmune disease, but proof is still lacking. According to one theory, the disease is initiated by an infection of the joint. Inflammatory cells and antibodies then move into the synovial cavity (Figure 6.13). Lysosomal enzymes released by the inflammatory cells damage the Fc region of IgG antibodies and create new antigenic determinants (neoantigens). In response to these neoantigens, antibodies of classes IgM and IgG appear, called **rheumatoid factor** (RF). RF reacts with the modified IgG, these complexes stimulate another round of chemotactic and anaphylatoxic reactions, and the disease is perpetuated as a series of cyclical exacerbations. Much more must be learned before it will be known if the theory has any merit. One of the problems with the theory is its failure to account for the fact that RF also reacts with IgG from some apparently normal people and even reacts with IgG from rabbits and other species. As a matter of fact, the ability of RF to react selectively with certain human IgG molecules was the way that Gm subgroups or allotypes were originally discovered. It is now known that rheumatoid factors also occur in other major immunoglobulin classes, but tests for the IgM class of RF are the only ones routinely performed in the clinical laboratory because of the much greater agglutinating capacity of IgM molecules. These tests for RF(IgM) tend to be inhibited by self-association of IgG molecules, and IgG may need to be removed from the serum (e.g., by gel filtration in acid buffers) before the RF (IgM) test is run. Rheumatoid factors revealed following gel filtration are called "hidden rheumatoid factors." Injecting RF into synovial sacs of healthy individuals does not provoke rheumatoid arthritis. It thus appears that RF is a product of the disease rather than its cause. Many other chronic inflammatory diseases also generate RF, including lupus erythematosus, bacterial endocarditis, tuberculosis, leprosy, syphilis, cancer, etc. Even apparently healthy individuals may have RF titers. In other words, the RF test is certainly not specific for rheumatoid arthritis. Rheumatoid factor has been detected in about 75 percent of clinically diagnosed cases of rheumatoid arthritis.

Serology and Immunology

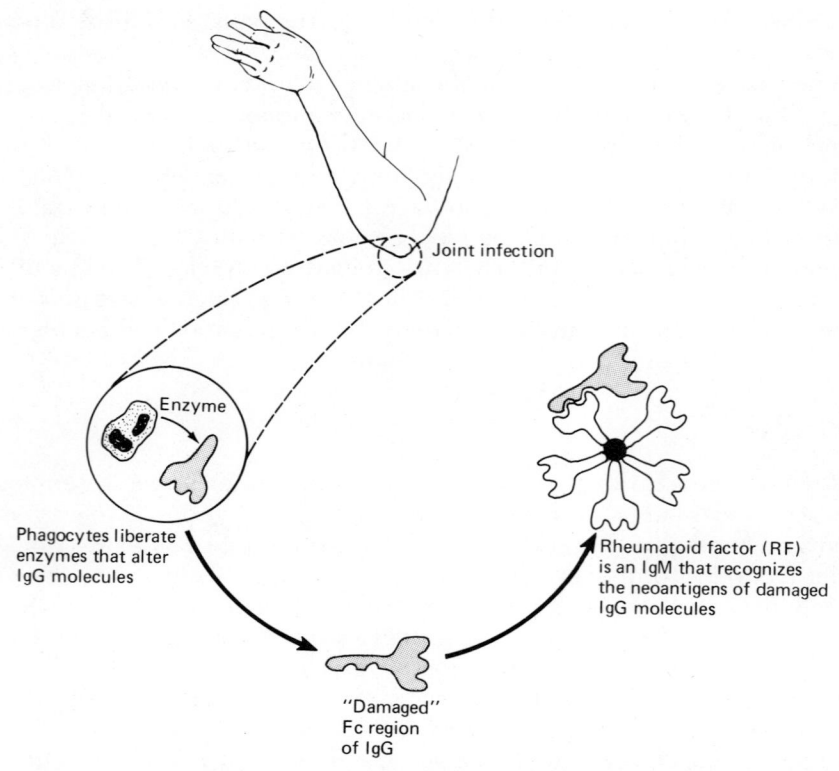

FIGURE 6.13. Diagram of one theory for the production of rheumatoid factor (RF). It is thought that RF is an IgM antibody against altered Fc portions of IgG molecules.

There is little correlation between the RF titer and the severity of the disease. Titers exceeding 1:80 are usually confirmatory of some current or recent RF-provoking disease, but titers of less than 1:20 are considered to constitute a negative test.

Test kits for RF are commercially available and contain a buffered saline diluent, positive and negative control sera, and an IgG-particle complex. IgG can be adsorbed or linked to latex particles. When RF (IgM) in the patient's serum combines by its Fab region to the Fc region of certain IgG molecules, the latex particle to which IgG is attached becomes passively agglutinated, indicating a positive test. Slide tests are usually read against a dark background so the light-colored latex aggregates can be more easily seen (Figure 6.14). A tube test on serially diluted serum can be employed for a quantitative test. All sera should be heated at 56°C for thirty minutes prior to the test to aid in inactivation of substances (including fraction C1q of complement) that tend to produce false positive reactions. Sheep erythrocytes coated with rabbit gamma globulin may also be used as an indicator particle. Latex tests are generally more sensitive but less specific than erythrocyte tests. High-titer heterophile hemagglutinins against sheep red cells give biological false positive reactions. If necessary, these could be removed prior to the RF test by absorption of the sera with native sheep cells, but this materially detracts from the utility (time, cost) of the test in the clinical laboratory.

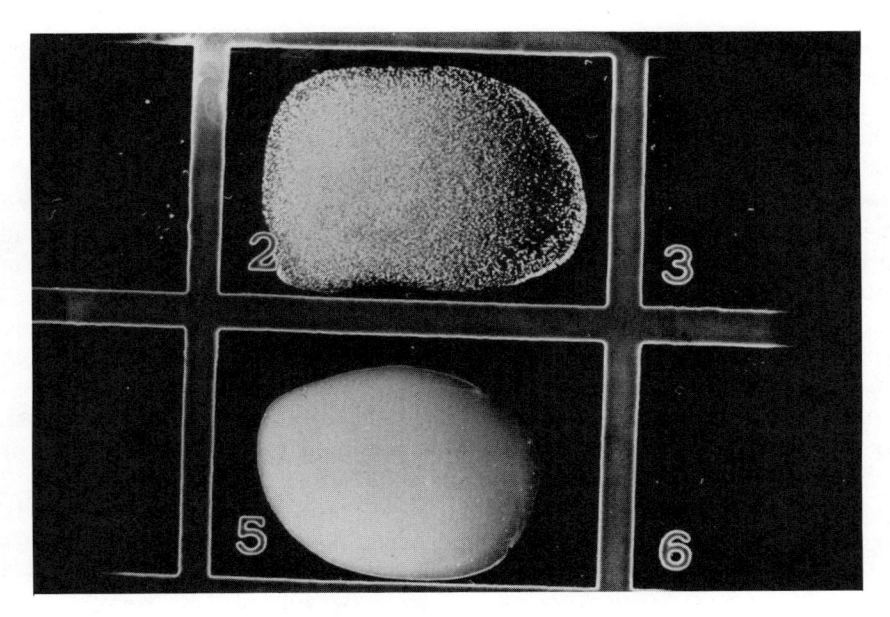

FIGURE 6.14. Passive agglutination of latex particles in a slide test for rheumatoid factor (RF). Positive and negative reactions are at top and bottom, respectively. [*Courtesy of Elliot Scientific Corp., New York City.*]

INHIBITION TESTS

Pregnancy Tests for HCG. Among its many jobs, the placenta has an endocrine function. Within ten to fourteen days after the first missed menses or about forty-one days after onset of the last menstrual period (LMP), the hormone human chorionic gonadotropin (HCG) can be detected in the urine of pregnant women. With rare exception, this hormone (hapten) is absent in nonpregnant women. Test kits employ a latex or red cell particle coated with HCG. The patient's urine is first incubated with anti-HCG. If HCG is present in the urine, it will bind to the anti-HCG and inhibit any further reactivity of the antibody. HCG-coated latex particles are then added. If no agglutination occurs, then it is inferred that HCG was present in the specimen (Fig. 6.15). If HCG was not present, then anti-HCG would be free to passively agglutinate the particles. The test may be done as a slide or tube method, and as a qualitative or quantitative procedure. A known positive serum control and a negative control (either serum or saline) should be run concurrently. A negative reaction would be expected if the specimen is obtained less than forty-one days after onset of LMP. The urine sample should be clear and not grossly contaminated with bacteria. One way to avoid bacterial contamination is to use a sterile bottle and obtain a "clean catch," i.e., intercept the urine flow in midstream without touching the bottle to any part of the body. False positive results can be expected if the sample contains blood, bacteria, or protein. Titers in excess of 1:64 prior to sixty days or over 120 days after LMP may suggest a pathological condition such as diabetes, toxemia of pregnancy, Rh sensitization, hydatidiform mole, or chorionepithelioma. Normal urine titers for pregnant women seldom exceed 1:16. Titers of HCG normally tend to fall

Serology and Immunology

toward zero in the second and third trimesters of pregnancy, but by then more obvious signs of pregnancy are available.

Drugs of Abuse. A wide variety of simple chemicals (haptens) can become immunogenic if covalently coupled to larger carrier molecules such as bovine serum albumin. Injection of hapten-carrier complexes into rabbits can produce antibodies reactive with the hapten. Red blood cells coated with drugs of abuse such as barbiturates can be used as indicator particles in a hemagglutination-inhibition (HI) test to detect and titrate their levels in human urine.

The urine is first incubated with specific antibody (e.g., anticocaine) and then exposed to red blood cells coated with cocaine. If "coke" was present in the patient's urine, it would inactivate the antiserum so that reagent red cells fail to agglutinate. Standards for each drug are available by which quantitation in terms of $\mu g/ml$ can be obtained on each specimen. The hemagglutination inhibition test is very sensitive, capable of detecting 2 $\mu g/ml$ of barbiturates in a urine sample. HI tests can detect as little as 10 nanograms (0.010 microgram) of morphine per milliliter of urine, whereas thin-layer chromatography (TLC) or gas-liquid chromatography (GLC) will normally detect it in the range of 500 ng/ml. Because of the close structural similarity of some of the narcotic drugs (Figure 6.16), cross-reactivity is commonly a problem. For example, codeine (a common component of cough medicines) may react equally or in some cases better than morphine in immunoassays for the latter. Morphine is a drug that (when detected in a urine sample) indicates the use of heroin or that a patient is receiving morphine as an analgesic (painkiller). Negative results from highly sensitive immunoassays for drugs of abuse may be considered reliable, but all positive results should be considered ambiguous and must be confirmed by some nonimmunological procedure.

Drugs of abuse, HCG, and rheumatoid factor are only three examples in a virtually endless list of substances that can be detected by passive aggluti-

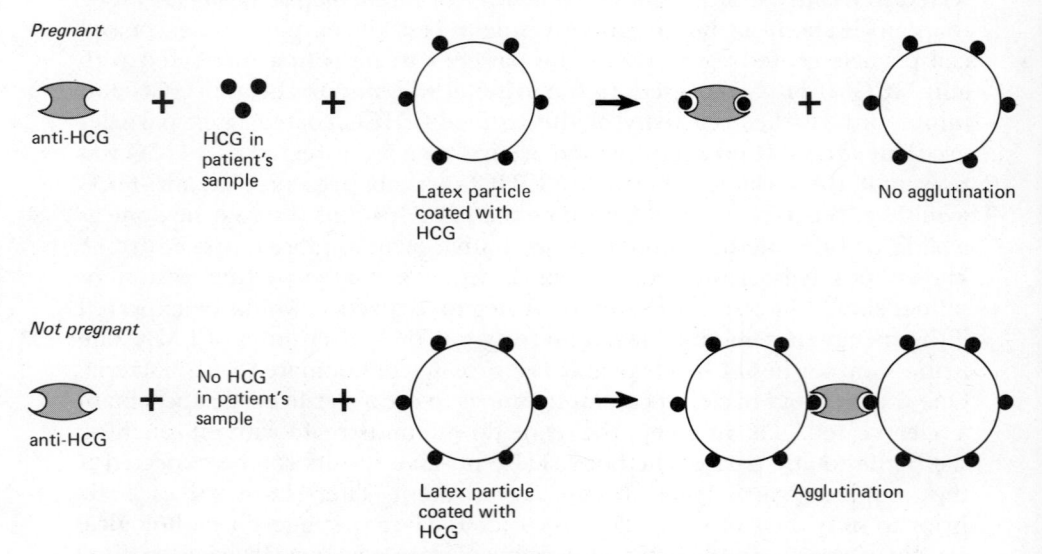

FIGURE 6.15. Hemagglutination inhibition test. Diagram of a pregnancy test based on the ability of the patient's HCG to inactivate the agglutinating properties of anti-HCG.

FIGURE 6.16. Structural similarity of heroin, codeine, and morphine.

nation or agglutination-inhibition techniques. Regardless of the specific hapten or antigen being assayed, the principle of the test is the same.

REVERSED PASSIVE AGGLUTINATION TESTS

One final modification of the indirect agglutination technique will be mentioned. If an antigen is being sought in the sample, and it is desired to avoid the preliminary antigen-antibody incubation of an inhibition test, then a **reversed passive agglutination** (RPA) test can be performed. In this technique it is antibody (rather than antigen) that is attached to the indicator particle. C-reactive protein was formerly detected by a precipitation test in capillary tubes. Now the method of choice is a reversed passive agglutination test with anti-CRP attached to latex particles (Figure 6.17). The reversed passive agglutination technique also lends itself to detecting almost any multivalent antigen for which a specific antibody is available to be attached to carrier particles.

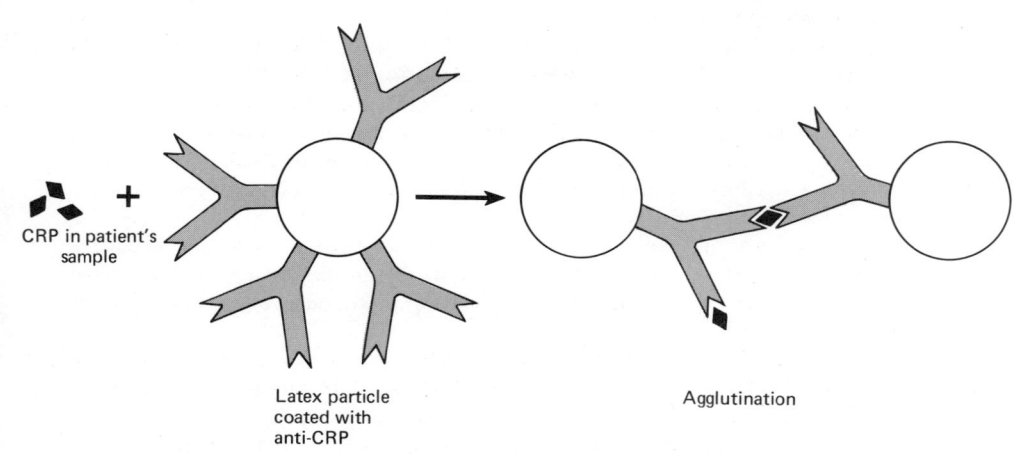

FIGURE 6.17. Example of a reversed passive latex agglutination test for CRP.

Serology and Immunology

SELF-EVALUATION

Terms

1. A serological category of antibodies often appearing in a patient after primary atypical pneumonia. (3 words)
2. Antibodies produced in response to one antigen, but cross-reacting with substances from unrelated sources (e.g., antibodies produced after infectious mononucleosis cross-react with sheep cells).
3. Agglutination test using *Salmonella* antigens.
4. An agglutination test for antirickettsial antibodies using *Proteus* antigens.
5. An antigen derived from beef heart used in the VDRL test for syphilitic reagin.
6. The most widely used kind of serological test for detecting antibodies to influenza, rubella, and certain other viruses that cause red cells to clump. (2 words)
7. A change in serological reactivity of a virus induced by mutation. (2 words)
8. The class of agglutination reactions in which a soluble antigen is coupled to an inert carrier particle prior to the test.
9. The class of agglutination reactions in which antibody is coupled to an inert carrier particle by its Fc fragment prior to the test. (2 words)
10. Any gain or loss of bacterial antigens (exemplified by S-R variation).

Multiple Choice. Choose the one best answer.

1. The sheep cell agglutinins associated with infectious mononucleosis are (a) absorbed by guinea pig kidney (GPK) antigen, but not by boiled beef cell extract (BC) (b) absorbed by BC, but not by GPK (c) absorbed by both GPK and BC (d) not absorbed by either GPK or BC (e) serologically unreactive with antigens of either GPK or BC
2. Flagellar antigens of bacteria are designated (a) F (b) H (c) K (d) O (e) R
3. Which of the following diseases would not be expected to generate febrile agglutinins? (a) rheumatic fever (b) typhoid fever (c) typhus (d) tularemia (e) brucellosis
4. Which of the following is not characteristic of the RPR test? (a) an agglutination test performed on a glass slide (b) specimen must be heated prior to the test (c) either serum or plasma may be used (d) antigen is mixed with charcoal particles (e) more than one of these
5. In addition to nonspecific cold hemagglutinins, patients with primary atypical pneumonia often have antibodies that agglutinate the MG strain of (a) *Brucella* (b) *Klebsiella* (c) *Streptococcus* (d) *Diplococcus* (e) *Shigella*
6. Before immunizing a woman for rubella, which of the following tests should be performed? (a) crossmatch (b) VDRL (c) ASO (d) HCG (e) RF
7. Which of the following is not part of the titration test for rubella antibodies? (a) absorption of natural hemagglutinins for chicken erythrocytes (b) doubling serial dilutions of the patient's serum (c) determination of the least amount of virus that can cause complete agglutination of the erythrocytes (d) incubation at 37°C (e) incubation at 4°C
8. Formalinized erythrocytes tend to make good indicator particles for a passive agglutination test because they (a) resist lysis (b) can be frozen or lyophilized (c) readily absorb protein haptens (d) tend to spontaneously aggregate (e) more than one of these
9. The conventional antigenic formula for *Salmonella* serotypes lists (1) somatic antigens, (2) phase 1 H antigens, and (3) phase 2 H antigens in the order (a) 1-2-3 (b) 1-3-2 (c) 3-2-1 (d) 2-3-1 (e) none of these
10. To be clinically significant, the minimal change in titer between paired sera should be (a) twofold (b) tripled (c) fourfold (d) sixfold (e) tenfold

True-False

1. Bacterial K antigens are usually present in R (rough) strains.
2. Suspensions of enteric bacteria are routinely heated before testing with agglutinating antisera against O antigens in order to destroy the inhibiting effects of the Vi antigen.
3. Specific aggregation of red cells by lectins is classified as a direct immune agglutination phenomenon.
4. The screener test for agglutinating heterophile antibodies requires that the serum be preheated to destroy complement.
5. The VDRL test is designed to detect specific antitreponemal antibodies of class IgM.
6. Agglutinations involving bacterial H antigens are expected to be more compact than those involving O antigens.
7. There is a strong correlation between reagin titer and the severity of syphilis.
8. Serological screening for narcotic drugs of abuse tends to lack specificity because of widespread cross-reactivity among them.
9. Encapsulated bacteria tend to be more resistant to phagocytosis than unencapsulated forms.
10. Most serological pregnancy tests are passive agglutination inhibition tests.

CHAPTER 7

Complement and Cytotoxicity

CHAPTER OUTLINE

The Complement System
   The Classical Pathway
   The Properdin Pathway
   Regulation of Complement Activity
   Specific Component Assays
Complement Fixation Tests
   Lytic CF Tests
      Hemolysin Titration
      Complement Titration
      Tests for Syphilitic Reagin
      Rice Test
   Nonlytic CF Test
Cytotoxicity
   Antistreptolysin Tests
   Potency of Toxins and Antitoxins
   Toxigenicity Tests of *Corynebacterium diphtheriae*
   Skin Tests for Immunity to Toxins
   Venoms
Self-evaluation

In 1894 Pfeiffer discovered a heat-labile cytolytic factor normally present in guinea pig serum that became activated by antibodies against cholera bacilli (*Vibrio cholerae*). Buchner named this factor **alexin** ("to ward off"). Bordet later found that alexin could also cause hemolysis in cooperation with antibodies against red blood cells. Ehrlich renamed it **complement** ("to make complete"). In those early days, complement was considered to be a single entity. Today, however, we know that complement consists of at least nine different proteins (C1, C2, . . . C9), all of which must be functional to produce cytolysis. Most of the complement components are easily denatured by heating serum at 56°C for thirty minutes, thus destroying the serum's cytolytic activity. Heat lability and antibody-initiated cytolytic activity were two classical hallmarks of the original complement concept.

Only immunoglobulins of classes IgM and IgG can activate the complement system. IgM is a much more efficient complement activator than IgG. Presumably complement must simultaneously bind to two adjacent immunoglobulin Fc regions in order to become activated. One IgM molecule furnishes the multiple adjacent Fc regions required to activate complement. It may require attachment of hundreds of times more IgG molecules on a cell in order to ensure that at least two of them would be close enough to bind a complement protein in common. Complement is not bound to an antigen-antibody complex to the same extent by all subclasses of IgG. The binding efficiency for complement (in order of diminishing affinity) is IgG3, IgG1, IgG2, IgG4; the latter weakly binds complement but fails to activate it. Not all IgM antibodies bind complement to the same extent, but this variability does not appear to be correlated with IgM subclasses. Antibodies of classes IgA, IgD, and IgE do not bind ("fix") complement in their native state. Prolonged heating of antisera to destroy complement would also diminish the antigen-binding capacity of IgD and IgE. This is an important consideration in preparation of sera for certain serological tests. The attachment site on IgM for complement is in its fourth constant domain on the heavy chain (C_H4); it is in the C_H2 domain of IgG near the hinge region. When antibody binds to antigen, it presumably undergoes a conformational change that exposes the complement-binding site. Likewise, the binding of the first complement protein (C1) to the antigen-antibody complex causes C1 to experience an **allosteric transformation** (shape change) that exposes a new site (allosteric site) by which it can react with another complement protein (C4). This changing of a nonenzymatic presursor (**proenzyme**) to an enzymatically active form is termed **complement activation.** From then on, a series of conversions from proenzymes to enzymes occurs, with other complement components behaving as substrates. The details of this **complement cascade** will be discussed in the next section of this chapter.

Some intermediates of the complement cascade have important biological functions of their own. Some of them (C3a and C5a) behave as **anaphylatoxins,** i.e., substances that degranulate mast cells. Recall that mast cells are the counterparts in tissues of basophils in blood and that their conspicuous cytoplasmic granules are rich in histamine and heparin. Anaphylatoxins stimulate mast cells to release these chemicals (degranulation). Histamine increases vascular permeability and thereby aids in (1) emigration of phagocytic leukocytes into the tissues, (2) passage of antibodies from the blood to the tissues, and (3) dilution of any bacterial toxins in the tissues. These are all potentially beneficial aspects of the inflammatory response, but they may also be accompanied by some undesirable effects. Increased vascular permeability produces **edema** (excess tissue fluid) that may be painful. Histamine also causes some smooth muscles to contract thereby producing allergic symptoms. For example, histamine may stimulate constriction of bronchioles in the lung, making breathing difficult (asthma, hay fever, etc.). Heparin is an anticoagulant also released by mast cell degranulation that alters normal blood clotting.

Some intermediates of the complement cascade qualify as **chemotaxins,** substances that attract leukocytes to migrate up the concentration gradient. Neutrophils are highly phagocytic leukocytes that are attracted by some of these chemotaxins. Mast cell granules also contain an eosinophilic chemotactic factor of anaphylaxis (ECF-A). Hence, when anaphylatoxin-stimulated mast cells degranulate, eosinophils would also be attracted to the site of release. This is why eosinophils are commonly seen in certain hypersensitivity reactions (especially in response to some allergies and parasites). At least one complement component behaves as an opsonin, a substance that modifies particles so as to facilitate their endocytosis by phagocytes. Still other complement proteins act as a "glue" in a phenomenon called **immune (serologic) adherence.** When particulate antigen, homologous antibody, and complement unite, the complex behaves as though it was "sticky," adhering indiscriminately to any surface, including blood vessel walls. Since phagocytic action is more efficient if the cell can trap the particle against a solid surface, immune adherence may also qualify as an opsonic phenomenon. Particles of many kinds may be nonspecifically trapped in immune adherence complexes including red cells, white cells, platelets, bacteria, yeast, etc. One of the complement components (C4) greatly enhances neutralization of viruses by homologous antibodies. The components of the complement system are discussed in the next section.

Serology and Immunology

The Complement System

The complement cascade is analogous to the coagulation cascade. Both systems consist of multiple proteins, some of which are proenzymes. Activation of the cascade depends on converting a proenzyme to a functional enzyme. Thereafter a series of such conversions, with some of the products serving as substrates for subsequent reactions, culminates in cytolysis or a blood clot (fibrin formation), respectively. There are three ways by which the complement cascade can become activated. The **classical pathway** is initiated when antibody unites with antigen. All nine major proteins of the complement system are involved in the classical pathway.

An alternate pathway (**properdin pathway**) is activated by a protein called **initiating factor** (IF). This factor may be identical to a gamma globulin called nephritic factor (NeF) found in the serum of patients with a nephritis that is associated with hypocomplementemia (subnormal levels of certain complement components in the blood). The properdin pathway (named for a relatively late-acting homotetrameric protein) may be nonspecifically stimulated by various complex lipopolysaccharides (many of which are derived from microbial cells). Three of the early-acting intermediates of the classical pathway are bypassed by other reactions; the later-acting components are common to both pathways.

A third pathway of complement activation begins with the conversion of **Hageman factor** (factor XII of the coagulation system) to its activated form. The stimulus that activates Hageman factor is unknown; possibly local trauma causes the release of tissue enzymes that activate it. Once activated, it results in the formation of plasmin. Plasmin is not only involved in both fibrin formation and fibrin digestion, but also in activation of C1 to initiate the complement cascade (same reactions as in the classical pathway). It is important to note that many of the protective functions of complement as well as some of the undesirable side effects commonly associated with the antibody-triggered classical activation pathway can also be produced in the absence of antibody (nonimmunological). For example, a patient with "hay fever–like" symptoms may not be responding immunologically to an allergen, but rather as a result of producing anaphylatoxins by nonserological activation of his complement system.

THE CLASSICAL PATHWAY

Attachment of antibody to antigen causes an allosteric structural change in the immunoglobulin, creating a complement receptor site. At least two of these receptors (on constant regions of heavy chains) must be in close proximity to bind and activate complement. These conditions are provided by a single IgM molecule. It usually requires relatively high concentrations of IgG to provide the same activating conditions. The first complement protein to attach is C1. This is a very complex molecule consisting of three subfractions designated C1q, C1r, C1s (Figure 7.1), held together by a calcium ion (Ca^{++}). Without calcium, the complex dissociates and activation does not occur. This is why plasma containing a calcium-binding anticoagulant is not a suitable specimen for a CF test. This also explains the use of calcium-enhanced saline as diluent for the CF test. The entire C1 protein is thought to consist of a single C1q molecule, two C1r molecules, and four C1s molecules. Fraction C1q has six immunoglobulin receptors and can bind up to six IgG molecules. Little is known about C1r other than it seems to act as an intermediate (perhaps also converted to an enzymatic form) between C1q and C1s in the activation process. C1s is a proenzyme in the native (unattached) C1 molecule. Upon attachment, an allosteric transformation presumably changes C1s into the active enzyme $\overline{\text{C1s}}$ (all activated complement components are designated by a bar over the symbol). C4 is the substrate for $\overline{\text{C1s}}$ (the symbols were assigned to the fractions before the order in which they reacted was fully known). A small inert fragment (C4a) is cleaved from C4; the remaining piece (C4b) is capable of binding to bacterial or erythrocyte membranes and to other antigens. If C4b cannot bind to a surface very near the antigen-antibody-$\overline{\text{C1qrs}}$ complex, no further reactions will occur. A characteristic of all enzymes is that they can catalyze a reaction over and over again without being consumed in the process. Therefore, $\overline{\text{C1s}}$ can cleave many C4 molecules, providing a tremendous biological amplification of complement-mediated phenomena. After C4b attaches to the surface, adsorption of C2 to C4b is aided by magnesium ions (Mg^{++}). This explains the need for magnesium salts in the diluent used in the CF test. The adsorbed C2 can now be split by the adjacent $\overline{\text{C1s}}$ into two large fragments. Therefore, the single enzyme $\overline{\text{C1s}}$ has two substrates (C4 and C2). Fragment C2a activates C4b into a functional enzyme called "C3 convertase" or $\overline{\text{C4b,2a}}$. Fragment C2b is apparently inert. C3 convertase then cuts C3 into two fragments (C3a, C3b). C3a has both chemotactic and anaphylatoxic properties but does not interact with other complement components. C3b joins C3 convertase to form a new enzymatic complex called "C5 convertase" ($\overline{\text{C4b,2a,3b}}$). Much of the enzymatic activity of both C3 convertase and C5 convertase is attributed to the C2a portion. C5 may then be split by C5 convertase into two fractions. The smaller fragment (C5a) is chemotactic and anaphylatoxic like C3a. The larger fragment (C5b) joins the complex and becomes the receptor for C6 and C7. The C5b,6,7 complex dissociates from the other complement components and attaches to the cell surface at a new site. The exact mechanism whereby cellular dissolution is accomplished is not known. When C8 joins the complex, however, Manfred Mayer proposes that the components of the C5b,6,7,8 assemblage arrange themselves in the lipid bilayer of the cell membrane to form a doughnut-shaped structure (Figure 7.2). The hole in the "doughnut" allows water and salts to flow into the cell. Cells bearing this complex will slowly lyse. The addition of C9 greatly accelerates lysis.

If the cell membrane was simply a semipermeable membrane, it would allow small molecules (water, salts) to pass through but prevent passage of large molecules (proteins). Given water, salts, and proteins on one side of a semipermeable membrane and only water and salts on the other side, a flow of water and salts would be expected through the membrane toward the side with the proteins. If this happened to a cell, it would swell until the membrane ruptures (a phenomenon known as the **Donnan effect**). Healthy cell membranes, however, do not behave as simple semipermeable structures. The cell has active transport mechanisms that pump substances through its membrane against concentration gradients by the expenditure of energy. However, when a cell membrane is damaged by complement, its properties become those of a semipermeable membrane. Water and salts (ions) flow into the cell causing it to burst (cytolysis). Through enzymatic

Serology and Immunology

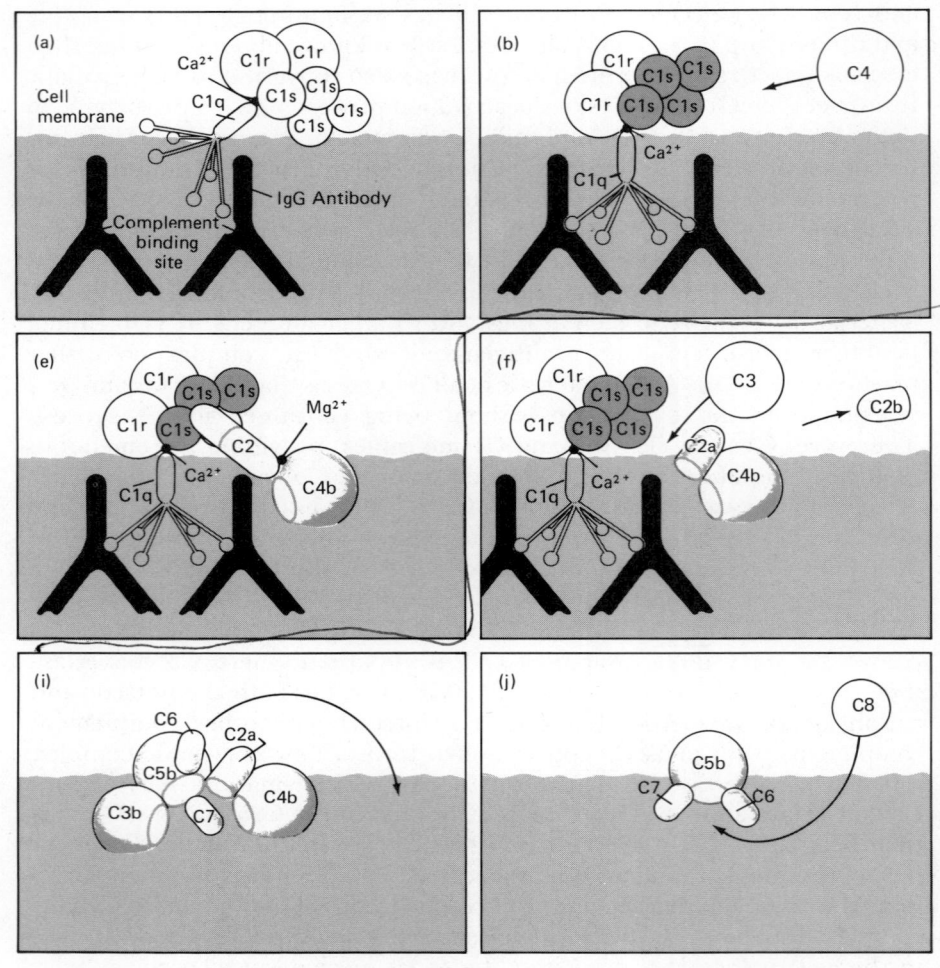

FIGURE 7.1. Diagram of the classical pathway of complement-mediated cytolysis. (*a*) C1 (consisting of three subunits C1q, C1r, and C1s connected by a calcium ion) can bind to adjacent immunoglobulin molecules following attachment of the antibodies to antigenic sites on the foreign cell. (*b*) Binding of C1q activates C1s to become a serine esterase enzyme (C$\overline{\mathrm{1s}}$). (*c*) C$\overline{\mathrm{1s}}$ splits C4 into two fragments (C4a and C4b). (*d*) C4b becomes attached to the cell surface nearby. (*e*) C2 is also cleaved into two fragments (C2a and C2b) by C$\overline{\mathrm{1s}}$. (*f*) C2a becomes attached to C4b with the help of magnesium ion and is converted into a proteolytic enzyme C$\overline{\mathrm{4b,2a}}$. (*g*) C3 is split into two fragments (C3a and C3b) by C$\overline{\mathrm{4b,2a}}$; C3b becomes attached to the cell surface. (*h*) If C3b is close to C$\overline{\mathrm{4b,2a}}$, this complex can bind and cleave C5 into two fragments (C5a and C5b). (*i*) C6 and C7 attach to C5b. (*j*) The C5b,6,7 complex dissociates from the C$\overline{\mathrm{3b,4b,2a}}$ complex and becomes attached to a different site on the cell and binds C8. (*k*) The C5b,6,7,8 complex assembles itself to form a small channel in the membrane through which some ions can pass. (*l*) The union of C9 to this complex greatly enlarges the channel and accelerates the passage of water and ions into the cell, resulting in osmotic cellular lysis. [From M. Mayer, "The Complement System," *Sci. Am. 229*, 54 (1973). Copyright © 1973 by Scientific American, Inc. All rights reserved.]

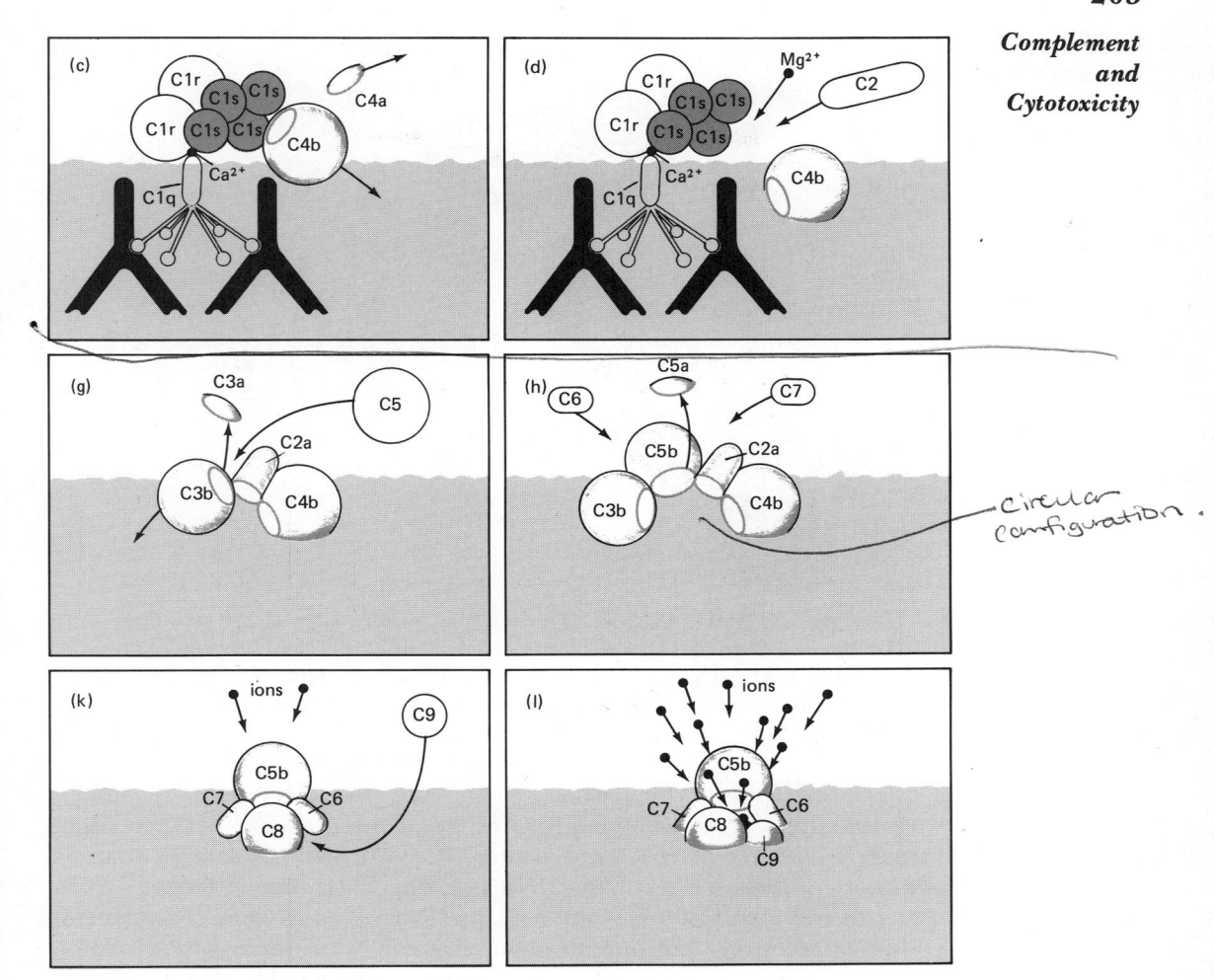

amplification of complement intermediates (e.g., one C$\overline{1s}$ molecule can cleave many C4 molecules), a single antibody attacking a cell may commonly produce multiple holes. It is not known how many "holes" must be made in a cell before it will lyse.

THE PROPERDIN PATHWAY

An alternative to the classical pathway for activation of the complement system involves a naturally occurring tetrameric plasma protein called **properdin** (Figure 7.3). This pathway can be activated in the absence of complement-binding antibodies (IgM, IgG) by a variety of naturally occurring particulate polysaccharides and lipopolysaccharides (LPS) including bacterial endotoxins as well as by IgA aggregates. The properdin pathway seems to provide a mechanism for promoting phagocytosis and for activating the inflammatory (chemotactic) and lytic properties of the complement system in the absence of immunoglobulins. It therefore may be an important component of early protection against bacterial invasion prior to the establishment of effective antibody levels.

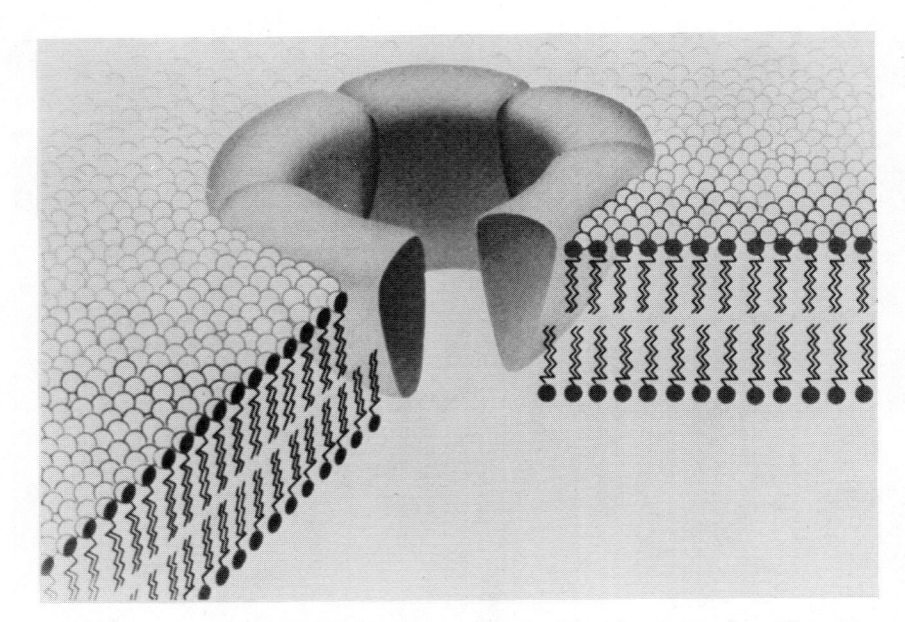

FIGURE 7.2. Mayer's model of a doughnut-shaped pore in the cell membrane created by the complement assemblage C5b,6,7,8,9. The cell membrane is a bilayer of lipid molecules stacked side by side with their polar heads facing outward and their nonpolar fatty-acid tails facing inward. [*From M. Mayer, "The Complement System,"* Sci. Am. *229,54 (1973). Copyright © 1973 by Scientific American, Inc. All rights reserved.*]

Five proteins have been identified in the properdin shunt: (1) initiation factor (IF), (2) factor B or proactivator (PA), (3) C3, (4) factor D or proactivator convertase (PAse), and (5) properdin (P). Initiation factor is a 7S dimer of two identical polypeptide chains. Proactivator is a β_1 glycoprotein consisting of a single polypeptide chain. Proteolytic activation of PA follows its cleavage into fragments Ba (inactive) and Bb ($\overline{\text{B}}$). The Bb fragment, formerly called C3 activator (C3A), is enzymatically active in cleaving C3, the same substrate as that for C2a (the classical-pathway counterpart of PA). Proactivator convertase (factor D) is an alpha globulin consisting of a single polypeptide chain. It functions as a serine esterase and is responsible for activating PA. The four polypeptide chains of properdin are of similar molecular weight and may be identical in primary structure.

Several possible mechanisms have been proposed for the initiation of the properdin pathway, only one of which will be discussed here. When IF contacts the activating particle (e.g., bacterial LPS), IF becomes activated ($\overline{\text{IF}}$) and interacts with PA (factor B), PAse (factor D), and C3 to produce a C3 convertase. This enzyme splits C3b from a free native C3 (not from the C3 portion of the enzyme); C3b then becomes deposited at sites on the particle nearby. Properdin can attach to closely associated particle-bound C3b fragments (properdin receptors) if factor B binds to these receptors. B then becomes activated by factor D and more firmly binds to the receptors. This bound-activated enzyme is a C3/C5 convertase ($\overline{\text{C3b}_n,\text{B}}$, where $n > 1$). This enzyme is able to activate properdin ($\overline{\text{P}}$) so that it too can become bound. The only role of properdin seems to be in stabilizing $\overline{\text{C3b}_n,\text{B}}$, converting it to the $\overline{\text{C3b}_n,\text{P},\text{B}}$ enzyme. This P-stabilized C5 convertase activates

```
                    Activating
                    particle          IF
                         \            /
                          \          /
                           ‾IF‾
                              \      C3, B, D, Mg⁺²
                               \      /
          C3                   ‾IF, B, C3‾  (IF-stabilized C3 convertase)
            \                       |
   Fluid     \                      |
   phase      \                     ↓
   positive   → C3b       B, D, Mg⁺²
   feedback        \       /
                    \     /
                  ‾C3b, B‾  (properdin receptor)
                       |
                       | P
                       ↓
                  ‾C3b, P, B‾ (stabilized C5 convertase)
                       |  C5, 6, 7, 8, 9
                       ↓
                  C5b-9 (membrane attack complex)
```

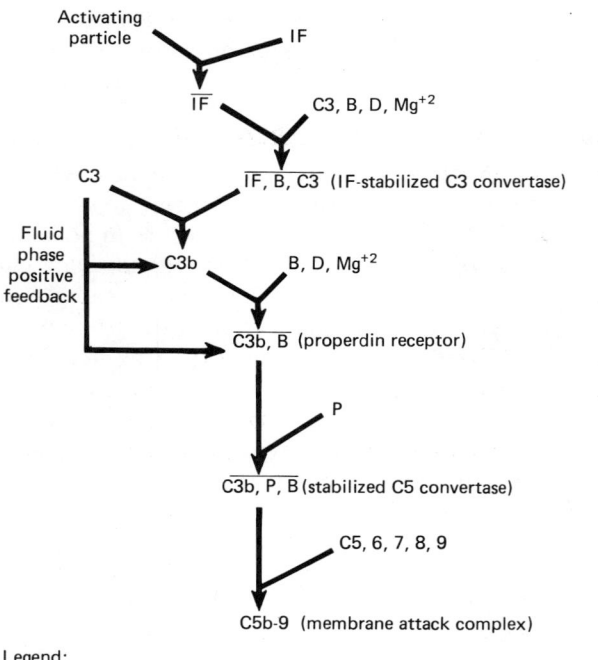

Legend:

IF = initiation factor
B = proactivator (PA); C3 proactivator (C3PA); GBG = glycine-rich beta glucoprotein
B̄ = C3 activator (C3A); fragment Bb
    B ⇌ Bb = B̄ (active)
        D ↘ Ba (inactive)
D = PAse; proactivator convertase
P = properdin; P̄ = bound (activated) properdin
‾C3b, B‾ = properdin receptor forming enzyme (PRFE); bound C3/C5 convertase, labile

FIGURE 7.3. The properdin pathway is an alternate pathway for activation of C3 and later-acting components.

C5, and self-assembly of the membrane attack complex (C5b-9) ensues. The properdin shunt and the classical pathway each produces its own kind of C5-activating enzymes (convertases), and from there on they use a common pathway in the formation of the C5b-9 complex. Enzymes that are structurally different but catalyze the same reaction are called **isozymes** or **isoenzymes.** Thus, the C5 convertase of the properdin shunt (C̄3̄b̄,P̄,B̄) and that of the classical pathway (C̄3̄b̄,2a,4b) qualify as isozymes.

REGULATION OF COMPLEMENT ACTIVITY

Several control mechanisms exist to modulate the complement cascade. An unregulated system, once activated, would continue until the critical intermediate was exhausted. Regulator substances of the complement system are classified as either inactivators or inhibitors. **Inactivators** are usually enzymes that destroy the primary structure (amino acid sequence) of complement components. **Inhibitors** do not break amino acid chains, but rather combine with complement components in ways that prevent their further interaction with other intermediates of the cascade. One inhibition mechanism is allosteric transformation. Another possibility is steric hindrance; the closer an inhibitor binds to the active site on the complement protein, the more likely it is to get in the way and physically prevent interaction with other components at the active site. A heat-labile glycoprotein in normal serum known as C$\overline{1}$ INH or C$\overline{1s}$ inhibitor combines only with activated C$\overline{1}$ in a 1:1 molar ratio. A deficiency of C1 INH is associated with **hereditary angioneurotic edema** (HANE), a disease characterized by symptoms of paroxysmal (sudden attacks of) edema. This inhibitor is labile above 60°C and may be inactivated by preheating sera prior to a CF test. An example of an inactivator is the enzyme C3b INAC found in normal serum. This enzyme hydrolyzes C3b, thereby terminating the complement pathway to all subsequent reactions. A protein in cattle serum called "conglutinin" (discussed later in this chapter in connection with the nonlytic complement fixation test, CCAT) combines with one of the fragments produced by C3b INAC. Because the CCAT depends on catalysis of C3b, this enzyme has also been called **conglutinogen activating factor** or KAF (from the German equivalent). Within limits, the activity of enzymes generally increases proportional to the temperature. An overnight incubation in the refrigerator is specified in the Kolmer complement fixation test. This allows antigen, antibody, and complement to combine with relatively little loss in complement activity due to catabolism by KAF and other inactivators. Rapid loss of complement activity at room temperature is largely attributed to degradation by inactivators.

The properdin pathway is regulated in at least three ways: (1) the C3/C5 convertases spontaneously decay, (2) the P-stabilized C5 convertase is actively disassembled by soluble C3b (possibly also by native C3), and (3) a serum enzyme termed properdin receptor-destroying enzyme (PRDE) causes inactivation of bound C3b and C3b,$\overline{P}$, thereby controlling the formation and function of $\overline{P}$-C5 convertase. PRDE may be identical with C3b INA.

SPECIFIC COMPONENT ASSAYS

Proteins of the complement system comprise about 10 percent of all serum globulins. Complement levels are not elevated as a result of immunization, but may be subnormal during certain diseases as a result of consumption by combative antibodies. Just as the strength of a chain is dependent on its weakest link, the hemolytic titer of complement in a patient's serum is dependent on the limiting component.

Determination of the component that is limiting or abnormal requires a specific serological assay. This may be helpful in determining how the patient is responding to a disease. For example, if specific component analyses reveal that levels of C1, C4, and C2 are normal, but C3 levels are subnormal, it indicates that an alternate pathway of complement activation is being used rather than the classical pathway. In other words, antibodies are probably not being utilized to combat the disease. As another example, a patient is suspected to be suffering from hereditary angioneurotic edema (HANE). Confirmation of this diagnosis would be provided by finding depleted levels of C4, C2, and C$\overline{1}$ INH. Radial immunodiffusion (RID) plates containing specific antisera incorporated into agarose are now commercially available for assay of some proteins of the complement system. As more associations become known between diseases and complement abnormalities, the workload of assays for specific complement components in clinical laboratories is expected to increase. These serological assays detect only the antigenic integrity of the molecule, not its functional (biological) activity. For example, when C3 becomes activated, only a small piece (3a) is removed. The remainder (3b) contains most of the antigenic activity of the entire C3 molecule. Likewise, when C3b is cleaved by C3b INAC (KAF), another small piece (C3d) is liberated, but most of the antigenicity remains in the other fragment (C3c). Radial immunodiffusion tests using anti-C3 antisera might detect normal antigenic levels of C3 even if it was in the form of C3b or C3c. A serum containing mostly C3c, however, would not have any hemolytic activity. Specific component assays for biological activity (rather than serological activity) are also becoming commercially available. These tests employ serums that are devoid of one specific complement protein, but possess all other components in normal amounts. A hemolytic test for biological function is performed by mixing the patient's serum with a serum of known deficiency and sensitized sheep red cells. Since all other components of the single deficiency serum are present in at least normal amounts, the lytic titer is indicative of the functional capacity of the specific component being measured in the patient's serum.

Complement Fixation Tests

Cytolysis requires cooperation of all nine major proteins of the complement system. But not all cells can be lysed by antigen-antibody-complement complexes. Among those most susceptible to lysis are erythrocytes, leukocytes, thrombocytes, and some gram-negative bacteria. Lysozyme in blood serum acts synergistically with complement to effect bacteriolysis of gram-negative bacteria. The lysozyme digests certain components of the cell wall, thereby allowing antibodies and complement access to membrane antigens. Gram-positive bacteria, most mammalian cells, plant cells, yeasts, and molds are resistant to complement-mediated cytolysis. The nature of the antigen-antibody complex is not important for complement binding as long as the immunoglobulin is of the proper class. Therefore, even though many cellular antigen-antibody complexes will not be lysed by complement, certain complement components will be bound, fixed, activated, or consumed.

The **complement fixation (CF) test** is designed to detect complement consumption in virtually any cellular or noncellular antigen-antibody reaction to which complement is bound. Complement is relatively nonspecific in its fixation property; i.e., it will combine with immunoglobulins of the same or different species. However, it does show some specificity in that mammalian complement reacts best with mammalian immunoglobulins, avian complement reacts best with avian antibodies, etc. Complement is found in all vertebrates phylogenetically higher than lampreys. Complement from certain species will fix some of its proteins to antigen-antibody complexes, but it may not be an efficient cytolytic agent. Serum from horses, cattle, sheep, and mice are essentially noncytolytic. Rabbit serum is the preferred source of complement in hemolytic tests for blood typing cattle erythocyte antigens. Guinea pig serum is the preferred source of complement for most clinical tests involving human antibodies (an exception is in human histocompatibility typing where human or rabbit complement is preferred). The reason why guinea pig complement is usually preferred is because the concentration of certain complement components in human and other mammalian sera is relatively low.

Complement is notoriously unstable. It is "inactivated" by heating serum at 56°C for thirty minutes. Many serological protocols specify this pretreatment of sera without any explanation as to why it is done. It may be assumed that in such tests one or more heat-labile proteins would interfere with the intended reaction. Recall that the VDRL test requires heating the serum before it is exposed to the antigen. Complement will rapidly lose its hemolytic activity within twenty-four hours at room temperature. It loses activity over three or four days under refrigeration but can be active up to one month if stored at −20°C and for at least six months at −40°C. It can be stored for even longer periods if lyophilized (freeze-dried). Technologists should always check the expiration date on commercially available lyophilized complement to be sure it has not expired. This is an important responsibility of medical technologists in all aspects of their work, viz., checking all reagents before use to be certain they are not older than the expiration date printed on the label by the manufacturer.

In addition to aging or heating, complement can also be nonserologically inactivated by vigorous agitation, various chemicals (acids, alkalies, alcohol, etc.), enzymes, yeast or bacterial cells, tissue extracts, and hemolysis. It is therefore important to ensure that all glassware used in CF tests is chemically and biologically clean (though not necessarily sterile). Likewise, when collecting serum for its complement content, aseptic procedures should be employed (certain bacteriostatic agents may also be added), and care should be taken to prevent the anticomplementary effects of tissue damage and/or hemolysis.

Some degree of complement reactivation may temporarily be regained within about a day following heat inactivation (spontaneous renaturation). Therefore, if repeated CF tests are required on a patient's serum over several days, it should be heat-inactivated immediately prior to each such test. The use of ice-cold diluents and buffers aids in maintaining complement activity in CF tests.

Complement fixation tests are among the most complicated and time-consuming serological tests presently available. Simpler tests with equal or greater degrees of sensitivities have largely replaced the complement fixation tests in hospital laboratories. However, complement fixation tests are still used in state and federal public health virology laboratories. A complement fixation test may be classified as either lytic or nonlytic. The more common lytic tests will be discussed first.

LYTIC CF TESTS

An "indicator system" is required to detect whether or not complement has been bound by interaction between the patient's serum and the antigen added to the complement fixation test. The indicator system usually consists of sensitized sheep erythrocytes, i.e., red blood cells to which anti-sheep rbc antibodies are attached. These antibodies are commonly produced by injecting rabbits with washed sheep red blood cells (SRBC). If an antiserum can activate complement and cause immune lysis of the SRBC, it is termed a **hemolysin.** It was also named **amboceptor** by Ehrlich to describe an antibody that possesses two different attachment sites (ambo = both). One site

(Fab) is specific for the homologous antigen. The other site (Fc) will bind complement after it attaches to antigen. Some of these antibodies are undoubtedly anti-Forssman if they are of rabbit origin. In the absence of complement, undiluted amboceptor behaves as a sheep red cell hemagglutinin. At high dilutions (low concentrations) the only demonstrable serological effect of amboceptor is fixation of complement. In the presence of complement, amboceptor behaves as a hemolysin. For the complement fixation test, amboceptor is commonly diluted 1:500 or greater. At these high dilutions, amboceptor has no hemagglutinating activity, but may still be hemolytic. Amboceptor (hemolysin) is a very stable antibody under refrigeration and therefore needs to be titrated only infrequently (perhaps only every six months).

Prior to performance of a complement fixation test, both amboceptor and complement must be titrated to determine their respective "units," i.e., the smallest amounts of each reactant that interact to completely lyse the quantity of SRBC that will be used in the complement fixation test. Once the units have been found for hemolysin and complement, the complement fixation (CF) test can be performed as a balanced system. Suppose that we are looking for antibodies against Q fever rickettsiae (*Coxiella burnetii*) in a patient's serum. The first step is to heat-inactivate the native complement in the patient's serum (56°C, thirty minutes) so that the only source of complement in the test will be exogenously added. We next incubate the patient's serum with Q fever rickettsia antigen and 1 unit of complement (Figure 7.4). The antibody combines with the antigen, and this complex binds (fixes) complement. Then sensitized sheep red cells are added as an indicator system (containing 1 unit of hemolysin). If all the complement is bound in the first reaction, none will be available to bind with hemolysin on the red cells. No lysis occurs, indicating a positive serum (i.e., antibodies against Q fever rickettsiae are present). In a negative test, no antibodies are present in the patient's serum. After incubating the serum with antigen and complement, the complement remains free (not fixed). When sensitized cells are added, the free complement can bind to the hemolysin causing lysis of the red cells. Lysis, in a CF test, indicates a negative serum (in this case, no anti-Q fever rickettsiae antibodies).

Hemolysin Titration. Hemolysin titration may begin with an initial dilution of 1:500 or 1:1,000 of rabbit anti-sheep cell serum (depending on prior experience with the source). Dilutions of the hemolysin are pipetted into tubes with sufficient diluent to measure the same in all tubes (e.g., 0.3 ml total in Table 7.1). The diluent, called **complement fixation saline,** is a physiological saline to which the cations calcium and magnesium have been added. These ions are important for binding certain components during the complement cascade. A surplus of complement is added to ensure that this is not a limiting reagent (e.g., 1:20 fresh or lyophilized guinea pig serum should be sufficient). A suitable dilution (2 to 5 percent) of washed sheep red blood cells suspended in saline is added. The mixture is shaken, incubated at 37°C for thirty minutes, centrifuged, examined macroscopically for the degree of lysis, and scored as in Figure 7.5. The smallest amount of hemolysin producing complete lysis constitutes **1 unit.** In the example of Table 7.1, the greatest dilution showing complete hemolysis is in tube 5. Therefore the unit of hemolysin is 0.06 ml of a 1:500 dilution. Note that for each antiserum the unit must be specified as

Serology and Immunology

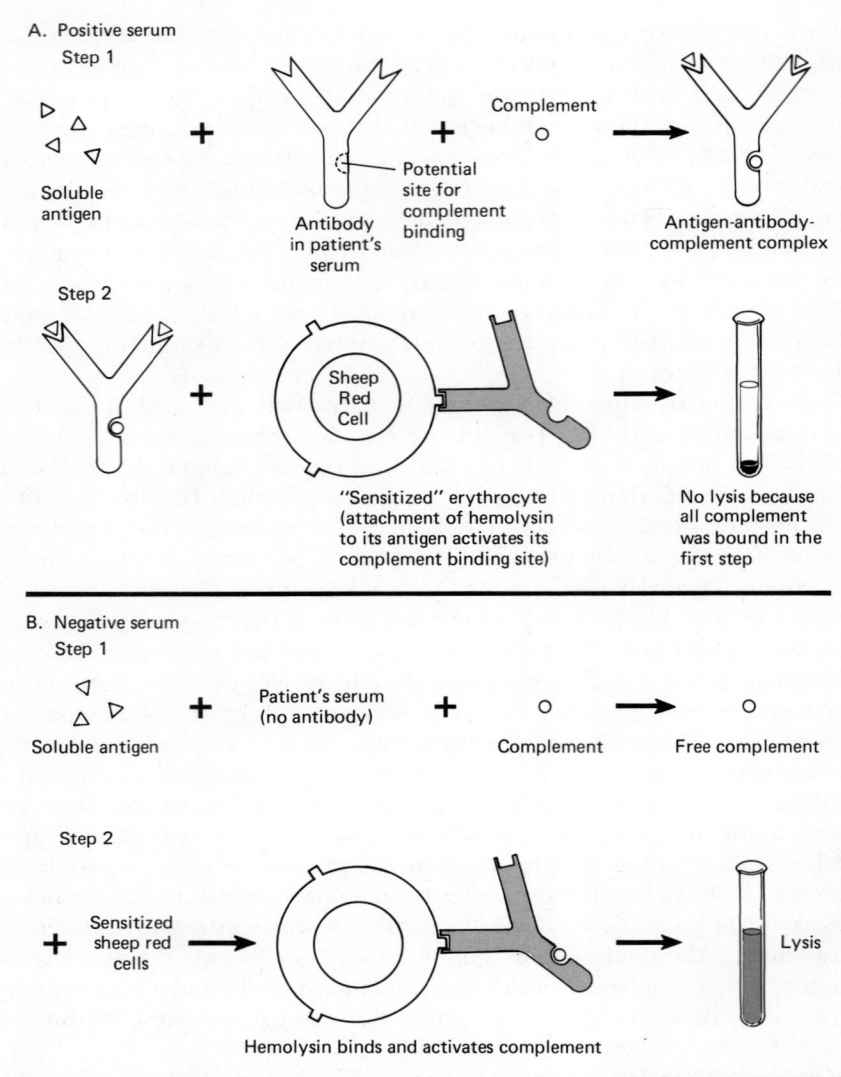

FIGURE 7.4. The complement fixation test. Diagram A is typical of a positive serum (containing the antibody); diagram B represents a negative serum (antibody absent).

a certain quantity of a certain dilution. In performing a complement fixation test, it is convenient to use a dilution of hemolysin that contains 1 unit in some easily measured volume (e.g., 0.1 ml). To calculate this dilution (using the previous example), a simple proportion is established; viz., if 0.06 ml of a 1:500 dilution contains 1 unit of hemolysin, then 0.1 ml of a weaker dilution $\left(\frac{1}{x}\right)$ will also contain one unit.

$$0.06 \text{ ml } (1/500) = 0.1 \text{ ml} \left(\frac{1}{x}\right)$$
$$0.06x = 50$$
$$x = 50/0.06 = 833.3$$

If we make a 1:833 dilution of hemolysin, each 0.1 ml of that dilution

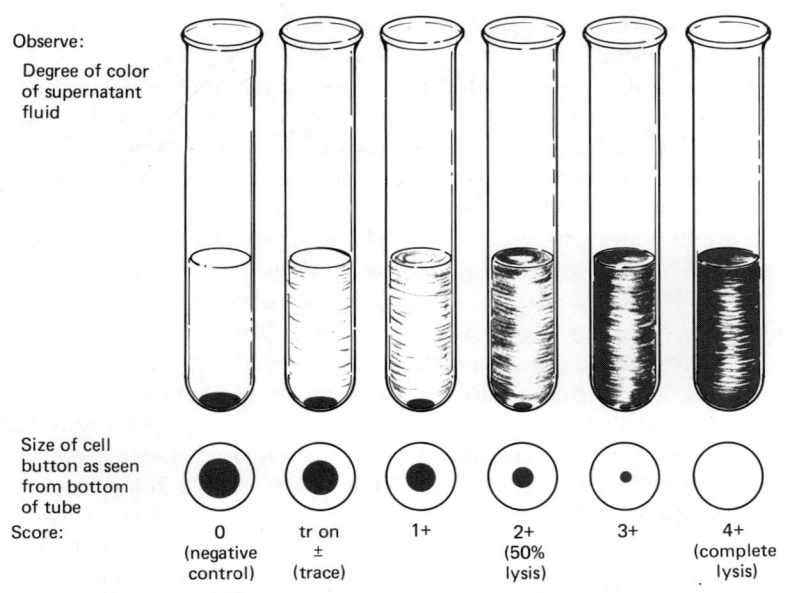

FIGURE 7.5. A guide for scoring lytic reactions following centrifugation.

Observe:
Degree of color of supernatant fluid

Size of cell button as seen from bottom of tube

Score: 0 (negative control) | tr on ± (trace) | 1+ | 2+ (50% lysis) | 3+ | 4+ (complete lysis)

should contain 1 unit. If multiple units of hemolysin are desired in any given volume, this can also be easily calculated. For example, suppose we want 3 units in 0.5 ml. If 0.06 ml of 1:500 dilution is 1 unit, then 3 times this amount (0.18 ml of 1:500) contains 3 units. Since we want 3 units in 0.5 ml, we set up the proportion:

$$0.18 \text{ ml } (1/500) = 0.5 \text{ ml} \left(\frac{1}{x}\right)$$
$$0.18x = 250$$
$$x = 250/0.18 = 1388.9$$

Table 7.1 EXAMPLE OF A PROTOCOL FOR HEMOLYSIN TITRATION AND HYPOTHETICAL RESULTS
Each tube receives 0.1 ml complement (1:20) and 0.1 ml sheep red blood cells (2%) and incubation at 37°C for thirty minutes

Tube	Amboceptor (1:500), ml	Saline ml	Lysis
1	0.10	0.20	+4
2	0.09	0.21	+4
3	0.08	0.22	+4
4	0.07	0.23	+4
5	0.06	0.24	+4
6	0.05	0.25	+3
7	0.04	0.26	+1
8	0.03	0.27	Tr
9	0.02	0.28	0
10	0.01	0.29	0
11	0.00	0.30	0

Therefore, if we prepare a 1 : 1,389 dilution of hemolysin, each 0.5 ml of it contains three units.

Neutral glycerin is often added as a preservative in a 1 : 1 ratio to commercial anti-sheep cell serum. If we wish to prepare a 1 : 500 dilution of hemolysin from such a glycerinated product, we could take 2 ml of it and add it to 498 ml diluent. In practice, much smaller quantities of diluted hemolysin are required. In order to be frugal with costly reagents, we could take the smallest amount of glycerinated hemolysin that could accurately be measured with our pipette (e.g., 0.1 ml containing 0.05 ml of hemolysin) and add it to 9.9 ml diluent. Now we have 0.05 ml hemolysin in a total of 10 ml fluid, equivalent to 1 part hemolysin in 200 total parts (1 : 200). The contents of the tube are mixed thoroughly by flushing them up and down through a pipette. The next dilution should be by a factor of 1/2.5 so that the final dilution is 1 : 500 (1/200 × 1/2.5 = 1/500). If 10 ml hemolysin is needed, we could take 4 ml of the 1 : 200 dilution and pipette it into 6 ml of diluent (4/10 = 1/2.5), resulting in 10 ml of a 1 : 500 hemolysin. These kinds of calculations are often required in the serological laboratory.

Care should be taken to wash sheep cells thoroughly so that no trace of redness (free hemoglobin) can be seen in the wash saline, as this might be confused with immune hemolysis in a lytic test. Cell washing is also required to remove chelating compounds such as ethylenediamine tetraacetic acid (EDTA) and sodium citrate, both of which are commonly used anticoagulants. These substances bind calcium ions (required for the coagulation reaction) and would inhibit the complement cascade. The last tube of a hemolysin titration contains only sheep red cells and diluent. It serves as a **RBC control** or **corpuscle control.** No lysis should be observed in the control tube. If lysis does occur, the cells may be autolysing because they are too fragile (typical of aged cells) or the diluent may not be isotonic with the red cells.

Complement Titration. Complement is so unstable that it must be titrated immediately prior to use in a complement fixation test. Guinea pig serum is diluted 1 : 10 to 1 : 40 and pipetted into tubes with complement fixation saline diluent (as in the protocol of Table 7.2). In order that hemolysin will not be a limiting factor, 2 units of hemolysin are commonly added to each tube together with a suspension of washed sheep red blood cells. If preferred, the red cells may be mixed with the hemolysin and added to the test as "sensitized cells." The tubes are shaken, incubated at 37°C for thirty minutes, centrifuged, and scored for hemolysis. Because there are two incubation periods in a complement fixation test, it may be desirable to do likewise in the complement titration. The first incubation period follows mixing of complement and saline; the second incubation follows addition of sensitized cells. The least amount of complement producing complete hemolysis constitutes 1 unit. In the example of Table 7.2, tube 2 was the last tube to show +4 lysis. Therefore, 1 unit of complement is 0.12 ml of 1 : 40.

A much more critical determination of end-point titers in both hemolysin and complement titrations is the 50 percent hemolytic end point. As can be seen from Figure 7.6, the degree of hemolysis is related to the amount of complement by a sigmoid (S-shaped) curve. Between approximately 30 and 70 percent lysis, the curve is almost linear, indicating that each increment of additional complement produces approximately equivalent increments of

Table 7.2 EXAMPLE OF A PROTOCOL FOR COMPLEMENT TITRATION

Each tube receives 0.1 ml of amboceptor (2 units) and 0.1 ml of sheep red cells (2%); incubation is at 37°C for thirty minutes following the addition of cells.

Tube	Complement (1:40), ml	Saline ml	Lysis
1	0.13	0.17	+4
2	0.12	0.18	+4
3	0.11	0.19	+2
4	0.10	0.20	±
5	0.09	0.21	0
6	0.08	0.22	0
7	0.07	0.23	0
8	0.06	0.24	0
9	0.05	0.25	0
10	0.04	0.26	0
11	0.03	0.27	0
12	0.02	0.28	0

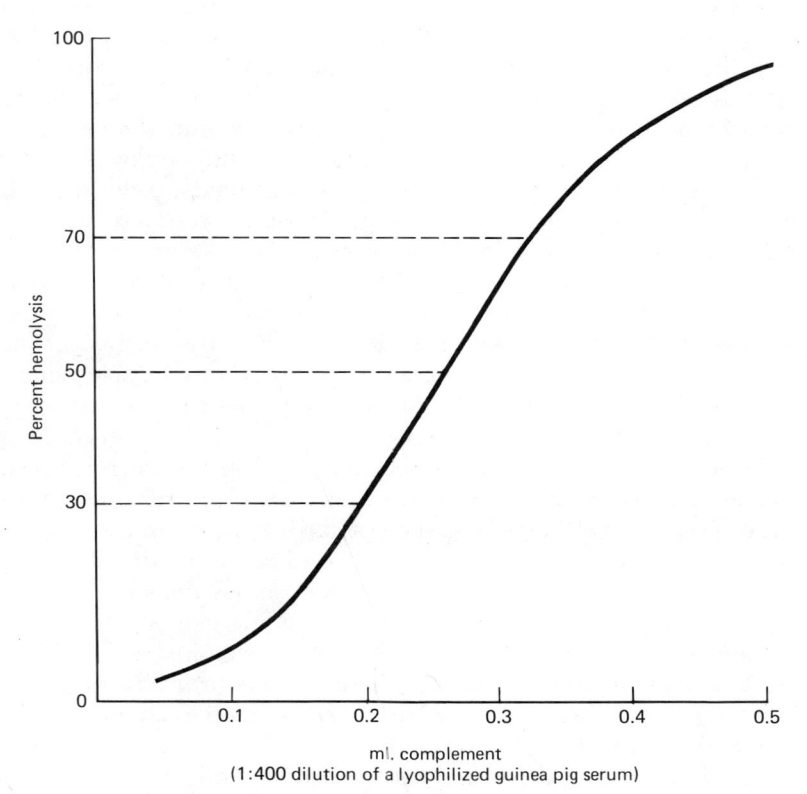

FIGURE 7.6. Example of the relationship between the amount of complement and percent hemolysis. The curve is essentially linear between 30 percent and 70 percent hemolysis. Red cells are sensitized with 2 units of amboceptor.

lysis. The upper limit of the curve is more nearly flat, indicating that addition of relatively large amounts of complement is required to obtain 100 percent hemolysis. Because the curve is steeper in its central region, much greater precision is obtained by measuring the 50 percent end point than the 100 percent end point. A reference standard is made by osmotically lysing half the amount of sheep red cells used in the test with distilled water. The degree of lysis in the standard and each tube of the test is then measured precisely in a spectrophotometer. Measurements from the tubes that bracket the 50 percent hemolytic end point can be used to determine the 50 percent hemolytic unit by interpolation. For example, if linearity exists between 30 percent and 70 percent hemolysis (corresponding to 0.2 and 0.34 ml of a 1:400 dilution of complement respectively), then 50 percent hemolysis should correspond to $0.2 + \frac{1}{2}(0.34 - 0.2) = 0.27$ ml of the diluted complement.

Tests for Syphilitic Reagin. Perhaps the best-known example of a complement fixation test is the Wassermann test for syphilitic reagin as modified by Kolmer. The Wassermann test originally employed as antigen liver extracts from stillborn fetuses maternally infected with syphilis. These extracts contained the causative agent of syphilis, *Treponema pallidum*. A substance in the patient's serum reacted with these extracts and bound complement. Later it was found that the patient's serum would also fix complement when exposed to a purified alcoholic extract of beef heart (**cardiolipin**). The substance in the serum was therefore not an antibody specific for the treponeme. It was called **reagin.** Unfortunately, the name reagin has also been given to the antibody of allergy, IgE. It is therefore best to qualify them as syphilitic (Wassermann) reagin and allergic reagin, respectively. Syphilitic reagin is now known to be an antibody of class IgM.

The titer of syphilitic reagin in a patient's serum tends to decline relatively rapidly if treatment is successful (syphilis usually responds very well to penicillin therapy). Titers of specific treponemal antibodies, on the other hand, tend to be detectable over relatively long periods after recovery from a disease. Reagin is also regularly produced in response to several diseases other than syphilis (especially malaria or leprosy). Because reagin declines after the patient is cured, monitoring reagin titers is of considerable value in following the patient's response to treatment. In untreated patients, reagin usually is detectable in serum within four or five weeks after infection. Its titer peaks after five or six weeks when secondary lesions (chancres) appear. Reagin tends to decrease after about two years, but often remains detectable for the remainder of life unless the patient becomes cured.

It has been suggested that reagin is an autoantibody to lipids released by tissue damage in generalized diseases such as syphilis and lupus erythematosus. Antibodies specific for the treponeme can be detected by using *T. pallidum* antigens prepared from rabbit testes infected with the organism. The titer of these specific antibodies tends to persist long after the patient is cured and hence is useful for determining if a patient has ever had previous contact with the treponeme.

Cardiolipin is a much cheaper and less hazardous antigen for detecting reagin in a complement fixation test than the original Wassermann antigen. Cardiolipin is exclusively used today as antigen in both the complement fixation test and the VDRL microflocculation test. Cholesterol is added to the beef heart extract to enhance reactivity and lecithin is added to reduce anticomplementary activity (nonimmunological binding of complement) of the antigen.

Commercial complement fixation test kits for reagin are available. These kits typically contain cardiolipin antigen, complement fixation saline, sheep red blood cells, lyophilized complement, hemolysin, and a positive control serum. When diluted according to the manufacturer's directions, both the complement and the hemolysin contain 1 unit in the amounts used in the test. The manufacturer has titrated the reagents and the kit is ready to use immediately. An example of the Kolmer qualitative complement fixation test is presented in Table 7.3. The test can easily be made quantitative by making dilutions of the patient's serum. Five controls are run simultaneously: (1) antigen control, (2) serum control, (3) hemolytic system control, (4) RBC control, and (5) positive control serum. The first two controls are designed to detect the possibility of nonspecific (nonimmunological) inactivation (binding) of complement by anticomplementary factors in the antigen or in the patient's serum. In the case of the antigen control, no patient's serum is present. In the case of the serum control, no antigen is present. If either of these fails to lyse completely, some nonspecific binding of complement has occurred. Many substances can inactivate complement including alkalies (e.g., soap residue on glassware), metal ions, dirt, bacterial con-

Table 7.3 EXAMPLE OF A KOLMER-WASSERMANN QUALITATIVE TEST KIT PROTOCOL

Tube	Serum, ml	Saline Solution, ml	Antigen, ml		Complement, ml		Hemolysin, ml	2% Sheep Cells, ml	
Test sample	0.2	None	0.5	Shake rack well, allow to stand at room temperature for 10 to 15 minutes	1.0	Incubate for 15 to 18 hours at 6° to 10°C Followed by 10 minutes at 37°C	0.5	0.5	Incubate at 37°C until the positive control serum shows the predetermined reactivity pattern
Serum control	0.2	0.5	None		1.0		0.5	0.5	
Antigen control	None	0.2	0.5		1.0		0.5	0.5	
Hemolytic system control	None	0.7	None		1.0		0.5	0.5	
Sheep cell control	None	2.2	None		None		None	0.5	
Positive control serum	0.2 of appropriate dilution	See manufacturer's instructions (Table 7.4)	0.5		1.0		0.5	0.5	

Serology and Immunology

Table 7.4 Protocol for a Positive Syphilitic Serum Used As a Control for a Kolmer-Wasserman Complement Fixation Test

Tube	Dilution	Lytic Reaction
1	1/2.5	0
2	1/5	0
3	1/10	+1 to +3
4	1/20	+4
5	1/40	+4

taminants, lipids, etc. Glassware should be scrupulously clean. Care should be taken to prevent bacterial contamination and growth in patient's serum and in reagents. When bleeding guinea pigs for their serum complement or sensitized rabbits for anti-sheep cell serum, the animals should be fasted a day before drawing blood to minimize its content of lipids. The hemolytic system control lacks serum and antigen and should lyse completely in a balanced system containing 1 unit each of complement and hemolysin. The red blood cell control should not lyse because only buffer is added. The kit also contains a lyophilized serum known to contain syphilitic reagin. It is serially diluted according to the manufacturer's directions and then treated identically to the patient's serum including heat inactivation prior to the test. A pattern of lysis should develop according to the manufacturer's specifications (Table 7.4). If this pattern fails to develop, or any of the other controls fail to show the expected responses, the test is invalid. The test may be read as soon as the prescribed pattern of lysis appears in the control serum. Careful note should be taken of the subtle difference in names between the "serum control" (patient's serum) and the "control serum" (manufacturer's serum).

Suppose that a qualitative test of a patient's serum produces +1 lysis, and that all controls are normal (including +4 in the hemolytic system control). Obviously, most (but not all) of the complement was bound immunologically by the serum. The degree of complement binding (expressed on a scale from 0 to +4) is +3. The report to the physician would be in terms of the complement-binding capacity of the patient's serum, not in terms of the degree of lysis observed. In a quantitative complement fixation test (Figure 7.7), the titer of course would be the reciprocal of the highest dilution that completely inhibited lysis. For example, if a one-sixteenth dilution of the patient's serum was the greatest dilution in which no lysis occurred, the titer is 16 or 16 dils (dilutions).

If the antigen used in a complement fixation test is anticomplementary (as are some bacterial antigens and lipid-rich antigens), it should be titrated. Serial dilutions of the antigen are prepared and incubated with a unit of complement and sensitized cells. The smallest amount of antigen that slightly inhibits hemolysis is considered the **anticomplementary unit.** This establishes the upper limit of antigen to be used in the CF test. The lower limit of antigen is determined by serially diluting it as before, but exposing it to constant amounts of a known positive homologous serum, 1 unit of

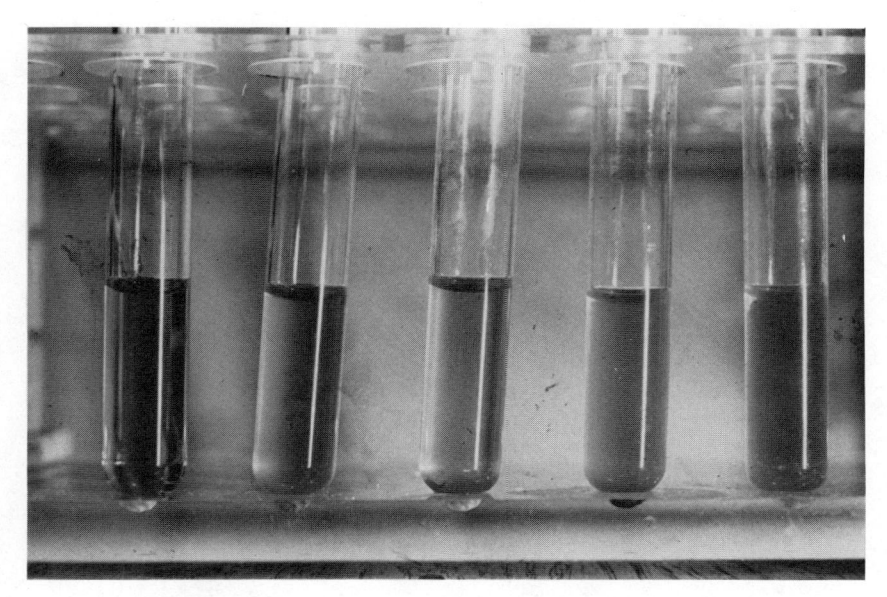

FIGURE 7.7. Quantitative complement fixation tube test. Varying reactions from complete hemolysis (negative) on the far left to complete absence of hemolysis (4+ positive) on the far right with varying degrees of partial hemolysis is between. [*Courtesy of Elliot Scientific Corp., New York City.*]

complement and sensitized cells. The smallest amount of antigen that completely fixes complement under these conditions is the **antigenic unit.** The dose of antigen chosen for use in a standard complement fixation test is intermediate between the antigenic unit and the anticomplementary unit.

If very precise titers are to be determined (as in research), 1 unit each of complement and hemolysin could be used, but sometimes controls do not react correctly under these limiting conditions. In most practical work (including clinical assays), 2 or more units are used to avoid the spurious results sometimes encountered under marginal conditions. If 2 hemolytic units of complement are used in the test, then the patient's serum must fix twice as much complement to give the same results (no lysis) as when only 1 unit is used. Highly accurate determination of titers generally is not necessary because the difference in results from paired sera tested under identical conditions is more meaningful than a single titration. Furthermore, titers of most antibodies correlate poorly with severity of the disease.

The complement fixation test is potentially adaptable to any antigen-antibody system. It is more sensitive than precipitation tests, about equal to bacterial agglutination tests, and less sensitive than viral neutralization, radioimmunoassay, and bactericidal tests. It is a costly and complicated test to perform. In California, the State Department of Public Health still uses it for some diseases (e.g., coccidioidomycosis), and especially in its viral laboratory (Figure 7.8). Other simpler and less expensive tests have largely replaced CF tests in most clinical laboratories.

Rice Test. Some antibodies react with homologous antigens but do not fix complement (e.g., IgA, IgD, IgE). To be certain that a negative CF test has not missed detecting a noncomplement-fixing antibody, a **Rice** or **indirect CF test** is performed as a control. The patient's serum is mixed with 1 unit of antigen and 1 unit of complement and is incubated (Figure 7.9). If the

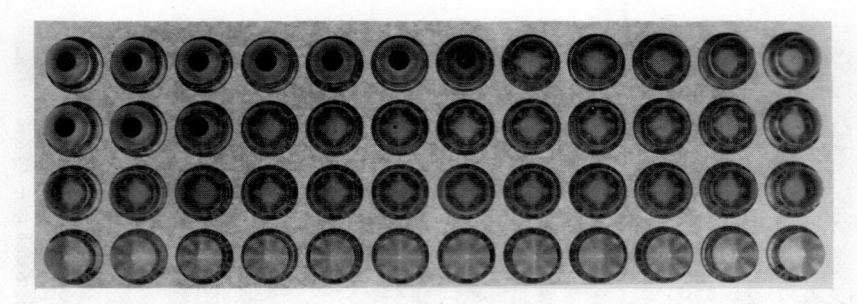

FIGURE 7.8. Significant diagnostic rise between a convalescent and an acute serum sample for virus complement-fixing antibodies as performed with Microtiter® system. The hemolytic end point for the convalescent serum (top row) is in well 6 from the left. No hemolysis is seen in wells 1 to 6. Well 7 is partly hemolyzed and wells 8 to 12 are completely hemolyzed. The end point for the acute specimen (second row) is in well 2. A negative serum (containing no antiviral complement-fixing antibodies) is in the third row. All wells are completely hemolyzed. Serums are serially diluted left to right. Microtiter plates are viewed from below by reflection in a mirror.

serum contains a non-complement-fixing antibody, it will bind some or all of the antigen but none of the complement. Next, a known complement-fixing antibody specific for the antigen is added. Since the antigen was in short supply to begin with, most or all of it has been bound by antibodies in the patient's serum. There is little or no antigen with which the CF antibody can unite; complement remains free. Finally, sensitized sheep red cells are added. The free complement attaches to the hemolysin causing lysis of the red cells. A lytic Rice test is indicative of a non-complement-fixing antibody in the patient's serum (a positive serum). On the other hand, if a patient's serum contains no antibody, both antigen and complement will remain free. Addition of a known CF antibody results in an antibody-antigen-complement complex. When sensitized sheep cells (indicator system) are added, there is no more free complement with which hemolysin can combine. The cells do not lyse. A nonlytic Rice test indicates that there were no antibodies homologous to the antigen in the patient's serum (a negative serum).

CF test positive → no further testing required

CF test negative ⟨ lytic rice test → positive serum
nonlytic Rice test → negative serum

NONLYTIC CF TEST

A beta globulin of bovine (cattle) serum, called **conglutinin,** combines rather nonspecifically with complex polysaccharides. At least one complement protein (C3) contains a polysaccharide moiety. Antigen-antibody-complement complexes are aggregated by conglutinin. It is this property that led to the development of the **conglutinating complement adsorption** test (CCAT, Figure 7.10). Suppose we wish to identify a certain antibody in the patient's serum. The serum is mixed with the homologous antigen and 1 unit of horse complement (containing sublytic quantities of C2). If the antibody is present, it combines with its homologous antigen and fixes complement. After incubation, sheep red cells are added together with normal bovine serum. All normal cattle sera contain conglutinin and a low-titer, nonhemagglutinating anti-sheep erythrocyte antibody. The anti-erythrocyte antibody combines with the red cells forming sensitized cells. Since the complement was fixed to the patient's antibodies in the first step, there is none left to react with the sensitized cells in the second step. No agglutination occurs with a positive serum (antibody is present). Conglutinin may cause aggregation (precipitation) of some immunoglobulins to which complement is bound, but they usually remain soluble and cannot be

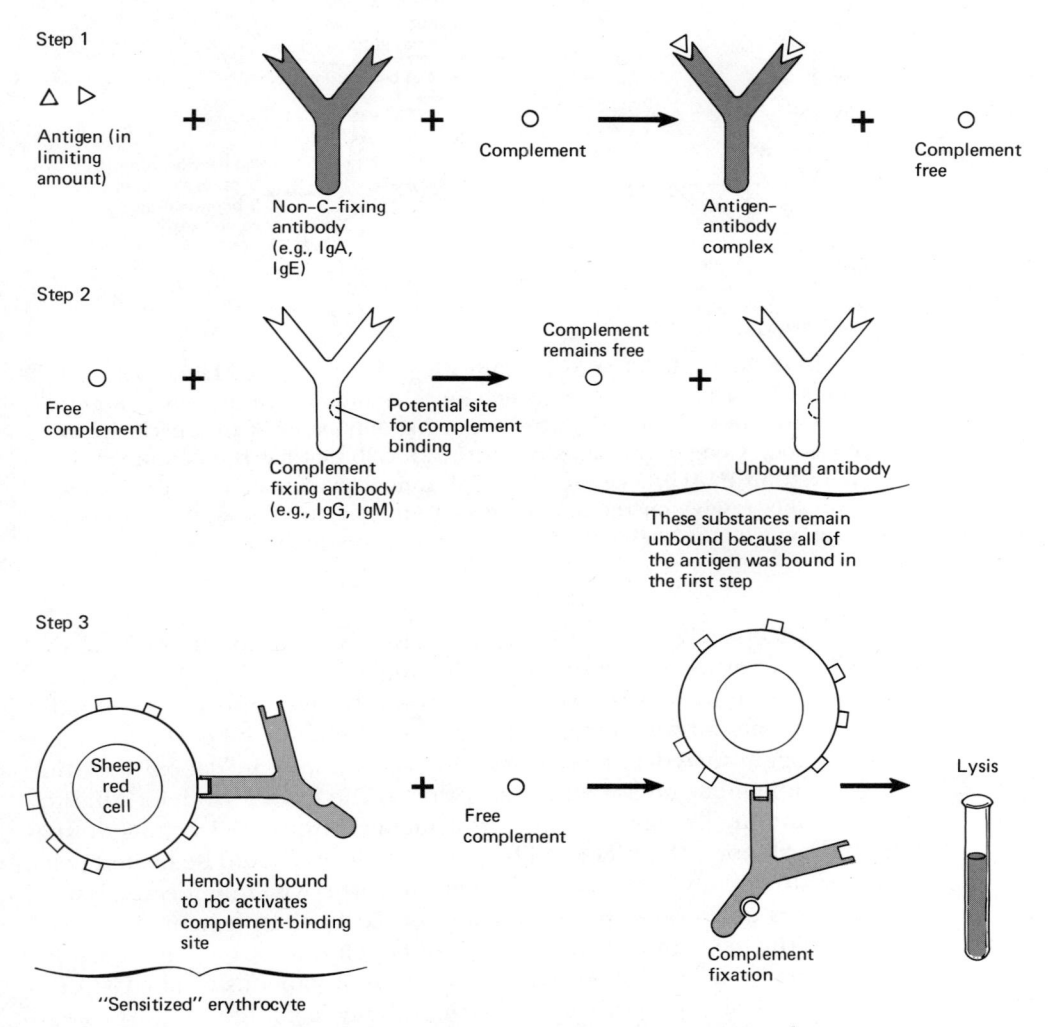

FIGURE 7.9. The Rice test. This diagram represents the expected events when the patient's serum contains a non-complement-fixing antibody specific for the antigen used.

Serology and Immunology

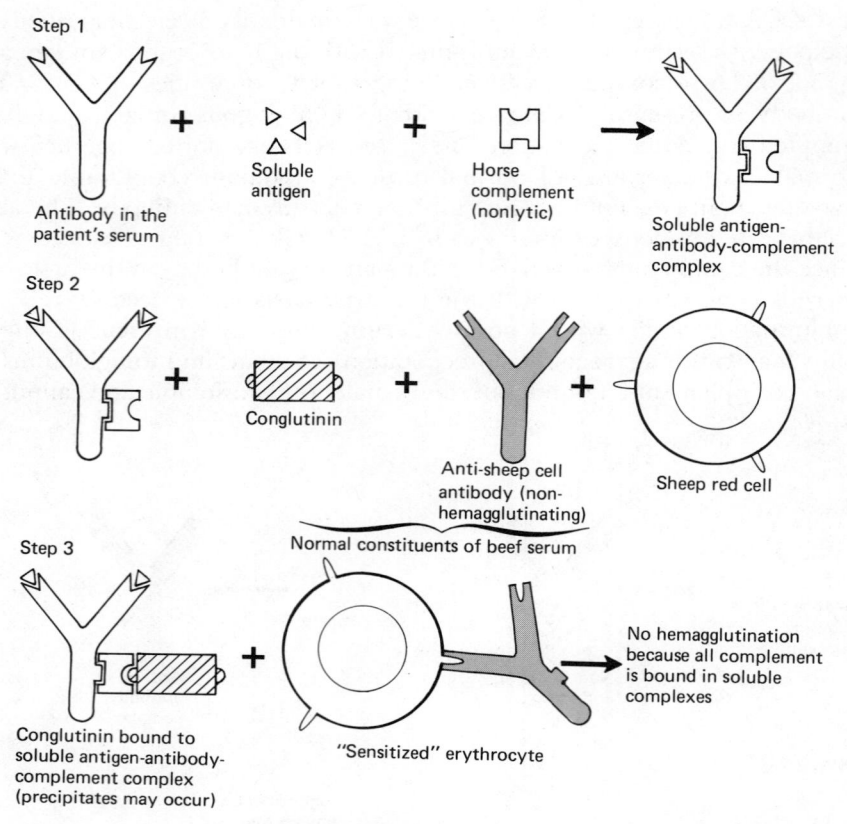

FIGURE 7.10. Model of a conglutinating absorption test. Left: Expected results for a positive serum (containing the antibody in question). Right: Expected results for a negative serum (no antibodies of the specificity in question). Conglutinin actually reacts with C3b that has been modified by KAF (C3b INAC). The modified C3b cannot participate in cell lysis and probably resides on the antigen very near its activating antibody rather than attached to the antibody as shown in this symplistic model.

seen macroscopically. Alternatively, if a patient's serum does not have the antibody in question, none of the complement is bound in the first step. Therefore, complement is free to bind to the bovine anti-sheep cell antibody, and conglutinin attaches to the complement. The red cells are passively agglutinated in a negative test (no antibody in patient's serum). Horse complement must be titrated prior to the CCAT to determine the unit, i.e., the smallest amount of complement that gives +4 hemagglutination in the absence of antibody. The patient's serum should be heated prior to the test to destroy human complement that otherwise might cause lysis of the red cells or provide an extraneous source of complement that could neutralize the hemagglutinating activity of conglutinin. Controls analogous to those used in a lytic CF test should be run simultaneously. The CCAT is reported to be slightly more sensitive than the lytic CF test. Nonlytic complement fixation tests are seldom used in clinical work, but they may be useful research tools.

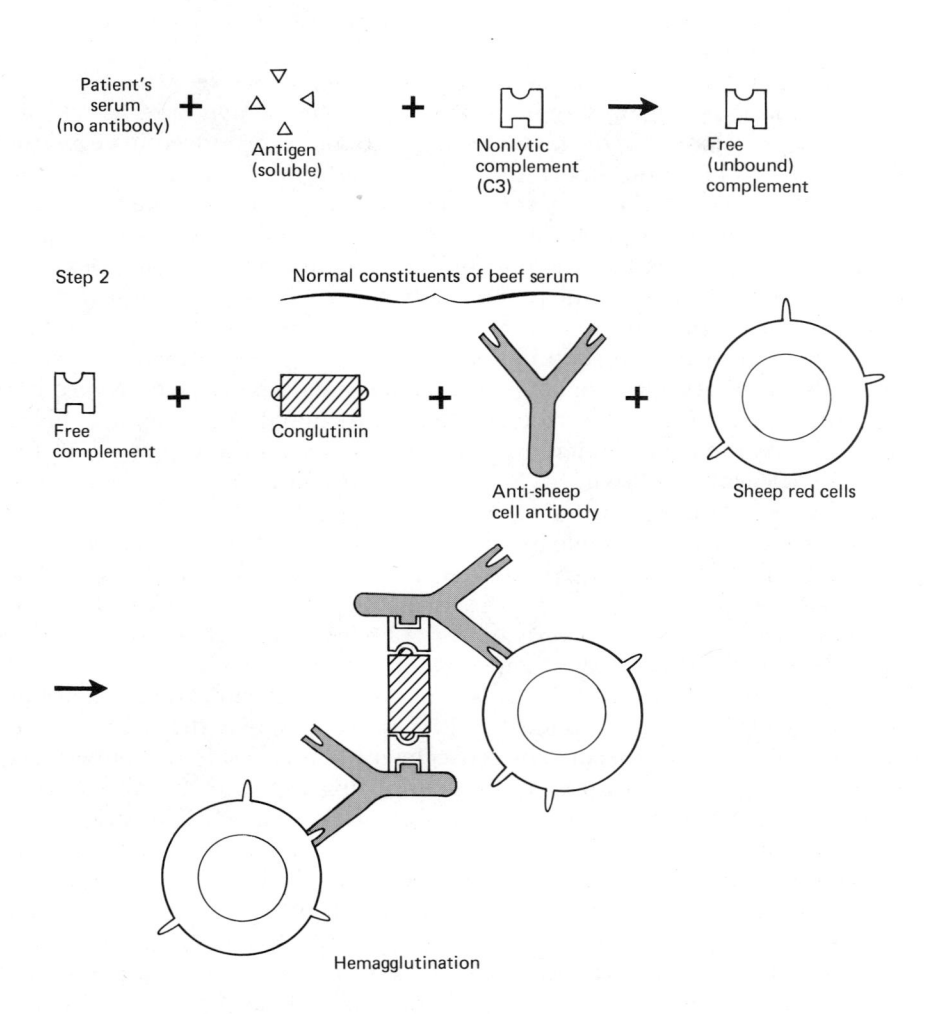

Step 1

Patient's serum (no antibody) + Antigen (soluble) + Nonlytic complement (C3) → Free (unbound) complement

Step 2

Normal constituents of beef serum

Free complement + Conglutinin + Anti-sheep cell antibody + Sheep red cells

→

Hemagglutination

Cytotoxicity

Antibodies against antigens of erythrocytes or leukocytes can activate the enzymes of the complement system and thereby cause changes in the membranes that result in cell death. Thus, hemolysins and leukocidins are potential cytotoxic agents. One of the lymphokine products of T lymphocytes is **lymphocytotoxin (lymphotoxin)** that causes lysis of target cells. Killer T cells therefore also qualify as cytotoxic agents. **Toxins** are defined as antigenic poisons. When unqualified, the term *toxin* is usually considered to be a bacterial enzyme. Bacterial toxins are broadly classified as either exotoxins or endotoxins. **Exotoxins** are heat-labile proteins (usually enzymes or enzyme inhibitors) released primarily by certain gram-positive bacteria. Exotoxins usually are highly antigenic and extremely poisonous (e.g. botulism, tetanus, and diphtheria). Exotoxins must be converted to nonpoisonous toxoids for safe use in stimulating immunity as vaccines. Chemical treatment of an exotoxin with formaldehyde, phenol, beta-propiolactone, or various acids usually detoxifies the molecule but does not destroy its antigenicity.

Antibodies made in response to a natural exposure to a toxin might contain antibodies against regions in or near the catalytic site as well as other antigenic portions of the molecule. Antibodies produced in response to an artificial immunization with a toxoid might not have specificities for the catalytic site of the corresponding toxin because that site has been modified in the toxoid molecule. It is not known how antitoxins neutralize their homologous toxins. One possibility is that an antitoxin combines with an antigenic region in or near the catalytic site of the toxin and thereby prevents interaction with the enzyme's substrate (susceptible target tissues) by steric hindrance. A second hypothesis proposes that antitoxin induces a reversible allosteric effect (change in secondary and higher levels of protein structure) that renders the catalytic site nonfunctional. A third possibility is that the toxin may be rendered incapable of entering the target cell if it is complexed with antitoxin. Whatever the mechanism, the neutralizing capacity of antitoxins is usually high for exotoxins.

Endotoxins are heat-stable lipopolysaccharides (LPS) associated with the cell walls of most gram-negative bacteria. Endotoxins do not have enzymatic properties because all enzymes are proteins. This class of toxin can resist temperatures of 60°C for several hours without losing its poisonous properties. **Boivin antigens** and somatic (O) antigens are sometimes used as synonyms for endotoxins. This is not exactly correct, however, because at least some of the toxic component of LPS appears to be in the lipid fraction whereas all of the O-specific antigenic determinants reside in the polysaccharide component. In general, the neutralizing capacity of antitoxins for endotoxins is therefore relatively poor because lipids are feeble antigens. If the steric hindrance hypothesis of antitoxin neutralization is correct, then the closer the polysaccharide antigen is located to the toxic lipid component in the cell membrane, the greater its neutralizing properties should be. Because endotoxins are poorly neutralized by their homologous antitoxins, any mixture of endotoxin-antitoxin is likely to be rather poisonous for experimental animals. Endotoxins become available as toxins only following death of the bacterial cell and degradation of the cell wall to reveal the LPS moieties. The polysaccharide component of LPS preferentially stimulates the production of IgM-neutralizing antibodies; the protein nature of exotoxins is more likely to stimulate neutralizing antibodies (antitoxins) of class IgG.

The rabbit pyrogen test for gram-negative bacterial contaminants is currently the only one acceptable by the United States Food and Drug Administration (FDA), Bureau of Biologics (BOB), for quality assurance of parenteral solutions, foods, and water. Endotoxins are also known as **pyrogens,** i.e., fever-producing agents. However, the *Limulus* amebocyte lysate (LAL) test may soon be accepted by the FDA as an alternate (or perhaps preferred) endotoxin assay. The LAL test is the most sensitive assay for bacterial endotoxins, reportedly capable of detecting as little as 0.003 ng/ml of *E. coli* endotoxin. Moreover, it is specific for endotoxins and much more economical than rabbit tests. The only circulating blood cells in the horseshoe crab (*Limulus polyphemus*) are amebocytes. When lysed, these cells release a proclotting enzyme that can be activated by endotoxin with the help of calcium and magnesium ions. The clotting protein or coagulogen in the plasma of the crab is cleaved by the activated enzyme and the larger fragments polymerize to form a clot. The LAL test can be quantitated by spectrophotometry or by nephelometry. The latter is a photometric technique based on light scattering (reflection) or turbidity (transmission) by particles or macromolecular complexes in solution such as LAL-polymerized coagulogen fragments, bacterial suspensions, or antigen-antibody precipitates. Nephelometry is reportedly more sensitive than spectrophotometry for quantitating LAL tests and has the potential to supersede most gel precipitation methods.

Exotoxins tend to attack specific targets, whereas endotoxins tend to produce more generalized damage. For example, tetanus exotoxin attaches to receptors in the neuromuscular junctions of voluntary muscles and to anterior horn cells of the central nervous system (CNS). The hemolytic toxins of certain streptococci attack vascular endothelium. Botulinum toxin is specific for certain peripheral motor nerve endings. Deaths due to diphtheria toxin are primarily caused by its action on heart muscle, but it also affects nerves, liver, adrenals, and skin. A broader range of tissues is affected by diphtheria toxin than is typical of most exotoxins. In this sense, it more nearly resembles the action of an endotoxin than an exotoxin. The major distinctions between exotoxins and endotoxins are summarized in Table 7.5.

Extracellular enzymes (exotoxins) are important contributors to the invasive properties of some pathogenic microorganisms. *Clostridium perfringens* liberates a collagenase that disrupts collagen (the major protein in white fibers of connective tissue) and a lecithinase that splits lecithin (essential constituents of animal and plant cells and especially abundant in myelin sheaths of nervous tissue). *Staphylococcus aureus* produces a coagulase that

Table 7.5 Distinguishing Characteristics of Exotoxins and Endotoxins

Characteristic	Exotoxin	Endotoxin
Chemical nature	Protein	Lipopolysaccharide
Bacterial source	Mainly secreted by living, gram-positive cells	Released following disintegration of gram-negative cells
Thermostability	Most are inactivated at 60–80°C	May resist 120°C for 1 hour
Target tissues	Usually specific	Generalized
Relative size of lethal dose	Small	Large
Detoxified by formaldehyde	Yes	No
Relative antigenicity	High	Variable
Relative neutralizing capacity of antitoxins	High	Low
Class of immunoglobulins usually involved in neutralization	IgG	IgM

stimulates fibrin formation, a fibrinolysin (kinase) that dissolves fibrin clots, and a leukocidin that lyses leukocytes. Some bacteria produce proteases, nucleases, or lipases that depolymerize proteins, nucleic acids, and fats, respectively. Some staphlococci and streptococci produce any of several hemolysins that lyse erythrocytes.

Patients that have been exposed to these hemolytic exotoxins are expected to develop homologous antitoxins. Among the most common serological tests for such antitoxins are the antistreptolysin tests.

ANTISTREPTOLYSIN TESTS

Serologic group A streptococci (*Streptococcus pyogenes*) release several important harmful agents. One of these is an "aggressin," a "virulence factor," or a "spreading factor" called hyaluronidase. This is an enzyme that solubilizes the ground substance of connective tissues, thereby enhancing the spread of the organism in the host. A skin rash–producing erythrogenic toxin is released by the lysogenic (infected with a bacterial virus) strains that cause scarlet fever. Streptolysin S (SLS) can cause lysis of mammalian erythrocytes and leukocytes. It is not immunogenic, but it is oxygen-stable. SLS causes a clear zone of beta hemolysis surrounding streptococcal colonies on blood agar plates. Streptolysin O (SLO) is a hemolysin with direct toxic effects on heart tissue. Unlike SLS, SLO is antigenic. The letter "O" designates that this toxin is "oxygen-labile."

The latent period required for the development of rheumatic fever symptoms coincides with the time required for the production of high titers of antistreptococcal antibodies. This and other facts suggest that these antibodies may be involved in the etiology of rheumatic fever. As a result of previous contact with streptolysin O, healthy people may have titers of antistreptolysin O (ASO) as high as 125 units. Therefore, a single titer on a patient is of little diagnostic value unless it is extremely high. Most patients with rheumatic fever have ASO titers of about 500 units. A fourfold rise in titer between paired sera taken two or three weeks apart is indicative of a current or recent streptococcal infection. Similarly a drop in titer from 250 to 125 units over a longer period of time is indicative of recovery. One type of ASO test involves inhibition of hemolysis by streptolysin O with the antitoxin, **antistreptolysin O** (ASO, ASLO). Streptolysin O can cause nonimmune lysis of red blood cells if unopposed by ASO. If the patient's serum contains ASO antibodies, they will combine with the antigen (toxin; streptolysin) and neutralize its hemolytic activity. Care must be taken to avoid agitation (aeration) of this toxin because it oxidizes readily and loses its hemolytic properties. The dried, powdered form of streptolysin O should not be rehydrated unless it is to be immediately added to an *in vitro* test.

Commercial kits are available that contain streptolysin O, a special buffer, 5 percent rabbit or human group O red cells, and an ASO reference standard. A protocol for setting up the test is shown in Table 7.6. The patient's serum is diluted with the buffer 1:10, 1:100, and 1:500 and delivered to twelve tubes according to the protocol. The tubes are gently shaken to mix buffer and serum. Then 0.5 ml of streptolysin O antigen is added to each tube. They are gently shaken and then incubated at 37°C for fifteen minutes. During this incubation the antitoxin (if present) will combine with

Table 7.6 EXAMPLE OF A PROTOCOL FOR AN ANTISTREPTOLYSIN O TITRATION TEST

	Tube Number													
	1	2	3	4	5	6	7	8	9	10	11	12	13	14
Serum Dilution	1:10				1:100					1:500			Controls	
Diluted serum, ml	0.8	0.2	1.0	0.8	0.6	0.4	0.3	1.0	0.8	0.6	0.4	0.2	0.0	0.0
Buffer solution, ml	0.2	0.8	0.0	0.2	0.4	0.6	0.7	0.0	0.2	0.4	0.6	0.8	1.5	1.0
	Shake tubes gently to mix													
Streptolysin "O" reagent, ml	0.5	0.5	0.5	0.5	0.5	0.5	0.5	0.5	0.5	0.5	0.5	0.5	0.0	0.5
	Again shake gently to mix, then incubate at 37°C for 15 minutes													
Rabbit or human "O" cells, 5% suspension, ml	0.5	0.5	0.5	0.5	0.5	0.5	0.5	0.5	0.5	0.5	0.5	0.5	0.5	0.5
Final serum dilution	1:12	1:50	1:100	1:125	1:166	1:250	1:333	1:500	1:625	1:833	1:1250	1:2500		
Todd unit value	12	50	100	125	166	250	333	500	625	833	1250	2500		

Shake tubes gently after addition of cell suspension and incubate at 37°C for forty-five minutes. (Shake tubes again after first fifteen minutes of incubation). After forty-five minutes' incubation, centrifuge tubes for one minute at 1,500 rpm.

Serology and Immunology

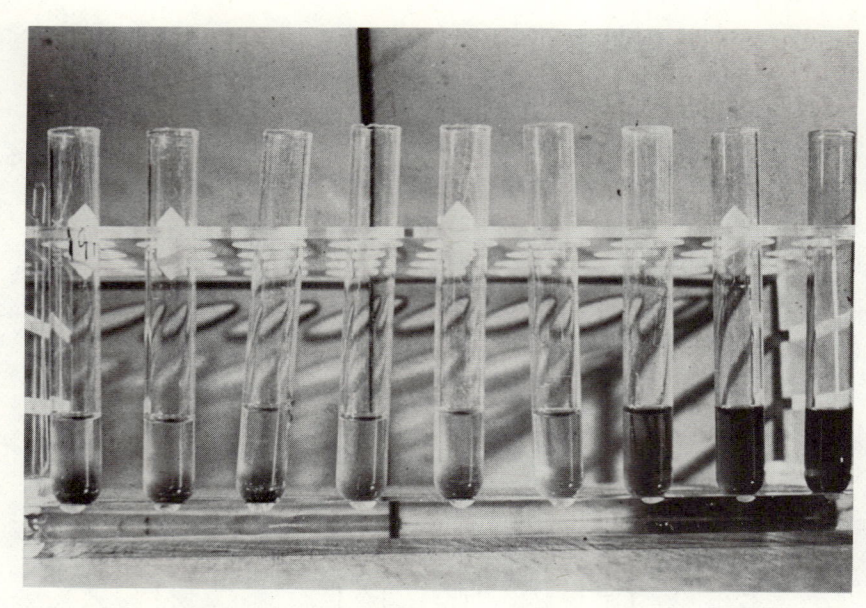

FIGURE 7.11. Antistreptolysin O titration. Left to right: Tubes 1 through 6 have completely inhibited streptolysin (no hemolysis); tube 7 shows partial streptolysin inhibition; tubes 8 and 9 did not inhibit streptolysin (complete hemolysis). End point is in tube 6. [*Courtesy of Elliot Scientific Corp., New York City.*]

the toxin and neutralize it so that it cannot react with red cells. The erythrocyte suspension is added, the tubes are gently shaken, and they are incubated again for forty-five minutes. During the second incubation any free toxin can attach to red cells and cause them to lyse. The tubes are centrifuged and read for the degree of hemolysis (Figure 7.11). In contrast to the "vin rosé" red lysis by complement, that induced by the toxin is a dirty purple color (or violet in weak lysis).

The end-point titer is the reciprocal of the greatest dilution showing no hemolysis. In tube 2 of Table 7.6, for example, initially 0.2 ml of a one-tenth dilution of serum is diluted with 0.8 ml buffer so that the final volume is 1 ml of some other dilution ($1/x$). Therefore,

$$0.2 \text{ ml } (1/10) = 1 \text{ ml } (1/x)$$
$$x = 50 \text{ or } 50 \text{ Todd units}$$

Each unit of titer is called a Todd unit, named for E. W. Todd who pioneered the test in 1933. Todd units refer only to ASO, not to any other kind of antitoxin. All other Todd unit values are calculated in a similar way.

Tube 13 is a red cell control that should not lyse. Tube 14 is a streptolysin control that should produce complete lysis. The ASO reference standard is usually a lyophilized antiserum of known ASO titer. When reconstituted with buffer according to the directions on the label, it may represent a 1:100 dilution. This reference standard would then be run in parallel with one or more unknowns as a series of five tubes (3 to 7) in the 1:100 dilution series. If the manufacturer claims that the titer of the reference standard is 166 Todd units, then no lysis should be seen in tubes 3, 4, or 5; some lysis is expected in tube 6 and more lysis is expected in tube 7. Only when all controls behave normally can the test of unknowns be considered valid.

The antistreptolysin test (ASLT) is the most common serological test for the detection of group A streptococcal infections. The neutralization of toxin by antitoxin is reflected in inhibition of hemolysis. In addition to this type of test, there are various agglutination tests for ASO antibodies. The toxin can be coated onto latex particles or onto aldehyde-fixed (nonlysable) sheep cells. It then may serve as an agglutinogen. In a slide agglutination test, the patient's serum is first exposed to streptolysin (both in appropriate dilutions). Next, the agglutinogen reagent is added, mixed with a clean glass rod, and rocked or rotated for a specified time. If there is more antitoxin than needed to bind all of the free toxin, some antibodies will be left to cause clumping of the toxin-coated particles. Usually these screening tests are designed to yield positive agglutination with sera that have an ASO titer (by hemolytic inhibition test) of 166 to 200 or greater because elevated ASO titers (>200 units) are detected in about 80 percent of patients with clinical symptoms of acute rheumatic fever. Single tests are not reliable. It is far better to obtain evidence of a rising titer on weekly or biweekly specimens through quantitative tests, but early treatment with antibiotics and/or the slow progress of streptolysin-induced glomerulonephritis may preclude obtaining paired acute and convalescent specimens. This disease will be discussed in greater detail in Chapter 9.

Some commercial companies offer agglutinogen reagents coated not only with streptolysin O, but also with one or more other streptococcal exoenzymes including streptokinase, hyaluronidase, deoxyribonuclease (DNase), and nicotinamide adenine dinucleotidase (NADase). When antihyaluronidase (AH) tests are run simultaneously with ASO tests, the number of positive sera can be increased to about 90 percent of those with rheumatic fever. Similarly, by testing simultaneously for anti-DNase and anti-NADase (ANAD) in addition to ASO and AH, at least one of these antibodies or a summation of two or more antibodies will show elevation (give a positive screener test) in approximately 95 percent of rheumatic fever patients. This type of combined screening test is of greater diagnostic value than tests for a single exoenzyme antibody such as ASO. The titer of a serum derived from a quantitative multiexoenzyme test should not be expressed in Todd units, because the contribution that ASO antibodies make to such a titer is unknown. Commonly, however, there is good correlation between ASO titer and multiexoenzyme titer. Agglutination tests can be performed much faster than the lytic inhibition (classical ASO) test. Cholesterol and beta lipoproteins tend to cause false positive titers in the classical ASO test; these substances do not interfere with the agglutination tests.

A feeble ASO response is generally observed after streptococcal infection of the skin (pyoderma). One of the anti-DNase tests has been shown to provide serological evidence of previous streptococcal infections in acute glomerulonephritis (AGN) resulting from pyoderma. Four biochemically and serologically distinct streptococcal DNases are known, designated A, B, C, and D. Antibodies against DNase-B (ADNase-B) are of the greatest clinical significance because the majority of group A streptococci produce easily detectable quantities of DNase-B, and other groups of streptococci (a few members of groups C and G excepted) do not produce DNase-B. In principle, the ADNase test is based on the fact that cognate antibody will neutralize the depolymerization activity of DNase on DNA. Enzyme activity is reflected in the color change of an indicator, e.g., blue or bluish-violet indicating lack of enzyme activity (i.e., enzymatic inhibition by antibody) and pinkish-violet indicating enzyme activity (lack of antibody inhibition). The anti-DNase response is age-dependent. Mean normal levels are as follows: preschoolers, 1 : 60; school age children, 1 : 170; adults, 1 : 85. A titer exceeding 1 : 250 is considered to be elevated regardless of age. Again, titer changes seen in biweekly samples are more meaningful than the absolute value of a single determination.

POTENCY OF TOXINS AND ANTITOXINS

Federal and state public health laboratories are charged with the responsibilities of determining the potency of toxins and antitoxins to be used as reference standards or (in the case of toxoids and antitoxins) as prophylactic and/or therapeutic agents. A large number of variables exist in the assay of a toxin including the species of animal used, the route of administration, the kind of toxin, the dosage, and the method employed in end-point determination. Humans, guinea pigs, and horses are susceptible to tetanus toxin, whereas dogs and chickens are resistant. Within a susceptible species, larger animals can generally tolerate higher doses of nonneurogenic toxins than smaller animals. Most toxins administered by mouth are destroyed by proteolytic enzymes of the gut. Botulinum toxin is a notable exception in this regard. If a toxin affects only certain target tissues, then the closer the target tissue is to the site of toxin entry, the faster the symptoms of toxicity should appear. Intravenous injection, of course, would distribute the toxin most rapidly to all parts of the body. Subclinical amounts of toxin probably do some damage. The damage tends to increase with the dosage up to the lethal dose. The time required for symptoms to appear tends to vary inversely with the dosage. All of these variables are usually standardized in an end-point assay such as the **minimum lethal dose** (MLD). This is defined as the smallest dose of toxin that kills all members of a group of test animals (of the same species) in a specified time, when administered by a specified route. The range of weights of the animals is also specified, usually a group selected for uniformity in this regard.

Another method that usually gives a sharper end point than the MLD is the **LD$_{50}$**. This is the amount of toxin required to kill 50 percent of a group of animals (species, weight, route, and time specified). The LD$_{50}$ is usually estimated from a semilogarithmic plot of cumulative mortality against dosage.

A **minimal reacting dose** (MRD) is the amount of toxin that produces minimal, but definite, "standard" focal inflammation in the skin of a series of susceptible test animals. These reactions include congestion and edema, induration, degenerative changes, and desquamation of epidermal cells that become apparent eighteen to twenty-four hours after intracutaneous injection of the toxin and reach a peak in about ninety-six hours.

Once the potency of a toxin has been established, the antitoxin can be standardized. The potency of an antitoxin is expressed in arbitrary units that only apply to that kind of antitoxin and cannot be equated with units for a different kind of antitoxin. For example, in the United States the official unit of diphtheria antitoxin is defined as a certain amount (weight) of a certain dried horse serum antitoxin maintained by one of the government agencies as a reference source for many years. By international agreements, some antisera are defined in terms of international units (IU), but in other cases individual countries may have their own units. For example, the American unit (AU) of tetanus antitoxin is twice the value of the IU. The guinea pig is the official test animal for testing the potency of diphtheria and tetanus antitoxins in the United States. Some other countries prefer to use the mouse because the results appear comparable and mice are less expensive.

The **L₊** dose of toxin (L = *Limes Tod;* German = death limit) is the smallest amount of diphtheria toxin that, when combined with 1 unit of diphtheria antitoxin and injected subcutaneously, kills any 250-gm guinea pig within four days. The **L₀** dose of toxin (*Limes Null;* German = zero limit) is the largest amount of diphtheria toxin that, when combined with 1 unit of diphtheria antitoxin and injected subcutaneously into any 250-gm guinea pig, fails to produce symptoms of toxicity. The difference between the higher L₊ and lower L₀ doses is not simply 1 MLD, but rather it is usually between 10 and 100 MLD. The reason for this can be explained by reference to Figure 5.1. Suppose that tube 3 in this figure represents a mixture of an L₀ dose of toxin with 1 unit of antitoxin. Adding a relatively small amount of toxin represented by 1 MLD would cause only a minor change in the antigen-antibody ratio. The additional toxin would be incorporated into the lattice. A considerable amount of toxin in excess of the original L₀ dose might be required before enough remained free to be lethal to the guinea pig.

In 1902, J. Danysz discovered that the toxicity of a mixture of toxin and antitoxin depends on the way the reagents are mixed as well as on their relative final concentrations. As an example, suppose that 10 parts each of toxin and antitoxin constitute a neutral mixture if allowed to incubate for ten minutes at room temperature prior to inoculation into a test animal. However, if 7 parts of toxin and 3 parts of antitoxin are placed in one tube and 7 parts of antitoxin and 3 parts of toxin are placed in a second tube, both tubes are incubated for ten minutes, then they are mixed and immediately injected, the test animal dies. If an additional ten minutes' incubation of the mixture had occurred prior to injection, the animal would have survived. The animal's death was caused by unneutralized toxin from the first aliquot; toxin in the second aliquot combined with more antitoxin than required for neutralization. Given more time to equilibrate before injection, the antigen-antibody complexes of the two aliquots dissociate and recombine in a new way that neutralizes all of the toxin. The **Danysz phenomenon** demonstrates that mixtures of toxin and antitoxin can combine in variable proportions and that these complexes can dissociate and recombine in new ways given sufficient time.

In 1909 Römer devised a method for titrating an unknown diphtheria antitoxin and a standard antitoxin in the same animal. This methodology circumvents the problem of variation between individuals that occurs when the unknown and the standard are tested in different animals or groups of animals. Römer found the smallest amount of diphtheria toxin that, when mixed with 1 unit of antitoxin and injected intracutaneously in the shaved skin of a susceptible guinea pig, produced a minimal local inflammatory reaction (erythma and/or edema). This is referred to as the **Lᵣ** dose or the "limes-reacting" dose. It is a highly sensitive assay method, capable of detecting as little as 1/50,000 unit of diphtheria antitoxin in 0.1 ml of serum. For all practical purposes, the L_r dose and the L_o dose are equivalent because a slight excess of toxin above the L_o dose results in a local skin response.

The L_f dose or "limes flocculation" dose is the amount of diphtheria toxin flocculating (precipitating) most rapidly with 1 unit of antitoxin in a Ramon titration test. This is a test of antigenicity, not toxicity of the toxin. The L_f value of a toxin can be calculated as follows.

$$L_f/\text{ml toxin} = \frac{(\text{antitoxin units/ml}) \times (\text{ml of antitoxin})}{\text{ml of toxin}}$$

As an example, if 0.15 ml of antitoxin containing 1,000 units/ml is the amount found to flocculate most rapidly with 2 ml of toxin, then

$$L_f/\text{ml toxin} = \frac{1,000 \times 0.15}{2} = 75, \text{ and 1 } L_f \text{ dose of toxin} = 1/75 = 0.0133 \text{ ml}$$

TOXIGENICITY TESTS OF *CORYNEBACTERIUM DIPHTHERIAE*

In order to prepare a toxoid, the exotoxin must be extracted and purified from a culture of the microorganism. Special culture conditions are sometimes required to induce the bacteria to produce the toxin. *C. diphtheriae,* for example, only produce diphtheria toxin in a neutral or alkaline medium containing a minute amount of iron. Not all isolates of this organism have the genetic instructions for making toxin. Only those strains that harbor a special temperate bacteriophage (bacterial virus; one carrying *tox* gene) integrated into the host chromosome (provirus) are potential toxin producers.

There are two major methods used to determine whether or not a given isolate of *C. diphtheriae* is a toxin producer. The serological (*in vitro*) method, also known as the **Elek test,** employs an agar medium enriched with peptones and rabbit serum (potassium tellurite is added to inhibit growth of most organisms other than corynebacteria). A *strip* of filter paper soaked with diphtheria antitoxin (500 units/ml) is placed on the surface of (or embedded in) the plate of agar. Each isolate of *C. diphtheriae* to be tested for toxigenicity is inoculated on the medium as a single line streak at right angles to the filter paper. The plate is incubated to allow bacterial growth and read daily for three days. If a culture has liberated diphtheria toxin, it will have diffused from the streak of growth and formed lines of precipitation radiating at 45-degree angles from the intersection of culture and filter paper as shown in Figure 7.12.

The second qualitative method for assaying the toxigenic state of a *C. diphtheriae* isolate is the animal (*in vivo*) method. Pure broth test cultures of *C. diphtheriae* are injected (0.2 ml) intradermally in a row of the upper half of a shaved area on the side of a rabbit. Four hours later, 1,000 International Units of diphtheria antitoxin are injected in the marginal ear vein. Each culture is then reinoculated in a row below the corresponding site in the upper row. The bottom row serves as neutralized controls for the tests in the upper row. After 48 hours the rabbit is inspected for signs of necrosis, edema,

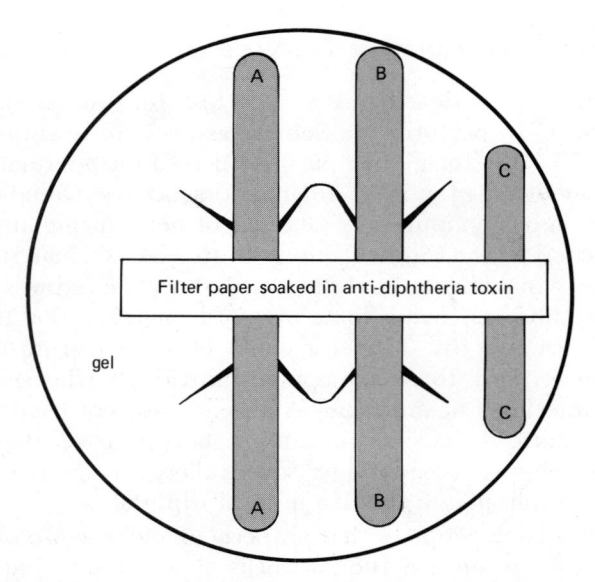

FIGURE 7.12. Toxin precipitation technique in gel (Elek test). *A* is a control culture streak of a known toxigenic strain of *Corynebacterium diphtheriae*. *B* is a streak of the culture under test. *C* is a negative reaction, indicating that this strain does not produce toxin.

or erythema at the test sites. Inflammation at the test site with no reaction in the control site indicates that the strain of *C. diphtheriae* is a toxin producer. Toxin produced by bacteria in the lower row is immediately neutralized by circulating antitoxin, thereby preventing tissue damage. Toxin produced by bacteria in the top row had up to four hours to cause tissue damage that cannot be reversed by the subsequent administration of antitoxin. The union of toxins with target cells is firm and undissociable. To be effective in neutralization, antitoxin must combine with toxin before it attaches to target cells. This is why it is extremely important that antitoxin be administered for effective passive immunity as soon after exposure to a toxin as possible. Five American units of diphtheria antitoxin is the therapeutic dose required to neutralize ten fatal doses of toxin intravenously administered to a rabbit if it is given within ten minutes. After thirty minutes, 2,000 AU is required; after ninety minutes, no amount of antitoxin can save the rabbit.

An alternative *in vivo* test of toxigenicity for an isolate of *C. diphtheriae* involves a pair of guinea pigs. Their abdomens are shaved and 500 units of diphtheria antitoxin are injected intraperitoneally into the control pig. Thirty minutes later, 0.2 ml of pure broth culture of the organism is injected subcutaneously on the side of both pigs. If the culture contains a toxin-producing strain, the unprotected pig will usually die within five days with a necrotic area at the injection site. The control pig, protected by passive immunity, should survive with no symptoms of illness. The rabbit assay has the test and the control in the same animal, thereby avoiding possible differences in sensitivities and responsiveness between individuals that may occur in guinea pig pairs.

SKIN TESTS FOR IMMUNITY TO TOXINS

In 1913, B. Schick developed a skin test for human immunity to diphtheria toxin. To perform the **Schick test,** 0.1 ml of diphtheria toxin (containing 1/50 MLD for guinea pigs) is injected intradermally on a convenient place such as the forearm. Inflammation occurs around the injection site if the person has no immunity (absence of neutralizing antibodies [antitoxins]). The test is read within twenty-four to thirty-six hours; the reaction usually reaches a maximum about the fourth day. The redness and induration gradually subside, leaving some brownish pigmentation that may last for three to four months. This test could be used during a diphtheria epidemic to determine those susceptible individuals who should receive prophylactic injections of antitoxin. Antitoxins are not used routinely in prophylaxis because (1) passive immunity is short-lived, (2) they are expensive, and (3) foreign sera may trigger severe allergic responses. The Schick reaction is not applicable to the diagnosis of diphtheria.

Before immunizing people with diphtheria toxoid, the **Moloney test** may be employed to determine if the patient is hypersensitive (allergic) to the toxoid. In the Moloney test, 0.1 ml of a one-tenth dilution of the toxoid is injected intradermally. If more than a minimal local reaction occurs, the immunizing dose of toxoid should be administered in fractions at suitable intervals to avoid triggering a severe hypersensitivity response.

The **Dick test** is a skin test for immunity to the erythrogenic (skin-reddening) exotoxin of certain strains of *Streptococcus pyogenes* (carrying a particular temperate phage) that is responsible for the rash and other symptoms of scarlet fever. A "skin test dose" is the smallest amount of the toxin that produces a typical reaction in fully susceptible individuals (no antitoxin titer). A skin test dose is injected in the forearm. Slight inflammation may be observed in immune patients. Therefore, a positive reaction (indicating lack of immunity to scarlet fever) is one in which the diameter of the erythma exceeds 1 cm. The reaction reaches a maximum in about eighteen to twenty-four hours and then fades rapidly. Some evidence supports the contention that the Dick reaction is at least partly a hypersensitivity response to streptococcal antigens induced by previous infections and that the toxin merely serves to exacerbate the test response. If the Dick reaction were solely a hypersensitivity phenomenon, a positive reaction (skin reddening) would indicate that some degree of immunity exists in the patient. Because this problem has not yet been resolved, the Dick test is considered unreliable and is seldom used today in the United States.

The rash of scarlet fever is difficult to distinguish from the rash of German measles or other rash-producing infections. It is possible to differentiate scarlet fever rash from the others by the **Schultz-Charlton test.** If scarlet fever antitoxin is injected intradermally into a reddened area of the skin of a patient with scarlet fever, a blanching of the rash should be observed at that site within five to six hours and usually persists until the rash over the rest of the body disappears. Blanching is indicative of toxin neutralization by the antitoxin.

At least three erythrogenic toxins (A, B, and C) have been demonstrated. Recovery probably confers lifelong type-specific immunity. Penicillin is normally used to kill all beta-hemolytic group A streptococci. The danger from the scarlet fever organism is not its toxin so much as the possibility of its spreading from the throat to cause serious infection of the middle ear, septicemia, osteomyelitis, or its persistence associated with secondary sequelae such as rheumatic fever or acute glomerulonephritis.

VENOMS

The poisonous fluid injected by the bites of certain snakes, and spiders, or the stings of scorpions, bees, wasps, and other animals is termed **venom** (venin, venene). Extreme pain and swelling at the bite site, vomiting, hemorrhages, shock (failing pulse), collapse, and shortness of breath are common symptoms of snake venom poisoning. Contrary to popular belief, the bite of a venomous snake is not inevitably poisonous. Perhaps up to 30 percent of snakebites are not effective in delivering poison into the victims. According to one study, there is considerable variation in efficiency of venom delivery from one species of snake to another and also between geographical areas (states). Rattlesnakes appeared to be slightly more efficient (18 percent of persons bitten were not "venomated") than copperheads or cottonmouth moccasins (approximately 25 percent of both escaped venomation). South Carolina's snakes are most infallible (only 13 percent of bitten patients escaped venomation), whereas those of Mississippi and Texas were least infallible (30 percent escaped venomation).

Suction at the injection site is effective in removing venom from experimental animals up to two hours after it is injected. If the venom is not removed promptly, however, the pain becomes more intense with time and the redness and congestion spread from the injection site. If no redness or congestion is seen within four hours after the bite, it may be concluded that the patient does not have "pit viper"* venomation.

One of the dangers in treating patients with antivenoms (antivenins, antivenenes) of animal origin is the possibility of a severe immediate hypersensitivity (allergic) reaction to the foreign serum proteins or a delayed reaction several days or weeks later (serum sickness). On the other hand, the effectiveness of antitoxins in general declines rapidly with time after the bite. Clearly, it is important to have a method available to efficiently and rapidly test patients at risk from toxins or venoms for preexisting sensitivities (allergies) to antitoxin (usually horse serum) protein. There are two major sites for conducting sensitivity tests to horse serum (horses are commonly used to produce antitoxins and antivenoms). A skin test consists of the intracutaneous injection of a small amount of diluted antivenom. If no reaction is observed within thirty minutes, a stronger dose is injected. If still no reaction is seen within another fifteen to thirty minutes, then the full-strength antivenom is injected. If the patient is already sensitive to horse serum, edema and redness will usually appear at the test site. In general, the shorter the interval between injection and the beginning of the skin reaction, the greater the sensitivity of the patient to horse serum. A second

---

* "Pit vipers" are members of the subfamily Crotalinae of the family Viperidae. They have a thermosensory pit between the eye and the nostril. All pit vipers are poisonous.

site for sensitivity testing is the conjunctiva of the eye. A drop of test serum is placed in the conjunctival sac of the lower eyelid. Dilation of the conjunctival vessels, itching, and edema of the conjunctiva and inner eyelid constitute a positive test (sensitivity). Even though these sensitivity tests appear negative, they do not entirely eliminate the possibility of either a severe immediate reaction upon administration of the antiserum or a delayed reaction (serum sickness). If the patient is sensitive to horse serum, then a different source of antivenom must be found; otherwise the risk of administering the antiserum must be weighed against the risk of withholding it.

If antivenom is used, it should be injected intramuscularly or subcutaneously at several sites above the bite on a limb. For a bite on the head, the antiserum should be injected around the bite. If a relatively long delay period exists between the bite and the administration of antiserum, it should be given intravenously. The smaller the body size of the patient, the larger the dose of antivenom required. Because children have less resistance and less body fluid with which to dilute the poison, they may require twice as much antivenom as adults. Upon arrival at a medical facility, the blood of the patient should be typed as soon as possible because of the potential for severe extensive destruction of red cells necessitating transfusions and because hemolysins present in the venom may alter blood proteins and thereby interfere with accurate cross-matching. Antibiotics and tetanus antitoxin may be prescribed by the physician as routine prophylactic measures for any puncture wound.

Most of the commercial "field kits" contain a lyophilized **polyvalent antiserum** with antibodies against the venoms of the most common pit vipers of North and South America. A polyvalent antiserum is required because one cannot predict by which species of snake he may be bitten.

In contrast to viper venoms, the venoms of bees, wasps, hornets, and yellow jackets are not cytotoxic agents. The stings of these insects cause anaphylactic reactions in hypersensitive people. Those individuals sensitive to bees may be advised to subject themselves regularly (perhaps daily) to a bee sting in order to maintain themselves in a "desensitized" state. Whole body extracts (WBEs) of the insects have been used both in skin testing for sensitivity and in desensitization. Obviously, the only relevant antigens are those in the venom. Up to 90 percent of all people skin-tested with WBEs produce "allergic" reactions, but such reactions are probably due to toxic components of the insect's body rather than allergic reactions to the venom. Bee venom should be used for skin testing and prophylaxis, but WBE is all that has been commercially available until just recently. The subject of desensitization to this and other forms of allergy is discussed in Chapter 9. As with all allergies, the best policy is avoidance of the antigen. Hymenopteran insects are attracted to flowers, perfumes, deodorants, hairsprays, and the like; so these should be avoided if possible, especially in spring and summer. If you are stung, the stinger should be promptly removed. If the venom sac has also been left with the stinger (as it usually is) it may continue to extrude venom for up to three minutes. Care should be taken to avoid squeezing additional venom from the sac when removing the sting. Epinephrine and an antihistamine should be kept available to counteract an anaphylactic reaction.

SELF-EVALUATION

Complement and Cytotoxicity

Terms

1. Any complement fragment that causes degranulation of mast cells.
2. Any substance that attracts leukocytes and inflammatory cells.
3. The propensity of particulate antigen-antibody-complement complexes to indiscriminately attach themselves to surfaces. (2 words)
4. A term commonly used to indicate that complement is bound, activated, or consumed.
5. Ehrlich's name for a complement-fixing antibody against sheep red blood cells that can participate in hemolysis; hemolysin.
6. An indirect complement fixation test used to detect the presence of a specific noncomplement-binding antibody.
7. A beta globulin of normal bovine serum that combines nonspecifically with complex polysaccharides and C3.
8. A protein involved in an alternate pathway of complement activation (other than the classical pathway) and for which the alternate pathway is named.
9. The toxicity of a mixture of toxin and antitoxin may depend on the manner in which they are mixed. (2 words)
10. The name of the skin test for immunity to diphtheria toxin.

Multiple Choice. Choose the one best answer.

1. Which of the following is a gel precipitation test for detecting toxin production by isolates of *Corynebacterium diphtheriae*? (a) Schultz-Charlton (b) Ehrlich (c) Donnan (d) Elek (e) Moloney
2. For most serological tests that employ complement, from which animal is it usually derived? (a) horse (b) guinea pig (c) sheep (d) cattle (e) rabbit
3. What two cations should be added to physiological saline for use in complement fixation tests? (a) calcium, magnesium (b) iron, zinc (c) iron, copper (d) phosphorus, calcium (e) manganese, copper
4. The first component of the classical complement cascade that can attach to antigens is (a) C1 (b) C2a (c) C4b (d) C5 (e) none of these
5. The properdin alternate pathway of complement activation converges with the classical pathway at (a) C1 (b) C2 (c) C3 (d) C5 (e) none of these
6. With which of the following diseases is a deficiency of $C\bar{1}$ inhibitor associated? (a) paroxysmal cold hemoglobinuria (b) systemic lupus erythematosus (c) thrombocytopenic purpura (d) hereditary angioneurotic edema (e) more than one of these
7. Which of the following is not characteristic of endotoxins? (a) heat-stable at 60°C (b) enzymatic properties (c) detoxified by formaldehyde (d) attacks specific target tissues (e) more than one of these
8. Which of the following is not a streptococcal exoenzyme for which a serological test is employed? (a) amylase (b) streptokinase (c) hyaluronidase (d) DNase (e) NADase
9. The amount of diphtheria toxin that, when mixed with 1 unit of antitoxin, precipitates most rapidly in a Ramon titration test is designated (a) L_+ (b) L_0 (c) MLD (d) L_r (e) L_f
10. ASO titers are specified in units named for (a) Ehrlich (b) Todd (c) Danysz (d) Römer (e) Schick

True-False

1. Antibody must bind antigen before it can bind complement.
2. C3 activation occurs only when an antibody (of a class that can fix complement) binds to an antigen.

Serology and Immunology

3. Heating serum at 56°C for thirty minutes destroys the hemolytic properties of complement.
4. Anticoagulants (such as EDTA or sodium citrate) render plasma unsuitable for complement activation.
5. Complete hemolysis in a qualitative complement fixation test (all controls behaving properly) indicates that the substance in question is present.
6. If lysis fails to occur in either the serum control or the antigen control of a complement fixation test, nonspecific complement inactivation has occurred.
7. A nonlytic Rice test indicates a positive serum (the unknown substance is present).
8. Normal biological functions of the complement system are assured if radial immunodiffusion tests indicate that all specific complement components are present in normal concentrations.
9. A positive Dick reaction (skin reddening at the site of injection) indicates that the patient lacks immunity to diphtheria.
10. Bee venom is a potent cytotoxic agent.

Tagged Reagents

CHAPTER 8

CHAPTER OUTLINE

Fluorescence Serology
  Qualitative Immunofluorescence Tests
    Direct Immunofluorescence Test
    Inhibition Immunofluorescence Test
    Indirect Immunofluorescence Test
    Complement-staining Immunofluorescence Test
    Fluorescent Antigens
  Quantitative Immunofluorescence Tests
    Fluorescence Quenching
Radioimmunoassay (RIA)
  Basic Principles
  Radionuclides
  Separation of Bound from Free Antigen
  Measuring Radioactivity
  RIA for Digoxin
  RIA for IgE
  Competitive Protein-binding Assays
Enzyme Immunoassay (EIA) or Immunoenzyme Techniques
  Qualitative Slide Tests
  Quantitative Tube Tests
    Heterogeneous EIA Methods
    Homogeneous EIA
Electron Spin Resonance (ESR) Immunoassay
Ferritin Labeling
Self-evaluation

This chapter will be concerned with antigen-antibody complexes that do not go beyond the first phase (antigen-antibody union) of a serological reaction. The first phase occurs almost instantaneously. The second phase involves building a lattice to form visible aggregates of precipitates or agglutinates, and this requires a longer time; e.g., most slide agglutination tests are allowed one to two minutes to fully develop. If either antigen or antibody is monovalent or in low concentration, only the first phase of the reaction occurs and visible aggregates do not form. Some of the major differences between the first and second phases of serological reactions are summarized in Table 8.1. A "label" or "tag" can be placed on either antigen or antibody so that the first phase of antigen-antibody complexes can be identified. Five types of labels will be discussed: (1) fluorescent, (2) radionuclide, (3) enzyme, (4) free radical (spin label), and (5) ferritin.

Fluorescence Serology

QUALITATIVE IMMUNOFLUORESCENCE TESTS

Direct Immunofluorescence Test. A **fluor** or **fluorochrome** is a chemical that can absorb electromagnetic energy of relatively short wavelength and almost instantaneously emit light at a longer frequency (lower energy level). In fluorescence serology, a fluor is chosen that can absorb ultraviolet or short-blue light (200 to 400 nm) and emit light in the visible part of the electromagnetic spectrum (400 to 700 nm). Some fluors can be covalently linked or conjugated to an immunoglobulin without materially affecting the

Table 8.1 COMPARISON OF THE FIRST AND SECOND PHASES OF SEROLOGICAL REACTIONS

Distinguishing Criteria	First Phase	Second Phase
Relative rate of reaction	Fast	Slow
Relative change in free energy	High	Low
Requires electrolytes	No	Yes
Monovalent antigen and/or antibody required	Yes	No
Aggregates develop	No	Yes

antigen-binding capacity of the antibody. These conjugates can then be used in an **immunofluorescence test,** also known as a **fluorescent antibody** (FA or FAB) **test** or **Coons test** (after A. H. Coons, a pioneer of this technique). Among the most popular fluorochromes for FA tests are fluorescein isothiocyanate (FITC), lissamine rhodamine B, and 1-dimethylaminonaphthalene-5-sulfonyl chloride (DANSYL). These fluorescent compounds can easily be covalently joined to free amino groups of proteins. FITC fluoresces in the yellow-green region of the spectrum, whereas rhodamines fluoresce in the orange-red region.

In a **direct immunofluorescence test** (Figures 8.1 and 8.2), an unknown antigen (as in a bacterial smear) is fixed to a slide and then exposed to a fluorescent-tagged antibody of known specificity. The antibody binds to the antigen and thereby also becomes fixed to the slide. The preparation is gently rinsed with buffer to remove any unattached fluorescent antibody and then is examined under a microscope. Ultraviolet light from a mercury lamp is directed at the specimen from below. A primary or excitation filter inserted between the lamp and the microscope removes light waves longer than 450 to 500 nm so that only UV and some blue light hits the specimen (Figure 8.3). The fluor becomes "excited" (electrons moving to new orbits) and releases photons of light almost immediately as its energy returns to the ground state (electrons jump back to original orbits). The emitted light is characteristic of the fluor itself, not of the excitation light. A suitable secondary (emission, barrier) filter is chosen and placed between the specimen and the eye of the observer to remove ultraviolet rays (damaging to the eye) and to allow only the emission characteristic of the fluor to pass.

A different type of microscope, called an **epifluorescence microscope,** has recently become available for viewing fluorescent antibody tests. In this instrument, the UV light enters the barrel of the microscope. The light passes through the excitation filter and is reflected from a dichroic mirror

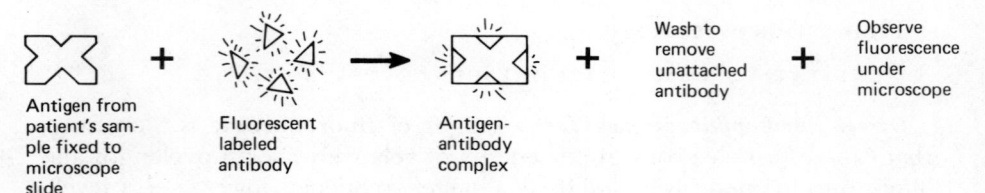

FIGURE 8.1. Model of a positive direct immunofluorescence test. [*Modified from Cherry, W. B., et al., 1960. Fluorescent Antibody Techniques in the Diagnosis of Communicable Diseases. Public Health Service Publication No. 729. U.S. Government Printing Office, Washington, D.C.*]

Tagged Reagents

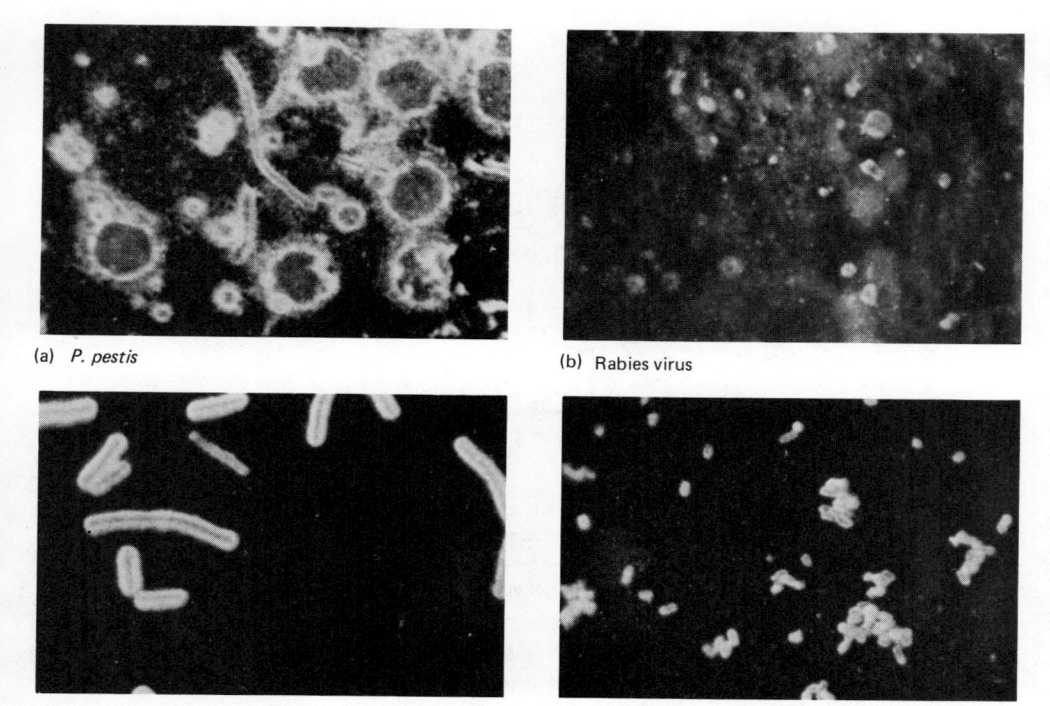

(a) *P. pestis*

(b) Rabies virus

(c) *B. anthracis*

(d) *E. coli*

FIGURE 8.2. Direct immunofluorescence staining. (*a*). *Pasteurella pestis* in smear of fluid aspirated from bubo of a fatal case of plague. Homologous antibody prepared by injecting whole-cell antigen. Note bizarre forms of plague bacilli and specifically stained soluble antigen surrounding tissue cells. (*b*). Rabies virus in impression smear of the brain of a mouse infected with street virus. Note the large aggregates of stained antigen (Negri bodies) and the numerous smaller particles that stain. (*c*). *Bacillus anthracis* in an impression smear from the liver of a mouse. Note both encapsulated and stripped forms. (*d*). *Escherichia coli* in feces from a case of infantile diarrhea. Stained with pooled antibodies for enteropathogenic types of *E. coli*. [Source: Cherry, W. B., M. Goldman, and T. R. Carski. *Fluorescent Antibody Techniques in the Diagnosis of Communicable Diseases.* U.S. Dept. of Health, Education and Welfare, Public Health Service, Bureau of State Services, Communicable Disease Center, Atlanta, GA. Public Health Service Publication No. 729, 1960.]

down through the objective lens onto the top of the specimen. Flourescent light from the specimen passes back up through the objective lens, through the dichroic mirror, through the barrier filter, and through the eyepiece. The dichroic "mirror" reflects UV light, but allows fluorescent light of longer wavelength to pass through it. Epifluorescence microscopes have at least three advantages over conventional microscopes: (1) no dark field condenser is needed, (2) the UV light source can be less intense and therefore the costly mercury lamp is likely to be longer-lived, and (3) thin specimens are not required because surface fluorescence can be examined on thick specimens.

An **autofluorescence control** should be run with the antigen alone. If more fluorescence is observed in the test than in the autofluorescence control, the test is considered positive; i.e., the antigen is present. Known posi-

Serology and Immunology

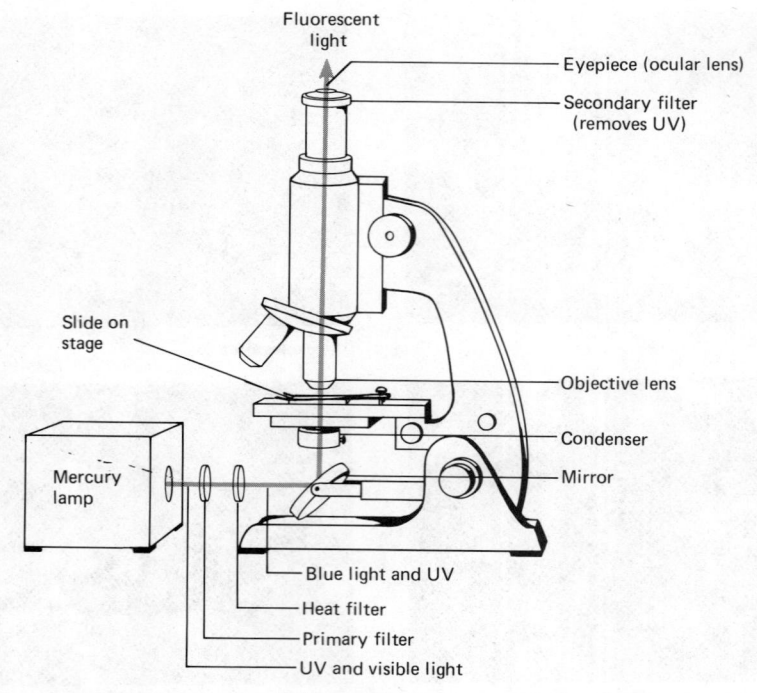

FIGURE 8.3. Diagram of instrumentation used in fluorescence immunomicroscopy. The primary filter allows only ultraviolet and blue light to pass; the secondary filter allows only the light characteristic of the fluor to pass.

tive and negative controls (with and without the antigen, respectively) plus the tagged antibody should be run simultaneously. Any fluorescence in the negative control greater than that in the autofluorescence control indicates incomplete washing that failed to remove the tagged antibody. A **blocking control** may also be used if an unlabeled homologous antibody is available. If the antigen is present and it is exposed to the unlabeled antibody before the labeled antibody is added, no fluorescence should be seen subsequently. The reason for this is that the unlabeled antibody would bind to the antigen first and thereby prevent the attachment of the fluorescent antibody. Washing of the slide prior to reading the test should remove all of the unattached labeled antibody.

A direct FA test is used to detect the presence of *Treponema pallidum* in tissue exudates from external syphilitic lesions (chancres) or in aspirates of regional lymph nodes. This test is called the **fluorescent-antibody dark field (FADF) technique.** A smear from a lesion or node is heat-killed and fixed to the slide. The antibody to be used in the test is absorbed with the nonpathogenic Reiter strain of treponeme to remove genus (group) specific antibodies that might cross-react with saprophytic spirochetes. This absorption aids in rendering the antiserum species-specific and greatly reduces the incidence of biological false positive reactions. When used in this way, the Reiter strain is called **sorbent** material. A fluor is then attached to the specific antibodies. When the fluor-antibody mixture is dialyzed against buffered saline, any unattached fluorochrome is removed, leaving only the conjugate of antibody and fluor inside the dialysis tube. The smear is exposed to the conjugate, incubated in a humidity chamber to prevent drying, and then washed with saline and distilled water. After being blotted with bibulous paper, the slide is examined with dark field microscopy for the fluorescence of organisms with the size and morphology (especially coiling) characteristics of *T. pallidum*. It has not been possible to grow this organism readily on laboratory media or in tissue culture, although it can be grown on the skin, testes, and scrotum of rabbits. The Reiter strain of treponeme can be cultivated on nonliving media, casting doubt on its original classification as *T. pallidum*. A traditional, though nonspecific, screening test for identification of *T. pallidum* is dark field examination of fresh smears showing live, wiggling spirochetes by reflected light. The FADF test has proven to be as accurate as dark field microscopy. It has the additional advantages of using dead organisms and being more serologically specific.

Although the *T. pallidum* immobilization (TPI) test is not a fluorescent antibody test, it is useful for detecting and titering immobilizing antibodies in serum or spinal fluid. The patient's sample is mixed with live, motile, virulent *T. pallidum* (Nichols strain) and guinea pig complement. Following overnight incubation at 37°C in an atmosphere of 95 percent nitrogen and 5 percent carbon dioxide, the mixture is examined by dark field microscopy for loss of motility as compared with serum controls treated in a similar fashion but containing inactivated complement. The TPI test is not performed in hospital laboratories, but only in state or federal public health laboratories as the treponemal test of reference. It does not distinguish between the treponematoses and it is not useful in assessing therapy, but it does remain reactive over long periods of time even though it is relatively insensitive in early syphilis.

Inhibition Immunofluorescence Test. The direct FA test is useful for detecting the presence of pathogenic agents (bacteria, fungi, protozoans, viruses) in cultures or tissues derived from a patient. When antibody is the unknown, a **FA inhibition test** can be used. Its principle is essentially the same as the blocking control of the direct FA test except that the antigen is the known reagent (Figure 8.4). After the known antigen is fixed to the

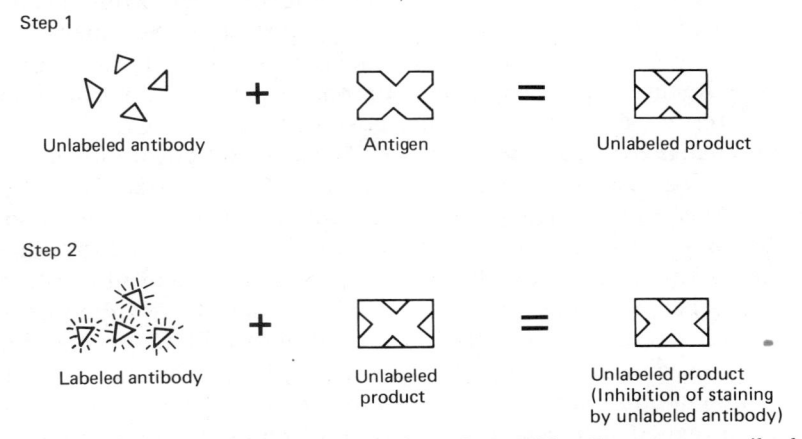

FIGURE 8.4. Schematic representation of a positive fluorescent antibody inhibition staining reaction. [*From Cherry, W. B., et al., 1960. Fluorescent Antibody Techniques in the Diagnosis of Communicable Diseases. Public Health Service Publication No. 729. U.S. Government Printing Office, Washington, D.C.*]

slide, it is flooded with the patient's serum. If the corresponding antibody is present in the serum, it will attach (fix) to the antigen. When specific fluorescent antibody reagent is added, it cannot become fixed because all of the antigenic sites are already occupied by the unlabeled patient's antibodies. The labeled reagent is removed by washing the slide. When the slide is examined through the microscope, the test shows no fluorescence. Of course, the negative control slide should fluoresce because there are no antibodies to inhibit the fixation of the labeled antibodies. A "two-step" inhibition test involves adding the patient's serum and the labeled reagent to the slide consecutively. An equilibrium would eventually be reached in which the patient's antibodies and the fluorescent antibodies would compete for the same antigen sites. Therefore, lower titers or false negative results may be obtained if the labeled antibody is allowed to react over too long a period of time before washing. A "one-step" inhibition test is performed by exposing the antigen to a mixture of the patient's serum and the tagged reagent. If the labeled antibody is in much higher titer than the unlabeled antibody of the patient, most of the antigen sites would be complexed with the tagged antibody and therefore would produce brilliant fluorescence (interpreted as a negative test).

Indirect Immunofluorescence Test. A fluor-labeled antiglobulin conjugate is employed in an **indirect fluorescent antibody** (IFA) **test.** This procedure may be used to detect either unknown antigen or antibody. As an example, consider an indirect fluorescent test for treponemal antibodies (FTA). In the first step of a FTA test, a loopful of dead *T. pallidum* (of the virulent Nichols strain) is spread on a slide, air-dried, and fixed with methanol or acetone. A small amount of patient's serum is added to the smear and incubated in a humidified chamber at about 35°C for thirty minutes. The slide is then rinsed and soaked in buffered saline for ten minutes, rinsed with distilled water to remove salt crystals, and dried. Fluorescent antihuman globulin is then added, incubated, washed, and dried as before. If the patient's serum contained antitreponemal antibodies, they would be fixed to the treponemes on the slide. Washing removes any unattached globulins. The tagged reagent reacts with the human immunoglobulins fixed to the antigen. Washing removes any unreacted reagent. Microscopic examination reveals fluorescence in a positive test (Figure 8.5). Specificity of the FTA can be improved by absorbing the patient's serum with the nonpathogenic Reiter strain of treponeme to remove group-specific antibodies. When the test is performed on Reiter-absorbed sera, it is called a **fluorescent treponemal antibody absorption** (FTA-ABS) **test.** The indirect test has several advantages over other types of FA tests. One fluor-labeled reagent serves to detect any antigen-antibody complex provided the antibody is from the same species as the immunoglobulins that were used to stimulate the production of the antiglobulins. For example, a labeled antihuman globulin is capable of detecting any antibody (monovalent or polyvalent) of human origin. Most of the materials cost of FA tests is in the preparation of the fluor-labeled reagents and the purified antigen. The use of a single labeled antiglobulin reagent for indirect tests can be cheaper than stocking a battery of tagged specific antibodies as required by the direct and inhibition techniques. If unknown antigens are being tested with known rabbit antisera, only one fluorescent reagent need be prepared, viz., fluor-labeled antirabbit globulin. Indirect tests are more sensitive than direct tests be-

Step 1

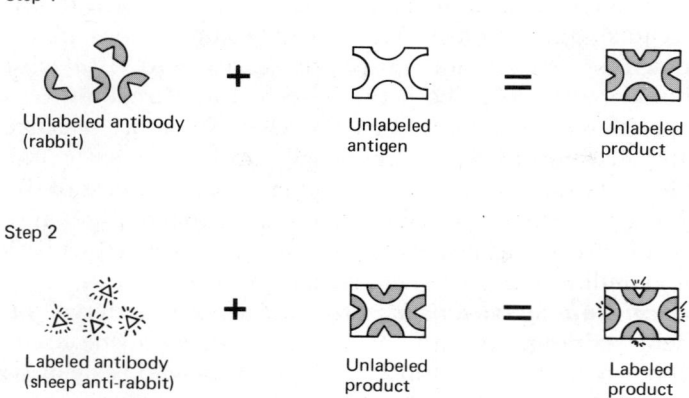

[Unlabeled antibody (rabbit)] + [Unlabeled antigen] = [Unlabeled product]

Step 2

[Labeled antibody (sheep anti-rabbit)] + [Unlabeled product] = [Labeled product]

FIGURE 8.5. Diagram of a positive indirect FA test. [*From Cherry, W. B., et al., 1960. Fluorescent Antibody Technique in the Diagnosis of Communicable Diseases. Public Health Service Publication No. 729, U.S. Government Printing Office, Washington, D.C.*]

cause for every antibody bound to antigen there can be binding of multiple fluorescent antiglobulins (Figure 8.6). The antigen-antibody-antiglobulin complex is referred to as an "immunologic sandwich." Since the labeled antiglobulin reagent reacts with antibodies rather than directly with the treponemal antigen, the indirect test is less specific than the direct test. It is also more complicated, takes more time, and requires more controls. For example, in the FTA-ABS test the following controls should be run with each batch of patients' sera. The antigen should be tested with the conjugate for the absence of nonspecific staining. The Reiter sorbent should not cause nonspecific staining of the antigen when mixed with the conjugate.

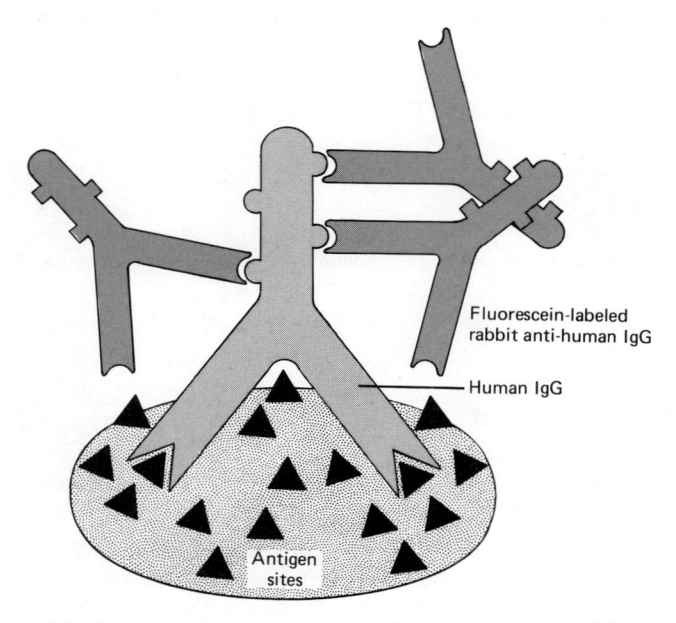

FIGURE 8.6. Sensitivity of the indirect FA test is increased by multiple binding of fluorescent antibodies to immunoglobulins of the patient.

Serology and Immunology

Reactive control serum, minimally reactive control serum (both syphilitic human serums), and a nonspecific control serum (a nonsyphilitic human serum known to demonstrate nonspecific reactivity to *T. pallidum,* Nichols strain) should be tested in both the absorbed and unabsorbed states for standard patterns of reactivity. The FTA-ABS test is more sensitive than the TPI during all stages of syphilis, especially in the very early and very late stages. It tends to remain reactive for a long time regardless of therapy, but fails to distinguish between syphilis and other treponematoses and is subject to false positive reactions (especially in diseases associated with elevated or abnormal globulins, lupus erythematosus, and pregnancy).

Complement-staining Immunofluorescence Test. A fourth type of FA test is **complement staining.** As with the indirect test, it can be used to detect either unknown antigen or antibody. The fluor-tagged reagent is a species-specific anticomplement. For example, in the first step an unknown rabbit serum and goat complement are mixed with known antigen fixed to the slide (Figure 8.7). After a suitable incubation period, the slide is washed to remove any unattached complement. A fluor-labeled antigoat complement is added in the second step, followed by washing and microscopic viewing. If the rabbit serum contained a primary antibody specific for the antigen, it would bind and complement would be fixed. Antigoat complement then can bind to produce a fluorescent antigen-antibody-complement-anticomplement immunological sandwich. Four controls should be run with a complement-staining FA test: (1) test serum control, (2) negative ("normal") serum control, (3) complement control, and (4) known positive serum control. Only the last control should fluoresce. The complement-staining technique has the advantage of being applicable to any antigen-antibody-complement system as long as the anticomplement is reactive with the species from which the complement was derived. Complement-staining FA tests for rickettsiae commonly produce end-point titers about 5 times as great as end points of hemolytic complement fixation tests and hence are more sensitive.

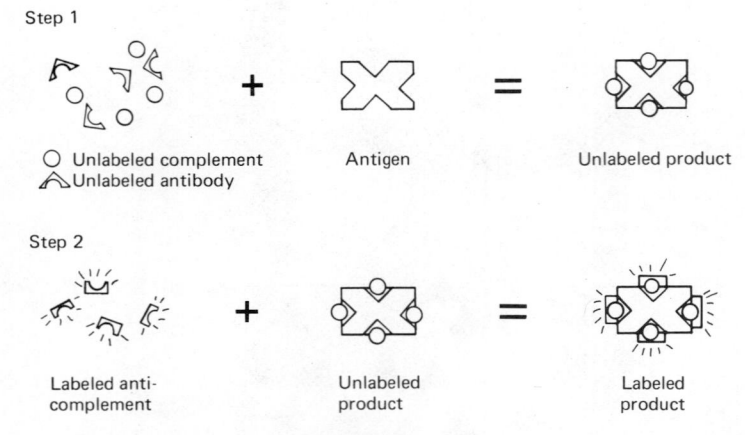

FIGURE 8.7. Example of a complement-staining FA test. [*From Cherry, W. B., et al., 1960. Fluorescent Antibody Techniques in the Diagnosis of Communicable Diseases. Public Health Service Publication No. 729, U.S. Government Printing Office, Washington, D.C.*]

A major disadvantage of all FA microscopy tests is the subjectivity in scoring the results and the difficulty in quantitating the tests. These tests must be read in a darkened room so that weak immunofluorescence can be more easily detected. A dark field condenser is commonly used on the microscope because fluorescent points of light are more easily seen against a black background. Light is refracted to the specimen at such an angle that none of it passes directly into the objective lens. With the exception of a small amount of light scattered from objects on the slide, only the light emitted by the fluor enters the objective lens.

Fluorescent Antigens. Protein antigens can also be fluorescent-labeled and used to detect antibodies by a direct test. This technique is not used for clinical tests, but has been used in research for detecting the location of antigens in various cells and tissues. Labeled antigen is injected into a sensitized animal, which is later sacrificed to provide tissue sections for analysis. Fluorescence may be seen (1) in lymphoid tissues where the labeled antigens have complexed with antibody-producing plasma cells, (2) inside phagocytic cells, and (3) as antigen-antibody complexes deposited in various places such as the glomeruli of the kidney.

QUANTITATIVE IMMUNOFLUORESCENCE TESTS

Some commercial kits are available that can quantitate antigen levels in biological fluids by an immunofluorescent technique. The following description applies to a kit for quantitating IgG concentration in serum, but in principle could be used with a wide variety of antigens. A lyophilized preparation of rabbit antihuman IgG covalently bonded to small hydrophilic derivatized polyacrylamide beads forms a solid-phase immunoadsorbent (Figure 8.8). The patient's serum is added to a tube containing this sorbent and incubated at 37°C for about one hour. All IgG molecules are bound because the immunoadsorbent is maintained in excess. FITC-labeled rabbit antihuman IgG is added and binds to IgG fixed to the sorbent. This creates an immunological sandwich of insoluble [anti-IgG]-[IgG]-[labeled anti-IgG] complexes. After another hour of incubation at 37°C, the tubes are centrifuged and washed to remove unattached labeled reagent. They are then read in a filter fluorometer or spectrophotofluorometer. Standards provided with the kit are treated the same way as the patient's samples. A typical standard curve is shown in Figure 8.9. Linearity along the entire range is an attractive feature of this technique when compared to curvilinear results of radial immunodiffusion and radioimmunoassay. As little as 100 ng/ml to as much as 200 mg/ml of IgG can be detected by the quantitative immunofluorescence test (compared with 20 μg/ml to 20 mg/ml in RID). It can be completed in four to six hours and is usually less expensive than RID plates.

Fluorescence Quenching. Antibodies to be fluorescently labeled should be highly purified because albumins, alpha globulins, and beta globulins become labeled more readily than gamma globulins. The antibodies of unpurified sera may be poorly labeled, resulting in low fluorescence, and the specimen may show nonspecific fluorescence of the contaminating labeled proteins. Many tissues autofluoresce in the blue-gray region, and these must be differentiated from the color characteristic of the specific fluoro-

Serology and Immunology

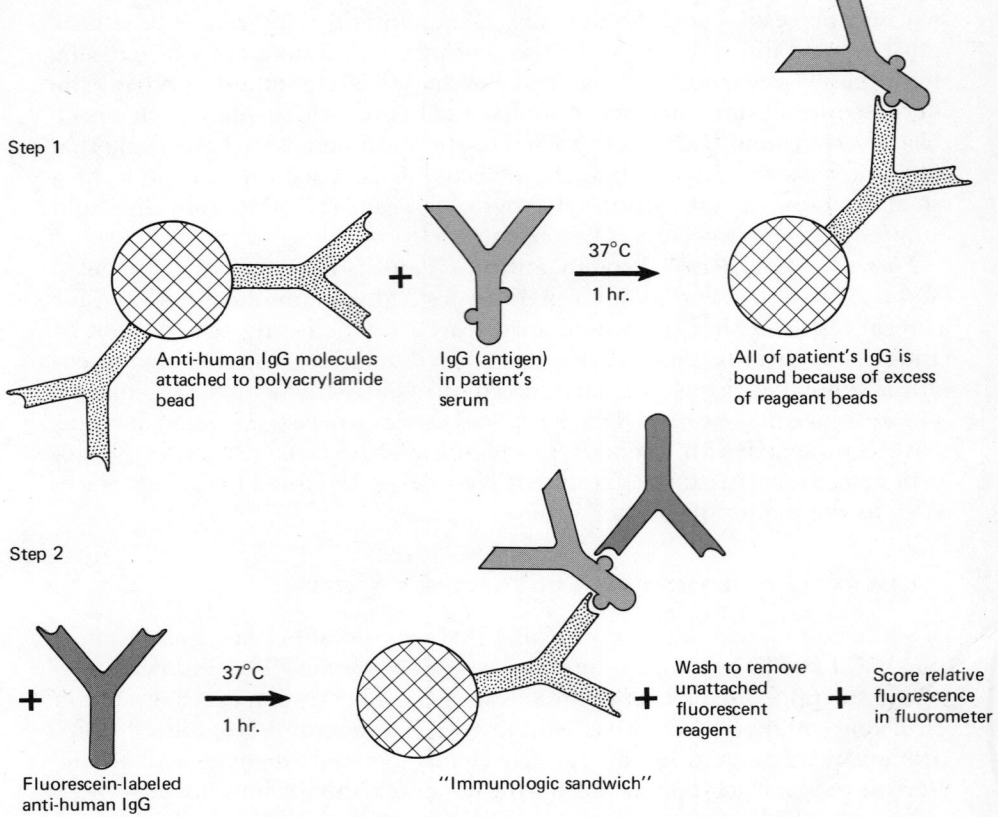

FIGURE 8.8. Example of a quantitative immunofluorescence test for human IgG.

chrome used. Nonspecific fluorescence staining can be diminished **(quenched)** by background staining of tissues with dyes such as Evans blue or Congo red. This tends to improve the contrast for observing specific immunofluorescence.

Almost all proteins will fluoresce when activated by UV light between 280 and 350 nm. They tend to be most fluorescent at about 330 to 350 nm; so the choice of exitation wavelength is about 280 nm. When an antibody combines with a hapten, its autofluorescence may be quenched, presumably by transferring some of the excitation energy to the hapten rather than into visible light. Some antigens do not make good acceptors of the excitation energy and hence are poor quenchers. A spectrophotofluorometer can be used to quantitate the degree of quenching, which in turn reflects the amount of hapten bound. Although the fluorescence-quenching technique is not used in the clinical laboratory, it has been used to determine the association constant that represents the intrinsic affinity of the antibody-combining site for the antigenic determinant (ligand). Only highly purified antibody can be used in this test and, of course, the haptens or ligands must have quenching properties.

Standards	Relative Fluorescence	Corrected Relative Fluorescence	IgG mg %
0	5	—	—
1	92	87	3470
2	64	59	2320
3	36	31	1165
4	16	11	500

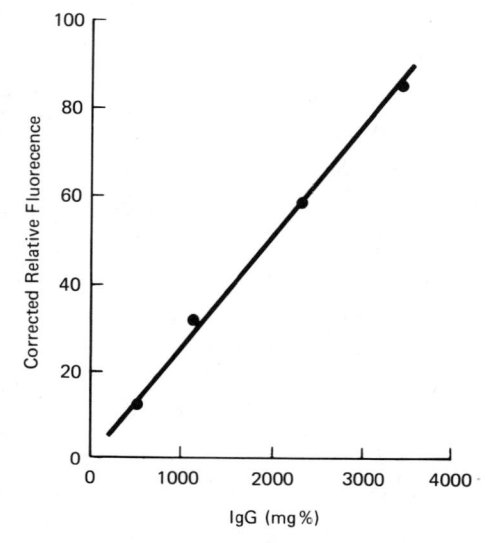

FIGURE 8.9. Typical standard curve for an IgG assay by quantitative immunofluorescence test.

Radioimmunoassay (RIA)

BASIC PRINCIPLES

Use of radioactively tagged reagents can detect nanogram (10^{-9}) or even picogram (10^{-12}) quantities of substances and are therefore among the most sensitive serological tests. It is extremely useful for monitoring the levels of hormones such as insulin, thyroxine, human growth hormone (HGH), thryoid-stimulating hormone (TSH), testosterone, estrogen, progesterone, etc. It is also used to detect vitamins (B_{12}, folic acid, etc.), viral antigens (e.g., hepatitis-associated antigen), therapeutic drugs such as digoxin, and abused drugs (opiates, barbituates, amphetamines).

In principle, the test is quite simple (Figure 8.10). An unknown quantity of antigen in a patient's serum is allowed to compete for antibody binding with a known quantity of the same antigen to which a radioactive isotope is covalently bonded. During incubation, the labeled and unlabeled antigens compete for a limited number of antibody combining sites. If unlabeled antigen is in higher concentration than the labeled antigen, more antigen-antibody complexes will not be radioactive. Free antigen is separated from the antigen-antibody complexes. The radioactivity in the bound phase and/or the free phase is quantitatively measured. By the use of standards containing known amounts of unlabeled antigen, a curve can be plotted relating the counts (disintegrations per minute, dpm) to concentration. The

Serology and Immunology

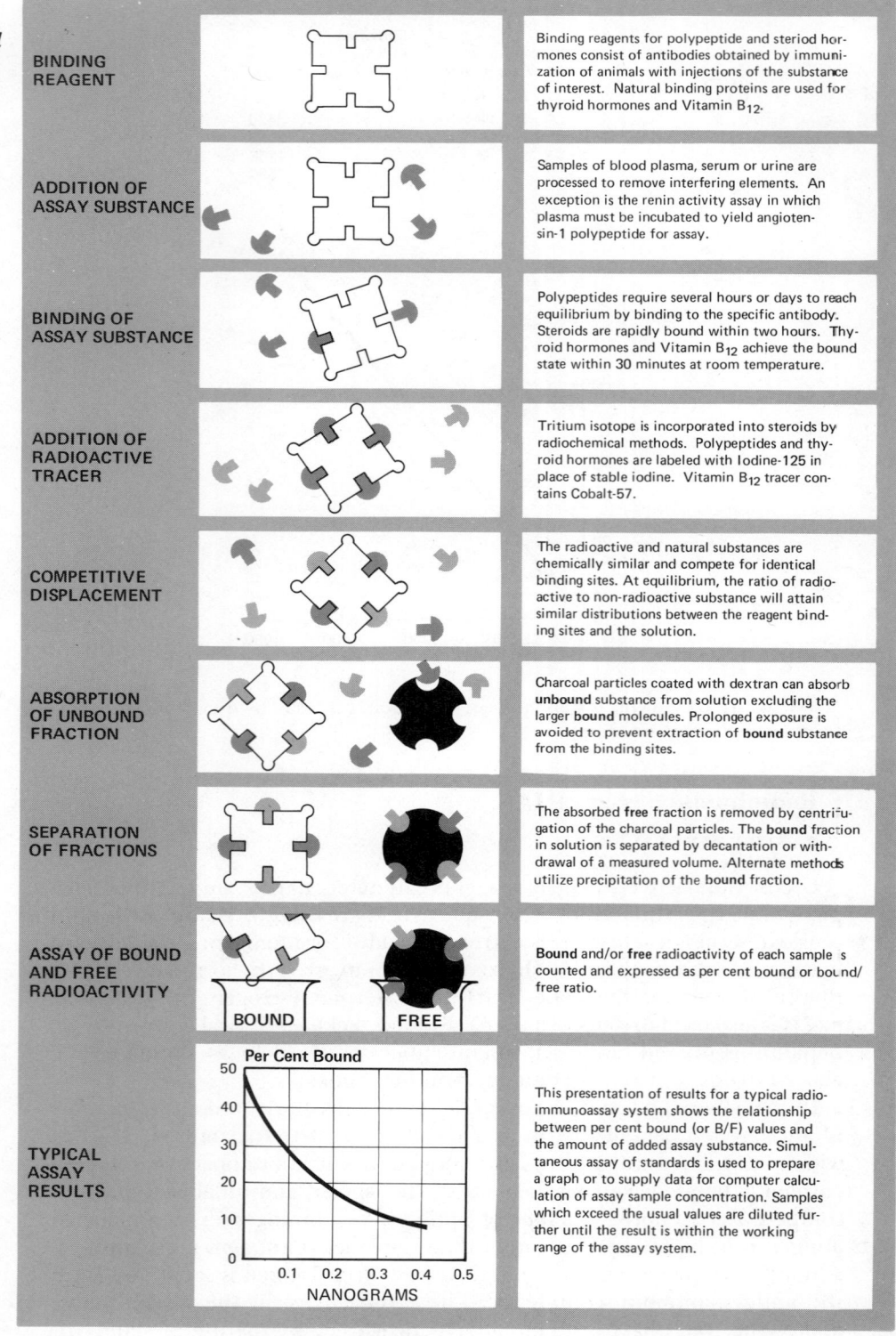

BINDING REAGENT	Binding reagents for polypeptide and steroid hormones consist of antibodies obtained by immunization of animals with injections of the substance of interest. Natural binding proteins are used for thyroid hormones and Vitamin B_{12}.
ADDITION OF ASSAY SUBSTANCE	Samples of blood plasma, serum or urine are processed to remove interfering elements. An exception is the renin activity assay in which plasma must be incubated to yield angiotensin-1 polypeptide for assay.
BINDING OF ASSAY SUBSTANCE	Polypeptides require several hours or days to reach equilibrium by binding to the specific antibody. Steroids are rapidly bound within two hours. Thyroid hormones and Vitamin B_{12} achieve the bound state within 30 minutes at room temperature.
ADDITION OF RADIOACTIVE TRACER	Tritium isotope is incorporated into steroids by radiochemical methods. Polypeptides and thyroid hormones are labeled with Iodine-125 in place of stable iodine. Vitamin B_{12} tracer contains Cobalt-57.
COMPETITIVE DISPLACEMENT	The radioactive and natural substances are chemically similar and compete for identical binding sites. At equilibrium, the ratio of radioactive to non-radioactive substance will attain similar distributions between the reagent binding sites and the solution.
ABSORPTION OF UNBOUND FRACTION	Charcoal particles coated with dextran can absorb **unbound** substance from solution excluding the larger **bound** molecules. Prolonged exposure is avoided to prevent extraction of **bound** substance from the binding sites.
SEPARATION OF FRACTIONS	The absorbed **free** fraction is removed by centrifugation of the charcoal particles. The **bound** fraction in solution is separated by decantation or withdrawal of a measured volume. Alternate methods utilize precipitation of the **bound** fraction.
ASSAY OF BOUND AND FREE RADIOACTIVITY	**Bound** and/or **free** radioactivity of each sample is counted and expressed as per cent bound or bound/free ratio.
TYPICAL ASSAY RESULTS	This presentation of results for a typical radioimmunoassay system shows the relationship between per cent bound (or B/F) values and the amount of added assay substance. Simultaneous assay of standards is used to prepare a graph or to supply data for computer calculation of assay sample concentration. Samples which exceed the usual values are diluted further until the result is within the working range of the assay system.

FIGURE 8.10. Principles of radioisotope assays for polypeptides, steroids, thyroid hormones, and vitamin B_{12}. [*Damon Medical Services Group, 115 Fourth Ave., Needham Hts., Mass. 02194.*]

concentration of antigen in the patient's serum can then be interpolated from the standard curve. Given 100 paratopes or antibody (Ab) combining sites, and 100 molecules each of labeled (*) and unlabeled univalent haptenic antigens (Ag), the expectations can be expressed by the formula,

$$100\ Ag + 100\ Ag^* + 100\ Ab \rightarrow 50\ Ab\text{-}Ag + 50\ Ab\text{-}Ag^* + 50\ Ag + 50\ Ag^*$$

If there were four times as many unlabeled as labeled antigens, the equilibrium formula would be

$$100\ Ab + 100\ Ag + 25\ Ag^* \rightarrow 20\ Ab\text{-}Ag^* + 80\ Ab\text{-}Ag + 5\ Ag^* + 20\ Ag$$

A dilution of antiserum that binds about 50 percent of the labeled antigen in the absence of unlabeled antigen is normally used. When unlabeled antigen is added, the amount of labeled antigen bound by antibody is proportionately reduced in a phenomenon variously called **competitive binding, displacement,** or **radioligand inhibition** (a ligand, in this case, being an antigenic site). The amount of radioactivity can be expressed as percent bound, percent free, or bound-to-free (B/F) ratio. A highly purified antigen is required for labeling and for production of a highly specific antiserum. A variety of purification techniques can be used including column chromatography, gel filtration, and ion exchange resins. The purified antigen should be labeled with a radioisotope having a high specific activity, i.e., producing a large number of counts per minute.

RADIONUCLIDES

The specific activity of a radionuclide is reflected in its half-life. One half-life is the time required for a radioisotope to lose one half of its radioactivity (half of its unstable atoms disintegrate). An isotope that has a half-life measured in days has a higher specific activity than one with a half-life measured in years. Of the commonly used radiolabels for RIA, iodine-131 has the highest specific activity, but its shelf life is so short that it is seldom used. It is also difficult to obtain ^{131}I in carrier-free form (i.e., uncontaminated by other radioisotopes). Carbon-14 has a specific activity too low for a sensitive assay. Its long half-life presents problems in storage of radioactive wastes. The two most useful isotopes on the basis of their specific activities are ^{125}I and tritium (hydrogen-3). Radioactive iodine can be coupled to tyrosine residues in protein or peptide antigens by reaction with either chloramine-T or lactoperoxidase. Antigens lacking a tyrosine residue can be reacted with tyrosine before labeling. Labeled antigen must be isolated immediately after the reaction is completed in order to avoid damage to the antigen by the chloramine-T or peroxides. The molar ratio of iodine to antigen should not greatly exceed unity because overlabeling can also damage the antigen.

Antibody for use in RIA tests must be high-titered, highly specific, and avid. The optimal dilution of antibody is the one that binds about 50 percent of the labeled antigen, i.e., where the B/F ratio is unity. At this point the bound labeled antigen should be able to produce 2,000 to 3,000 counts per minute. The sensitivity of the assay is usually enhanced by adding reagents in the following order: antibody first, unlabeled antigen second, and labeled antigen third. Incubation should be no longer than needed to establish equilibrium. This may require minutes or several days. Many clinical RIA tests can reach equilibrium in thirty minutes to two hours. Prolonged incubation can lead to antigen deterioration in the presence of high concentrations of plasma proteins. Incubations longer than six hours should be at about 4°C. At low temperatures, antigen-antibody complexes are more stable, but their rate of formation is decreased. Antigen may nonspecifically bind to glassware and introduce large errors into RIA tests. This problem can be minimized by using plastic tubes and buffer solutions containing serum albumin.

SEPARATION OF BOUND FROM FREE ANTIGEN

Separation of antibody-bound radioactivity (bound label) from free label can be accomplished by a variety of techniques. One of the most popular methods, because of its simplicity and availability in commercial kits, is the **solid-phase method.** The manufacturer has physically adsorbed specific antibodies to the inner bottom surface of polystyrene test tubes. Following incubation, the contents of the tube are decanted, leaving only bound antigen (both labeled and unlabeled). Other solid-phase substrates for physical attachment of antibodies include polyacrylamide discs and resin beads, but these must be centrifuged and washed if bound label is to be counted. Antibody can be covalently coupled to polyacrylamide particles or to cellulose, Sepharose, or Sephadex. This is preferable to physical adsorption of antibody because the latter may dissociate from its substrate and cause loss of radioactivity (sensitivity) in the test. Cross-linked dextrans (Sepharose, Sephadex) entrap the antibody in their matrices, but permit smaller antigen molecules to diffuse through their pores.

A second method (applicable to nonglobulin antigens) for isolating bound label is by salt or solvent precipitation. Addition of saturated solutions of ammonium sulfate (Farr technique) or water-miscible solvents such as methanol or dioxane causes chemical precipitation of globulins and thereby renders the antigen-antibody complex insoluble.

A third way to separate bound label is by use of the **double-antibody technique.** The first antibody is the one specific for the antigen being assayed. The second antibody is a precipitating antiglobulin specific for the species from which the primary antibody was derived. An immunological sandwich is formed by the antigen–primary antibody–antiglobulin complex. Antiglobulin can bind to epitopes in the Fc region of the primary antibody without affecting the antigen-binding capacity of the primary antibody. Complexes can be separated by centrifugation or by filtration through a suitable membrane. There are two variations of the double-antibody method. In the preprecipitate technique, the antiglobulin is allowed to react with the primary antibody before antigen is added. In the postprecipitate technique, the antiglobulin is added after the union of primary antibody with its antigen.

A fourth method for separation of antibody-bound antigen from antibody-free antigen involves the nonspecific adsorption of free antigen (either labeled or unlabeled) onto dextran-coated charcoal particles, finely divided silica or talc, or ion exchange resins. Following centrifugation or filtration of these particulate adsorbents, antibody-free labeled antigen is associated with the adsorbent, whereas antibody-bound labeled antigen is found in the supernatant fluid or the filtrate.

MEASURING RADIOACTIVITY

Radioactivity can be measured on either the supernatant fluid or the precipitate or both depending on the method of separation. A scintillation counter is used to detect products of radioactive decay. High-energy gamma-ray emissions from ^{125}I or ^{131}I are detected by a crystal scintillation counter. The test tube is placed inside a sodium iodide–thallium crystal. When the crystal absorbes gamma rays, it becomes excited and subsequently fluoresces. Minute pulses of fluorescent light are detected and amplified by photomultiplier tubes. The size and geometry of the crystal determine its sensitivity or efficiency of detection. The number of scintillations (light pulses) per minute is proportional to the rate of gamma emissions and the light intensity (number of photons per pulse) is proportional to the energy of the gamma ray.

Tritium emits beta particles ("rays"). Electrons (either negatrons or positrons) are classified as beta particles. Gamma rays have very high penetration but low ionization properties. Beta particles have low penetration and medium ionization properties. Consequently, the higher detection efficiency of the liquid scintillation technique is required for beta-emitting isotopes.

Liquid scintillation involves a series of energy transfers mediated by an aromatic solvent and fluorescent substances called phosphors. The kinetic energy of the beta particle is used to excite the solvent molecules, which in turn transfer the energy to the phosphor molecules or "primary scintillator." If the detector does not function efficiently at the wavelength output characterisitc of the primary scintillator, a second fluorescent substance is also used. This "secondary scintillator" receives energy from the primary scintillator and emits light with a wavelength optimal for the detection equipment. Components of the scintillation medium ("cocktail") are selected to provide considerable overlap of the fluorescence spectrum of the solvent and the excitation or absorption spectrum of the primary scintillator. The same is true of the primary and secondary scintillators. A liquid scintillation cocktail usually contains an aromatic solvent such as toleune, benzene, or xylene and a primary scintillator such as diphenyloxazole (PPO) or a substituted oxadiazole (PBD or butyl-PBD). Scintillation efficiency is the ratio of the fluorescent energy released by the cocktail relative to the energy of the exciting beta particles. The efficiency rises with increases in concentration of phosphors up to a maximum, beyond which it falls due to self-quenching of the excited molecules. Any foreign materials in the sample tend to reduce scintillation and lower the apparent detection sensitivity. This is due to fewer collisions between the exciting particle and the scintillator molecules, interaction of the foreign material with the excited molecules, or absorption of fluorescence by the foreign matter. Ideally, the sample should be colorless and completely dissolved in the cocktail, but the system can work even when conditions are far from ideal. If the sample is soluble in toluene, it can be directly incorporated into the cocktail. Samples that are insoluble in organic solvents can often be incorporated by use of a solubilizing agent (usually a nonionic surfactant or detergent). If all else fails, solid samples can be prepared as a suspension using a thixotropic agent, i.e., one that liquefies when stirred but gels when undisturbed.

Scintillations are detected, converted to electrical current, and greatly amplified by the photomultiplier tubes. The signal is sent to a pulse height analyzer consisting of two precision-variable resistors, called **discriminators,** that set the upper and lower limits desired. The voltage difference between the discriminators is called the **counting window.** Since each isotope has its own characteristic emission spectrum, the counting window can be used to screen out extraneous emissions. After passing the window, the signal is transmitted to a counting device called a **scaler** and displayed as digital readout. Since the counting efficiency is affected by the sample matrix and the energy of the emitted radiation, counts must be converted by a mathematical formula to represent disintegrations per unit time. This would be important if comparisons were being made between different tissues and/or when different radioisotopes were used.

RIA FOR DIGOXIN

Two substances frequently monitored by RIA are digoxin and digitoxin. These cardiac glycoside drugs are administered to patients with congestive heart failure, atrial flutter or fibrillation, supraventricular paroxysmal tachycardia, and before cardiac surgery. They increase the force and efficiency of cardiac contractions. They stimulate the vagus nerve to slow the heart rate and also slow conduction of impulses through the AV node to the ventricles. There is a very narrow margin between therapeutic and toxic doses of these drugs. Consequently, their levels must be measured at frequent intervals. A typical commercial RIA kit for digoxin provides the following reagents:

1. Glycoside-free buffer. This reagent is also devoid of heavy metal ions such as magnesium or calcium that may enhance the damaging effects of certain enzymes and plasma proteins. It contains no substances structurally related to the digoxin antigen.
2. Glycoside-free human serum. This reagent is pooled serum from normal people not on a digitalis maintenance schedule. Its use assures that all tubes contain essentially the same concentration of serum proteins and thereby minimizes any between-tubes variations caused by nonspecific adsorption.
3. Tritium-labeled digoxin. When diluted according to the instructions, it will produce about 3,000 counts per minute in the antibody-bound fraction in the absence of unlabeled digoxin.
4. Digoxin antiserum. This specific reagent is usually lyophilized. After being reconstituted to the specified volume, it is able to bind about 50 percent of the labeled digoxin in the absence of unlabeled digoxin.
5. Dextran-coated charcoal. A buffer suspension of this adsorbent is used to bind free digoxin at the end of the incubation period.
6. Digoxin standards. These reference standards contain known amounts of unlabeled digoxin. From them, a standard curve will be constructed, relating counts per minute to digoxin concentration. Some kits may provide a single standard that must be serially diluted to produce a range of appropriate concentrations.

7. Tritiated toluene. This reagent is used only with the liquid scintillation technique to determine the quench correction factors for different samples. Quench refers to anything in the scintillation cocktail that prevents transmission of photons from sample to photocathode of the photomultiplier tube. Since different samples may contain different foreign substances, the tritiated toluene control for each sample allows the counts per minute to be "quench-corrected."

Table 8.2 lists the sequence in which the reagents are added in performance of a digoxin RIA. Two control tubes are run simultaneously with the test: (1) zero control and (2) background control. The zero control tube contains no unlabeled digoxin (no patient's serum or digoxin standard). After the first incubation it should contain the maximum amount of antibody-bound label. Since dextran-coated charcoal is used to adsorb free digoxin, all of the antibody-bound label should be in the supernate following centrifugation. The only active reagent in the background control tube is labeled digoxin. Therefore, if any free label is found in the supernate after the second incubation, it represents inefficiency of the adsorbent in binding all free antigen molecules. Each tube is run in duplicate and the average counts per minute is calculated. In order to correct for extraneous sources of radiation, the average count of the background tubes is subtracted from each of the average counts of all other tubes. This gives the corrected counts per minute (cpm). Sample data for five standards and two controls are presented in Table 8.3. The percentage of labeled standard A antigen (0.5 ng/ml) bound to antibody is calculated as follows:

$$\% \text{ bound labeled Ag at 0.5 ng/ml} = \frac{\text{corrected cpm standard A}}{\text{corrected cpm zero control}} \times 100$$
$$= \frac{1,715}{2,062} = 83.2$$

Similar calculations are made for each of the other four standards and plotted on special graph paper to linearize the data as shown in Figure 8.11. Counts per minute of unknowns can then be interpolated from the standard curve into concentration of digoxin in ng/ml.

Table 8.2 BASIC PROCEDURAL STEPS IN THE PERFORMANCE OF A DIGOXIN RIA

Step/Additions	Standard Tubes	Sample Tubes	Zero Tube	Background Tube
1. Glycoside-free buffer	x	x	x	x
2. Standards	x	No*	No	No
3. ^{3}H-digoxin	x	x	x	x
4. Glycoside-free serum	x	No	x	x
5. Digoxin antiserum	x	x	x	No
6. Incubation (25°C)	x	x	x	x
7. Charcoal-dextran	x	x	x	x
8. Incubate	x	x	x	x
9. Centrifuge (1,500 G)	x	x	x	x

* Samples are introduced into these tubes at this step.

Serology and Immunology

Table 8.3 SAMPLE RIA DATA FOR FIVE DIGOXIN STANDARDS AND TWO CONTROL TUBES

Sample Data	CPM	Avg CPM	Corrected CPM
Background control	155	158	—
	161		
Zero control	2,221	2,220	2,062
	2,219		
Standard A	1,874	1,873	1,715
0.5 ng/ml	1,871		
Standard B	1,572	1,586	1,428
1.0 ng/ml	1,599		
Standard C	1,160	1,162	1,004
2.0 ng/ml	1,164		
Standard D	785	784	626
4.5 ng/ml	783		
Standard E	510	516	358
8.0 ng/ml	522		

RADIOIMMUNOASSAY STANDARD CURVE

PER CENT BOUND $\left(p = \dfrac{100}{1 - e^{-l}}\right)$

LOGIT $\left(l = \ln \dfrac{p}{100 - p}\right)$

CALCULATION OF % BOUND Ag*

% bound Ag* at 0.5 ng/ml = $\dfrac{\text{corrected CPM Standard A}}{\text{corrected CPM Standard O}} \times 100$

SAMPLE DIGOXIN STANDARD CURVE

Standards	ng/ml	% Bound
O = zero control	0.0	100.0
A	0.5	83.2
B	1.0	69.3
C	2.0	48.7
D	4.5	30.4
E	8.0	17.4

CONCENTRATION

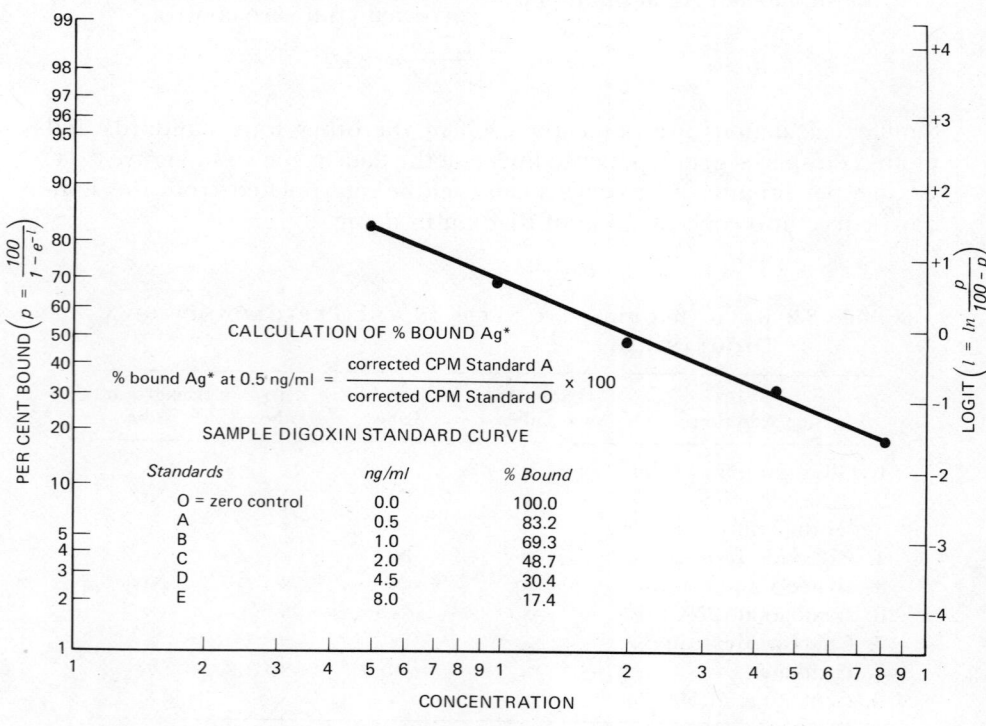

FIGURE 8.11. Semilog logit plot of RIA data from digoxin standards.

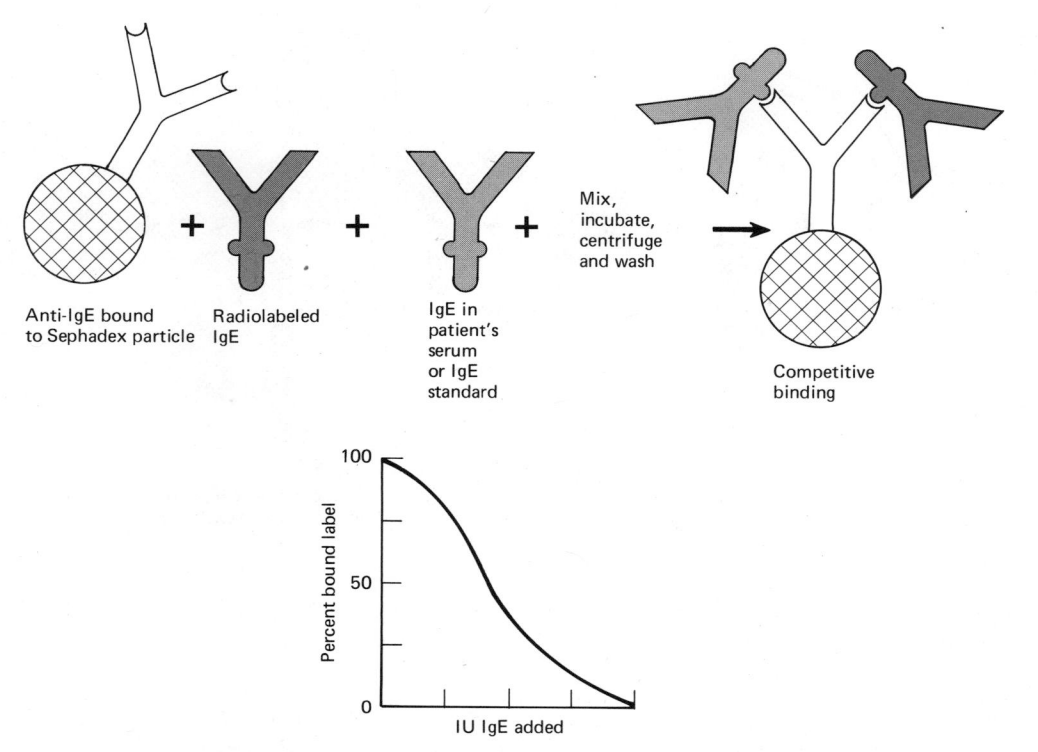

FIGURE 8.12. Diagram of an indirect radioimmunosorbent test for quantitating total IgE.

RIA FOR IGE

Immunoglobulin E (IgE) is normally present in serum in nanogram-per-milliliter quantities, and its quantification therefore requires the high sensitivity of radioimmunoassay. Patients suffering immune allergies commonly have elevated serum IgE levels, but not all allergies are IgE-mediated. Many parasitic infections produce extreme elevations of serum IgE levels together with a marked eosinophilia. Three RIA techniques are commonly employed to measure total serum IgE levels: (1) indirect radioimmunosorbent test (RIST), (2) direct radioimmunosorbent test, and (3) radioimmunoprecipitation (RIP) assay. A fourth method, radioallergosorbent test (RAST), is employed to quantitate a specific IgE antibody.

The **indirect radioimmunosorbent test** (RIST) is a **competitive binding assay.** Anti-IgE is covalently coupled to cross-linked dextran particles (Sephadex). A constant amount of radiolabeled (usually ^{125}I) IgE is added to each tube and allowed to compete for antibody receptor sites with IgE in the patient's serum sample or with standards containing known quantities of IgE (Figure 8.12). Following incubation, the tubes are centrifuged and washed three times with buffer. Decantation after the last wash leaves a pellet of complexes consisting of [Sephadex bead]-[anti-IgE]-[IgE]. Emission of gamma rays per unit time is counted and a standard curve constructed. The higher the concentration of IgE in the patient's serum, the lower the number of counts in the pellets. As with all competitive binding assays, the indirect RIST is subject to nonspecific inhibition by unknown

Serology and Immunology

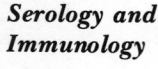

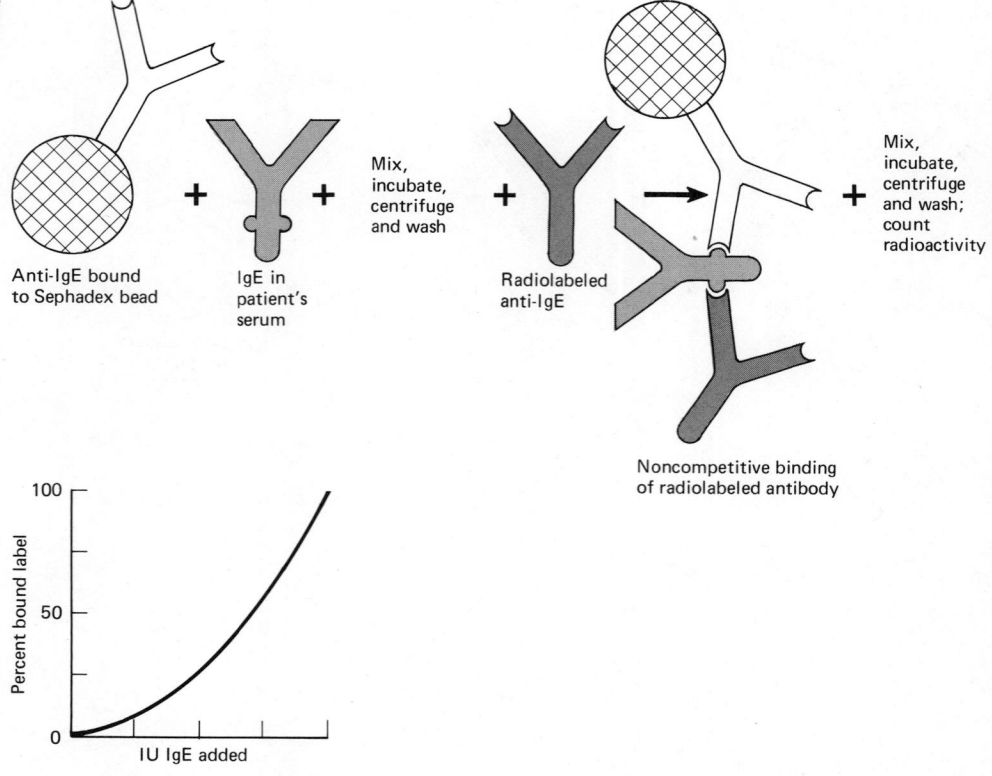

FIGURE 8.13. Diagram of a direct radioimmunosorbent test for quantitating total IgE.

serum factors. Its sensitivity (5 ng/ml) and precision (CV* = 18%) are moderate. It is a costly test because the radioactive antigen must be obtained from a rare IgE myeloma patient.

In a **direct noncompetitive binding radioimmunosorbent test** (direct RIST), no radiolabeled IgE is required. Anti-IgE is rendered insoluble by being coupled to Sephadex beads and incubated with patient's serum or IgE standards. Next the tubes are centrifuged and washed three times to remove any free antigen (IgE). A radiolabeled anti-IgE is then added, followed by incubation, centrifugation, and thorough washing to remove any unattached labeled reagent (Figure 8.13). Binding of the radiolabeled anti-IgE in the insoluble immunological sandwich is directly related to the IgE content in the patient's serum. The direct RIST is highly sensitive (as low as 10 pg/ml) and has excellent precision (CV < 5 percent). It is minimally affected by nonspecific serum factors. Because a second incubation period is required, it takes about twice as long to complete the direct RIST as the indirect RIST.

The currently most popular method is the **radioimmunoprecipitation (RIP) assay** because it is unsurpassed in precision (CV ≃ 5 percent) and reproducibility (CV = 10 percent). Sensitivity of RIP is about 1 International Unit (IU) IgE per milliliter (1 IU is equivalent to approximately 2.4

---

* CV is the coefficient of variation (see Appendix).

ng of IgE protein). Unlike the solid-phase RIST assays, RIP employs a soluble second antibody to precipitate the bound antigen (double-antibody technique). It is a competitive binding assay and therefore is susceptible to interference by serum factors at high serum concentrations, but in practical clinical work this seldom causes problems. A reference standard or patient's serum is mixed first with rabbit antihuman IgE and second with radiolabeled IgE myeloma protein (Figure 8.14). After incubation, the soluble IgE-antiIgE complexes are precipitated with goat antirabbit gamma globulin. The addition of a pretitrated amount of normal rabbit serum (or purified rabbit gamma globulin) before introduction of goat antirabbit gamma globulin contributes to the formation of larger aggregates, diminishes loss of soluble complexes, and thereby increases the sensitivity of the test. All tubes are incubated, centrifuged and washed thoroughly to remove unbound label, and counted. The standard reference curve is plotted with the logarithm of added IgE being a function of maximal binding (B_o = binding observed in the absence of unlabeled IgE). IgE concentration

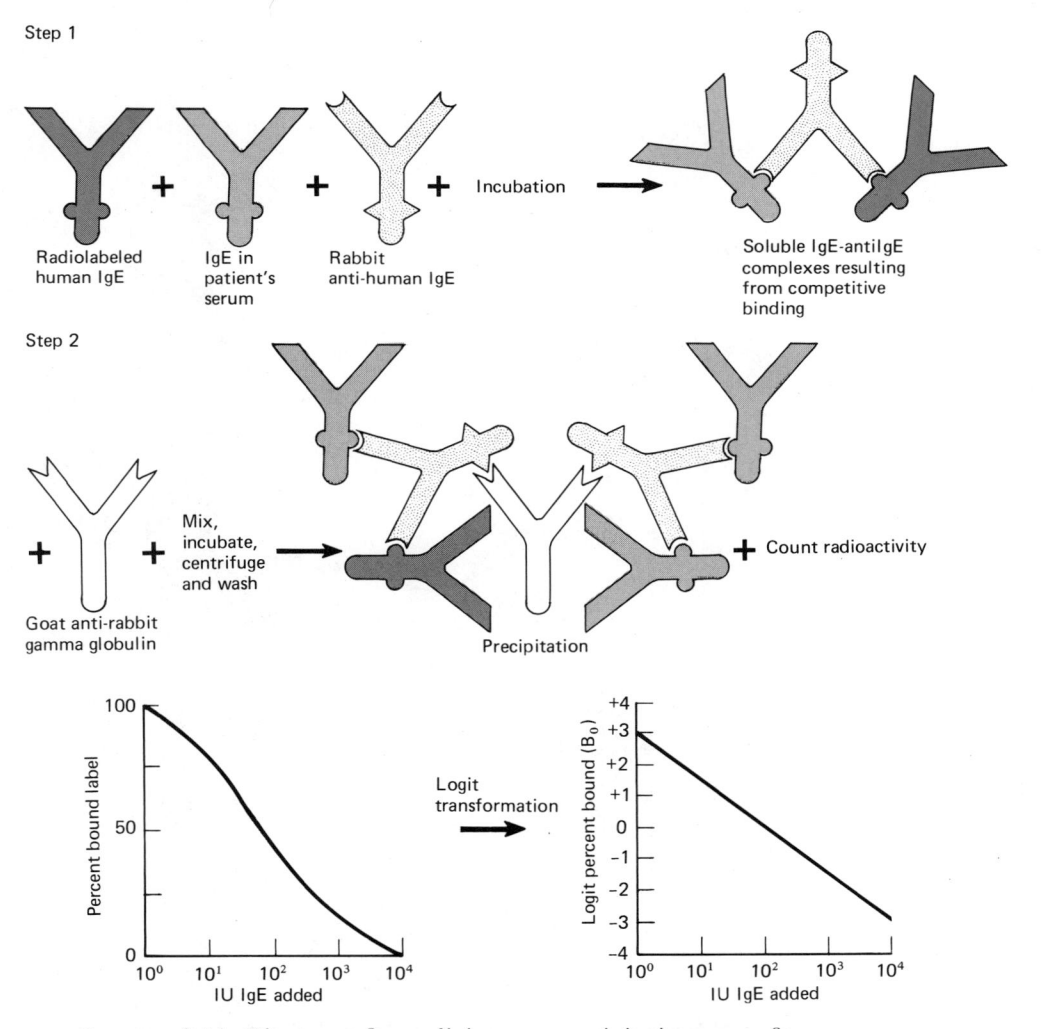

FIGURE 8.14. Diagram of a radioimmunoprecipitation assay for quantitating total IgE.

Serology and Immunology

in unknowns is then interpolated from the sigmoid curve of %B_o or from a linear curve obtained by plotting the data on special graph paper.

The **radioallergosorbent test** (RAST) is a method for assaying the level of a specific IgE in a patient's serum. This test employs a sorbent for allergen (antigen involved in allergy) insolubilization. Commercial kits use paper-disc sorbent, but a carbohydrate matrix sorbent (Sephadex, agarose, cellulose) can be used if maximal sensitivity is required. RAST is performed by incubating specific allergen-coated particles with the patient's serum. Homologous antibodies of all Ig classes may be bound to the allergen-sorbent. The tubes are centrifuged, and the sorbent is washed to remove all IgE molecules except those specific for the allergen. A radiolabeled anti-IgE antibody is then allowed to incubate with the complexes followed by centrifugation, washing, and counting (Figure 8.15). Quantitation of the RAST can be obtained if the patient's curve (obtained by making dilutions of the patient's serum) parallels the dilution curve of the reference serum.

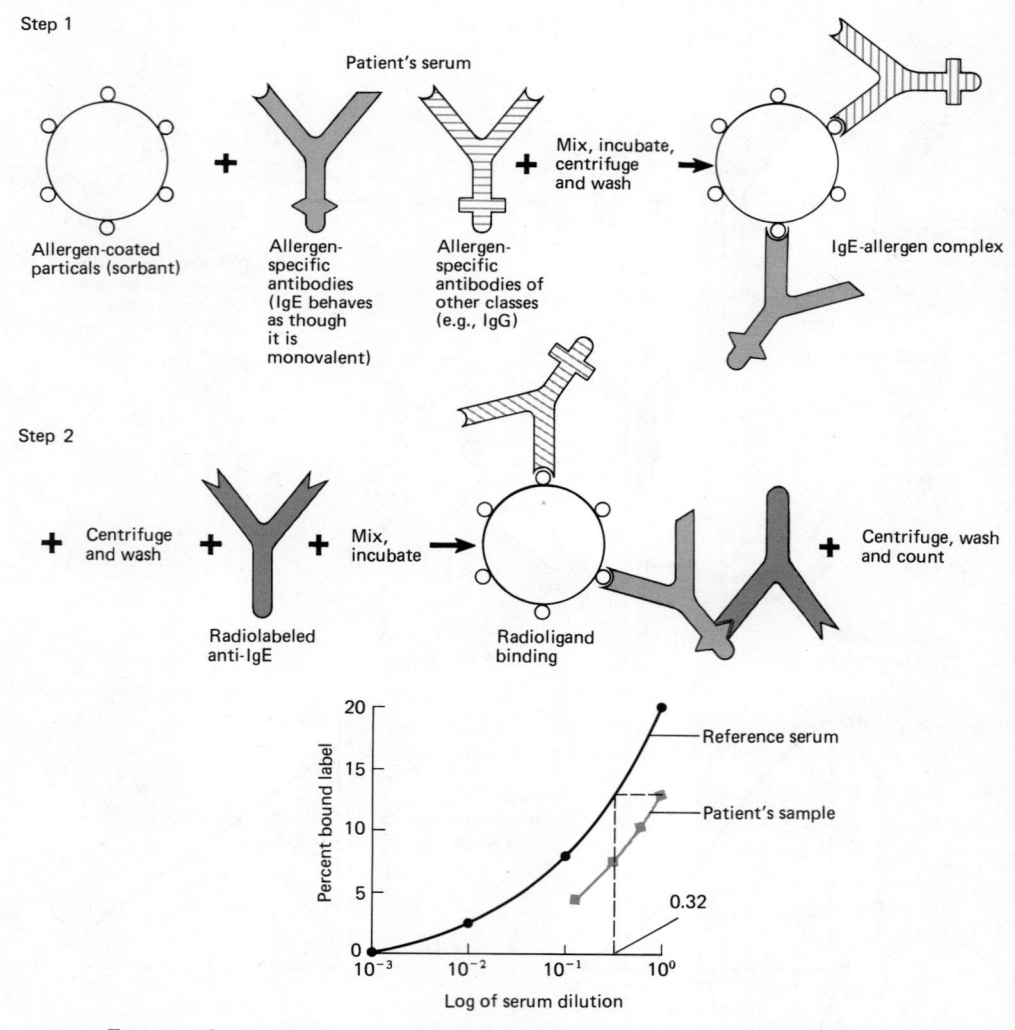

FIGURE 8.15. Diagram of a radioallergosorbent test for quantitation of allergen-specific IgE.

For example, in Figure 8.15 the serum dilution curves of patient and reference are almost parallel. If the reference serum is assumed to contain 1,000 arbitrary units of specific IgE, then any plot point of the patient's serum can be used to estimate its relative potency from the parallel portion of the reference curve. The titer of the patient's serum in Figure 8.15 is determined by the following formula:

$$\begin{bmatrix} \text{Arbitrary units} \\ \text{in patient's sample} \end{bmatrix} = \begin{bmatrix} \text{equivalent dilution} \\ \text{of reference sample} \end{bmatrix} \times \begin{bmatrix} \text{arbitrary units} \\ \text{in reference sample} \end{bmatrix}$$
$$= 0.32 \times 1,000 = 320 \text{ arbitrary units}$$

The reference serum provided with a commercial RAST kit may not be specific for the test allergen. For example, a birch pollen reference serum may be in a kit for ragweed pollen–specific IgE. Five hundred arbitrary units of ragweed pollen–specific IgE might be considered a high-titered serum for that allergen, but a low-titered serum for birch pollen allergen. In other words, the interpretation of the RAST is highly dependent on experience. Each laboratory must derive its own correlations between specific IgE titers and skin test results or other clinical data by which to interpret RAST results. The current difficulty in transforming RAST results into levels of clinical sensitivity that are meaningful to the physician has greatly limited its usefulness. Procedures are available for standardization of RAST reference sera in weight/volume terms (e.g., ng/ml). Once the absolute antibody concentrations of reference sera become commercially available, this technique will become more useful to clinicians.

COMPETITIVE PROTEIN-BINDING ASSAYS

A nonimmunological alternative to RIA is a competitive protein-binding assay (CPBA). CPBA is essentially similar to RIA, but substitutes a specific binding protein (usually a serum transport protein) in place of antibody. Biologically inactive derivatives of human chorionic gonadotropin tend to impair specificity in RIA tests for HCG. At least one company has developed a **radioreceptor assay** (RRA) that still utilizes the principle of competitive binding but increases specificity by replacing antibody with a highly specific receptor (bovine corpora lutea cell membranes). This receptor binds only the biologically active form of the hormone. The sensitivity of this test is reported to be 0.2 International Units (IU) HCG per milliliter of serum, corresponding to the average level attained at about the tenth day after conception.

Corticosteroid-binding globulin from humans or dogs is the transport protein used to measure human corticoid and progestin concentrations; progesterone-binding protein of guinea pig plasma is used to measure progesterone levels; thyroxine-binding globulin (TBG) is used for thyroxine; and human sex steroid–binding globulin or testosterone-binding protein is employed for assays of androgens and estrogens. RIA tests for these hormones are potentially more sensitive (hence requiring smaller sample volumes) and usually offer greater specificity than CPB assays. In both RIA and CPBA, the patient's serum must be deproteinized to release the hormone from its transport protein and to prevent nonspecific binding (NSB) to other serum proteins. For example, in a thyroxine (T_4) assay, the serum can be treated with acid or basic inorganic chemicals (e.g., 8-anilo-1-naphthalene-sulfonic acid = ANS, thimerosal, or diphenylhydantoin) or boiled to inactivate proteins and release all thyroxine in free form. Radioisotope-labeled thyroxine and exogeneous TBG (or antibody in a RIA) are added, and competition for binding sites occurs between the exogenous and endogenous thyroxine molecules. The more endogenous thyroxine present in the patient's serum, the more exogenous labeled thyroxine will be displaced from TBG. Bound thyroxine is separated from free thyroxine by adsorption of the free molecules to resin, silicates, or charcoal. Standards are provided with CPBA kits from which a calibration curve can be constructed.

Free T_4 is maintained in a narrow physiological range by hypothalamic-pituitary feedback mechanisms. It is the free T_4 (< 0.05 percent of the total) rather than the TBG-bound fraction that activates this control mechanism. If TBG is overproduced in a euthyroid (normal free thyroid level) patient, total T_4 (determined by either CPBA or RIA) is increased. The fraction of total T_4 that is free is reduced, and free T_4 concentration is normal. Therefore, some index of the number of unoccupied TBG sites is required to differentiate thyroid disease from variations in TBG production. This can be accomplished by exposing exogenous labeled T_3 to TBG in the patient's serum sample.

Triiodothyronine (T_3) is a precursor of thyroxine (T_4). Normally the T_3 level in serum is about one seventieth that of T_4, primarily because of the lower binding affinity of plasma thyroid-hormone binding proteins for T_3 than for T_4. Serum T_3 levels are of little use in discriminating the hypothyroid from the euthyroid patient. However, T_3 concentrations are almost always elevated in patients with hyperthyroidism. Radiolabeled T_3 is incubated with the patient's serum (containing TBG) and is bound in proportion to the degree of unsaturation of the TBG binding sites. Dextran-coated charcoal or resin particles are then added. The free, non-TBG-bound fraction of the T_3 tracer becomes bound to these particles. The tubes are then centrifuged and the supernatant fluid is removed by aspiration or decantation. This leaves the charcoal-bound labeled T_3 in the tube for scintillation counting. The results are interpreted in accordance with Table 8.4.

Free T_4 can also be directly estimated by the solid-phase RIA technique. A 50-μl sample (about five times larger than for a total T_4 assay) is pipetted into the bottom of a tube to which anti-T_4 antibody is fixed. The larger

Table 8.4 INFERENCES DRAWN FROM RESULTS OF A TOTAL SERUM T_4 TEST AND CHARCOAL ABSORPTION OF LABELED T_3 BY TBG IN PATIENT'S SERUM

Patient's Total T_4	Relative Uptake of Labeled T_3 by TBG of Patient	Relative Absorption of Free Labeled T_3 by Charcoal After Incubation with Patient's TBG	Inference
High	Low	High	Hyperthyroid
Low	High	Low	Hypothyroid
High	High	Low	Elevated TBG
Low	Low	High	Depressed TBG
Normal			Euthyroid

sample is required for a free T_4 assay than for a total T_4 assay because free T_4 is only a fraction of the total T_4 (most of which is bound to transport proteins and therefore cannot combine with the antibody). Buffer is added and the tube is incubated to allow free T_4 to bind to the antibody. The tube is then decanted to remove all T_4 that is unattached to antibody. A standard amount of buffer containing ^{125}I-labeled T_4 is then added. During subsequent incubation, the labeled T_4 is allowed to proportionately displace the unlabeled patient's T_4 from the antibody. All fluid is thoroughly decanted or aspirated from the tube. The radioactivity is then counted in a gamma scintillation counter. The higher the counts, the less free T_4 was in the patient's sample.

Because T_3 concentrations are normally so low, a RIA for T_3 requires a sample size about five times larger than for T_4 assays. If dextran-coated charcoal is used to separate bound from free labeled T_3, the concentration of charcoal must also be increased. The results of the T_3 and T_4 assays can be used to mathematically calculate a T_7 (or free thyroxine index, FTI) value that compensates for the elevated TBG levels (high total T_4 and low T_3 charcoal uptake) that commonly accompany pregnancy and contraceptive medication. Other conditions or drugs can also alter these hormone levels, and these should be considered in the interpretation of the test results.

Enzyme Immunoassay (EIA) or Immunoenzyme Techniques

QUALITATIVE SLIDE TESTS

Enzymes are biological catalysts that hasten biochemical reactions without being consumed in the process. A single enzyme molecule can convert millions of substrate molecules into product molecules. This huge amplification effect allows detection of minute quantities of enzymes and is utilized in highly sensitive immunoenzyme serological techniques. An immunoenzyme is an antibody labeled with an enzyme, and it is used as a reagent to detect a specific antigen.

As an example of a qualitative immunoenzyme test, let us consider a slide assay for antinuclear antibodies (ANA). Antibodies against DNA-histone complexes (nucleoproteins) or to DNA alone can be generated by a variety of autoimmune and connective tissue diseases. They may also be drug- or physician-induced (iatrogenic) as in procainamide-induced lupus. **Systemic lupus erythematosus** (SLE) is an inflammatory disease of unknown etiology that can affect connective tissues in almost any part of the body. It is strongly suspected to be an autoimmune disease. Certain people seem to be genetically predisposed more than others. Because SLE is more prevalent in certain families than others (familial incidence), a genetic predisposition to develop this disease may be inherited. For unknown reasons, it is primarily a disease of young women. SLE can cause death by cardiac failure and/or renal insufficiency. One of its external signs is a red butterfly- or wolfshead-shaped rash across the nose and upper cheeks, from which the name *lupus erythematosus* (red wolf) is derived. At least two laboratory tests can help establish a diagnosis of SLE. One of these is the hematological identification of the LE cell (Figure 8.16), and the other is the serological finding of LE factors in the serum. **LE factors** are antibodies (usually of

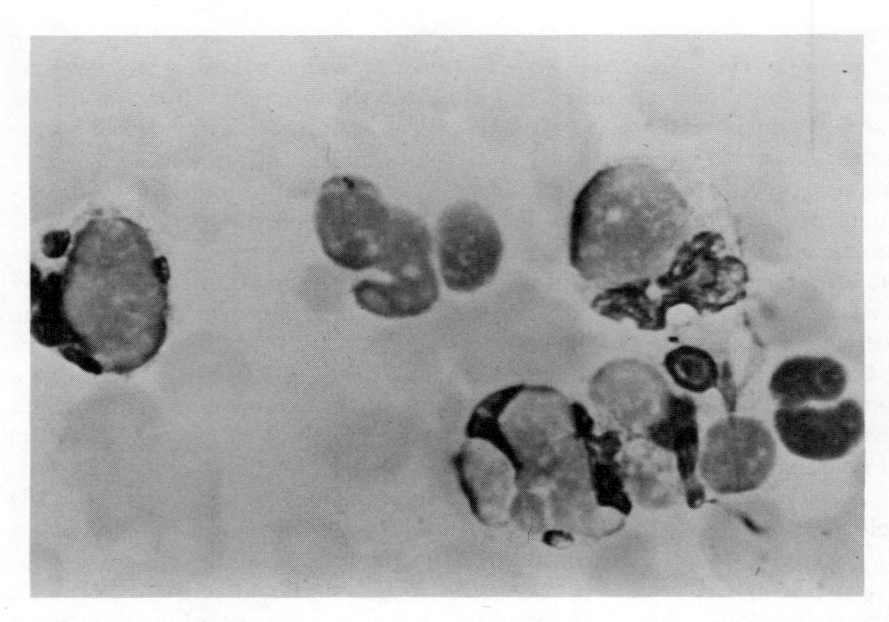

FIGURE 8.16. A positive LE cell preparation from peripheral blood. [*Courtesy of Elliot Scientific Corp., New York City.*]

class IgG) against DNA, RNA, or nucleoproteins. No autoantibodies to lymphocyte surface antigens have been found in SLE patients. However, it is thought that when some normal leukocytes become slightly damaged by mechanical or other means, LE factors can enter the cell. These antinuclear antibodies interact with nuclear antigens, causing the nucleus to become swollen. These damaged cells can then be attacked by phagocytic cells (usually neutrophils). If the cell is engulfed by a neutrophil, its cytoplasm is digested leaving a pale-staining nucleus as an inclusion body. The phagocytic neutrophil, containing remnants of the engulfed lymphocyte, is called an **LE cell.** Extrusion of a free nuclear body **(LE body)** from the phagocyte is common. A rosette of several attacking neutrophils around a central lymphocyte may also be observed. Since LE cells are found in less than 75 percent of active disease cases, they are not reliable diagnostic aids. They may also be associated with hepatitis, drug sensitivity, and rheumatoid arthritis.

The extent to which LE factors contribute to SLE disease is not known. Complexes of ANA and nucleic acid and/or nucleoproteins from various possible sources (such as viruses, mitochondria, red cells, platelets, etc.) tend to lodge in the kidney and contribute to glomerulonephritis. The presence of ANA in a patient is typical, but not diagnostic for SLE. However, failure to find ANA in a patient tends to rule out SLE. The concentration of ANA tends to increase with age and may be caused by loss of suppressor T cells. Titers of ANA less than 1 : 20 are considered negative; titers between 1 : 40 and 1 : 160 are positive and suggestive of disease. A titer greater than 1 : 160 is highly suggestive of SLE, but clinical evaluation and other tests are needed to exclude other autoimmune diseases.

Some laboratories may prefer to dilute the patient's serum greater than 1 : 160 for use in a screening type of qualitative slide test. Microtome sections of rat or mouse kidney are commonly used antigens in the clinical laboratory because they are always readily available and are not subject to interference by cross-reacting human blood group antibodies. The tissue section is fixed to a microscope slide in acetone. These sections can be stored indefinitely in the freezer. To perform an immunoenzyme test, slides are removed from the freezer, thawed, and flooded with an appropriate dilution of the patient's serum. Slides for positive and negative control sera should be run simultaneously. The slides are incubated in a moist chamber at room temperature for thirty minutes and then gently rinsed and soaked in phosphate buffered saline (PBS) to remove all unattached human serum. Next they are drained, blotted to remove excess fluid, and immediately exposed to a drop of enzyme-labeled antihuman globulin. A popular enzyme label is horseradish peroxidase. This enzyme is covalently coupled to AHG in such a way that both the catalytic site and the antibody-combining sites remain reactive. After a thirty-minute incubation period, the slides are washed in PBS to remove any unattached enzyme reagent. After draining, the slides are submerged in a solution containing substrate for the enzyme.

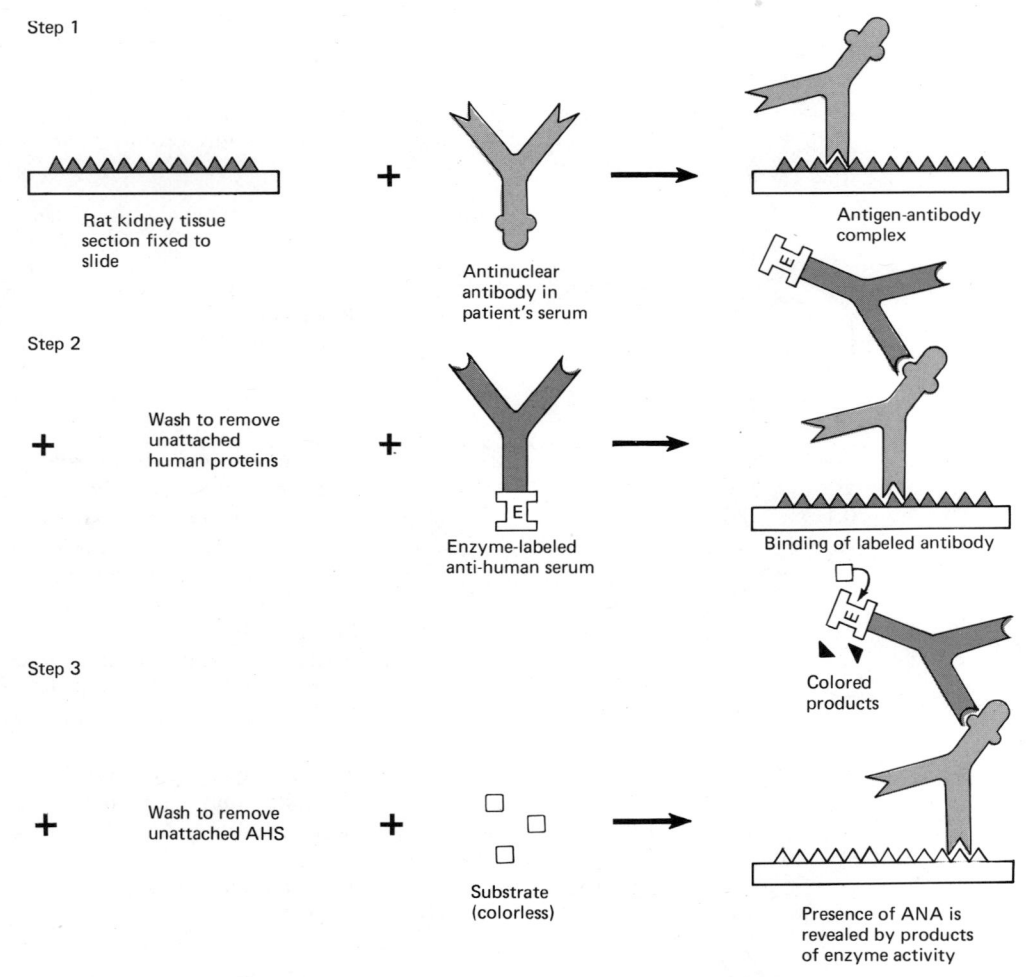

Tagged Reagents

FIGURE 8.17. Diagram of a positive qualitative immunoenzyme test for antinuclear antibodies.

Serology and Immunology

In the case of peroxidase, the substrate is 3-3′ diaminobenzidine (DAB). This substrate is carcinogenic and a search is underway for a suitable substitute. After ten minutes the slides are removed from the substrate solution, rinsed with PBS, dehydrated in ethanol, and may be counterstained (optional) with light green to enhance the contrast. They are then cleared in xylene and dried or coverslipped and sealed with Permount. When examined under the light microscope, a brownish, insoluble reaction product is seen in the regions where enzyme-labeled AHG was immunologically fixed to the kidney antigen–patient serum complex. If counterstain is used, light

Table 8.5 IMPLICATIONS OF ANTINUCLEAR ANTIBODY STAINING PATTERNS

	Nuclear Staining Pattern	Implications
1.	Solid or homogeneous	1. Often seen in SLE; involves antinucleoprotein (DNA-histone complex) antibodies
2.	Rim or peripheral	2. Associated with severe SLE; anti-DNA antibodies
3.	Nucleolar	3. Common in scleroderma; anti-RNA antibodies; rare in SLE or rheumatoid arthritis (RA)
4.	Speckled	4. Common in scleroderma and in connective tissue diseases such as SLE; involves extractable nuclear antigens (ENA) such as the Smith (Sm) antigen and ribonucleoprotein (RNP). Sm antigen is on a carbohydrate-containing acidic protein in the nucleus and is free of nucleic acid. Sm and RNP are usually absent in drug-induced lupus. High RNP titer suggests mixed connective tissue disease (MCTD)
5.	Thready	5. May be seen in SLE, but not RA

brown complex staining and light green tissue staining are observed. The major features of the ANA immunoenzyme test are summarized in Figure 8.17. Five types of positive ANA nuclear staining patterns are known: (1) solid or homogeneous, (2) rim or peripheral, (3) nucleolar, (4) speckled, and (5) thready. The implications of these various ANA staining patterns are summarized in Table 8.5.

Antinuclear antibodies may also be detected by a variety of other techniques including the indirect FA test, double gel diffusion, electroimmunodiffusion, passive agglutination, and RIA.

QUANTITATIVE TUBE TESTS

EIA slide tests are not easily quantitated because the amount of enzyme product seen in the light microscope is too subjective for uniform agreement among different technologists. Tube tests, however, can be easily quantitated in a spectrophotometer set to detect the amount of colored product of the enzyme reaction, usually as an increase in light absorbance. For example, if the enzyme is a bacterial glucose-6-phosphate dehydrogenase (G-6-PD), the substrate is glucose-6-phosphate. Nicotinamide adenine dinucleotide (NAD^+) is added to the substrate and becomes reduced to NADH when G-6-PD dehydrogenates its substrate. The concentration of NADH is correlated with increased optical density when measured spectrophotometrically at 340 nm.

When egg white lysozyme is the enzyme bound to the specific antibody for use in an EIA and the substrate is a bacterial suspension, the amount of antigen in the sample is correlated with an increase in light transmission or a decrease in optical density (absorbance). The reason for this is that lysozyme causes dissolution of the bacterial cells and thereby tends to reduce the turbidity of bacterial suspensions and thus decreases the absorbance. Any immunoassay method that requires physical separation of bound and unbound antigen is termed a **heterogeneous immunoassay** (e.g., RIA). If no separation of bound and free antigen is required, the method is a **homogeneous immunoassay**.

Heterogeneous EIA Methods. Four kinds of heterogeneous EIA methods are available for quantitating various clinically important antigens. One method is a competitive binding assay called an **enzyme-linked immunosorbent assay** (ELISA). A specific antibody is coupled to particles such as dextran beads or to the bottom of plastic tubes, forming a solid-phase immunosorbent (Figure 8.18). An unknown amount of the homologous antigen in the patient's sample is allowed to compete with a known amount of an antigen-enzyme complex for binding sites on the antibodies. After a suitable incubation period, the tubes are centrifuged and washed to remove any unbound antigen. Substrate for the enzyme is added, and the amount of product is measured in a spectrophotometer by the degree of change in optical density (absorbance) at the wavelength for maximal detection of the colored product. The more antigen present in the patient's sample, the less enzyme-antigen will be bound to the immunosorbent. Therefore, if very little "color" (OD) change is detected, a large amount of antigen is inferred to exist in the patient's sample. A calibration curve is constructed by running a series of several concentrations of a reference standard simultaneously with each run of unknowns. Reagents from

Serology and Immunology

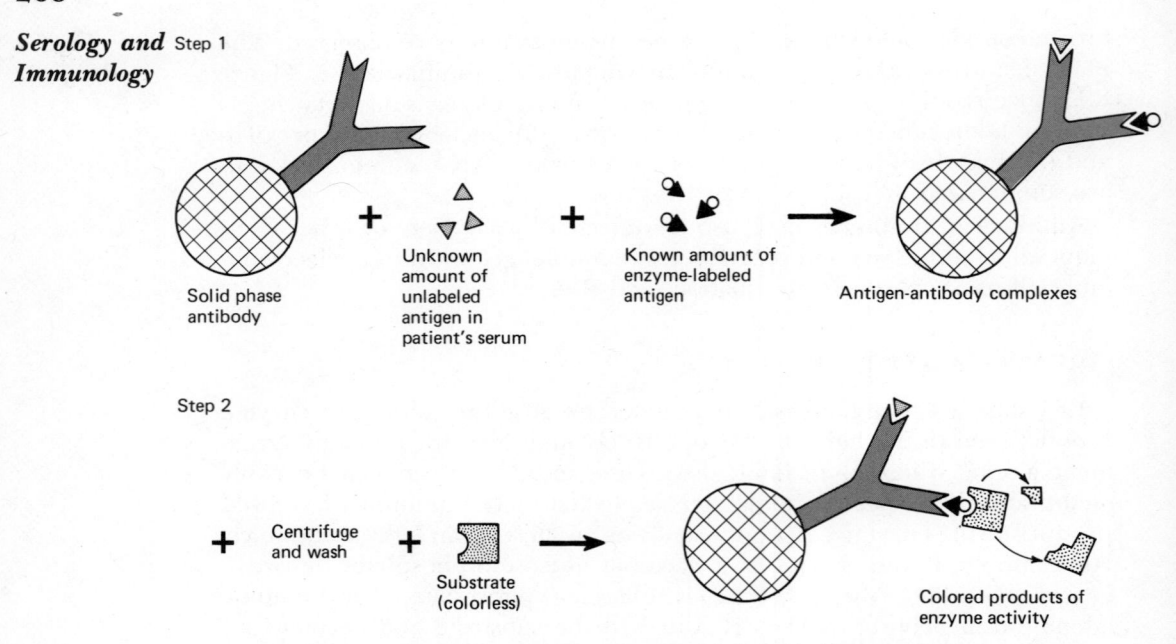

FIGURE 8.18. Diagram of an enzyme-linked immunosorbent assay (ELISA).

different kits should never be mixed because there can be large differences in reactivity of components from different lots or with different shelf ages.

A second kind of heterogeneous EIA is the **immunoenzymometric test** (Figure 8.19). An excess amount of enzyme-labeled antibody is added to the patient's specimen. If any homologous antigen is present in the specimen, it becomes bound to the antibody. Next a solid-phase antigen is added and adsorbs any antibodies with at least one free binding site. Centrifugation causes all immunosorbent particles to rapidly settle to the bottom of the tube. Only antibodies with all their combining sites occupied by patient's antigen will be extracted in the supernatant fluid. Substrate for the enzyme is added to the supernate, and product formation is monitored spectrophotometrically. The more antigen in the patient's sample, the more enzyme-linked antibody will be present in the supernate. This in turn will be reflected by a greater change in light absorbance as more colored product is made.

A third type of heterogeneous EIA is an immunological sandwich technique with patient's antigen serving as the "meat" of the sandwich. Step 1 (Figure 8.20) involves mixing an excess amount of solid-phase antibody with the patient's sample containing an unknown amount of homologous antigen. It should be noted that this technique works only if the antigen is at least bivalent (multivalent). A measured amount of enzyme-labeled antibody is then added, followed by incubation, centrifugation, and washing of the precipitate to remove any unadsorbed antibody. Substrate is added, and color change is measured by spectrophotometer and converted to antigen concentration by means of calibration standards. The more antigen in the patient's sample, the more enzyme-linked antibody will be bound to the sorbent, the more substrate will be catalyzed, and the greater the change in OD.

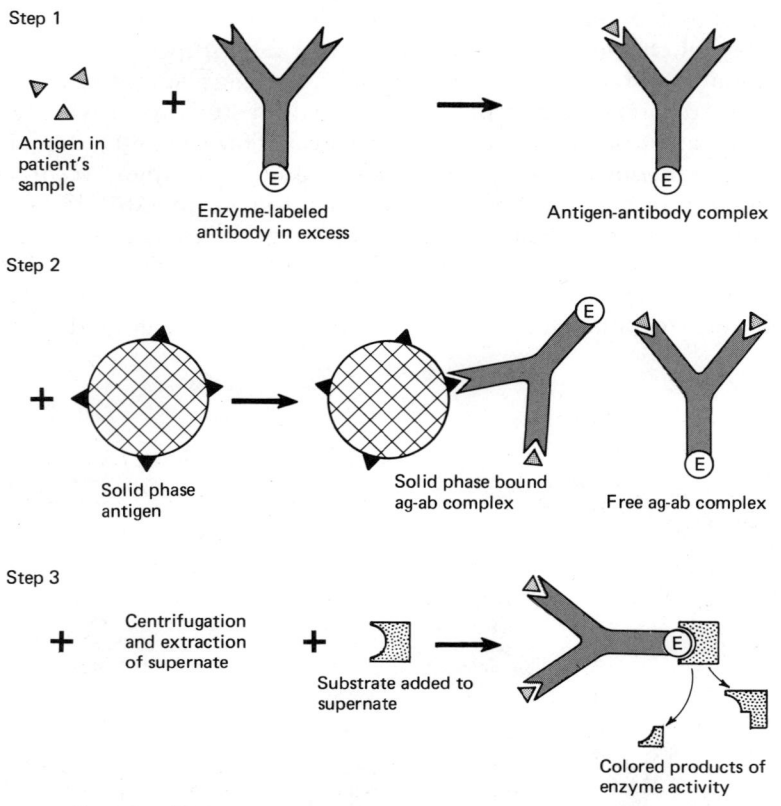

FIGURE 8.19. Diagram of an immunoenzymometric test.

A fourth variation of heterogeneous EIA involves the use of antiglobulin (Figure 8.21). An unknown quantity of multivalent antigen in a sample is mixed with solid-phase homologous antibody (e.g., derived from a goat). A second homologous antibody from another species (e.g., rabbit) is added, forming an immunological sandwich. To this point, the test is identical to the antigen sandwich method with the exception that the second antibody is not enzyme-labeled. The tubes are then centrifuged and washed to remove any unadsorbed rabbit antibody. Next is added an enzyme-labeled antirabbit gamma globulin (e.g., derived from a sheep). Centrifugation and washing are now required to remove any unadsorbed enzyme-labeled antirabbit immunoglobulin. Substrate can then be added and color change evaluated by a spectrophotmeter. The quantity of antigen in the patient's sample will be directly correlated with change in absorbance.

Homogeneous EIA. This method employs an antigen attached to an enzyme in such a way that the substrate cannot enter the catalytic site if the enzyme-antigen complex is bound to antibody. Presumably the antibody sterically blocks substrate-enzyme interaction when it is part of the complex. When the patient's sample (usually serum or urine) is mixed with antibody and the enzyme-labeled antigen, free antigen molecules from the sample will compete with the enzyme-labeled molecules for a limited number of antibody-combining sites (Figure 8.22). The more antigen in the sample, the more enzyme will remain unbound and catalytically active. After adding substrate to the mixture, the free enzyme converts it to a "colored" product that changes the optical density at a rate proportional to the concentration of unbound enzyme. Typically, these measurements are made with a spectrophotometer especially designed for studying enzyme kinetics, possessing a temperature-stabilized microscale flow cell and a digital readout or printout device for easy handling of multiple samples. Accuracy and precision can be enhanced by use of a semiautomatic pipettor/dilutor and a timer/printer or programmable calculator integrally connected to the spectrophotometer. For large volumes of EIA, an automated spectrophotometer system can be used. Homogeneous EIA tests are very popular because bound and free antigen do not have to be physically separated.

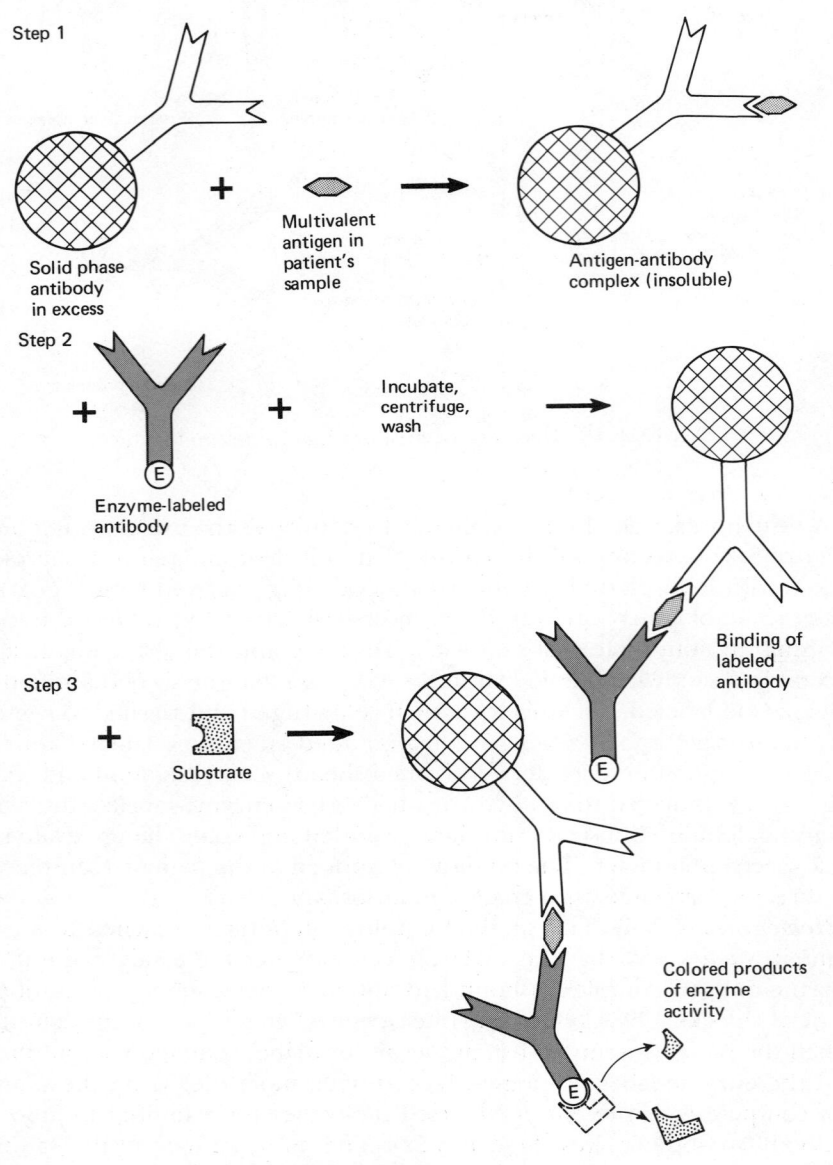

FIGURE 8.20. "Antigen sandwich" EIA.

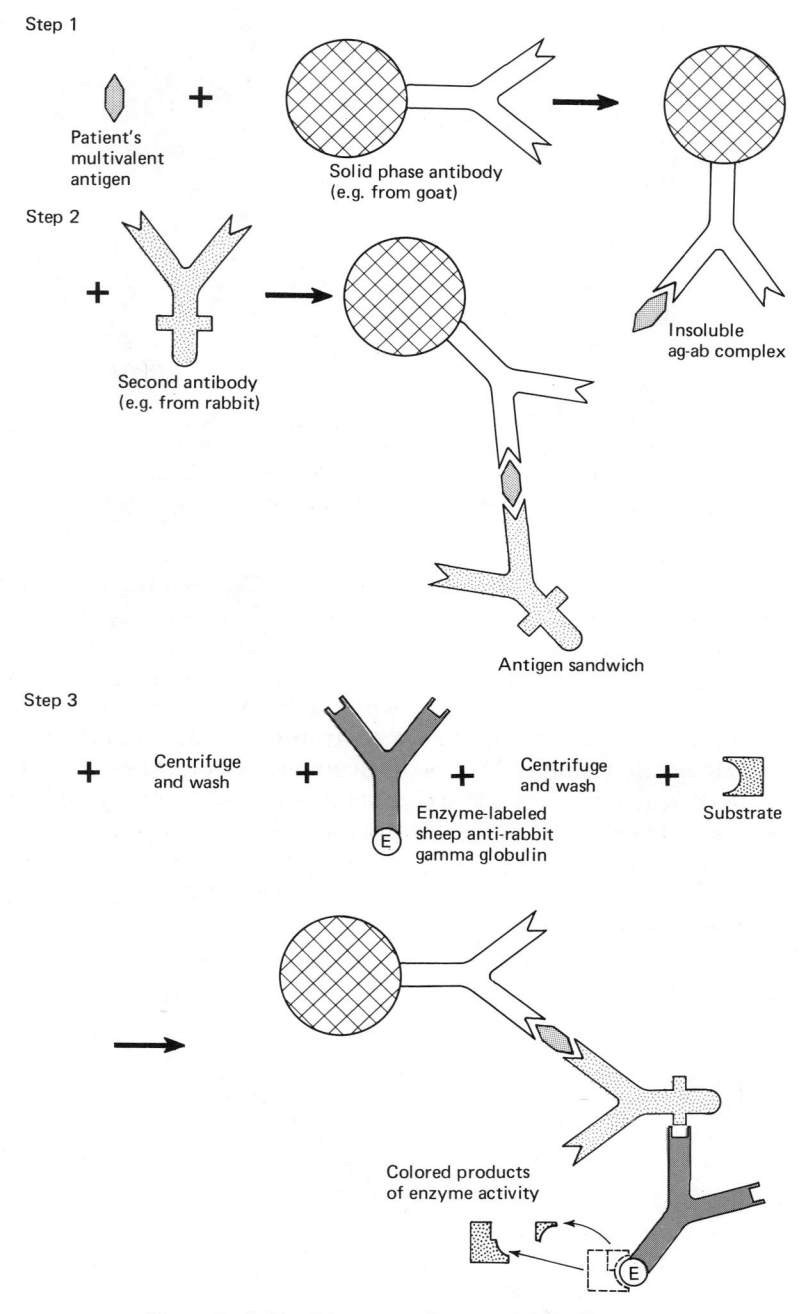

FIGURE 8.21. Diagram of an antiglobulin EIA.

Typically, the assay mixture is aspirated into the spectrophotometer flow cell maintained at 37°C. To ensure the proper temperature, the instrument should be turned on fifteen to twenty minutes prior to the test. A short ten to fifteen-second delay is commonly allowed for temperature equilibration of the sample within the spectrophotometer. An automatic timer triggers both an initial OD reading and a second reading after a prescribed interval

Serology and Immunology

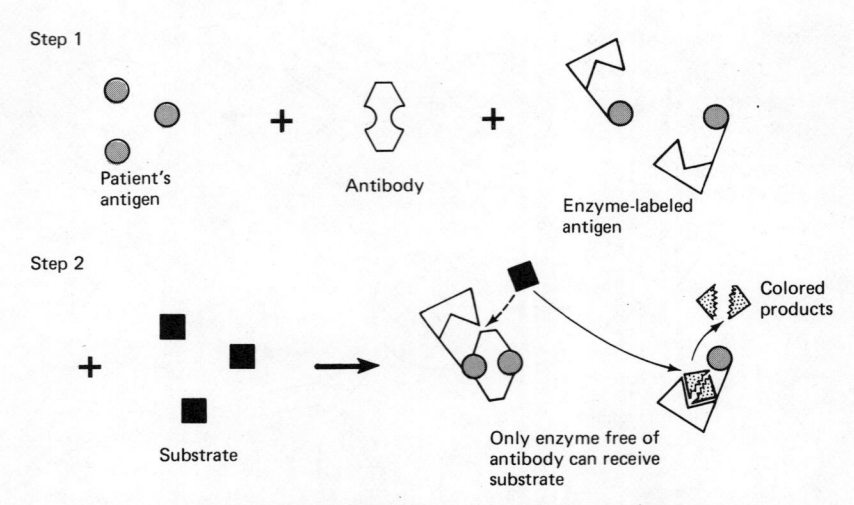

FIGURE 8.22. Diagram of a homogeneous enzyme immunoassay.

(usually about one to one and one-half minutes). Two readings are printed for each sample (including standards of known concentration). The technologist then calculates the absorbance (optical density) change (ΔA or ΔOD) during the test interval for the standards and plots the results on special semilog graph paper supplied with the kit (Figure 8.23). By interpolation from the standard curve, the concentration of antigen in the patient's sample can be determined. If the instrument is equipped with a programmable calculator, all of these computations can be done automatically and no graph paper is required. The sample number is printed together with its antigen concentration. Obviously the first samples sent through the spectrophotometer on any given run would be the standards against which the unknowns would be interpreted.

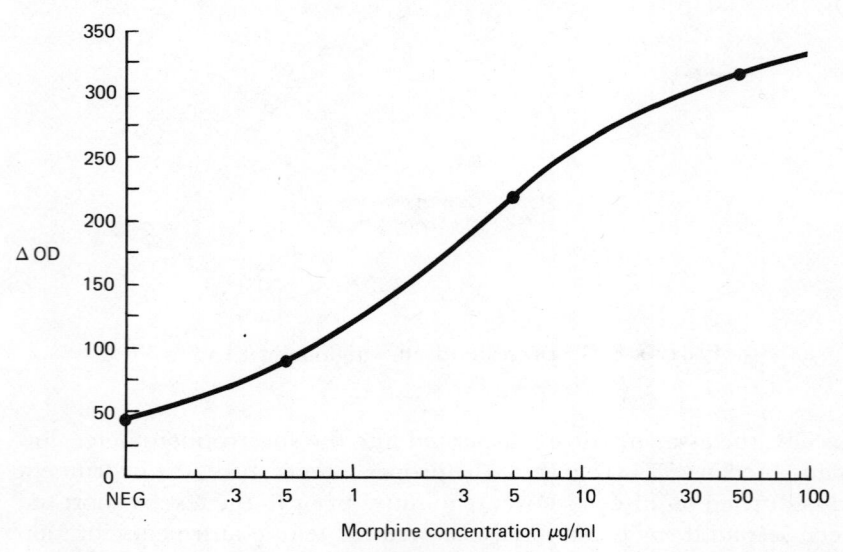

FIGURE 8.23. Typical standard curve of a homogeneous EIA for morphine.

Most EIA techniques have several advantages including (1) high degree of sensitivity, (2) short run times (usually less than two to three minutes), (3) simplicity of sample handling, (4) ease of automation, (5) moderate shelf life of reagents, (6) economy, and (7) avoidance of the hazards of working with radioactive substances. Because of these advantages, EIA tests are likely to supplant RIA tests for many analyses. For example, EIA kits are now available from Syva Corporation, Palo Alto, California, for assay of drugs including digoxin, theophylline, antiepileptic drugs, and drugs of abuse under the trade name EMIT (enzyme-multiplied immunoassay technique). Theophylline is an antiasthmatic drug commonly administered with such adjunctive bronchodilating agents as ephedrine. As with digoxin therapy, there is a narrow margin of safety between effective and toxic dosage levels. High-dosage theophylline treatment requires regular blood level measurements to maintain dosage within the therapeutic range. Previously the slow and complicated high-pressure liquid chromatography process was the only available clinical assay for this drug. Essentially the same problems formerly existed for monitoring the levels of anticonvulsant drugs (e.g., diphenylhydantoin, phenobarbital, etc.) used to treat epilepsies. Until recently, gas-liquid chromatography (GLC) was the most common analytical methodology for antiepileptic drug (AED) assays. Although GLC is accurate and sensitive (if properly performed), it is still complex, time-consuming, and quite sensitive to skills of the technician and sample preparatory procedures. All of these problems have virtually disappeared with the introduction of EIA test kits.

Electron Spin Resonance (ESR) Immunoassay

An electron spin resonance spectrometer is used to measure the energy absorbed by unpaired electrons of free chemical radicals as they "flip" from a stable to a meta-stable position in a magnetic field. Each free radical requires a characteristic energy for this transition to occur. For small molecules that tumble rapidly in solution, all field positions are averaged to produce a high, narrow spectrum (Figure 8.24). If a small, free radical becomes bound to a much larger antibody molecule that tumbles very slowly, spectral averaging no longer occurs, and the resulting spectrum is low and broad. By attaching a stable free radical (such as a nitroxide) to a low-molecular-weight antigen, the latter acquires a "spin label." The height of the ESR peak then becomes a direct measure of the amount of immunologically unbound antigen. This method has also been called a **free-radical assay technique** (FRAT). Since no physical separation of bound from free antigen is required, this homogeneous immunoassay is very rapid once the sample has been mixed and equilibrated with antibody and spin-labeled antigen. Unknowns are quantitated by comparison of their ESR peaks with a curve generated from standards of known concentrations. Figure 8.25 is a typical standard curve for ESR immunoassay of morphine. ESR spectrometers are very expensive and are seldom available in hospital laboratories.

The lowest levels of opiates detectable by EMIT are about 0.3 μg/ml; this is comparable to the lowest amounts of opiates detected with the FRAT system. There is good agreement between EMIT and RIA determinations

Serology and Immunology

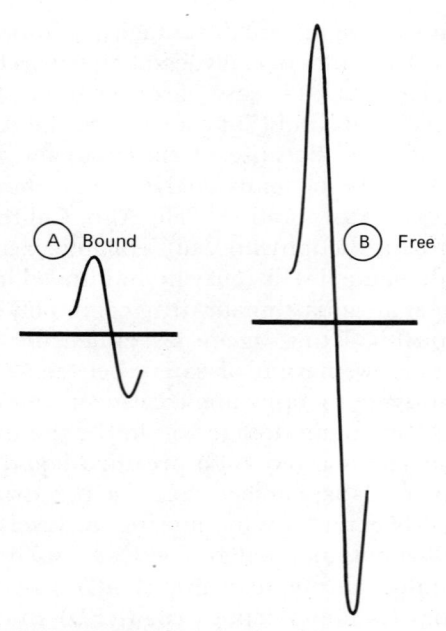

FIGURE 8.24. ESR (electron spin resonance) spectra of free-radical-labeled morphine in a FRAT (free-radical assay technique). *A*, Antibody-bound labeled morphine; *B*, antibody-free spin-labeled morphine.

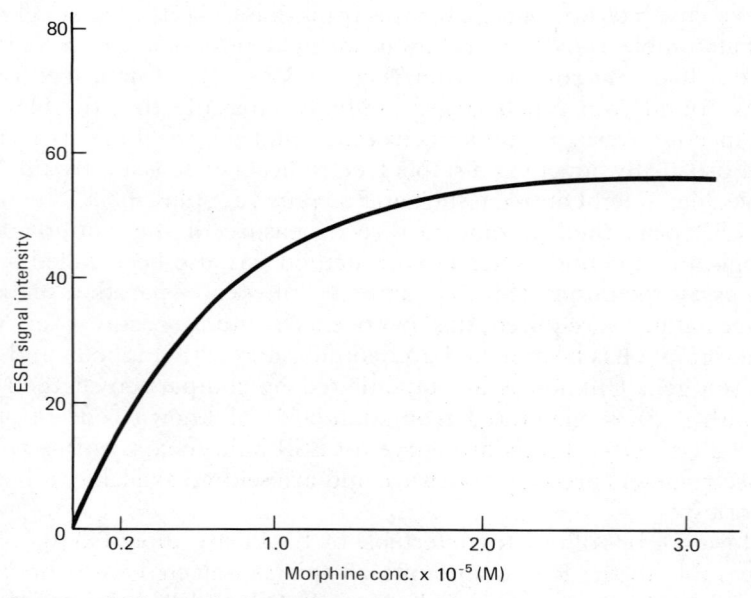

FIGURE 8.25. Typical standard curve for morphine assay by FRAT.

of digoxin in samples containing 1 to 2 ng/ml. Radioimmunoassays are the most sensitive immunoassays; e.g., RIA for progesterone have been made at 30 pg.

Ferritin Labeling

Ferritin is an electron-opaque protein containing nearly 23 percent iron. Its biological function is the transport of iron. When antibodies are tagged with ferritin through a diazotization reaction, they hinder the passage of electrons, can be detected by the electron microscope (EM), and appear on micrographs as dark spots. Obviously this is a research tool, not one for the clinical laboratory. Experimentally, ferritin-labeled antibodies have been used to detect the target tissues attacked by an antiserum and are especially useful for locating viruses within tissues. Bacterial and mycotic antigens have also been revealed within the body by this ferritin-labeling technique. For example, ferritin-labeled toxin of *Clostridium botulinum* has been injected into mice and detected in electron micrographs at neuromuscular junctions, especially in the motor end plates of the intercostal muscles. This information correlates with the fact that death by botulism is usually due to respiratory failure.

SELF-EVALUATION

Terms

1. Any substance that absorbs relatively high-energy photons and emits light of lower frequency.
2. A serological test for specific antibodies against the causative organism of syphilis, indicated by cessation of motility. (3 words)
3. The diminution of fluorescence of antibodies as a consequence of their union with homologous haptens.
4. General term for any specific binding agent, such as antibodies, transport proteins, cell receptors, etc., used in serological tests.
5. The kind of instrument required for the detection of beta-emitting radioisotopes. (2 or 3 words)
6. The term applied to any immunoassay in which separation of bound from free antigen is not required.
7. The specificity of autoantibodies commonly accompanying systemic lupus erythematosus.
8. A class of nonimmunological reactions employing a specific ligand other than antibody, but otherwise similar in principle to RIA. (4 words)
9. A radioimmunoassay designed to quantitate the amount of a specific IgE. (2 words)
10. An iron-rich protein used as a label for antibodies so that they can be detected with an electron microscope.

Multiple Choice. Choose the one best answer.

1. Which of the following is not considered to be a substance for "tagging" antibodies? (a) complement (b) FITC (c) ^{131}I (d) enzyme (e) ferritin
2. Which of the following tests is read by means of a microscope? (a) CPBA (b) RIA (c) EMIT (d) FTA (e) ESR

Serology and Immunology

3. Which of the following tests is not concerned with diagnosis of syphilis? (a) RPR (b) FADF (c) RIP (d) TPI (e) RPCF
4. Which of the following is not used to separate bound from free antigen in RIA techniques? (a) antibody-coated tubes (b) transport proteins (c) dextran-coated charcoal particles (d) saturated ammonium sulfate solution (e) antiglobulin
5. The most popular radionuclide for RIA and CPBA used in crystal scintillation counters is (a) ^{14}C (b) ^{131}I (c) ^{125}I (d) ^{3}H (e) none of these
6. Which of the following tests for IgE involves a "sandwich" technique (antigen between two antibodies)? (a) indirect RIST (b) direct RIST (c) RIP (d) RAST (e) more than one of these
7. Anti-RNA antibodies are most likely to cause an immunoenzyme staining pattern termed (a) solid (b) rim (c) nucleolar (d) speckled (e) thready
8. The kind of instrumentation required for free radical assay tests is (a) ESR spectrometer (b) ultracentrifuge (c) mass spectrometer (d) electron microscope (e) gas-liquid chromatograph
9. The kind of enzyme immunoassay that employs immunoglobulin from three different sources is (a) ELISA (b) immunoenzymometric test (c) antiglobulin EIA (d) EMIT (e) more than one of these
10. Which of the following is not an attribute of the first phase of serological reactions (relative to the second phase)? (a) slow rate of reaction (b) high change in free energy (c) requires electrolytes (d) formation of aggregates (e) more than one of these

True-False

1. It is possible to excite a substance with red light (650 nm) and cause it to fluoresce as a yellow color (575 nm).
2. A serological reaction is prohibited from attaining the second phase if either antigen or antibody is monovalent.
3. The emitted light of a fluor is characteristic of the excitation light, not of the fluor itself.
4. The FADF test requires a live spirochete antigen.
5. In an inhibition immunofluorescent test, the antigen is of unknown specificity.
6. A quantitative immunofluorescent test need not be washed before addition of the labeled antibody as long as the immunoadsorbent is maintained in excess.
7. The optimal dilution of antibody for use in RIA is the one that binds about 50 percent of the labeled antigen.
8. Albumin is sometimes added to RIA tests to enhance the union of antigen and antibody.
9. If relatively little or no OD change occurs in an ELISA, a small amount of antigen is inferred to exist in the patient's sample.
10. When lysozyme is the enzyme used in a positive quantitative immunoenzyme assay, the amount of antigen in the sample is positively correlated with a decrease in optical density.

Immunopathology

CHAPTER 9

CHAPTER OUTLINE

Immunoproliferative Diseases
   Multiple Myelomas
   Heavy Chain Diseases
   Dysfunctional Suppressor T Cells
Immunological
Dysfunction/Deficiency Diseases
   Accessory Cell Dysfunctions
   Complement Deficiencies and
   Defects
   T Cell Deficiencies
   B Cell Abnormalities
   Combined B and T Cell Deficiencies
Hypersensitivities
   Type I (Immediate)
   Hypersensitivities
     Allergies
     Chemical Mediators
     Desensitization
     Allergy Tests
     Anaphylactic Reactions
   Type III Hypersensitivities
   (Immune Complex Diseases)
     Arthus Reaction
     Serum Sickness
   Type IV (Delayed)

Hypersensitivities
   Tuberculin Reaction
   Contact Dermatitis
   Lymphokines
     Interforons
   "Killer" Cells
Autoallergic (Autoimmune) Diseases
   Immunoglobulin-associated
   Autoallergic Diseases
     Systemic Lupus Erythematosus
     Glomerulonephritis
     Rheumatic Fever
     Autoimmune Hemolytic
     Anemia
     Thrombocytopenic Purpura
     Other Diseases with
     Autoantibodies
   T Cell–associated Autoallergic
   Diseases
     Allergic Encephalomyelitis
     Sympathetic Ophthalmia
     Aspermatogenesis
     Hashimoto's Hypothyroiditis
Self-evaluation

Diseases associated with the immune system are known as immunopathological conditions. Unchecked growth of cancerous cells in many cases can be attributed in large measure to a dysfunctional immune response on the part of the host. This aspect of immunopathology is treated separately in Chapter 10.

Immunoproliferative Diseases

MULTIPLE MYELOMAS

Overproduction of immunoglobulins (immunoproliferation) can result from a plasma cell neoplasm. Multiple myeloma is a disease resulting from unrestricted proliferation of one or more clones of plasma cells (Figure 9.1). When a single clone is involved, a single kind of antibody is synthesized in excess, resulting in a nearly monophoretic protein that appears as a tall, narrow spike in the γ or γ-β region of an electrophorogram. This homogeneous protein is called the **M (myeloma) protein** and the disease is referred to as a **monoclonal gammopathy.** If more than one clone of plasma cells is

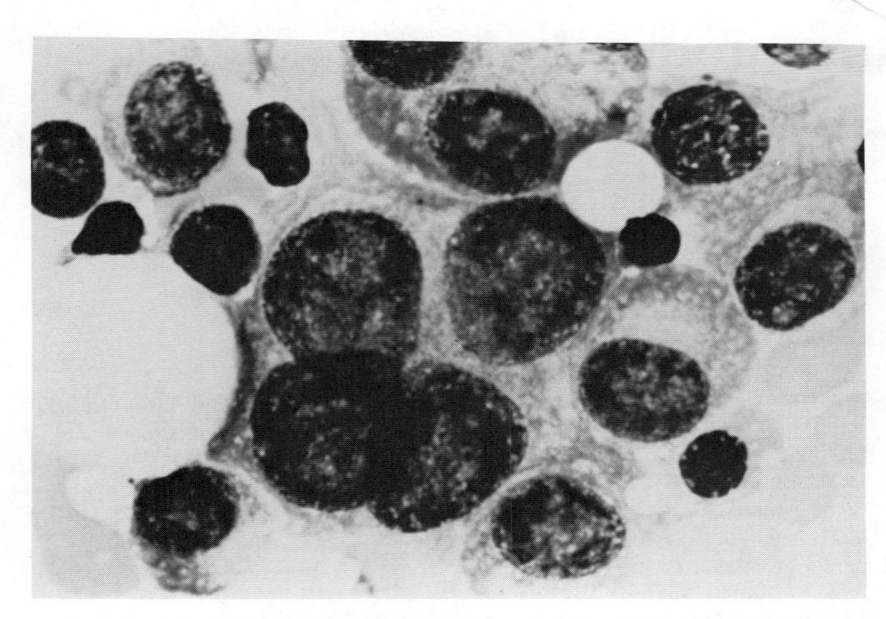

FIGURE 9.1. Massive proliferation of plasma cells associated with multiple myeloma. [*Courtesy of Elliot Scientific Corp., New York City.*]

involved (a **polyclonal gammopathy**), several portions of the beta-gamma globulin region or perhaps the entire gamma globulin region is elevated. A single class (e.g., IgG, IgA, IgM, etc.) of immunoglobulin is made by a plasma cell clone. In patients with multiple myelomas, plasma cells infiltrate dense bones and cause their erosion. Radiographic examination of hard bone tissue reveals the discrete holes that may so weaken them that they fracture easily. Biopsy of bone marrow or other lymphoid tissue reveals an excessive number of plasma cells. Some of the plasma cells possess a swollen cytoplasm containing inclusions of immunoglobulin called **Russell bodies.** A myeloma that produces IgM immunoglobulins is termed **Waldenström's macroglobulinemia.** There appears to be a hereditary predisposition to Waldenström's macroglobulinemia as it occurs more often than expected by chance in certain families. Regardless of the class of immunoglobulin produced, many myeloma patients have in their blood and excrete in their urine Bence-Jones proteins. These are immunoglobulin L chains as either monomers or dimers. About 10 percent of all myelomas produce only Bence-Jones proteins (no complete immunoglobulins).

HEAVY CHAIN DISEASES

Heavy chain diseases (Franklin's disease) are also overproduction diseases, classified as malignant lymphomas rather than multiple myelomas. Patients with heavy chain diseases apparently fail to make enough light chains, causing their plasma cells to overproduce heavy chains and excrete them into the blood and/or urine. Complete heavy chains are seldom found. Most common is α chain disease in which the heavy chain portion consists of the entire Fc and hinge region (approximately 75 percent of the α chain) as dimers of 3S to 4S. Patients with α chain disease commonly suffer malabsorption syndrome, diarrhea, steatorrhea (fatty stools), weight loss, and abdominal pain. Heavy chain diseases are known to involve γ chains and less frequently μ chains; no heavy chain diseases involving delta and epsilon chains have yet been found. Sharp electrophoretic peaks are not characteristic of heavy chain diseases. Diagnosis is aided by serum immunoelectrophoresis that reveals proteins in the beta and/or gamma regions that react with anti-IgA (or antibodies specific for other classes of immunoglobulins), but do not react with antisera to light chains.

DYSFUNCTIONAL SUPPRESSOR T CELLS

It is also possible that some kinds of unnecessary chronic immunoglobulin synthesis may result from a failure of suppressor T cells (T_S) to terminate the B cell response following the conquest of a microbial infection. Other kinds of T cell–B cell interactions or T cell–T cell interactions may be responsible for some forms of immune-associated diseases. For example, failure of a humoral response to a specific antigen may be attributed to a deficiency or absence of appropriate helper T cells (T_H) required for B cell activation rather than to a deficiency of cognate B cells themselves. Ironically, most immunological deficiencies result from medical treatment for other diseases. Adrenocorticotropic hormone (ACTH) is a potent anti-inflammatory agent, but its prolonged use seriously depletes the patient of T cells and in the long run may thereby allow infections to become fatal. Chemotherapy and x-ray treatment of cancers indiscriminately inactivates all rapidly dividing cells including those of the lymphoid system. Immunosuppressive drugs are also commonly used to prolong survival of tissue or organ transplants. Many of these patients die from infections that would have normally been prevented in an immunologically uncompromised host. Diseases caused by medical treatment (drugs) are called **iatrogenic diseases.**

Immunological Dysfunction/Deficiency Diseases

ACCESSORY CELL DYSFUNCTIONS

Immunopathology may also involve components of the immune system other than T cells and B cells. The role of phagocytic cells in antigen processing and stimulation of B cells is well documented. Dysfunctional phagocytes therefore can interfere with the afferent limb of the immune response. Abnormal phagocytic functions may be expressed in a variety of forms. Phagocytes may fail to exhibit motile responses to known chemotactic factors. The range of microorganisms phagocytized may be restricted or the phagocytes may be unable to kill endocytosed microorganisms. If the phagocyte is unable to generate hydrogen peroxide, this can be detected *in vitro* by use of the redox-sensitive dye nitroblue tetrazolium (NBT). This test may be used clinically to diagnose patients with **chronic granulomatous disease** (CGD; also called **congenital dysphagocytosis**) or those with **Job's syndrome.** CGD is inherited as a sex-linked recessive trait; hence it mainly appears in males. Job's syndrome is inherited as an autosomal recessive trait and therefore appears with equal frequency in males and females. In both

Serology and Immunology

diseases, neutrophils fail to switch from the anaerobic glycolytic pathway to oxidative metabolism (via the hexose monophosphate or pentose phosphate shunt) following phagocytosis. The oxidative pathway is normally used to make hydrogen peroxide (H_2O_2), which in turn is required to generate singlet oxygen (O^-) and hydroxyl (OH^-) radicals. One or both of these products seem to be the final bactericidal weapons or belong to the pathway of the true killing agent(s). Halide ions (chloride, iodide) are cofactors of the myeloperoxidase system by which toxic singlet oxygen is generated from hydrogen peroxide. The so-called "iodination of microorganisms" is the participation of these halide cofactors in the production of potent oxidizing agents.

Normal neutrophils produce peroxide and reduce NBT to its insoluble blue form that may then be observed as clumps in the cytoplasm. Peroxidase-deficient neutrophils do not stain with NBT. Female carriers (heterozygous) of the gene for Job's syndrome have about half the NBT reduction capacity of normal individuals. Both CGD and Job's syndrome are usually fatal in childhood. Paradoxically, it is usually opportunistic pathogens (such as *Escherichia coli, Enterobacter aerogenes, Serratia marcescens,* and *Staphlococcus epidermidis*) that cause these deaths rather than the common pathogens of childhood diseases (e.g., *Streptococcus pyogenes, Streptococcus pneumoniae, Neisseria meningitidis,* and *Hemophilus influenzae*). Some of the common pathogens produce peroxide, but lack the catalyase enzyme to destroy it, thereby creating a microenvironment hostile to their own survival. The opportunistic pathogens involved in CGD and Job's syndrome produce catalase that detoxifies peroxide into water and oxygen. The weak peroxide production of the defective phagocytes in these patients is easily detoxified by the catalase of these opportunistic pathogens, allowing the bacteria to survive and multiply. However, both *N. meningitidis* and *H. influenzae* produce catalase; so factors other than this must operate to account for the higher death rate by opportunistic pathogens in children with CGD or Job's syndrome.

Patient's with a deficiency of glucose-6-phosphate dehydrogenase (G-6-PD) also have neutrophils that are unable to destroy engulfed microorganisms. This enzyme is the one that diverts metabolism from the glycolytic pathway to the hexose monophosphate shunt. Consequently, little peroxide is made, making it easier for both catalase-positive and catalase-negative microbes to survive.

Both peroxide and the enzyme myeloperoxidase are required for protection against many pyogenic (pus-forming) bacteria. Patients with a deficiency of this enzyme suffer with severe acute infections. Their phagocytic cells manufacture peroxide, but little or no singlet oxygen production occurs, and therefore the killing of bacteria is depressed. Patient's with CGD produce sufficient myeloperoxidase but too little peroxide. Both appear to be necessary for "iodination" (singlet oxygen production) and killing of microbes.

A hereditary disease called **Chediak-Higashi syndrome** is characterized by phagocytes possessing normal endocytosis but their lysosomes are abnormally large and fuse sluggishly with phagosomes. It is inherited as an autosomal recessive disease and is commonly fatal in childhood as a consequence of increased susceptibility to pyogenic infectious diseases.

COMPLEMENT DEFICIENCIES AND DEFECTS

Hereditary deficiencies in some of the components of the complement system have been identified. Complement deficiencies are usually associated with a lowered resistance to bacterial infections and/or an elevated incidence of hypersensitivity diseases. A deficiency of Cl esterase inhibitor is inherited as an autosomal dominant genetic trait and is responsible for a disease called hereditary angioneurotic edema (HANE). This inhibitor is one of the substances that modulates the activity of the complement cascade. Without the inhibitor, complement reactions continue to function long after they are needed, producing recurrent episodes of local acute inflammation at the sites of activation. As a consequence, blood vessels become dilated and fluid transudates into the tissues, especially those of the skin, gastrointestinal (GI) tract, and upper respiratory tract. Severe edema in the throat may cause death by suffocation. Hereditary angioneurotic edema can also be caused by a mutation in the gene for $\overline{C1s}$ inhibitor that produces a nonfunctional protein antigenically identical to the functional inhibitor. This and other nonfunctional proteins such as Bence-Jones proteins (that are serologically cross-reactive with their functional counterparts) are classified as **paraproteins.** Their presence in blood is termed **paraproteinemia.**

T CELL DEFICIENCIES

The possible roles of dysfunctional suppressor T cells and helper T cells in "overproduction diseases" and deficient antibody responses, respectively, have already been discussed. Whenever T cells are deficient in number or in function, the patient is expected to be highly susceptible to a wide variety of viral, bacterial, and fungal (mycotic) diseases. Such patients often cannot combat even feeble pathogens. Vaccination with attenuated microbes may result in a fatal infection of such patients. A nonspecific diminution or absence of delayed-type hypersensitivity (T cell–mediated) to potent allergens (e.g., 2,4-dinitrochlorobenzene, DNCB) is termed **anergy** and typifies T cell–deficiency diseases. Failure to reject allografts (from genetically different members of the same species) also is a hallmark of T cell–deficient patients. However, this allograft test cannot be justified for routine clinical use because it would stimulate the recipient to histocompatibility antigens and make it more difficult to obtain a compatible donor should he later need one. T cell deficiencies that result from absence or dysfunction of a thymus can sometimes be rectified by transplants of embryonic thymus.

Assessment of T cell function can be made by a variety of *in vivo* techniques including skin response to DNCB, X ray of thymic shadow, histological and immunofluorescence studies of lymphoid morphology following exposure to diphtheria or tetanus toxoids, and studies of thymic morphology from biopsies. T cell function can be assayed *in vitro* by their response to known mitogens, foreign cells, or potent antigens. Only T cells form spontaneous "rosettes" with sheep erythrocytes (E rosettes).

Two congenital T cell–deficiency diseases involving the thymus are well known in humans. In the **Di George syndrome,** faulty embryogenesis of the third and fourth pharyngeal pouches results in the virtual absence of the thymus and parathyroid glands. The latter endocrine organ normally regulates calcium levels in the blood. Without the hormones of the parathyroids, the newborn infant develops hypocalcemia and experiences tetany (muscle spasm). If the parathyroid hormones can be exogenously supplied, the patient may later exhibit a wasting disease similar to that observed in neonatally thymectomized rodents. No hereditary basis has been established for the development of Di George syndrome.

The **Nezelof syndrome,** on the other hand, is inherited as an autosomal recessive trait. In this disease, both the thymus and T cells develop abnormally but the associated embryological defects of Di George syndrome are lacking. The **nude** mouse is, in some ways, the analog of Nezelof syndrome in humans. It too is inherited as an autosomal recessive trait. In addition to the nude mouse being hairless, its thymus is almost devoid of lymphocytes. There is no stem cell defect in either case, only a defect in the maturation of the stem cells. The nude mouse also has immunoglobulin levels lower than normal, making it an example of a combined immunodeficiency disease. Since the T cell defect is so much more severe than the humoral defect, it may be considered as mainly a T cell–deficiency condition.

Several acquired (not congenital) diseases are known to markedly affect T cell immunity. Certain lymphoproliferative diseases such as Hodgkin's disease, sarcoidosis, and thymoma exhibit secondary ramifications in the T cell arm of the immune system. **Hodgkin's disease** is a cancer of lymph node cells. Although the malignancy may be limited to a single node, a deficiency of T cell functions is exhibited throughout the body. The etiology of the loss of T cell function is unknown. **Sarcoidosis** is a systemic granulomatous disease of unknown origin. Lymphocytes from sarcoid patients are not stimulated by PHA but transform when exposed to the Kveim "antigen." The nature of this "antigen" is unclear. It is present in extracts from human sarcoid tissue. Following the intradermal injection of Kveim antigen, the sarcoid patient develops a papulated lesion at the injection site after about a month. Normal individuals are unresponsive to this **Kveim test.** T cell functions are also aberrant in leprosy, chronic mucocutaneous candidiasis (moniliasis), and episodic lymphopenia with associated lymphocytotoxin.

B CELL ABNORMALITIES

B cell function is usually assayed *in vitro* by quantitation of either total immunoglobulins (by the method of single radial immunodiffusion) or specific antibodies to previously administered antigens (diphtheria, tetanus, polio) by microhemagglutination titration. Tests can also be made for surface markers characteristic of B cells. Antibody tagged with a fluorochrome can be used to detect membrane-bound immunoglobulins (mIg). An immune complex tagged with a fluorochrome can detect receptors for the Fc region of IgG molecules; alternatively, Fc receptors can be detected by rosette formation with IgG antibody–coated erythrocytes. Complement receptors can be detected by rosette formation between B cells and erythrocytes coated with certain complement components.

A sex-linked recessive gene produces a congenital deficiency of plasma cells called **infantile sex-linked agammaglobulinemia** or **Bruton's disease.** Immunoglobulins are not totally absent, but their levels are expressed in micrograms (per 100 ml blood) rather than milligrams. Therefore, the term "hypogammaglobulinemia" is more accurately descriptive of the disease. At about six months of age, children with Bruton's disease begin to succumb to pyogenic bacterial infections of the skin and respiratory tracts. By this time, placentally transferred maternal immunoglobulins have disappeared. Treatment with antibiotics and hyperimmune human gamma globulin have been successful.

Acquired dysfunctional B cell diseases are also known but their causes are obscure. Some cases of acquired "agammaglobulinemia" have an abnormal class of suppressor T cells (T_s cells) that prevents stimulation of antibody synthesis in B cells. Selective dysgammaglobulinemias are also known that involve only one or a specific combination of immunoglobulin classes.

COMBINED B AND T CELL DEFICIENCIES

A "primary immunodeficiency disease" is one that stems from defects that originate in the primary lymphoid organs (e.g., spleen, thymus). A "secondary immunodeficiency disease" is one in which the lymphoid tissues acquire defects as a consequence of malfunction in other tissues or organs (e.g., endocrine organs) or as a consequence of exposure to immunosuppressive drugs, ionizing radiations, or other harmful environmental agents. If the cause of the immunodeficiency is unknown, the disease cannot properly be classified as of either "primary" or "secondary" origin.

Excessive secretion of cortisone and cortisol from the adrenal cortex characterizes **Cushing's disease.** These hormones are potent anti-inflammatory agents that cause direct lysis of most T and B lymphocytes. As the disease progresses, the patient becomes highly susceptible to infections, especially to those normally controlled by T cells. This is an example of a "secondary immunodeficiency disease."

A disease called **ataxia telangiectasia** results in loss of muscle coordination (ataxia) and highly dilated, tortuous small veins (tel = end; angio = vessel; ectases = stretching out). Immunological defects begin to appear at about five years of age. IgA levels become severely depleted and IgE levels may also be depressed. The thymus is alymphoid in these patients. They appear to have acquired a defective DNA repair system unable to correct X-ray damage to genetic material. However, it is not known if the X-ray sensitivity of these patients has any relationship to the etiology of this disease. An autosomal mode of inheritance seems to be part of its etiology.

Specific loss of IgM synthesis and T cell–mediated immunity with development of thrombocytopenia and eczema characterize the **Wiskott-Aldrich syndrome.** Thrombocytopenia indicates a loss of platelets (initiators of blood clotting) and eczema is an inflammatory condition of the skin associated with an inappropriate response of IgE to antigen. Patients with this disease are born normal but begin to develop problems at an early age; they begin to bleed easily, develop a skin rash, and later lose T cell functions. It is inherited as a sex-linked recessive disease. Life expectancy for boys rarely exceeds ten years unless successfully reconstituted with a histocompatible bone marrow transplant.

A congenital combined B cell and T cell deficiency characterizes the **Swiss-type agammaglobulinemia** (so named for the initial studies in Switzerland). This disease is also known as thymic alymphoplasia, thymic dysplasia, alymphocytosis, and hereditary thymic dysplasia. It may be inher-

Serology and Immunology

ited as either a sex-linked recessive trait or as an autosomal recessive character. Afflicted children cannot defend themselves against even weak pathogens and develop a wasting disease similar to that seen in experimental animals neonatally deprived of their thymuses. Lethality of the disease may be prevented by transplants of histocompatible fetal thymus and bone marrow to repopulate the patient with the missing T and B cells. This appears to be an example of a "primary immunodeficiency disease."

Hypersensitivities

The harmful effects of the immune responses are generally classified as hypersensitivities; the beneficial effects are termed immunity. Lymphocytic choriomeningitis virus (LCM), which infects rodents and occasionally man, causes inflammation of the choroid membrane of the third and fourth lateral ventricles of the brain and the meninges that cover the brain. Be-

Table 9.1 Distinguishing Characteristics of Immediate and Delayed Hypersensitivities

Characteristic	Immediate Hypersensitivity	Delayed Hypersensitivity
Response time following challenge dose of antigen	Visible within minutes; diminishes within a few hours	Gradually rises to peak at 24–72 hours; fades over several days
Responsible cellular and chemical agents	B cell products = immunoglobulins (IgE, IgG) trigger release of vasoactive amines from mast cells, basophils, and platelets	T cell products = lymphokines
Passive transfer via	Serum	T lymphocytes
Chemotherapy	Antihistamines and adrenergic compounds	Steroids (anti-inflammatory compounds)
Target tissues	Primarily smooth muscles; organ(s) involved varies with species; vascular tissues common	No special targets; generalized response
Histology of skin response	Erythema, edema, and wheal formation; granulocytes predominate in early response; mononuclear cells increase in later response	Erythema and induration; little edema; no wheal; mononuclear cells predominate
Tissue death	Common	Uncommon
Relative ease of desensitization	Easy; via formation of blocking antibodies	Difficult; mechanism unknown

cause virus-specific antigens commonly appear on the surfaces of viral-infected cells, killer T cells attack and destroy these virus-infected cells and thereby cause neurological damage. LCM infection does not cause lethality in thymectomized (and therefore immunologically compromised) hosts. This illustrates the principle that the beneficial aspects of immunity are sometimes not possible without concomitant potentially undesirable hypersensitivity reactions.

Two systems for classification of hypersensitivities are widely used. The older system (Table 9.1) distinguishes humoral (immunoglobulin-mediated) hypersensitivities from cellular (T cell) hypersensitivities. The newer system of Gell and Combs (Table 9.2) consists of four categories emphasizing the kind of immunopathological damage incurred.

The older system of classification recognized that some hypersensitivity reactions occur almost immediately (or within minutes) following the shocking dose of antigen. Responses to other antigens appeared hours or days later. This observation led to an artificial separation of "immediate" hypersensitivities from "delayed" hypersensitivities. We now know that the consequences of antigen-antibody interactions are primarily responsible for immediate hypersensitivities, and that the effects of T cell functions are primarily involved in delayed hypersensitivities. This is somewhat of an oversimplification because both B and T cell responses commonly are made to most antigens, but in many cases the effector mechanisms of one or the

Table 9.2 GELL AND COOMBS CLASSIFICATION OF HYPERSENSITIVITY REACTIONS

Characteristic	Type I	Type II	Type III	Type IV
Synonym	Anaphylactic	Cytotoxic; cytolytic	Immune complex	Delayed; T cell–mediated
Immunoglobulin class	IgE	Mainly IgG	IgG, IgM	None
Cellular involvement	Mast cells, basophils	RBC, WBC, platelets	Host tissue cells	Host tissue cells
Complement involved	No	Yes	Yes	No
Chemical mediators	Histamine and other vasoactive amines	Complement cascade	Immune complexes deposit in vessels, joints, or other tissues	Lymphokines
Type of antigens involved	Heterologous	Isoantigens or hapten-modified autoantigens	Heterologous or autologous	Heterologous or autologous
Examples	Allergies, anaphylaxis	Transfusion reactions, Rh disease thrombocytopenic purpura, autoimmune hemolytic anemia	Serum sickness, poststreptococcal glomerulonephritis, Arthus reaction, systemic lupus erythematosus	TB skin reaction, contact dermatitis, graft rejection, Hashimoto's hypothyroiditis

other predominate as the harmful agents. Indeed, some types of B cell activation require interaction with T_H cells; so it is really incorrect in a functional sense to attempt to separate the activities of B cells from those of T cells.

Four types of hypersensitivity reactions are recognized by the classification scheme of Gell and Coombs (Table 9.2). Types I, II, and III are mainly immunoglobulin-mediated; type IV is mediated by T cells and is synonymous with delayed hypersensitivity. Type I reactions include allergies and anaphylactic reactions induced by IgE antibodies attached to mast cells. Complement is not involved. Antihistimines can be effective in preventing or diminishing this class of hypersensitivity reactions. Type II hypersensitivities are complement-dependent cytotoxic reactions induced by IgG (and perhaps other immunoglobulins). Transfusion reactions and Rh disease of the newborn are examples discussed in earlier chapters. Type III reactions result from deposition of immune complexes in blood vessels, kidneys, and other tissues. Chemotactic complement components activated by these immune complexes cause most of the damage. Autoimmune diseases against self-antigens may be of types II, III, or IV.

TYPE I (IMMEDIATE) HYPERSENSITIVITIES

The hallmark of immediate hypersensitivities is their ability to be passively transferred from a sensitive individual to a nonsensitive individual via the serum. Early studies of this phenomenon were made by two Germans (Prausnitz and Küstner) in 1921. Küstner was allergic to cooked fish, but Prausnitz was not sensitive to this allergen. Küstner's serum was injected into the skin of Prausnitz. The next day, an extract of cooked fish was injected into the same site. Within minutes an inflammatory local allergic reaction developed around the injection site. The speed of the reaction and its ability to be passively induced via serum from a sensitive person qualifies the Prausnitz-Küstner (P-K) test as an immediate-type hypersensitivity. Because of the danger of transmitting serum hepatitis virus, this test is clinically employed with humans only when necessary to avoid multiple skin tests in seriously ill patients or babies. The rhesus monkey can be used in a P-K test for detecting the presence of skin-sensitizing IgE antibodies in human serum. The RAST is an *in vitro* technique for quantitating specific IgE antibodies (Chapter 8).

Allergies. **Allergies** are altered states of reactivity to antigens or haptens and considered to be synonymous with type I (immediate) hypersensitivites. The antigens or haptens involved in allergies are called **allergens** and the antibodies are **reagins.** The most common allergies are sensitivities to pollens, mold spores, certain foods, animal hair or sloughed skin cells (danders) from animal pets, feathers, dust, wool, insect bites and stings, some antibiotics, etc. **Hay fever** (allergic rhinitis) is a mild form of allergy with symptoms of itching and running nose, sneezing, watery reddened eyes, and respiratory distress. The term **atopy** (meaning foreign, unusual, or out of place) was formerly applied to such allergies. Because parents with specific allergies tend to have children who develop similar allergies, atopic diseases were thought to have a hereditary basis. The constellation of antigens to which an individual can respond is now thought to be genetically determined mainly by **immune response** (Ir) **genes** and by structural genes for variable regions (idiotypes) of immunoglobulin molecules. Still other genes are involved in regulation of the level of immunoglobulins. Therefore, all kinds of immunities and hypersensitivites ultimately have a hereditary basis.

In the case of hay fever, an individual contacts an allergen to which he is hereditarily predisposed to respond. In this initial contact, the allergen may be disposed without development of clinical symptoms but can leave that person sensitized (hypersensitive). The next time the same allergen is contacted, a supply of specific antibodies and memory cells is available to trigger an immediate hypersensitivity reaction. The humoral factors responsible for hay fever–type allergies were originally called "reagins" (allergic reagin should not be confused with syphilitic reagin). Now we recognize that reaginic antibodies of class IgE are responsible for these allergies. These antibodies are heat-labile. They behave as though they are monovalent and cannot be detected by tests requiring lattice formation; hence, they are called "nonprecipitating" antibodies. IgE antibodies do not fix complement and therefore cannot be detected by complement fixation tests. Because of these properties of IgE and the very low concentration of IgE in plasma, highly sensitive binding tests are required for its assay (such as RIST for quantitation of total circulating IgE and RAST for quantitation of antigen-specific IgE).

IgE antibodies have nonspecific affinity for mast cells and basophils, attaching to receptor sites on these cells via their Fc regions. Antibodies that attach nonspecifically to mast cells or basophils in this manner are called **cytotropic antibodies.** Binding of antigen to cytotropic IgE on receptor sites of mast cells somehow inactivates membrane-bound adenyl (adenylate) cyclase, the enzyme that converts ATP (adenosine triphosphate) to cyclic 3,5-AMP (adenosine monophosphate). When the intracellular level of cyclic AMP is lowered, it somehow stimulates mast cell degranulation. The large granules in the cytoplasm of mast cells and basophils contain histamine and heparin (Figure 9.2). The released histamine causes local smooth muscle contraction. When venules constrict, a compensatory capillary expansion occurs and plasma fluids are forced to transudate into the tissues causing edema. Edematous tissues in the upper respiratory tract contribute to the runny nose and swollen membranes of hay fever. Constriction of smooth muscles surrounding bronchioles produces part of the respiratory distress in hay fever victims.

Allergies form a spectrum of debilitations from the relatively mild hay fevers to life-threatening anaphylactic reactions. In some asthma victims, the bronchioles become so constricted that hypoxia becomes potentially lethal. Portier and Richet in 1902 exposed dogs to sublethal doses of sea anemone toxins in an attempt to build experimental prophylactic immunity. Instead of being refractory to a subsequent exposure to the same antigen, the dogs went into a state of shock. Richet coined the term **anaphylaxis** to denote the antithesis of prophylaxis in this reaction. Widespread dilation of capillary beds throughout the body causes a drop in blood pressure that may interfere with brain function and contribute to collapse and/or death. Smooth muscles in certain tissues of the body are more prone to histamine activation than others. These tissues are referred to as **shock tissues (organs).** In the dog, the major shock tissues appear to be the hepatic venules. Anaphylactic shock in dogs produces engorgement

Serology and Immunology

of the liver with blood. Over half of the shocked dog's total blood volume may be backed up in the liver, and death ensues as a consequence of inadequate blood volume. Constriction of the pulmonary arterioles is characteristic of anaphylactic shock in the rabbit. The inferior vena cava and right side of the heart become congested with blood and contribute to heart failure. In the guinea pig, the major shock tissue is the bronchiolar smooth muscle. Autopsy of lethally shocked guinea pigs reveals lungs swollen with trapped air that could not be expelled. In all of these animals, urination and defecation are commonly observed anaphylactic symptoms

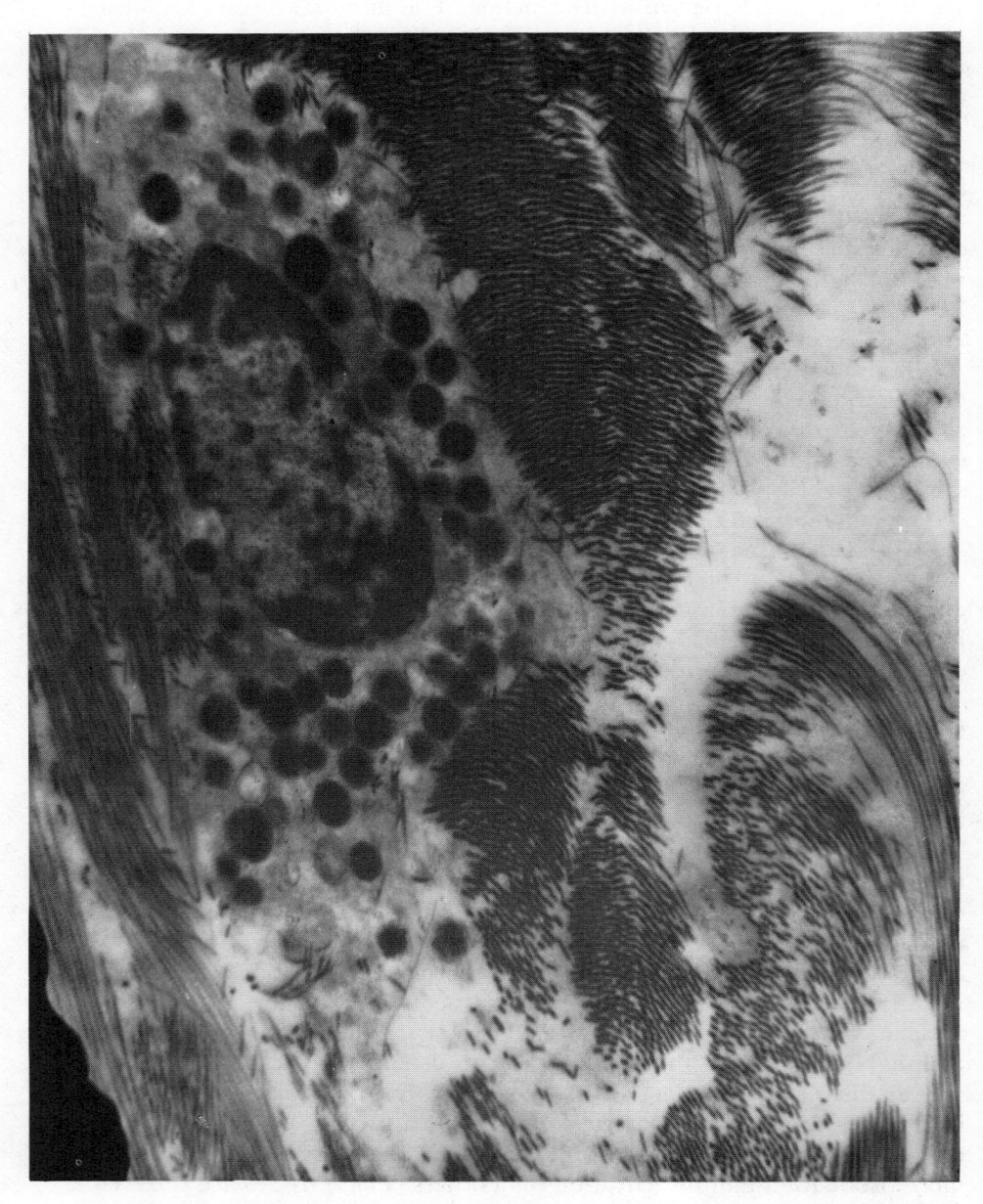

FIGURE 9.2. Electron micrograph of human mast cell from breast tissue with connective tissue collagen fibers surrounding it. [*Courtesy of David Hill.*]

indicating the systemic (referring to many parts of the body) contraction of smooth muscles. Anaphylactic shock in humans is more like that of the guinea pig than the dog or rabbit because the major shock tissues are in the lung and upper respiratory passages.

Chemical Mediators. Epinephrine (adrenaline) and other **adrenergic drugs** (those that mimic the actions of the sympathetic nervous system) help alleviate anaphylactic shock and milder allergies by dilating bronchiolar smooth muscle. The terms **sympathomimetic drug** and **catecholamine** are used synonymously with adrenergic drug. Antihistamine drugs such as chlorpheniramine, tripelennamine, diphenhydramine, etc., also help if given before an attack of allergy. The antihistamines compete with histamine for receptor sites on nerve endings. They neither combine with histamine nor prevent its release from mast cells. Consequently, antihistamines are relatively ineffective in the treatment of allergies once mast cells have been triggered to release histamine. In humans, antihistamines are generally better antagonists of edema and pruritus (itching) than in preventing bronchoconstriction. Sedation may be an undesirable side effect of many antihistamines. Theophylline is a drug that blocks the phosphodiesterase enzyme that hydrolyzes cyclical AMP to AMP, thereby contributing to elevated intracellular levels of cyclical AMP and prevention of histamine release from mast cells. Methyl xanthines such as theophylline, theobromine, and caffeine also are smooth muscle relaxants and useful as bronchodilators. Their diuretic qualities produce undesirable side effects.

Several chemical mediators of immediate-type hypersensitivities other than histamine are known. **Serotonin** (5-hydroxytryptamine) appears to be the most important mediator of anaphylactic shock in rodents. Tissues of the brain and gastrointestinal tract of most mammals are rich in serotonin, but it is not present in human mast cells. Its pharmacological effects are similar to those of histamine. Lysergic acid derivatives inhibit constriction of smooth muscles by serotonin but are seldom used because of their hallucinogenic side effects.

Bradykinin (*brady*=slow; *kinin*=to move) is a short peptide of nine amino acids that causes slow contraction of smooth muscles. It is a potent vasodilator and increases capillary permeability. Kinins are not produced by mast cells. Rather, their synthesis begins with activation of Hageman factor (factor XII) of the plasma coagulation system, followed by activation of four proenzymes to their functional counterparts. This synthetic pathway can be initiated *in vivo* by antigen-antibody complexes, or nonserologically *in vitro* by a variety of substances, including soft glass, carbon particles, colloidal silica, etc.

A substance called SRS-A **(slow-reacting substance of anaphylaxis)** causes prolonged contraction of certain smooth muscles and increased vascular permeability. Its chemical nature remained a mystery until 1979 when it was discovered to belong to a new class of prostaglandins called leukotrienes. Originally discovered in and named for the prostate gland, prostaglandins are found in many tissues. They typically are fatty acid compounds of about twenty carbon atoms. Because this new class of prostaglandins was originally found in leukocytes, it was named leukotriene. The "triene" portion of the name is indicative of the presence of three double bonds. The triene nature of these molecules produces a characteristic fluorescence in ultraviolet light that distinguishes them from other prostaglandins. SRS-A is now known as leukotriene C. Antigen-antibody reactions on cells probably cause a release of arachidonic acid that becomes enzymatically converted to leukotrienes. If this is true, it may be possible to develop new drugs to inhibit these enzymes and thereby reduce the contributions that SRS-A makes to allergic reactions. Presently, release of SRS-A and histamine from mast cells may be prevented by inhalation treatment with cromolyn sodium (disodium cromoglycate). This drug apparently has no effect on the cyclical 3,5-AMP system; so the way it prevents degranulation of mast cells is different from that of theophylline.

Complement can be activated by antigen-antibody complexes involving either IgG or IgM; it cannot be activated by IgE. Complement fractions C3a and C5a are anaphylatoxins. An **anaphylatoxin** is any substance that can cause histamine release from mast cells and basophils. Atopic allergies usually cannot be passively transmitted from a mother to her baby because IgE molecules do not cross the placenta. Antibodies of class IgG do cross the placenta and may contribute to "allergic" reactions via production of complement anaphylatoxins. The complement system can also be activated nonimmunologically through the alternate pathway. "Allergies" mediated by either the classical pathway or the alternate pathway of complement activation are of relatively minor importance compared to those allergies mediated by IgE antibodies. Much larger concentrations of complement-activating antibodies are required to affect release of active amines from mast cells.

A low-molecular-weight peptide called **eosinophilic chemotactic factor of anaphylaxis** (ECF-A) is present in mast cell granules. As the name implies, this factor is probably responsible for the accumulation of eosinophils in tissues experiencing allergic reactions. The role of eosinophils in the inflammatory allergic reaction is not well known.

Once a mast cell has degranulated, its supply of histamine and other mediators of allergy is depleted. It may require several days to replenish the cytoplasm with histamine-filled granules. For a short period of time following an allergic attack to an antigen (A), the patient may be refractory (**anergic**) to challenge with the same antigen. However, some cells that by chance were not complexed with IgE specific for antigen A may be complexed with IgE specific for a different antigen (B). If the patient is challenged with antigen B, those cells would be expected to degranulate and initiate another allergic episode. A given allergic reaction eventually subsides as histamine is inactivated by enzymatic conversion to either methyl histamine or imidazolacetic acid. Likewise, serotonin is eventually converted to 5-hydroxyindole acetic acid by monoamine oxidase. Other mediators of immediate hypersensitivities are probably enzymatically destroyed in a similar manner.

An **anaphylactoid reaction** mimics anaphylactic shock but is not an immunological phenomenon. Most of the substances that induce anaphylactoid reactions are not antigenic and do not behave as autocoupling haptens. Intravascular administration of india ink, acetic acid, starch, agar, organic iodine, bromphenol blue, gum tragacanth, etc., in sufficient dosage can induce anaphylactoid reactions at first encounter. These substances may directly activate basophils, mast cells, and the kinin system of the blood, causing the release of histamine, kinins, serotonin, and other pharmacological mediators of anaphylactic-type reactions. Since the complement system can be nonimmunologically activated by the alternate pathway, this may also provide a mechanism for some anaphylactoid reactions.

Desensitization. Attempts to "desensitize" an allergic individual are only sporadically effective. The term "desensitization" is actually a misnomer because once an individual has encountered an antigen and become sensitized, there is no known way to erase immunological memory. In one method of desensitization, the patient is first given antihistamines. Then a small dose of antigen is injected, resulting in a small amount of histamine release that soon is metabolized to an inert product. A second, slightly larger dose is given, and after any signs of histamine shock have subsided, the process is repeated with increasing dosage until the patient can tolerate therapeutic doses of the injectable antigen without experiencing allergic reactions. The entire process is completed within several hours. This method probably gradually degranulates susceptible mast cells and neutralizes IgE antibodies specific for the antigen (i.e., all paratopes on this species of IgE are complexed with antigen). All desensitizations are only temporary. After about a week, new (unneutralized) specific IgE has been made, degranulated mast cells have recovered, and so the patient is ready to participate in another allergic episode if cognate antigen becomes available.

Lymphocytes programmed to make IgE, unlike those that make IgG or other classes of immunoglobulins, are comparatively rare in the spleen and most lymph nodes. They are much more frequently found in tonsillar tissue, Peyer's patches, and other locations near the gastrointestinal and mucosal surfaces. Therefore, when antigens enter the body across a mucous membrane, they tend to stimulate high serum levels of IgE. Antigenization via muscular, subcutaneous, or intravenous routes is more likely to stimulate classes of immunoglobulins other than IgE. These other noncytotropic antibodies may function as blocking antibodies, combining with the allergen and thereby preventing its further reaction with cell-bound IgE. This forms the immunological rationale for a second method of desensitization involving gradually increasing booster doses of antigen over several weeks (rather than hours) via a route other than transmucosal. Hyperimmunization in this fashion is likely to produce some cytotropic IgE as well as noncytotropic, blocking antibodies of other classes (e.g., IgG). If a high concentration of these blocking antibodies can be developed, the offending antigen should have a statistically better chance of combining with free, circulating blocking antibody than with cell-bound IgE and thereby the antigen is prevented from triggering an allergic reaction. Desensitization by this technique may be extended over an entire pollen season by administration of antigen-adjuvant mixtures that continuously release small amounts of boosting antigen to maintain high levels of blocking antibody. Desensitization techniques are not always successful and are highly variable in the duration of their effective time limits.

Attempts are currently being made to synthesize a portion of the Fc region of IgE molecules that bind to mast cells. If successful in this regard, the synthetic IgE fragments could be administered to allergic patients as blocking agents. These fragments would compete with endogenous IgE for receptor sites on mast cells and thereby nonspecifically diminish or abolish many kinds of atopic reactions.

Desensitization is much more clearly related to circulating levels of IgG blocking antibody for bee venom than for hay fever or asthma. This is because the sting introduces the antigen at a site from whence it should rapidly enter the bloodstream and be neutralized by blocking antibody. In contrast, when allergen enters the nasal and lung tissues, they are nearer the source of IgE antibodies and less likely to be blocked by IgG antibodies.

Allergy Tests. Skin tests for allergies are highly sensitive, qualitative, *in vivo* assays. The P-K test is a passive skin test in that the reaction occurs in an individual other than the one who made the allergin. **Passive cutaneous anaphylaxis** is another skin test involving IgE antibodies. Serum from a sensitized person or animal is injected intradermally into another member of the same species. A latent period is allowed for fixation of the antibodies to mast cells and for diffusion of non-cell-fixed antibodies away from the injection site. Homologous challenging antigen is then mixed with a dye such as Evans blue and injected intravenously at some other convenient site. The union of cell-fixed antibody with antigen causes histamine release, resulting in increased local capillary permeability. Plasma containing the dye leaks out of the vessels at that point, resulting in a blue spot on the skin (most easily seen in an animal by sacrificing it and examining the inner surface of the skin). The size of the spot indicates the severity of the immune reaction. Very little IgE is required. PCA can be prevented by prior administration of antihistamine drugs because histamine release is involved. Complement is not required. The P-K test differs from the PCA test in that both antibody and antigen are injected intradermally at the same site in the P-K test.

Skin tests for active immunity are much more commonly used than those for passive immunity to detect sensitivities to specific allergens. A physician specializing in allergic diseases is called an **allergist.** An atopic test for a specific allergen is performed by introducing an aqueous suspension of the antigen into a scratch or prick (puncture) in the skin or by injecting the antigen intradermally (intracutaneously). Scratch or prick testing is much less sensitive than intradermal testing. Within minutes a so-called "triple response" is usually seen in the sensitive patient. Two of the three components of the "triple response" are wheal and flare. A **wheal** is an acute, circumscribed, transitory area of edema of the skin as seen in **urticaria** (hives). **Flare** or **erythema** is a reddening of the skin due to capillary engorgement. The third component of the "triple response" appears to be a redundancy. Some authorities say that erythema is caused by local dilation of capillaries due to smooth muscle contraction in postcapillary venules, whereas a flare or flush results from arteriolar dilatation produced by a local nerve reflex. Other authorities make a distinction between localized wheals and more extensive edema.

Multiple skin tests for different allergens can be made simultaneously on the arm or back of an individual. If an individual shows a positive skin test to one or more of the battery of antigens used, the most expedient treatment is simply to avoid the offending allergen(s) if possible. For example, if a patient has positive skin tests for fish extract and dog danders, he could give up eating fish and try to keep dogs out of his immediate environment. If the patient is allergic to a particular pollen widespread in his environment, it may necessitate his moving to a location where the plant does not grow. Many people move to desert regions because species diversity of plants is much more restricted there. If the allergen cannot be avoided, perhaps allergic attacks can be avoided or controlled through judicious timing of the use of antihistamines and/or desensitization techniques.

The **basophil degranulation test** is an alternative to skin testing. It is an *in vitro* counterpart of a P-K test. The *in vivo* P-K test involves **homocytotropic antibody,** i.e., antibody from an individual of the same species as the one providing the mast cells. In the *in vitro* test, the serum is of human origin and the mast cells are of animal origin; hence the antibodies are **heterocytotropic.** Rabbit or rat basophils are incubated with the patient's serum and the suspected allergen. If the patient is sensitive to the allergen, his IgE will attach to the mast cells, combine with the allergen, and trigger degranulation of the mast cells. This degranulation can be observed under the microscope. Positive and negative controls should also be run for each allergen tested.

Opthalmic testing for allergies is performed by placing a drop of the suspected allergen on the conjunctiva. A rapid reddening of the vascular bed in the white of the eye and inner lining of the eyelids constitutes a positive test. It is about as sensitive as intradermal testing, but it is less likely to elicit systemic anaphylactic reactions. Since most people have only two eyes, only two allergens can be tested at the same time.

Anaphylactic Reactions. Severe systemic forms of antibody-mediated allergies are called anaphylactic reactions and can be lethal. They typically result from injection of allergens, whereas the milder atopic diseases generally result from allergens that enter the body through mucous membranes of the respiratory or GI tract. Natural injections such as bee stings may be merely painful to nonsensitive people, but to those who are exquisitely sensitive the allergic response may lead to fatal shock. One of the most common forms of iatrogenic allergy is hypersensitivity to penicillin. Hundreds of people die each year from acute systemic anaphylactic shock to injections of this antibiotic drug. Penicillin itself is not antigenic. In the body, it is degraded to several products that can spontaneously form covalent bonds with proteins of the patient. It is these **autocoupling haptens** that are the anaphylactinogens. Penicilloic acid derivatives complexed to proteins are the most potent of these new antigens (**neoantigens**). Among those who are allergic to penicillin, some are much more sensitive than others; this is a reflection of their ability to respond to smaller doses of the drug rather than a function of the rate of hapten-protein conjugate formation.

Skin tests can be used to determine if an individual is hypersensitive to penicillin. Those found to be allergic by skin test or those with previous histories of reactivity could then be treated with antibiotics other than penicillin. The use of haptenic metabolites of penicillin for skin tests is undesirable for several reasons. These haptens may induce hypersensitivity in an unsensitized individual or they may cause shock rather than a mild skin reaction in a highly sensitive person. Unless the hapten becomes coupled to a protein carrier, it is usually a poor detector of sensitivity. Free hapten may complex with antibody, blocking the union of antibody with hapten-protein conjugates formed within the patient, and thereby produce a false negative skin test. Most of these problems can be alleviated by using hapten-protein conjugates for skin testing. This technique would not depend on *in vivo* conjugate formation, a phenomenon that varies considerably from one individual to another. However, it is possible to become sensitized to the protein carrier of the conjugate. Obviously, proteins commonly encountered such as egg albumin or milk casein should not be used as carriers. A synthetic protein carrier called poly-D-lysine can be used as a hapten carrier without inducing sensitivity. Furthermore, it is a very sensitive detector of penicillin hypersensitivity.

Experimentally, systemic anaphylaxis can be dramatically illustrated by sensitizing a guinea pig with an intraperitoneal injection of a small dose of foreign protein such as egg albumin. After about two weeks, cytotropic antibodies have developed and become attached to mast cells. A large challenging dose of the same antigen is then given intravenously so that it becomes rapidly distributed to all parts of the body. A systemic reaction involving contraction of many smooth muscles throughout the body usually begins with fifteen seconds to a minute. An early sign of the shock reaction is the elevation of neck hair in response to contraction of the arrectores pilorum muscles connected to the hair follicles. Scratching of the nose and coughing or sneezing are signs of respiratory distress. Voiding of urine and feces is commonly observed. Breathing becomes extremely labored and the animal soon collapses and may die within five minutes after administration of the shocking dose. Upon autopsy, the lungs are found to be swollen with air trapped by the constriction of smooth muscles of the bronchioles. Apparently the animal has a more powerful mechanism for inspiration than expiration. If antihistamines are given to a sensitive guinea pig thirty minutes to an hour before injection of the challenging dose of antigen, anaphylactic shock can be prevented or diminished. The waiting period is required to allow the antihistamine drug to circulate and become attached to and block histamine receptors on smooth muscles throughout the body. Intracardial injection of pure histamine to a guinea pig usually results in a violent systemic reaction that mimics an immunologically induced systemic anaphylaxis. These observations led to the early conclusion that histamine or histamine-like substances were pharmacological mediators of anaphylactic hypersensitivities.

An *in vitro* correlate of an *in vivo* anaphylactic reaction is the **Schultz-Dale test.** W. H. Schultz and H. H. Dale demonstrated that a segment of ileum from the small intestine of a sensitized guinea pig could be induced to contract when isolated *in vitro* and exposed to the homologous antigen. The tissue is washed free of contaminants and mounted in a smooth muscle water bath (37°C) containing a highly nutritive Tyrode solution through which oxygen is bubbled. One end of the muscle is attached to the bottom of the reaction vessel and the other to a transducer connected to a physiograph. After a base line of normal peristaltic movement is recorded, a heterologous antigen (one to which the guinea pig had not been sensitized) can be added to the vessel as a control. No response should be observed. Then the homologous antigen is added and within ten to fifteen seconds the muscle exhibits a tetanic contraction as antigen unites with cell-bound IgE and degranulates mast cells (Figure 9.3). The Schultz-Dale reaction serves as a model to vividly illustrate some of the typical symptoms of milder food allergies: cramping, nausea, diarrhea, and gaseous distention of the intestines. Inflammatory, crusting skin reactions called **eczema** with itching wheals called **urticaria** (hives) are also commonly seen in food allergies. Respiratory problems may also arise as part of a systemic allergic response to certain foods. Among the most common of food allergens are fish, milk,

*Immuno-
pathology*

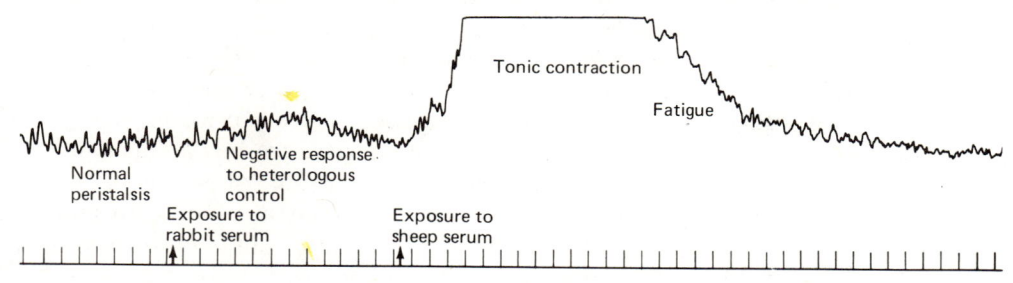

FIGURE 9.3. Physiograph tracing of a Schultz-Dale test using ileum of a guinea pig sensitized to sheep serum. The tissue was first exposed to rabbit serum as a heterologous control. Within less than ten seconds after challenge with homologous sheep serum, the tissue began to contract. The plateau on the contraction curve is an artifact of limitation of movement afforded the recording stylus.

eggs, strawberries, chocolate, nuts, citrus fruits, cereals, tomatoes, and wheat products.

TYPE III HYPERSENSITIVITIES (IMMUNE COMPLEX DISEASES)

Arthus Reaction. The prototype reaction of type III hypersensitivities is the **Arthus reaction.** In 1903, Maurice Arthus induced a localized inflammatory skin reaction in a previously sensitized rabbit by intradermal injection of cognate antigen. The reaction is easily seen if the hair is shaved from the site (Figure 9.4). A small bleb of injected material is immediately created

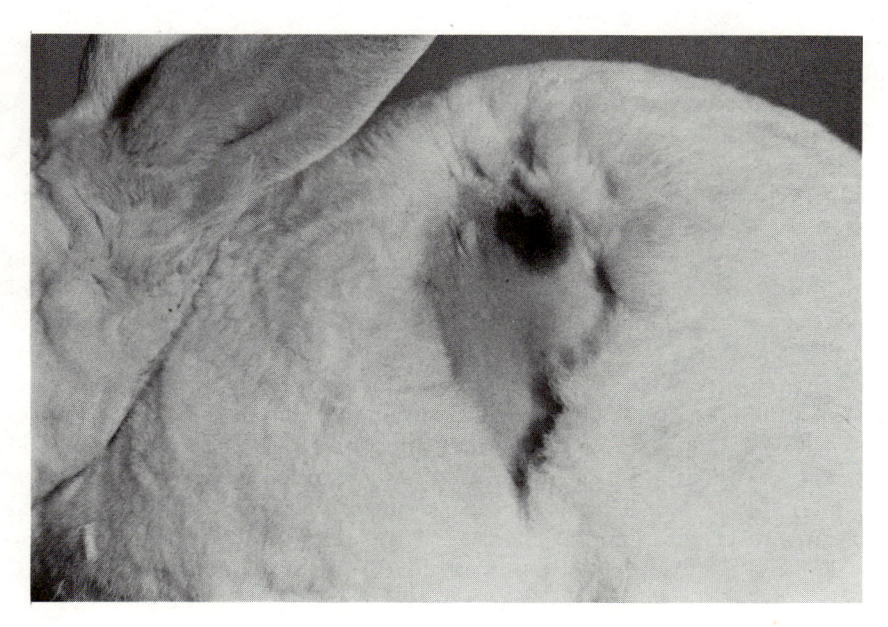

FIGURE 9.4. Arthus reaction after twenty-four hours on rabbit actively sensitized to horse serum. An intradermal challenge injection of horse serum was made at the top of the shaved area. Below it was a control injection of physiological saline (no skin reaction observed).

if the antigen is correctly administered intradermally. Several hours elapse before inflammation becomes visible at a gross level. This is longer than a typical immediate hypersensitivity but shorter than a typical delayed hypersensitivity. Nonetheless, it is classified as an immediate hypersensitivity reaction because the responsible antibodies can be passively transferred by serum. Antigen-antibody complexes form and adhere to the vascular endothelium. The complement system is activated, and some of its chemotactic (leukotactic, leucotactic) intermediates (C3a, C5a) attract neutrophils to the site as part of the inflammatory response. These same complement components are also anaphylatoxins that degranulate mast cells. Histamine release causes constriction of arterioles and retards the blood supply to that area. Platelets are stimulated by the immune complex to initiate the coagulation cascade, resulting in fibrin deposits. Eventually the vessels become plugged with thrombi and accumulated cells, causing an exudation of fluid into the surrounding tissues (edema). The tissues served by these vessels become deprived of a blood supply resulting in ischemic necrosis. Only precipitating (multivalent) antibodies can elicit the Arthus reaction (mainly IgG). Furthermore, relatively large amounts of antigen are also required. From these two facts it may be inferred that intravascular precipitates are the immune complexes that trigger the Arthus phenomenon.

In the **reversed passive Arthus** (RPA) reaction, antibody from a sensitized animal is injected intradermally and antigen is injected intravenously. No latent period is required because Arthus reactions are largely mediated by noncytotropic IgG-antigen complexes. In contrast to IgE-mediated local reactions such as the P-K test and passive cutaneous anaphylaxis, relatively large amounts of IgG antibodies are required for the Arthus reaction. Complement is involved in Arthus hypersensitivities but not in IgE-mediated hypersensitivities. Antihistamines are not effective in preventing Arthus reactions because they are primarily caused by intravascular precipitates and thrombi rather than by degranulation of mast cells. A comparison of RPA, PCA, Arthus, and P-K tests is summarized in Table 9.3.

The classical Arthus reaction is artificially induced. It has a natural counterpart in a group of human lung hypersensitivity diseases variously called immune complex pneumonitis, allergic pneumonitis, or hypersensitivity pneumonitis. These diseases are commonly associated with particular occupations from whence come names such as farmer's lung, pigeon breeder's lung, mushroom worker's lung, malt worker's lung, etc. All of these occupations are in dusty environments laden with either fungal spores or animal danders and excretory products. Inhalation of these antigens stimulates both IgG and IgE antibodies. Once sensitized, a person contacting these antigens typically displays a biphasic response. The earliest response is by IgE already affixed to mast cells. Sneezing, nasal discharge, and respiratory distress are common atopic symptoms. Several hours later, IgG-mediated symptoms begin to appear including a dry cough, shortness of breath, fever, and general malaise. If the individual is isolated from the occupational environment, these symptoms will disappear in a few days. Reexposure to the antigens triggers another attack. Histological examination of the lungs of patients suffering allergic pneumonitis reveals the same kinds of lesions that characterize an Arthus skin reaction: accumulations of IgG precipitates, neutrophils, platelets, and fibrin in the capillaries. Antihistamines may relieve the early symptoms but cannot prevent the later IgG-mediated symptoms that are the most distinguishing features of immune complex pneumonitis.

Serum Sickness. Patients receiving large doses of foreign serums (e.g., horse antitoxins against tetanus or antilymphocyte serum for immunosuppression of tissue transplants) commonly develop a disease called primary **serum sickness.** About a week or ten days following the initial exposure to a foreign serum, the patient develops malaise, fever, nausea, vomiting, edema, lymphadenopathy, muscle and joint pain, and hives. This single massive dose of foreign antigen serves both to stimulate the production of antibodies and later on also serves as the challenging dose. The reason for this is that all of the antigen has not been removed (degraded, cleared) from the body by the time antibodies begin to appear in the circulation. Immune complexes begin to form between these antibodies (primarily of class IgG) and the residual antigen. These complexes become deposited in various locations throughout the body including the joints, kidneys, and blood vessel walls (Figure 9.5). An immune complex nephritis is a common symptom of serum sickness. Leukotaxins generated by activation of the comple-

Table 9.3 DISTINGUISHING CHARACTERISTICS OF HYPERSENSITIVITY SKIN TESTS: REVERSED PASSIVE ARTHUS (RPA), PASSIVE CUTANEOUS ANAPHYLAXIS (PCA), ARTHUS REACTION, AND PRAUSNITZ-KÜSTNER (P-K) TEST

Characteristic	RPA	PCA	Arthus	P-K
Type of immunity	Passive	Passive	Active	Passive
Relative quantity of antibody required in the injection	Large	Small	—	Small
Cytotropic antibody required	No	Yes	No	Yes
Class of antibodies involved	IgG, IgM	IgE	IgG, IgM	IgE
Latent period (after serum transfer) required before antigen challenge	No	Yes	—	Yes
Complement participation	Yes	No	Yes	No
Histamine release	No	Yes	No	Yes
Reaction inhibited by antihistamines	No	Yes	No	Yes
Method of induction	Inject antibody into skin; challenge immediately with antigen intravenously	Inject antibody into skin; wait 24 hours; challenge intravenously with antigen (dye optional)	Sensitization by any of several routes (IM, IV, etc.); active sensitization develops over several weeks; challenge with antigen intradermally	Inject antibody into skin; wait 24 hours; challenge with antigen in the same site

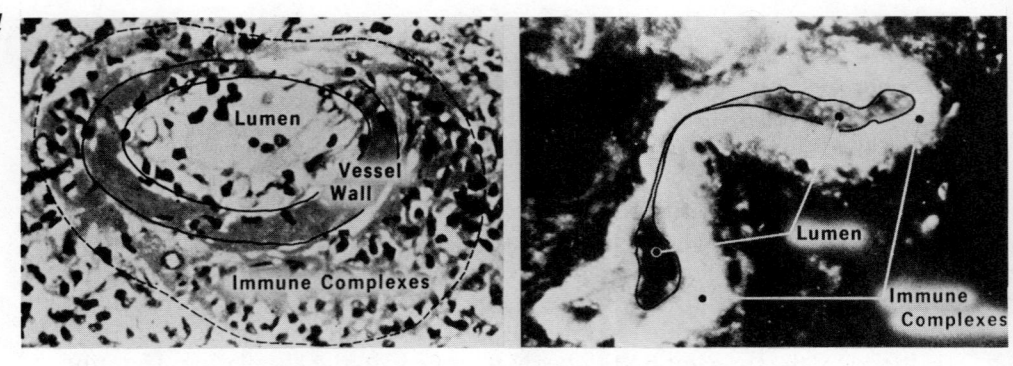

FIGURE 9.5. Histological characteristics of patients with generalized serum sickness-type reactions. Left: Hematoxylin-and-eosin-stained section displaying hyaline, amorphous material within the outer broken circle. This material contains immune complexes and is also present in the wall of the arteriole and in the perivascular connective tissue. The numerous nuclei in the surrounding tissue (as well as in the lumen of the arteriole) are mainly those of inflammatory cells. Right: Fluorescent micrograph of a similar vessel, stained with an antibody to human gammaglobulin. The vessel is partly collapsed. Note the immune complexes in the vessel wall. [From Hill, R. B., et al., 1973. Basic pathology series; immune complexes and disease (S-2951). National Audiovisual Center (GSA), Washington, D.C.]

ment system attract neutrophils and eosinophils toward the immune complexes. Some components of the complement cascade are anaphylatoxins that degranulate mast cells and release histamine, kinins, ECF-A, etc. Neutrophils release lysosomal enzymes that contribute to the local inflammation. Each antibody, after release from a plasma cell, is free to complex with antigen and complement, thereby making a small contribution to the disease. In this way, a sudden release of massive quantities of pharmacological mediators is avoided. Serum sickness is therefore a more chronic and less lethal disease than IgE-mediated anaphylaxis. IgE antibodies are probably also involved in serum sickness, but their role is a comparatively minor one.

Once a person has been sensitized to a foreign serum, a second contact with the same antigens may provoke an accelerated serum sickness reaction with symptoms appearing within two to five days. This is merely another example of the shorter latent period in an anamnestic (secondary) immunoglobulin response. Serum sickness is a systemic disease whereas the Arthus reaction is a localized disease, this difference being due to the route of antigenic challenge. They are both immune-complex (type III) diseases.

TYPE IV (DELAYED) HYPERSENSITIVITIES

In contrast to the immediate hypersensitivities that appear within minutes, delayed hypersensitivities usually require twenty-four to seventy-two hours to reach maximal reactivity. Despite the fact that serum sickness only develops several days after antigenic challenge, it is still classified as an immediate-type hypersensitivity because it can be passively transferred by serum and is therefore antibody-mediated. Delayed hypersensitivities do not depend on antibodies, but rather on T lymphocytes and their products. Type IV hypersensitivities can be passively transferred only via sensitized T cells. As summarized in Table 9.1, delayed hypersensitivities exhibit more generalized tissue involvement than just the smooth muscles affected in immediate hypersensitivities. Therefore, antihistamines and smooth muscle relaxants offer little relief from delayed hypersensitivities. Steroids and other anti-inflammatory substances are the main agents that have been found to combat T cell hypersensitivities, but even these are not always effective in this respect. Desensitization to delayed hypersensitivities is much more difficult than for antibody-mediated allergies and no clear immunological rationale exists for T cell desensitization.

Tuberculin Reaction. The tuberculin skin test is the prototype reaction for delayed (T cell-mediated) hypersensitivities. Formerly **old tuberculin** (OT) was used as the challenge antigen. Old tuberculin is produced by growing *Mycobacterium tuberculosis* in a special broth, concentrating it on a steam bath, and removing the mycobacteria by filtration. The filtrate is OT. A small protein called **purified protein derivative** (PPD), obtained by trichloroacetic acid precipitation from OT, is more stable when dried and is now more popular for skin testing than OT. The test antigen can be rubbed into scarified skin (von Pirquet technique) or into multiple punctures (tine test), injected intradermally (Mantoux test), or impregnated on paper and taped to the skin (Vollmer patch test). A positive reaction of erythema and induration (hardening) of the skin gradually develops, peaking after about forty-eight to seventy-two hours, and then subsiding. Edema and/or necrosis are rarely seen. This is a classical delayed hypersensitivity reaction mediated by T cells, indicating that the patient has previously contacted the antigen and has become sensitized. A positive test does not necessarily indicate that an active infection is in progress because delayed hypersensitivities, once attained, generally persist throughout life.

Similar skin tests are used to detect present or past infection with other pathogenic organisms. Coccidioidin is the antigen used in an intradermal skin test for coccidioidomycosis, a fungal granulomatous disease of the upper respiratory tract caused by *Coccidioides immitis*. Antibodies are also produced by contact with these pathogens but are not involved in the delayed hypersensitivity reaction. *In vitro* tests based on these antibodies may sometimes be used in place of or in conjunction with skin tests. For example, latex particles sensitized with coccidioidin are used as the indicator in a latex agglutination test for these antibodies.

An intradermal injection of histoplasmin is used to test for sensitivity to the fungus *Histoplasma capsulatum,* the causative organism of histoplasmosis. Histoplasmin is a crude culture filtrate of the fungus. Histoplasmosis is primarily a common benign infection of the pulmonary tract. Infections with fungi causing cryptococcosis and blastomycosis generate antibodies that cross-react with histoplasmin so that *in vitro* tests for histoplasmosis lack specificity. Skin testing with histoplasmin prior to serological testing elevates the titer of complement-fixing antibodies, making the complement fixation test unpredictable. A positive immunodiffusion test with histoplasmin and the patient's serum consists of several precipitin bands, only one of which is not influenced by previous skin testing.

Extracts of many other pathogenic organisms are available for skin tests of delayed hypersensitivities including lepromin for leprosy, brucellergen for infections with bacteria of the genus *Brucella,* and lygranum for the venereal disease lymphogranuloma venereum (Frei test). The delayed hypersensitivities to these and many other organisms were formerly referred to as **allergy of infection.** However, not all allergies to infectious organisms are of the delayed type, but it is so common that the two terms are often used interchangeably. For example, a combination of immediate and delayed hypersensitivity reactions can be seen in the skin test for the parasitic disease trichinosis. Extracts of the dried larvae are injected intradermally. An antibody-mediated immediate wheal-and-flare reaction reaches its maximum in ten to twenty minutes. After about twenty-four hours a cell-mediated delayed hypersensitivity reaction develops consisting of a red raised area with central blanching as seen in a positive tuberculin test. The Casoni skin test for *Echinococcus granulosus* uses sterile hydatid fluid from hydatid cysts of sheep, pigs, cattle, or humans as the antigen. A rapid wheal-and-flare response indicates prior contact with the parasite. A delayed response may also develop later, but the immediate reaction is the one of primary diagnostic importance in this case.

Contact Dermatitis. Many industrial chemicals and low-molecular-weight natural compounds can induce a delayed hypersensitive reaction on contact with skin. These substances behave as autocoupling haptens, forming neoantigens when complexed with proteins of the skin. Perhaps the best known of this group is **urushiol,** a group of four catechols found in the sap of the poison ivy plant (*Rhus radicans*). These catechols are easily oxidized to quinones, which, when autocoupled to proteins, become the sensitizing antigens. Catechols are also involved in delayed skin reactions to poison oak (*Rhus diversiloba*) and poison sumac (*Rhus toxicodendron*). A contact dermatitis is characterized by papular and vesicular lesions with later oozing, crusting, and desquamation over a period of a week to ten days. Pruritus (itching) is an almost universal symptom. In some cases, the lesions seem to gradually spread over the body, contributing to the erroneous idea that poison ivy is a contagious disease. What actually happens is that those exposed areas of the skin that received the larger doses of antigen break out first, and those with lighter doses develop lesions somewhat later. Unless urushiol is immediately removed by thorough washing with Fels naphtha soap, it can be disseminated more widely over the skin, even to previously unexposed areas, by the rubbing action of clothing or by the hands. One need not contact the plant directly in order to develop hypersensitivity. It can be acquired by touching urushiol on clothing or by contacting aerosols containing volatile oils released into the air when the shrub is burned.

Contact dermatitis often appears to be associated with certain occupations. Poison oak is more likely to be contacted by forestry workers, farmers, telephone linemen, and others in field-type occupations or by those whose avocation is hiking, camping, mountain climbing, etc. Workers in chemical plants are prone to develop "allergies" to specific chemicals, including dyes, insecticides, formaldehyde, and metals. Some people are allergic to the metals in jewelry, coins, watches, and watchbands. Certain women are allergic to specific chemicals in cosmetics, hair dyes, perfumes, lotions, hairsprays, depilatories, etc. The topical (local) application of penicillin and other drugs to the skin or mucous membranes may also provoke a delayed-type contact dermatitis. In all of these cases, the best prophylaxis is avoidance of the allergen. Perhaps this may require changing jobs, but in other cases it may involve simply wearing gloves to prevent the skin from contacting the allergen. Steroids and other anti-inflammatory therapeutic treatments for suppressing T cell activities have too many undesirable side effects to be used over long periods of time.

The rejection of tissue and organ grafts may also be considered a delayed hypersensitivity (type IV reaction) mediated by T cells. The grafted tissue serves as both the sensitizing dose and the shocking dose of antigen because the antigen is not cleared from the system by the time the primary immune response produces the effector agents. In this sense, transplant rejections may be considered to be the analog of serum sickness mediated by antibodies. Transplantation immunology is discussed in Chapter 10.

Lymphokines. Cell-mediated immunity and hypersensitivity reactions require that immunocompetent T cells contact cognate antigen and become activated (sensitized, primed) and mature into effector cells. In this process, certain genes become derepressed (become active in transcription of RNA and translation of RNA into protein), the cell **transforms** from a small lymphocyte into a large blast cell (Figure 9.6), mitosis is stimulated, and soluble effector molecules called **lymphokines** are released. Some of the distinguishing characteristics of lymphokines are listed in Table 9.4. Most lyphokines identified to date are low-molecular-weight polypeptides. They usually react with other host cells rather than with antigens. They are not generally present in lymphocytes prior to the cell's contact with antigen. The various lymphokines serve several major functions: (1) recruitment of uncommitted (unprimed) T cells, (2) retention of T cells and macrophages at the reaction site, (3) amplification of "recruited" T cells, (4) activation of the retained cells to effector status, and (5) cytotoxic effects against cells bearing foreign antigens (including foreign tissue grafts and cancer cells). Some lymphokines behave as chemotactic factors (CF) that attract and retain mononuclear cells (monocytes, macrophages, and lymphocytes) or neutrophils. For example, migration inhibition factor (MIF) serves to pre-

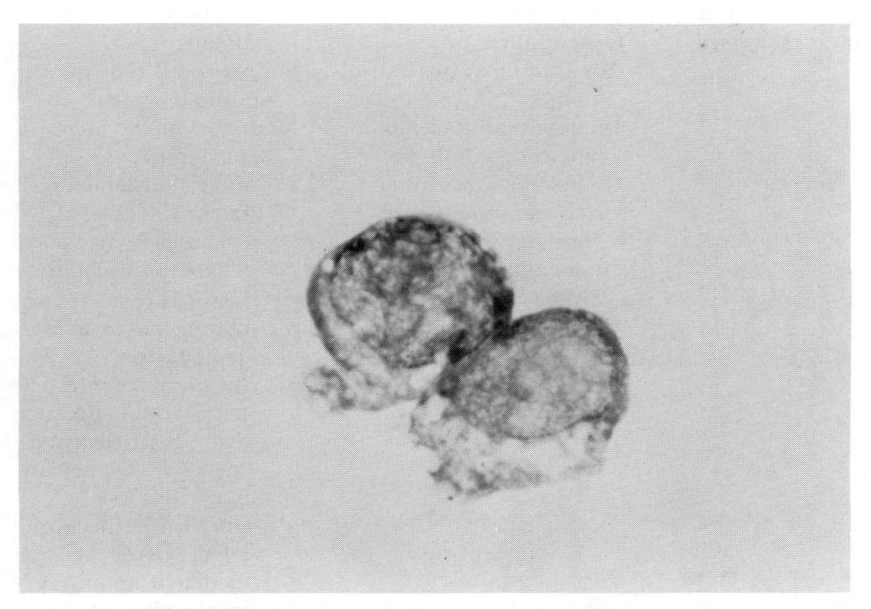

FIGURE 9.6. Blastic transformation of lymphocytes induced specifically by cognate antigen or nonspecifically by phytohemagglutinin. [*Courtesy of Elliot Scientific Corp., New York City.*]

Table 9.4 Distinguishing Characteristics of Antibodies and Lymphokines

Characteristics	Antibodies	Lymphokines
Cellular source	B lymphocytes	T lymphocytes (mainly)
Number of products per cell	Only a single class and specificity of Ig molecule is synthesized at a time by a given B cell	It is not known if one or several types of lymphokines may be produced simultaneously by a given T cell
Chemical nature:	Immunoglobulins; well known	Mainly relatively low-molecular-weight proteins; poorly known
Molecular weight	160,000–950,000 daltons	<60,000 daltons
Gross structure	Basic structure is a tetramer of two identical light chains and two identical heavy chains	They probably will be shown to have no common structural features and consist of single polypeptide chains rather than multiple chains
Serological classes	IgG, IgM, IgA, IgD, IgE	None
Relative concentration in serum	High: e.g., 800–1600 mg% in plasma for IgG	Very low: produced locally mainly in tissues where T cells encounter antigen
Biological half-life	2–3 days to 2–3 weeks	Unknown
Primary function	Specific binding of antigen	Regulates activities of host cells

Mechanisms by which the primary function is expressed	Agglutination
	Precipitation
	Opsonization
	Toxin or virus neutralization
	Immobilization of motile microorganisms
	Complement activation and immune lysis of foreign cells
	"Immediate" hypersensitivities
	"Humoral" immunity to pathogens
		Activates B cells (helper function to foreign antigens)
		Suppresses B cells (to self or autoantigens)
		Mediators of the inflammatory response
		  —migration inhibition factor (MIF)
		  —chemotactic factor
		  —leukocyte inhibitory factor (LIF)
		  —blastogenic or mitogenic factors
		Specific target cell destruction (by lymphotoxin)
		  —tissue graft rejection
		  —"delayed" hypersensitivity reactions
		  —elimination of virus-infected cells (cell-mediated immunity)
		  —immunological surveillance for neoplastic cells

vent macrophages from migrating away from the inflammatory site. Likewise, leukocyte inhibitory factor (LIF) retards the egress of polymorphonuclear leukocytes such as neutrophils. Blastogenic factors (BF) or mitogenic factors (MF) induce blast cell transformation of lymphocytes, a condition indicative of hyperactive metabolism (rapid synthesis of DNA, RNA, and protein). Lymphotoxin (LT) is a lymphokine causing destruction of target cells such as foreign tissue grafts and malignant cells. The action of LT on foreign cells rather than with host cells is an unusual property for a lymphokine.

A lymph node permeability factor (LNPF) can be extracted from guinea pig lymph nodes. It increases vascular permeability when injected into rat skin. Its chemical nature is unknown because it is unaffected by proteolytic enzymes, DNAse and RNAse. Furthermore, it is present in lymphocyte-poor tissues and it appears to be as abundant in normal lymphocytes as in those from animals with delayed hypersensitivities.

It may also be premature to classify transfer factor (TF) as a lymphokine. Delayed hypersensitivity to a specific antigen can be passively transferred by TF to an unsensitized person. TF is obtained by repeated freezing and thawing of lymphocytes from a sensitized donor. Sensitized lymphocytes incubated with cognate antigen secrete TF into the culture fluid. TF is sensitive to heat, but resistant to DNAase, RNAase, and trypsin. If transfer factor is double-stranded RNA, this would account for these peculiarities because these enzymes do not degrade double-stranded RNA molecules. Moreover, TF-induced delayed hypersensitivity may persist for as long as two years and therefore appears to have limited self-perpetuation properties. Since both delayed hypersensitivity and immunity to fungal, viral, and oncogenic diseases is mostly T cell–mediated, in theory TF should be capable of conferring passive immunity to specific diseases. Some degree of success has been reported in this regard, but much more study is needed.

INTERFERONS. Other chemicals produced by T lymphocytes are known to have well-defined physiological effects but perhaps should not be classified as lymphokines. Interferons, for example, are produced most actively by T cells, but many other cell types (spleen, liver, lung) also release interferons when invaded by viruses. Interferons (IF) have not been rigorously defined, but they are known to have nonspecific antiviral properties. They do not react directly with the virus particle, nor do they prevent attachment and penetration of virions to host cells. Rather, they somehow prevent the replication of viruses within infected cells. According to one theory, a virus enters a host cell and sheds its protein coat (capsid) thereby exposing its genetic material. It appears that the double-stranded RNA myxoviruses are the most potent natural inducers of interferons. The double-stranded RNA molecules attach to host repressor proteins that normally complex with the host operator gene for interferon. An allosteric transformation occurs in the repressor protein, rendering it unable to bind to host DNA. The interferon gene becomes derepressed, and very soon interferon RNA is transcribed and translated into interferon protein. Interferon proteins leave the infected cell and enter neighboring cells where they derepress a different operon, causing the production of a new protein referred to as **translation inhibitory protein** (TIP). TIP somehow inhibits the translation of viral mRNAs, but does not inhibit the translation of host mRNAs (Figure 9.7). This aspect of the theory requires an explanation. Another aspect of the

Serology and Immunology

theory requiring an explanation is the fact that many different substances can induce interferon production, including some bacteria, rickettsiae, malarial and other intracellular animal parasites, exotoxins and endotoxins, phytohemagglutinin, and synthetic polynucleotides.

Although TIP is produced by the originally infected cell, it usually appears too late to interrupt the production of progeny viruses in that same cell. A detectable titer of interferons can be found within a few hours after infection, and these interferons contribute to early (almost immediate) protection against many viral diseases until the immune response generates specifically activated T cells and antibodies several days later.

Recall from Chapter 1 that the beneficial aspects of the immune response sometimes cannot be achieved without concomitant detrimental hypersensitivity reactions. T lymphocytes are believed to be especially important to viral immunity against noncytolytic viruses that mature at cell membranes (rather than those that lyse the host cell). Sensitized lymphocytes interact with the sites of viral maturation on host cells and release cytotoxins that destroy virally infected cells. They also release chemotactic factors that recruit and activate phagocytes, making them more motile, "sticky," and phagocytic. These lymphocytes also generate more interferon that aids in limitation of the virus to previously infected cells.

Antibody-mediated viral immunity, on the other hand, is less likely to be

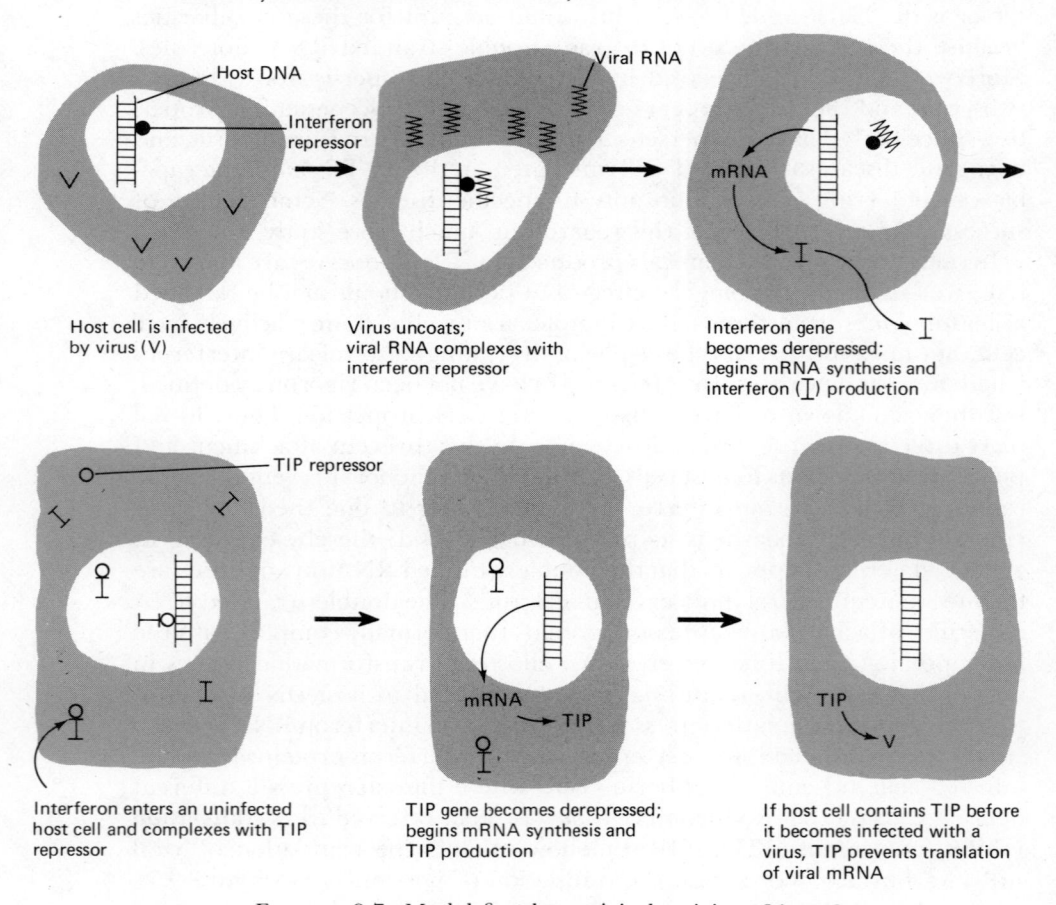

FIGURE 9.7. Model for the antiviral activity of interferon.

accompanied by undesirable hypersensitivity reactions. The mechanism whereby antibodies "neutralize" viruses is not well understood. Presumably antiviral antibodies combine at or near receptor sites on the capsid by which the virus would otherwise attach to and thereby gain entry into the host cell. Thus by steric hindrance or by allosteric transformation, antibodies may prevent viral infection of host cells. Immunoglobulin-mediated antiviral immunity is usually highly effective against viruses that spread through the body extracellularly (in tissue fluid, lymph, or blood). Intracellular viruses that spread from cell to cell without an extracellular phase (e.g., vaccinia, herpes simplex) are protected from antibodies outside the host cells. Recovery from established infection by these kinds of viruses depends on the activities of T lymphocytes (cell-mediated immunity or delayed hypersensitivity). Indeed, some of the more obvious clinical signs of certain viral diseases (such as the rash of measles) are probably due to a cell-mediated attack on virally infected skin cells.

The protective action of interferons is not viral-specific; interferons produced by infection with a specific virus can also prevent replication of a wide range of unrelated viruses or other intracellular parasites. Unless continually stimulated, however, host cells do not persist in the manufacture of interferons. Fortunately, about the time that the interferon titer is dropping, the titer of viral-neutralizing antibodies begins to rise, thus providing early and continuing protection. Although interferons are not viral-specific, they have some degree of host specificity. The protective activity of interferons of a given species of mammal is always greater within that same species than between different species. Thus, the best source of interferons for treatment of human viral diseases is from humans themselves. Interferons are proteins with considerable heterogeneity of size (monomeric forms may associate into polymeric forms) and are produced in very small quantities. These and other problems have made it difficult to obtain purified quantities of interferon at reasonable cost for therapeutic use. By genetic engineering techniques, it has recently been possible to incorporate genetic material coding for interferon into bacteria. By cloning these recombinant bacteria, it is hoped to make interferon production economically feasible.

Although no virus has yet been proven to cause human cancer, some tumors seem to be associated with infection by specific viruses. For example, women with genital disease caused by the herpes type II virus are more likely to develop cervical cancer than those who are free of this virus. Cancer researchers are eager to obtain sufficient quantities of IF to initiate large scale field trials of both its antiviral and potential antitumor properties. Recombination DNA techniques are also being applied in the production of thymosin alpha-1, a hormone that stimulates the human immune system. It has shown some promise in the treatment of brain and lung cancers.

A more recent theory of interferon activity proposes that interferon (acting like a hormone) binds to a specific receptor site on the host cell membrane and triggers the synthesis of at least two enzymes that mediate the antiviral effect. Perhaps these two enzymes correspond to the translation inhibitory protein (TIP) of the earlier theories. One of these enzymes is a protein kinase that transfers a phosphate group to a specific subunit of the initiation factor eIF-2. This initiation factor (along with at least one other protein) is required to stabilize the "initiation complex" (consisting of mRNA, the smaller subunit of the ribosome, and the initiator tRNA) whereby translation of mRNA into protein is started. The phosphorylated form of eIF-2 does not stabilize the initiation complex, so that translation of viral mRNA cannot begin. The protein kinase induced by interferon, however, is in an inactive form. It has been suggested that the single strand of viral mRNA loops back on itself to form double-stranded regions, and this form of mRNA serves as the activator of protein kinase. Following activation, the enzyme first phosphorylates itself (autophosphorylation) and then phosphorylates eIF-2.

The second enzyme induced by interferon is a synthetase that polymerizes adenine nucleotides into a chain called 2,5-oligoadenylic acid. This simple polymer activates a ribonuclease enzyme normally present in the cell. The activated ribonuclease selectively degrades the viral mRNA, but not the host cell mRNA. It is assumed that only the viral mRNA has the double-stranded regions that can activate protein kinase. Unless a mRNA is rapidly complexed to ribosomes (forming polysomes), it is subject to degradation by ribonuclease. Being uninhibited in forming stable initiation complexes, host cell mRNA usually becomes quickly covered with ribosomes "reading" the message from the 5' to the 3' end. The viral mRNA does not become complexed with ribosomes and hence is vulnerable to attack by ribonuclease.

This theory is bolstered by the fact that phosphorylation of eIF-2, triggered by a deficiency of hemin (a form of heme), is known to inhibit protein synthesis in bone marrow reticulocytes (immature red blood cells). This regulatory system functions to prevent the wasteful synthesis of globin protein when there is insufficient heme with which to combine to form hemoglobin.

"Killer" Cells. At least three types of cells (other than phagocytes) are known to have cytotoxic properties. Target cells may be destroyed by contact lysis (rather than by phagocytosis) involving target cell–bound antibodies and effector cells of the monocyte-macrophage lineage. This type of **antibody-dependent cell-mediated cytotoxicity** (ADCC) is independent of the complement system. In ADCC, the predominant effector cells, called **killer (K) cells,** are distinct from LT-producing cytotoxic killer T lymphocytes (T_c). Direct contact of the killer T cell with the target cell histocompatibility receptors (Chapter 10) is considered to be required for expression of cytotoxicity. K cells must also contact target cells, but K cells are known to react with the Fc portion of immunoglobulins attached to target cells. A minor role in ADCC may also be played by some "killer" B lymphocytes or by "natural killer" (NK) **null lymphocytes** (having neither beta nor theta antigens detectable on their surfaces). K cells are presumably triggered by attachment to the Fc portion of antibody-coated target cells and release of cytotoxic factors in a manner analogous to the release of LT lymphokines from T_c cells.

AUTOALLERGIC (AUTOIMMUNE) DISEASES

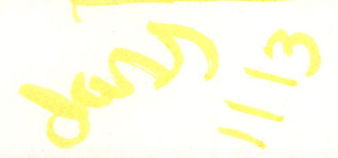

The word "immunity" implies a beneficial protective phenomenon; so the term "autoimmune disease" is a misnomer. Normally the body has an aversion to producing an immune response to its own (self) antigens. This is the essence of Paul Ehrlich's dictum "horror autotoxicus." For this reason, the term **autoallergic disease** is more accurately descriptive and therefore is the term of preference. How then can the body recognize self components (autoantigens) as foreign? One way is by release of self components that normally do not circulate. Such components are referred to as **hidden, occult, inaccessible,** or **sequestered antigens.** Antigens associated with thyroglobulin, proteins of the eye lens, milk casein in women, sperm of the male, etc., normally do not circulate and hence are not available to lymphoid tissues during that critical stage in development when self antigens are recognized as such. A second possible means of becoming sensitized to one's own antigens is by the production of neoantigens. Mutations in the genetic material may lead to the appearance of new antigenic determinants on cell membranes. Autocoupling haptens (previously discussed under the heading of contact dermatitis) or viruses may elicit a hypersensitive response directed partly against the host protein carrier antigens. Even physical agents such as light (visible or ultraviolet) and changes in temperature might be responsible for restructuring a self molecule to reveal new antigenic determinants. A third mechanism by which autoallergic disease may be triggered becomes operative when complex exogenous antigens contain some components that are similar or identical to self antigens. In responding to the foreign components, some immunological cross-reactions may inadvertently occur to the shared structures. A fourth possibility is mutation in an immunocompetent cell that abolishes self-tolerance to one or more autoantigens.

Bacteriologists follow **Koch's postulates** if they wish to establish the etiological (causal) relationship of a specific microbe with a specific disease and **Rivers' postulates** for specific viruses with specific diseases. Ideally, immunologists attempt to follow **Witebsky's postulates** for correlating immunological phenomena with specific human diseases. These include: (1) a prescribed set of autoallergic symptoms must be regularly associated with the disease, (2) an animal model must be available in which a mimic of the human disease can be induced, (3) both the natural human disease and the experimentally induced animal disease should possess similar immunopathological characteristics, and (4) passive transfer of the autoallergic disease should be possible by serum or lymphoid cells from a diseased donor animal to a normal recipient animal. Good animal models for many suspected human autoallergies are not currently available, seriously limiting the scientific demonstration of the immune system's role in these diseases.

Most autoallergic diseases share one or more common immunological symptoms: (1) T lymphocytes with demonstrable reactivity against autoantigens, (2) appearance of autoantibodies, (3) hypergammaglobulinemia, (4) generalized hypocomplementemia or subnormal levels of specific complement components, and (5) elevated chemotaxis and other complement-mediated activities in diseased tissues to which complement and immunoglobulins are bound. Serological tests for these and other immunological conditions are useful to the physician in early and provisional diagnoses of autoallergic diseases or as confirmatory evidence for a diagnosis based on other clinical signs. Both cellular and humoral responses are commonly observed in autoallergic conditions, and it is difficult to ascertain their relative contributions to a given disease. In some diseases, the T cell branch of the immune system appears to be mainly responsible for the apparent

Serology and Immunology

immunological damage, whereas in other diseases the humoral branch seems to predominate. It is often difficult to establish cause-and-effect relationships. For this reason, autoallergic diseases are said to be immunoglobulin-associated or T cell–associated.

Immunoglobulin-associated Autoallergic Diseases. SYSTEMIC LUPUS ERYTHEMATOSUS. Systemic lupus erythematosus (SLE) was discussed in Chapter 8 under the topic of immunoenzyme techniques. Antinuclear antibodies that attach indiscriminately to nuclei from almost any source are usually found in sera of SLE patients. Rheumatoid factor (RF) and anticytoplasmic antibodies are also commonly associated findings. Immune complexes tend to be filtered out in the kidney, producing a glomerulonephritis. These immune complexes can easily traverse the glomerular endothelium, but tend to become trapped and accumulate diffusely between the endothelium and the basement membrane (Figure 9.8). These clues plus presence of the LE cell are usually sufficient to justify a diagnosis of SLE. At least two good animal models for SLE are known. Hybrids between the New Zealand black (NZB) and the New Zealand white (NZW) strains of mice show symptoms typical of SLE including antibodies to DNA and RNA, immune complex glomerulonephritis, etc. It is hypothesized that a progressive loss of suppressor T cell activities accompanies the murine disease and is responsible for unregulated B cell synthesis of immunoglobulins and the subsequent appearance of autoantibodies and macroglobulinemia. The other animal model of SLE involves the dog, but in this case it is believed that a viral stimulation of lymphoid tumors is responsible for the abnormal antibodies.

GLOMERULONEPHRITIS. Glomerulonephritis associated with SLE and serum sickness is caused by autologous antibodies complexed with nonglomerular antigens that become trapped in the walls of capillaries. Fixation of complement generates chemotaxins and anaphylatoxins that indirectly contribute to local tissue damage. Two other forms of

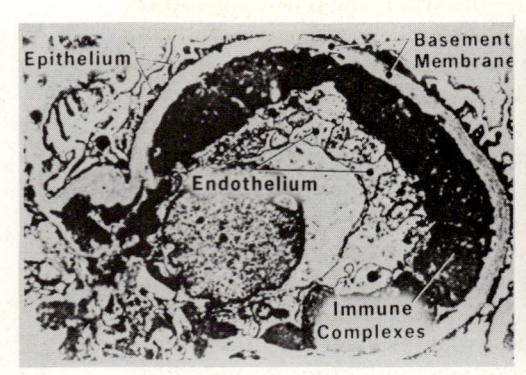

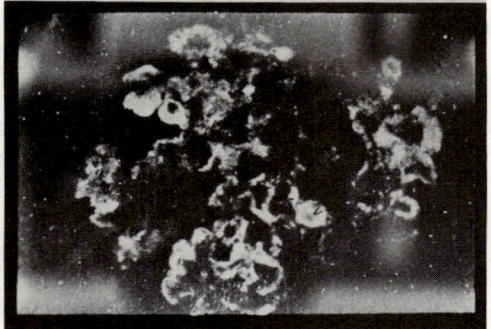

FIGURE 9.8. Immune complexes deposited in the kidney of patients with systemic lupus erythematosus. Left: Electron micrograph of portion of a glomerulus showing electron dense accumulation of immune complexes deposited diffusely between the basement membrane and the endothelium. Right: Fluorescent micrograph of a whole glomerulus specifically stained to reveal the presence of the gammaglobulins in these immune complexes. [*From Hill, R. B., et al., 1973. Basic pathology series; immune complexes and disease (S2951). National Audiovisual Center (GSA), Washington, D.C.*]

glomerulonephritis mediated by "self" antigen-"autoantibody" reactions are known. **Masugi nephritis** is induced experimentally in animals by injection of a heterologous antikidney serum. The antibodies attach directly to the glomerular basement membrane, activate complement, and cause a nephrotoxic (type II) nephritis. A natural autoallergy in humans called **Goodpasture's disease** is a Masugi-type nephritis involving autologous antibodies directed against antigens of the glomerular basement membrane. The other forms of glomerulonephritis (type III) involve cross-reactive antibodies. Rheumatic fever is a frequent sequela of many types of group A streptococcal infections. Poststreptococcal glomerulonephritis (PGN) is a less frequent complication following infection with group A streptococcus of type 12. Nonetheless, PGN may be the most widely known of the immune complex diseases. It usually appears about two weeks after infection with *Streptococcus pyogenes*. The antigen appears to be some component of the M protein of that organism. This is a type-specific cell-surface antigen present only in virulent members of group A β-hemolytic streptococci. It is an important antigen for inhibiting phagocytosis. Antibodies reactive with M protein tend to have a protective effect through opsonization. There are also glycoprotein antigens in the cell wall of the streptococcus that may be similar or identical to those in the basement membrane of the glomerulus. In responding immunologically to the M protein and/or glycoprotein antigens on the cell wall of the microorganism, some antibodies are made that cross-react with one or more identical or structurally similar antigenic determinants in the host's kidney. In contrast to SLE, the immune complexes of PGN tend to accumulate nonhomogeneously on the other side of the glomerular basement membrane (Figure 9.9). These immune complexes activate complement and contribute to the inflammatory response.

RHEUMATIC FEVER. Cross-reacting antibodies are also considered to be primarily involved in the etiology of rheumatic fever. Apparently one or more antigenic determinants present in more than fifty types of streptocci of group A are also present in heart tissue. Macrophages and lymphocytes aggregate around fibrinoid deposits in heart tissue damaged by streptococci, forming histologically distinctive complexes called **Aschoff's bodies** that are virtually pathognomonic for rheumatic fever. IgG and complement are deposited in Aschoff's bodies in the sarcolemma and in the perivascular connective tissue of the heart. Streptolysin O is known to have a direct cytotoxic effect on heart tissue. Hyaluronidase is a streptococcal enzyme that digests connective tissue ground substance. These and other toxins and enzymes of group A streptococci may contribute to the inflammatory process in cardiac tissues independently of the immune complex-induced damage. Antistreptolysin O and antihyaluronidase antibodies aid in neutralizing these toxins or enzymes.

AUTOIMMUNE HEMOLYTIC ANEMIA. Most autoimmune hemolytic anemias are **idiopathic** (cause unknown). Some of these anemias appear following primary atypical pneumonia, infectious mononucleosis, or drug treatment. It is hypothesized that neoantigens are formed by autocoupling of haptens from infectious microorganisms, viruses, or drugs to red cells of the host. Antibodies produced in response to these neoantigens may be cold agglutinins that readily bind to erythrocytes at about 4°C, but are eluted at 37°C. Most cold agglutinins are of class IgM. The presence of cold-reacting immunoglobulins or complement components on red cells can be detected

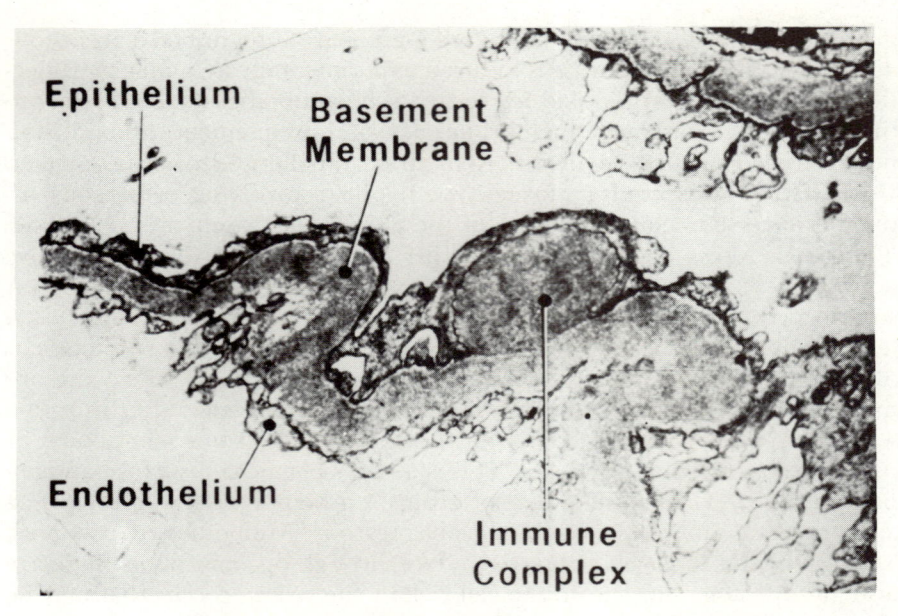

FIGURE 9.9. Electron micrograph of kidney section from patient with poststreptococcal glomerulonephritis. Notice the electron-dense immune complexes deposited in humps between the basement membrane and the foot processes of the podocyte. [*From Hill, R. B., et al., 1973. Basic pathology series; immune complexes and disease (S-2951). National Audiovisual Center (GSA), Washington, D.C.*]

by a direct Coombs test using a broad-spectrum antihuman serum. Warm agglutinins may also be associated with autoimmune hemolytic disease. They tend to be relatively weak as agglutinators or as complement fixers. These warm agglutinins are commonly of class IgG and reactive with an antigen of the Rh system, but they are seldom found in severe hemolytic episodes. Some autoantibodies of class IgG can bind to erythrocytes at low temperatures and then activate complement at body temperature to function as hemolysins. This explains why a patient with **paroxysmal cold hemoglobinuria** experiences a severe hemolytic episode following a cold shock. The autoantibody in this case is usually against the P blood group antigen and is a common complication of tertiary syphilis.

THROMBOCYTOPENIC PURPURA. Autocoupling of haptenic drugs to platelets is believed to be responsible for the disease called **thrombocytopenic purpura.** Thrombocytopenia is a subnormal platelet count that alters the blood-clotting mechanism, resulting in localized petechial (dotlike) hemorrhages in the skin (purpura) and other tissues of the body. When the drug is withdrawn from the patient, the disease subsides; upon reinitiation of therapy with the same drug, the symptoms reappear. This evidence strongly supports the theory of iatrogenic etiology for this disease. In a serological test for thrombocytopenic purpura, fresh patient's serum is mixed with human platelets and the suspected drug hapten. If specific antibodies are present, they will attach to the hapten-platelet complex, fix complement, and cause dissolution of the platelets. If the patient's serum is preheated to destroy complement, the platelets may be agglutinated by the same antibodies. Another theory proposes that the drug does not bind directly to platelets but rather to some carrier molecule (a serum protein) and this complex is then adsorbed to the platelet. Babies can also suffer this disease by passive transfer of IgG "antiplatelet" antibodies and drug from the mother across the placenta.

OTHER DISEASES WITH AUTOANTIBODIES. Antimyoid antibodies and antibodies against acetylcholine receptors are associated with some cases of myasthenia gravis; anti-IgG antibodies are associated with some cases of rheumatoid arthritis; etc. In these and numerous other diseases, antibodies are sporadically present, presumably as a consequence of the disease rather than as its cause. Serological tests for these antibodies may aid in diagnosis of the disease, but are not diagnostic alone.

T Cell–associated Autoallergic Diseases. ALLERGIC ENCEPHALOMYELITIS. One of the problems following the use of Pasteur's rabies vaccine was the relatively rare appearance of encephalomyelitis. The early vaccines were crude antigen preparations from phenolized spinal cords of rabbits with experimentally induced rabies. In addition to the inactivated virus, this vaccine contained many antigens of the rabbit's central nervous system (CNS). Apparently basic myelin proteins of the CNS are sequestered antigens that do not circulate and hence have not been recognized as self components. Rabbit and human myelin proteins share common antigens; so an immune response to these rabbit proteins in the rabies vaccine results in a cross-reactive autoallergic response to one's own CNS myelin proteins. Postvaccinal encephalomyelitis is no longer a problem with the rabies vaccines used today because the virus is grown in tissues of chicken or duck embryos devoid of cross-reactive neural tissues. Both humoral and cellular immune responses are produced to rabbit myelin proteins, but only the latter seem to be involved in etiology of the disease. Experimental allergic encephalomyelitis (EAE) can be induced in a variety of laboratory animals by injecting them with brain extracts (from any mammal) in Freund's adjuvant.

Symptoms similar to those of postvaccinal encephalomyelitis are sometimes noted following immunization with smallpox virus or after infections with measles, mumps, chickenpox, and other viruses with neurotropic tendencies. These viruses are hypothesized to stimulate an autoallergic response by one or more of several possible mechanisms. If the virus becomes integrated into the host chromosome, it may code for a new antigenic protein in the cell membrane. Some viruses enclose themselves with an envelope of host membrane as they emerge from the cell, thereby possibly creating new complex antigens. Some viruses may also directly damage cell membrane antigens and myelin, thereby revealing new antigen determinants.

SYMPATHETIC OPHTHALMIA. Injury to one eye can release lens proteins that stimulate immunological damage in the other healthy eye within several days or a few weeks. Lens protein is a sequestered antigen that does not normally circulate and to which tolerance has not been established. Mononuclear cells invade the uveal pigment, but antilens antibodies can seldom be detected in sympathetic ophthalmia. This disease can be experimentally induced in animals and responds to treatment with steroids. Delayed-type skin reactions to lens protein can be provoked in animals. These facts suggest that T cells are probably the primary etiological agents. Surgical removal of a cataract can sometimes provoke a postoperative complication called phacoanaphylaxis (phaco = lens). Lymphocytes and macrophages invade the lens, but the patient displays immediate-type skin reactions to lens protein suggesting that perhaps both cell-mediated and humoral responses may be involved.

ASPERMATOGENESIS. Sperm are not produced until relatively late in life and are usually sequestered from the lymphoid centers. Hence the male's immune system is not tolerant of sperm antigens. Guinea pigs or rats injected with autologous testis extracts in Freund's complete adjuvant soon fail to produce sperm. Very little generalized tissue damage is seen. Antibodies develop and anaphylactic hypersensitivity can be demonstrated, but the condition is passively transferred only by cells, not by serum. This indicates that experimental aspermatogenesis is T cell–mediated. Normal sperm production is gradually restored after about a year. Injections of sperm are as effective as testis extracts in provoking this hypersensitivity. Application of this phenomenon to humans offers hope of developing a temporary male sterility form of birth control.

Some infertile women possess high titers of circulating antibodies against sperm antigens. It might also be possible to develop a vaccine for women that would stimulate production of sperm agglutinating and immobilizing antibodies. The class of antibodies most likely to be effective in preventing pregnancies is secretory IgA because the antibodies must enter the female reproductive tract to complex with sperm. Animal experiments with this method of birth control have had some degree of success, but its efficiency must be greatly improved before it can be considered for routine use in humans.

HASHIMOTO'S HYPOTHYROIDITIS. Thyroglobulin is a sequested antigen to which the body normally has no tolerance. Experimentally, a cell-mediated autoallergy against this protein can be induced in laboratory animals by injecting autologous thyroid gland extracts in Freund's complete adjuvant. The thyroid is a bilobed structure in mammals. One lobe can be removed for preparation as the antigen and the other lobe can be left intact to assay the hypersensitive response. The gland becomes enlarged and infiltrated with plasma cells and lymphocytes. Colloid-filled vesicles containing the thyroid hormone disappear. Antithyroglobulin and antibodies against other thyroid gland antigens are produced. The role of these antibodies in the natural human equivalent of these animal models, Hashimoto's hypothyroiditis, is probably a minor one because the disease is difficult to passively transfer by serum. On the other hand, the disease can readily be passively transferred by sensitized lymphocytes. Furthermore, the intensity of delayed hypersensitivity skin reactions to thyroglobulin correlates with the severity of the disease. This is strong evidence that this form of thyroiditis has a T cell etiology. How the disease is initially triggered in humans is unknown.

Two animal models of autoimmune hypothyroiditis appear to have a predominantly humoral rather than a cellular etiology. In the Buffalo strain of rat, delayed-type skin reactions to thyroid gland extracts are negative and no MIF can be detected in the serum of affected individuals. In the obese strain of chickens, bursectomy reduces the severity of the disease. B lymphocytes are the predominant mononuclear cells invading the thyroid. Thymectomy exacerbates the disease in affected chickens. Perhaps abnormal suppressor T cell activities are responsible for the predominance of B lymphocyte functions in this case. This serves to exemplify the potential fallacy of attempting to classify autoallergic diseases into cell-mediated or antibody-mediated categories.

SELF-EVALUATION

Terms

1. A genetic deficiency of Cl esterase inhibitor. (3 words)
2. An adjective applied to diseases that have no known cause.
3. A term applied to diseases induced by drugs or other medical treatments.
4. A redox-sensitive dye used clinically to diagnose patients with CGD. (2 words)
5. A nonspecific diminution or absence of delayed-type hypersensitivity to potent allergens.
6. Name of the mutation that produces a nonfunctional thymus in the mouse.
7. A test for IgE-mediated immediate hypersensitivity in which immune serum is injected intradermally followed by antigen a day later into the same site. (2 words)
8. A test for type III hypersensitivity in which antigen is injected intradermally into a previously actively sensitized individual.
9. A trichloroacetic acid precipitate of OT, widely used in TB skin tests. (3 words)
10. A soluble substance capable of passively transferring delayed hypersensitivity when extracted from sensitized lymphocytes by repeated cycles of freezing and thawing. (2 words)

Multiple Choice. Choose the one best answer.

1. Which of the following is a congenital T cell deficiency disease? (a) Franklin's disease (b) iatrogenic disease (c) Job's syndrome (d) Chediak-Higashi syndrome (e) Di George syndrome
2. Which of the following is not considered to be a combined B and T cell deficiency disease? (a) Cushing's disease (b) Goodpasture's disease (c) ataxia telangiectasia (d) Wiscott-Aldrich syndrome (e) Swiss-type agammaglobulinemia
3. Which of the following is not a general characteristic of immediate hypersensitivities? (a) passively transferred by immune serum (b) treatment with antihistamines (c) mediated primarily by T cell products (d) specific target tissues (e) desensitization easier than for delayed hypersensitivities
4. In the Gell and Coombs classification of hypersensitivities, which class corresponds to the "delayed" group? (a) I (b) II (c) III (d) IV (e) more than one of these
5. Which of the following is not characteristic of passive cutaneous anaphylaxis? (a) no latent period required for challenge dose (b) small amount of IgE required (c) prevented by antihistamine (d) complement is not involved (e) antibody is injected intradermally and antigen is injected intravenously
6. Which of the following is not characteristic of lymphokines? (a) relatively low-molecular-weight proteins (b) low concentrations in serum (c) specific antigen-binding properties (d) some are responsible for graft rejection (e) some are mitogenic for lymphocytes
7. Which of the following is not a common immunological symptom shared by most autoallergic diseases? (a) autoantibodies (b) hypergammaglobulinemia (c) generalized hypocomplementemia (d) blocking antibodies (e) T cells reactive with autoantigens
8. Which of the following is classified as a T cell–associated autoallergic disease? (a) systemic lupus erythematosus (b) poststreptococcal glomerulonephritis (c) rheumatic fever (d) thrombocytopenic purpura (e) allergic encephalomyelitis

Serology and Immunology

9. Which of the following is not an explanation for the origin of autoallergic diseases? (a) deficiencies of complement inhibitors (b) occult antigen release (c) neoantigens (d) autocoupling haptens (e) mutation of an immunocompetent cell
10. The immunological rules for establishing the autoimmune nature of a disease were established by (a) Koch (b) Witebsky (c) Pasteur (d) Roux (e) Masugi

True–False

1. Interferons nonspecifically combine with viruses and prevent them from infecting host cells.
2. The Schultz-Dale test is a skin test for delayed hypersensitivity to a specific allergen.
3. Anaphylactoid reactions are considered to be nonimmunological.
4. Babies are commonly born passively sensitized to the IgE-mediated allergies of their mothers.
5. Antihistamines are usually effective in preventing type III hypersensitivities if taken early enough.
6. Functionally monovalent antibodies cannot induce an Arthus reaction.
7. Reaction to poison oak is classified as a delayed hypersensitivity.
8. Serum sickness is an immunological disease that can develop in a previously unsensitized individual after only one dose of an antigen.
9. Paroxysmal cold hemoglobinuria is a common complication of streptococcal infections.
10. A positive TB skin test (erythema) indicates that the patient has some degree of immunity to that organism.

Transplantation and Oncoimmunology

CHAPTER 10

CHAPTER OUTLINE

Graft Rejection
Graft-vs.-Host Reaction
Histocompatibility Antigens
  Mouse
  Human
Histocompatibility Typing
  Serological Tests
  Compatibility Tests

Immunosuppression
Immunological Privilege
Oncoimmunology
  Cancer Etiology
  Serological Indicators of Cancer
  Prophylactic Possibilities
Self-evaluation

The problems encountered in attempting to transplant tissues or organs from one human to another are well known even to the general public. Antigens present on cells of the donor's tissues are recognized as foreign by the recipient and the graft is immunologically rejected sooner or later. The tissue antigens involved in this rejection phenomenon are called **histocompatibility antigens.** They are produced by corresponding histocompatibility genes (loci). Therefore, the closer the genetic relationship between recipient and donor, the better the chance that they will share common antigens, and therefore, the greater the probability that the graft will "take" (be accepted, tolerated). A piece of one's own tissues can be removed and replaced in its natural location (an **orthotopic graft**) or in a different anatomical region **(heterotopic graft)** on the same individual. These **autografts** or autogeneic grafts should be permanently accepted because they contain no foreign antigens. The best chance of finding a match of compatible tissue from another individual is among members of the recipient's family (parents, children, siblings). No immunological barrier exists to impede the transplantation of tissues or organs between **identical twins.** These **monozygotic twins** develop from a single fertilized egg and hence share identical heredities and therefore also have identical histocompatibility antigens. Grafts between individuals with identical heredities are called **syngrafts** or syngeneic grafts. Cloning is the production of multiple individuals with identical heredities. Identical twins represent a clone of size two. The nine-banded armadillo regularly produces clones of size four (identical quadruplets). By intensively inbreeding laboratory mice (e.g., brother-sister matings) for many generations, man has been able to produce strains with essentially identical heredities (genotypes). Within such an inbred strain, tissue transplants between any two members present no immunological barriers. However, transplants between strains differing with respect to histocompatibility genes and antigens are not likely to be permanently accepted. The term **allograft** (or allogeneic graft) is applied to transplants involving genetically different members of the same species. Such is the case involving transplants between **fraternal** (dizygotic, or two-egg) **twins.** Fraternal twins of the same sex are no more likely to share common genes than are like-sex siblings (brothers, sisters) born at different times. Siblings are 50 percent genetically related, (i.e., they share about 50 percent of their genes in common). The same degree of genetic relationship exists between a parent and its offspring. Half-sibs (siblings sharing only one parent in common) have a genetic relationship of 25 percent; in cousins it is 12½ percent, etc. In theory, the probability of graft survival should increase with the degree of genetic relationship, although some histocompatibility genes seem far more important than others. In the early days of transplantation (1950s) grafts between different species were attempted (e.g., grafts of baboon kidneys to human recipients). Transplants involving different species are termed **xenografts** or xenogeneic grafts. It was soon learned that a xenograft cannot be maintained for even short periods of time without the continuous use of steroid drugs or other agents that suppress the immune responses of the recipient. These immunosuppressive agents have harmful side effects that become counterproductive to the welfare of the patient in heavy, continuous dosages. Pigskin is sometimes used on burn patients to temporarily protect the patient from excessive loss of tissue fluids and electrolytes and to help prevent infections. Synthetic skin membranes may temporarily be used for the same purposes without stimulating the immune responses of the patient. Aside from this, xenografts are of little practical use in medicine. In order to shift emphasis from the immunological to the more fundamental genetic aspects of the problem, a new terminology for transplantation work has supplanted the older terms derived from blood banking. A comparison of the new with the old terminology is given in Table 10.1.

Graft Rejection

On first contact with foreign histocompatibility antigens, an allograft recipient usually exhibits what is called a **first-set rejection** phenomenon. The graft initially appears to "take"; i.e., it revascularizes, looks healthy, and regains its biological functions (e.g., a kidney graft would excrete urine, an endocrine gland would secrete hormones, etc.). After about one week, however, the allograft becomes infiltrated with several kinds of mononuclear cells (lymphocytes, monocytes, tissue macrophages, plasma cells), and blood

Table 10.1 Comparison of New Transplantation Terminology with Obsolete Nomenclature

Type of Graft		Obsolete Term	Donor-Recipient Genetic (Antigenic) Relationship
Noun	Adjective		
Autograft	Autogeneic	—	Same individual
Syngraft	Syngeneic	Isograft	Genetically identical individuals
Allograft	Allogeneic	Homograft	Genetically dissimilar, same species
Xenograft	Xenogeneic	Heterograft	Different species

clots begin to form. A combination of specific and nonspecific cytotoxic events together with loss of blood supply to the allograft usually results in its necrosis and rejection in eleven to seventeen days. T lymphocytes appear to be the major source of the specific recognition of the foreign graft antigens. After T cells have contacted these antigens, they are thought to release lymphokines that recruit other uncommitted lymphocytes and macrophages. These recruited cells become "hyperirritable" or "angry" and attack the grafted cells. The cytotoxic reaction does not require constant contact between the T lymphocyte and the target cell. A brief contact period seems to be all that is required. A family of proteins called **lymphocytotoxins** or **lymphotoxins** (LT) are released by the T cells, and these products cause cell membrane damage and eventual death of target cells. Little is known at present why LT damages only the foreign cells and not the cells of the host. Other lymphokines that might aid in the rejection response function to stimulate mitotic division of other lymphocytes (blastogenic or mitogenic agents), attract and hold leukocytes and macrophages in the vicinity of the T cell–target cell interaction (e.g., chemotactic factor), and make macrophages more phagocytic, more mobile, and more cytocidal (macrophage-activating factor, MAF). Antibodies may also play a minor role in graft rejection. There is an antibody-dependent, cell-mediated cytotoxicity (ADCC) reaction attributed to nonphagocytic cells of the monocyte-macrophage lineage. If antibody coats the target cells, certain cells (B cells or undifferentiated lymphocytes, neutrophils, monocytes) will attach to determinants on the Fc portion of the cell-bound immunoglobulins and somehow become responsive against the foreign cells.

As a result of prior exposure to foreign antigens in the first-set rejection, the recipient now has a large population of committed T lymphocytes. If at some later time the host receives a second graft from the same donor (or another donor with the same antigens as that of the original donor), a **second-set rejection** occurs. In many ways, the second-set response is akin to the anamnestic antibody response. Again, T cells apparently are the major source of the cytotoxic reactions, but ADCC reactions may also be involved. Typically, the second-set phenomenon is an accelerated rejection in which the graft never looks healthy. It does not vascularize (white graft), it does not regain biological functions, and it is sloughed in three or four days.

The rapidity of the second-set rejection phenomenon can be utilized experimentally in selecting from a group of potential donors those whose tissues are most likely to be compatible with those of the intended recipient. In lieu of a solid tissue graft, easily obtained lymphoid cells of the recipient are injected into the skin of an unrelated individual (called the "third man" or "third person") and serve to sensitize the volunteer against histocompatibility antigens of the intended recipient. After the first-set rejection occurs in the third man, he receives an injection of lymphocytes in the skin from several potential donors. The third man is expected to show an accelerated inflammatory skin reaction (as an analog of a second-set graft rejection) against donor lymphocytes that bear histocompatibility antigens in common with the intended recipient (to which the third man has been previously sensitized). Therefore, the best match of tissues for the recipient from among the potential donors tested is the one whose lymphocytes elicited the strongest second-set reaction in the third man (Figure 10.1). The "third-

Serology and Immunology

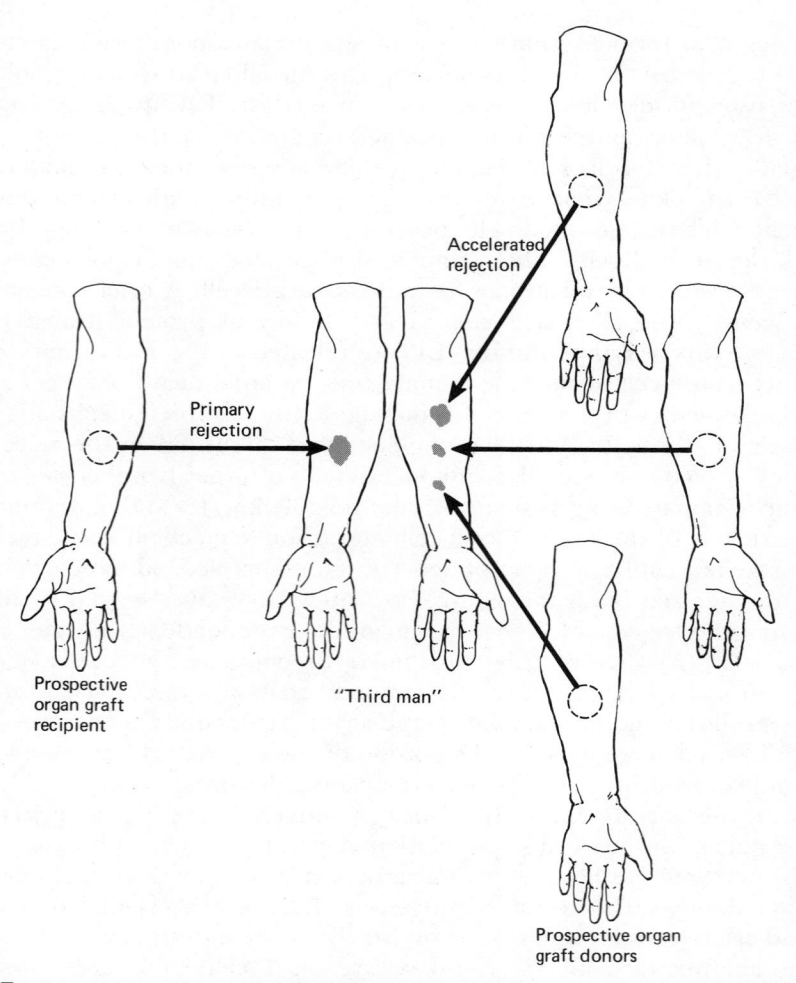

FIGURE 10.1. The "third-man" test for screening tissue or organ graft donors. A "third" person unrelated to either the intended recipient or potential donors is sensitized to histocompatibility antigens of the intended recipient. After the first-set (primary) rejection has occurred, the third person receives primary skin grafts from a group of potential donors. The graft that is rejected most rapidly indicates the donor that shares the strongest histocompatibility antigens with the intended recipient.

man test" is seldom used to match tissues in human transplantation work because it is difficult to find an unrelated volunteer to serve as the "third man." In addition, sensitizing the "third man" to many different histocompatibility antigens by this method will make it just that much more difficult to find a compatible donor for him if he ever should need a transplant. Some of the *in vivo* methods for detecting histoincompatibilities (such as the third-man test) are clinically impractical because of ethical and legal considerations; some tests also require several weeks. Nevertheless, they illustrate important immunological principles and are presented here for that purpose.

Graft-vs.-Host Reaction

We normally think in terms of a graft being rejected by the host (a host-vs.-graft or HVG reaction). However, in some special instances, it is possible for a graft to reject the host (GVH reaction). Such a graft would need to contain immunologically competent cells and the recipient would need to be immunologically compromised in some fashion. Perhaps the recipient might be a newborn whose immune system is relatively immature or it might be a genetically/congenitally immunodeficient individual or an adult whose T cell responses have been neutralized by radiation or other forms of immunosuppression. A GVH reaction can be easily demonstrated with inbred strains of mice (Figure 10.2). If nonlymphoid cells from strain A are injected (or a skin graft is made) into a newborn of strain B, the latter will usually accept the cells (graft) as his own. First exposure to foreign cells at a later time is likely to result in rejection because by then the animal has learned to recognize self from nonself. Subsequent grafts of tissues from A to B should be accepted as readily as an autograft. This is the phenomenon of **immunological tolerance.** If a piece of skin is transplanted from strain A into a tolerant individual of strain B, the graft would normally be permanently accepted. However, if after the graft has taken we inject immunolog-

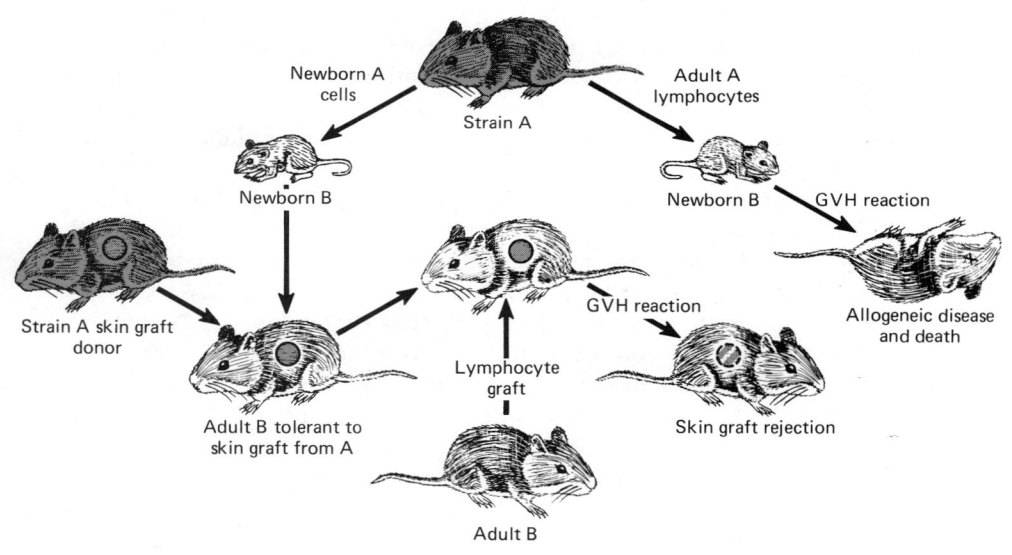

FIGURE 10.2. A scheme for induction (in mice) of graft-vs-host (GVH) reaction, induction of immunological tolerance, and breakage of tolerance by grafted lymphocytes. Two highly inbred strains of mice (A and B) are used with corresponding differences in histocompatibility antigens. Injection of immunologically competent adult A lymphocytes into newborn B results in a GVH reaction that stunts the growth and eventually kills B as a juvenile (allogeneic disease). Injection of incompetent fetal or newborn A cells into newborn B results in immunological tolerance. B matures as a chimera or mosaic of A and B cells. As an adult, B will be tolerant of a skin graft from any adult of strain A. After the graft "takes," an injection of lymphocytes from a nontolerant B adult (or from one previously sensitized to A cells) results in a GVH attack on the A graft by the injected cells.

ically competent adult T lymphocytes from strain B into the tolerant animal, a GVH reaction (actually a graft-vs.-graft reaction) will ensue. The immunologically competent T lymphocytes of the graft would recognize the antigens in the skin graft from strain A as foreign and mount a localized GVH reaction against them. A first-set rejection of the skin graft would occur. Now if we take immunologically competent adult T lymphocytes from strain A and inject them into a newborn mouse of strain B, a systemic GVH reaction would occur. A newborn mouse is relatively immunologically defenseless against a large graft of foreign T cells. The grafted A lymphocytes mount an immunological attack in many parts of the B body resulting in stunting of growth and eventual death. This is variously termed **runting disease, wasting disease,** or **allogeneic disease.** This is the reason why it has been difficult to transplant immunologically competent thymus tissue into babies born without a functional thymus (congenitally athymic) or to give bone marrow transplants from healthy individuals to those who have been immunologically compromised. If a graft containing immunologically competent T lymphocytes is transplanted into an immunologically competent host, both HVG and GVH reactions are expected. The outcome of this mutual incompatibility depends on such factors as the numbers of antagonistic cells in graft and host, the difference in strengths of histocompatibility antigens, etc. Since the numbers of T cells in a graft are usually much smaller than the numbers in the host, the battle usually is won by the HVG reaction (graft rejection). The transfer of immunologically competent cells from a sensitized individual to an unsensitized one is termed **adoptive immunity.** It is a special form of passive immunity with little practical application in medicine. However, some cases of acute leukemia and malignant lymphoma in humans have responded favorably to a combination of bone marrow grafts and active immunization. The adoptively transferred tissue has little chance of surviving unless it is histocompatible with the recipient or the recipient is immunologically suppressed or tolerant.

In addition to the first-set and second-set rejections, there also exists the possibility of an **acute** or **hyperacute rejection** dependent on "sensitivity factors" existing prior to contact with the graft. One of the most important factors in this regard is ABO blood group system incompatibility of donor and recipient. If the grafted tissue is donated from an individual of blood group A and the recipient is blood group B, then the "naturally present" anti-A of the host would immediately attack the A antigens of the graft. By activating the complement system and phagocytic cells, cytotoxic tissue destruction results in very rapid graft rejection similar to a second-set rejection phenomenon. In some organ grafts involving surgical connection of major blood vessels, blood flow slows, the organ becomes engorged with blood, and perhaps blood clots begin to form within minutes of being sutured into place. It is almost immediately obvious that the graft will not take and must be removed. For this reason, all potential organ transplant donors must be initially matched with the recipient for compatibility in the ABO blood group system. Of course, incompatibility in other blood group systems or preformed antibodies to histocompatibility antigens might also contribute to a hyperacute graft rejection, but in this case the irregular antibodies would have been acquired as a result of one or more previous incompatible blood transfusions (or pregnancies). A blood transfusion is a graft of a tissue containing cells dispersed in a liquid medium (plasma).

Antigens of the ABO system are on virtually all body cells, but histocompatibility antigens are not present on enucleated cells (mature erythrocytes). Therefore, histocompatibility typing cannot be performed on red cells. Blood leukocytes are a convenient source of cells for histocompatibility tests. Antibodies can participate to some extent in rejection of solid-tissue grafts, but they are much more important than T cells in rejection of incompatible blood transfusions.

Histocompatibility Antigens

The immunological basis of graft rejection resides in the glycoprotein surface antigens of foreign cells (**histocompatibility antigens**) and their interactions with antibodies or killer T cells. Since grafting is not a common natural process, the evolution of histocompatibility antigens could not be dependent on this phenomenon. Rather, they must have evolved because they conferred some survival (fitness) advantage on the host. It has been suggested that they evolved as important components of the **immunological surveillance system** by which the animal body rids itself of virally infected cells and cancer cells (both of which commonly bear foreign antigens). Killer T cells appear unable to attack virus-infected mouse cells unless the lymphocyte and the target cell share at least one histocompatibility antigen in common. The same is also true in mice concerning cancer cells. Killer lymphocytes cannot attack mouse cancer cells if the tissue culture medium is first incubated with antibodies against the shared histocompatibility antigens. Presumably, the antibody sterically masks the histocompatibility antigens on the cancer cells so that killer T lymphocytes can no longer recognize them. This blocking phenomenon has also been implicated in prolonging the life of certain grafts. In graft rejection, the histocompatibility antigens are the foreign anigens. Antibodies to these antigens can prevent their recognition by killer T cells and thereby prolong the survival of the graft. **Immunological enhancement** is the name given to the phenomenon whereby the life of incompatible grafts (or foreign cells of any kind) is extended by antibodies to histocompatibility antigens.

A major difference between graft rejection and immunological surveillance is that the histocompatibility antigen is a foreign substance to killer T cells in graft rejection, but it serves as a common recognition signal in immunological surveillance. There are two major hypotheses concerning the manner by which killer T cells recognize histocompatibility antigens in immunological surveillance. These two hypotheses are epitomized in the one-receptor and two-receptor models of Figure 10.3. According to the one-receptor model, the killer T cell has only one site by which it recognizes a hybrid antigen consisting partly of the foreign (tumor or virus) antigen and partly of the histocompatibility antigen. Alternatively, the two-receptor model attributes two binding sites to a killer T cell. One receptor binds the histocompatibility antigen and the other attaches to the tumor or virus antigen. Protein molecules embedded in the cell membrane may be highly mobile. By reacting the histocompatibility antigen and the abnormal antigen with different fluorescent-labeled antibodies, they were found to form aggregates in the same region; these aggregates eventually fuse at one position on the cell to form a fluorescent cap. The results of this "capping"

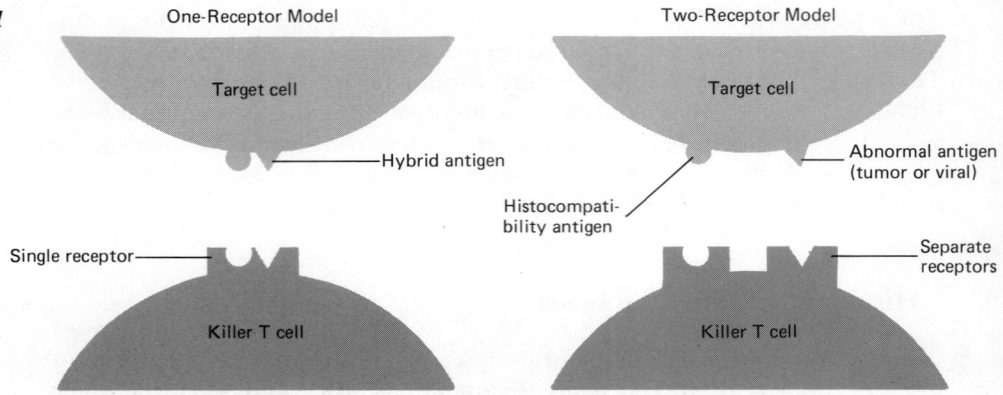

FIGURE 10.3. Two models representing the nature of the receptor site(s) by which killer T cells recognize target cells.

experiment indicate (but do not prove) that both antigens are close together.

Not all histocompatibility antigens elicit equivalent immunological responses. The strongest antigens in the mouse belong to the **H-2 system,** and the corresponding antigens in man belong to the **HLA system.** Each of the these systems is genetically controlled by a **major histocompatibility complex** (MHC), a closely linked group of genes involved with histoincompatibility and other immunological functions. Several weaker (minor) histocompatibility antigens exist, but little is known of their genetic control. If a graft bears a MHC antigen different from the recipient, it is likely to be rejected "acutely" within about two weeks. Incompatibilities involving only minor H antigens would usually take much longer to affect graft rejection ("chronic rejection").

Weak histoincompatibility antigens of mice do not always follow the same rules applicable to the strong antigens. For example, minor H loci cannot be ranked for potency of their antigenic products without specifying the particular interallelic combination involved. Allelic dosage effects are demonstrable for some of these combinations; i.e., homozygous grafts are rejected more rapidly than grafts heterozygous for the same foreign allele. The weaker the immunogenetic disparity between donor and recipient strains, the greater the variation in survival times of individual skin grafts. For grafts involving strong histoincompatibilities, there is a detectable inverse relationship between graft size (antigen dosage) and its expected survival time; small grafts tend to survive longer than larger grafts. However, for grafts involving only weak histoincompatibilities, small grafts may be rejected chronically whereas larger grafts may survive indefinitely under similar experimental conditions. In contrast to strong H antigens, weak H antigens may act synergistically; i.e., the mean survival time (MST) of skin grafts differing by two histocompatibility factors may be significantly shorter than when graft and host differ by only one such factor.

The MHC of the mouse has been much more extensively studied than the MHC of humans because experimentation with humans has ethical and legal restraints. Moreover, genetic studies are much easier in a multiparous animal such as the mouse where controlled breeding can be performed. If brother-sister matings are made for many generations, highly inbred lines

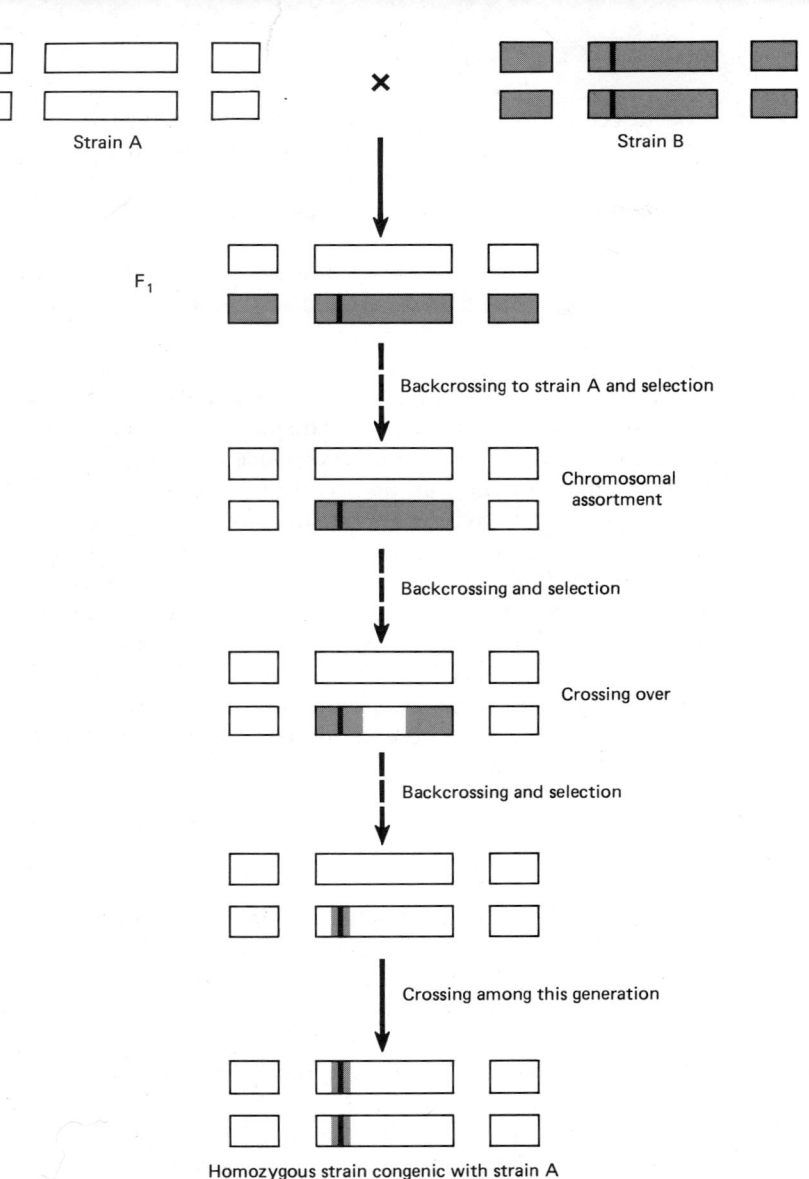

FIGURE 10.4. A plan for creating congenic strains of mice (differing only in traits governed by a small segment on one pair of chromosomes). Two highly inbred (genetically uniform) strains (A and B) are crossed. The F_1 is then backcrossed to strain A, and only those progeny that possess the desired B trait are saved (the desired trait might be the antigens of the H-2 locus, represented genetically by the dark band on the longest chromosome). Several generations of backcrossing to strain A and selecting the character will produce individuals that differ genetically from strain A only in the H-2 region of one chromosome. Crossing among these individuals is expected to produce about 25 percent homozygotes for the H-2 genes of strain B. Breeding among only the homozygotes maintains this congenic line. Although the diagram shows that during backcrossing there is first loss of all B chromosomes other than the one bearing the H-2 locus by chromosomal assortment and then further loss of B genes on the H-2 chromosome by crossing over (recombination), actually these two processes are likely to occur simultaneously. The mouse has twenty pairs of chromosomes and the H-2 locus is on chromosome 17.

of mice can be developed. By selective breeding (Figure 10.4), **congenic** strains of highly inbred mice differing from one another in only one or a few chosen traits can be produced. The advantages for immunological studies of congenic strains of mice differing only by one MHC antigen are obvious.

Suppose, for example, that two congenic mouse strains differ by only one histocompatibility antigen. Strain C has the C antigen and strain D has the D antigen; all other antigens are common to both strains because of identical heredities at all other genetic loci. Strain C cannot donate tissues to strain D or vice versa (Figure 10.5). However, the CD hybrid offspring from mating these two strains is able to accept transplants from either parental strain because no new antigens are being introduced. Hybrid tissue cannot be grafted back to either of the parents; strain C would react against the foreign D antigen of the CD hybrid and strain D would reject the hybrid graft because of the foreign C antigen. Matings between hybrid mice produce an F_2 generation, all individuals of which could donate tissue back to the F_1 hybrids. It is expected that one quarter of the F_2 would be homozygous for the C gene and hence exhibit only the C antigen on tissues. One half of the F_2 would be heterozygous CD like the F_1. Another one quarter would be homozygous for the D allele and consequently have only the D antigen on tissues. This model can easily be extended to multigenic situations by application of basic Mendelian laws.

MOUSE

In the mouse, the MHC or H-2 complex resides on chromosome 17. It consists of four closely linked regions designated K, I, S, D, which genetically map in that order (Figure 10.6). Major histocompatibility antigens are governed by genes in the K and D regions. It is not known how many genes or multiple alleles exist within the K and D regions. Until the situation becomes clarified, it is convenient to refer to each region as though it were a single gene with multiple alleles, each allele specifying a different H-2 antigen. At least ten antigens have been discovered in inbred strains in each of the H-2K and H-2D loci. Hundreds of antigenic variants of these loci are thought to exist in wild outcrossed populations.

Chemically the H-2 antigens of the K and D regions are glycoproteins, but the polysaccharide moeities apparently are not involved in the antigenicity of the entire molecule. Two methods have been used to remove H-2 antigens from cell membranes: (1) detergent and (2) the proteolytic enzyme papain. Detergent-extracted H-2 antigens appear to be tetramers each consisting of two long (heavy) polypeptide chains and two short (light) chains. The gross structure of the tetramer is remarkably similar to that of an immunoglobulin (Figure 10.7), but it is questionable that the tetrameric structure exists *in vivo*. Light chains are held to heavy chains by noncovalent bonds; heavy chains in detergent solution are covalently bonded to one another. All of the carbohydrate of the H-2 antigen is associated with the heavy chains. H-2 antigens cleaved from the membrane by papain appear to consist of a dimer of one heavy and one light chain. This dimer is designated F_s because it is a fragment soluble in water. The heavy chain portion of F_s is designated F_H. A much smaller fragment of the heavy chain remains

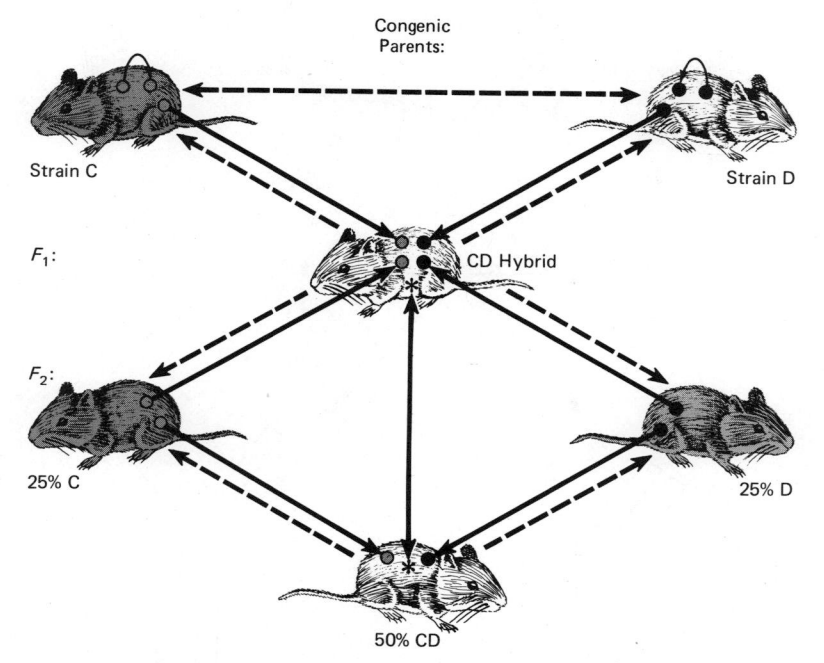

FIGURE 10.5. Basic principles of transplantation genetics demonstrated in congenic mouse strains. Solid lines indicate compatible transfers; broken lines are incompatible grafts.

embedded in the membrane and is designated F_m (fragment, membrane). There is no clear evidence for covalent bonds between heavy chains when the antigen is attached to the membrane (not in detergent solution). Therefore, H-2 antigens of the K and D regions probably exist on the cell surface only as a dimer of one heavy and one light chain.

The light chain of an H-2 antigen is synonymous with the beta-2-microglobulin. This protein is manufactured by almost every nucleated cell of the body in all vertebrate animals. Its name is derived from its electrophoretic migration with the beta globulins and its relatively low molecular weight (11,500). There appears to be little variation in the amino acid

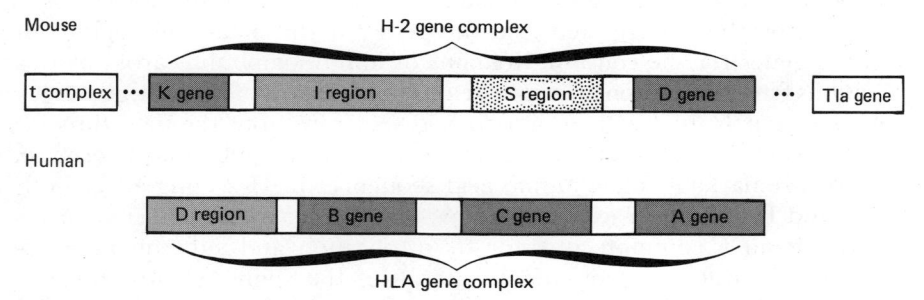

FIGURE 10.6. Comparison of the major histocompatibility complexes (MHC) in mouse (H-2) and human (HLA). Homologous regions are the same shade. The *t* and *Tla* (*TLa*) genes of the mouse are closely linked to the H-2 gene complex and may be functionally related to H-2 genes. The *t* complex is known to regulate development of the tail. The *Tla* locus produces distinctive T cell antigens in mice with thymus-derived leukemia.

Serology and Immunology

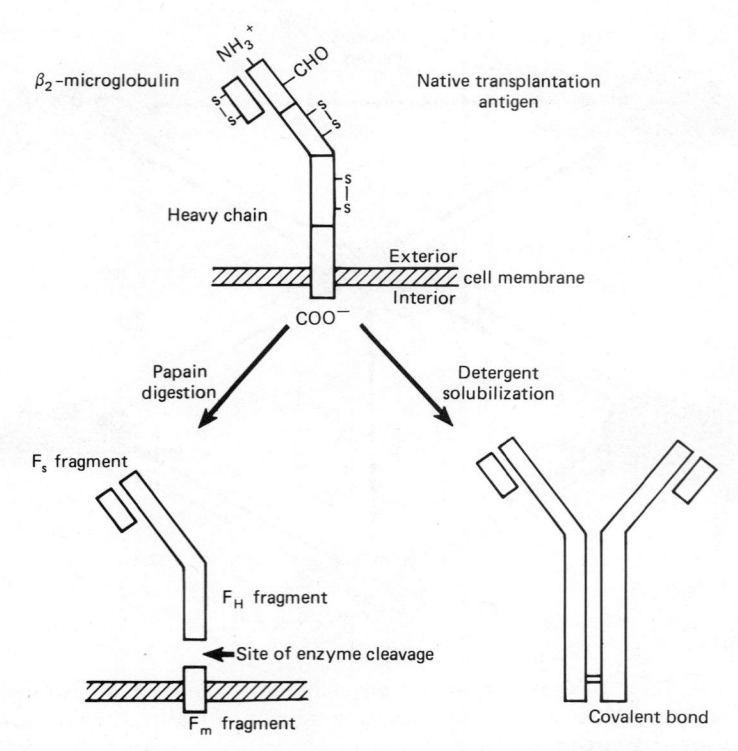

FIGURE 10.7. Basic structure of transplantation antigens (H-2 antigens) in the mouse. H-2 antigens can be separated from the cell membrane by treatment with the enzyme papain or by detergent. When cleaved by papain, a small part of the heavy chain remains membrane-bound (F_m fragment); the rest of the H-2 antigen is soluble (F_s fragment) consisting of most of the heavy chain (F_H fragment) and all of the beta-2-microglobulin. Entire H-2 antigen molecules are released from the membrane by detergent treatment, forming covalently bonded dimers. A carbohydrate group (CHO) is attached to the N terminal domain of the heavy chain.

sequences of beta-2-microglobulins either within a species or between species. There is a striking resemblance in structure of the beta-2-microglobulin to the constant domains of immunoglobulin molecules. It has therefore been suggested that the gene for the beta-2-microglobulin and the genes for the constant domains of immunoglobulins arose by duplications from a common ancestral gene. Heavy chains of H-2 antigens have only been partly analyzed for amino acid sequences, but the data thus far show no convincing similarities to any of the immunoglobulins. There are, however, remarkably close amino acid sequences in H-2 antigens of both the K and D regions, leading to the hypothesis that their respective genes evolved from a common ancestor by duplication and subsequent modification by different mutations. Because the light chains (beta-2-microglobulins) are virtually invariate in composition, all of the antigenic specificity of the H-2 antigens resides in the variable amino acid sequences of the heavy chains. The role played by light chains in self-recognition is still a mystery. However, the close homology between light chains and the C_H3 domain of IgG (which binds complement) suggests that light chains may contribute to binding of complement on cell surfaces.

The **I** or **Ir** (immune response) region of the mouse MHC is located adjacent to the H-2K region. This region contains genes that govern the ability to make an antibody response to some synthetic polypeptides. An inbred strain of mice, possessing the appropriate Ir gene, can respond to one of these synthetic antigens; other strains that do not have this same Ir gene cannot make an immune response. Genes in the Ir region have also been found to control specific humoral responses to some natural antigens (e.g., erythrocyte antigens, bacterial lipopolysaccharides, and mouse thymocyte antigen). It is not known how this region controls immune responsiveness. There are, however, some **Ia** (I region–associated) antigens that are controlled in some way by genes in the I region, even though the antigens themselves appear not to be Ir gene products. These Ia antigens are found on B lymphocytes, but are absent (or in very low concentration) from T lymphocytes. The functions of Ia antigens are unknown. Some evidence supports the hypothesis that Ia antigens might behave as T cell receptors on B cells and thereby allow T cell–B cell interactions (helper or suppressor functions).

The S region of the mouse MHC is located between the I and D regions. At least one gene in this region is known to synthesize a beta globulin of the complement system (C4). Complement interacts with antigen-antibody complexes in bacteriolysis, hemolysis, and lysis of grafted cells. Hence all four regions of the mouse MHC are involved in immune functions.

HUMAN

The MHC of humans is the HLA **(human leukocyte antigen)** gene complex, a group of closely linked genes on chromosome 6 (Figure 10.7). There are four major regions in the HLA complex (HLA-A, HLA-B, HLA-C, and HLA-D). The first three regions (A, B, C) contain genes responsible for histocompatibility antigens and therefore are functionally the equivalent of the H-2K and H-2D regions of the mouse MHC. Region HLA-D appears to be the functional equivalent of region I in the mouse, governing humoral immune responsiveness. The D region of humans has its DR-associated antigens, which appear to be the counterparts to the Ia antigens of the mouse. Much less is known of the detailed structure of HLA antigens than of H-2 antigens. Nevertheless, the protein sequences available so far indicate that the structures of the HLA antigens of humans are very similar to the H-2 antigens of the mouse. Early in the analysis of the human MHC, it was thought to be composed of only two genetic regions. The antigens of these regions were originally designated as belonging to either the LA or four series. Now these series have been renamed HLA-A and HLA-B, respectively. As with the mouse H-2 regions, it is convenient to consider each region as a single gene with multiple alleles even though it is quite probable that more than one locus exists within each region. Much more is known of the A and B regions than of the C and D regions. Because the A and B genes are so closely linked, the gene pairs on a parental chromosome are almost invariably transmitted as a unit to offspring. For this reason, it has become common practice to specify the corresponding pairs of antigens as a **haplotype** (i.e., the antigenic products of the HLA genes found in a gamete). Each antigen of the A and B series is numbered (e.g., A1, A2, A3, etc.; B5, B7, B8, etc.). If the genes determining A1 and B5 are on one chromosome of an individual, then its haplotype is A1, B5. If the homologous chromosome of this individual contains the genes for antigens A2 and B7, then the other haplotype is A2, B7. A complete antigenic description for an individual would consist of its two haplotypes (e.g., A1, B5 / A2, B7). Since each HLA gene has many alleles, there are so many antigens and haplotypes possible that any one haplotype is rare except within a family lineage. The number of possible phenotypes with n alleles is found from the equation $\frac{1}{2}(n^2 - n + 2)$. If there are 15, 21, 7, and 10 alleles for the A, B, C, and D antigens, respectively, there are approximately twenty million possible phenotypes. Therefore, if it can be shown that a child possesses the same haplotype as that of a putative father (the haplotype being absent from the mother), then this constitutes strong evidence of paternity. Recall that blood group antigens can be used to exclude paternity, but do not offer more than suggestive evidence of parentage. Because of this limitation, HLA antigens are very likely to replace blood group antigens for use in cases of disputed paternity. An example of how HLA antigens are genetically inherited is given in Table 10.2.

Some remarkable correlations have been found between certain HLA antigens and some diseases presumed to have an immunological origin. For example, in ankylosing spondylitis (a kind of rheumatoid arthritis of the spine) about 88 percent of afflicted individuals possess antigen HLA-B27, whereas it is present in only 8 percent of unafflicted control individuals. Strong correlations of this kind can be of considerable diagnostic aid to the physician. Medical laboratory technologists can therefore expect to be performing histocompatibility typing in the future on individuals not necessarily being typed for grafting operations. Weaker and therefore less useful diagnostic correlations have been found between antigen HLA-B8 and myastenia gravis and Graves' disease. Approximately 55 percent of individ-

Table 10.2 An Example of Inheritance of HLA Antigens

Individuals	HLA-A Antigens						HLA-B Antigens				
	1	2	3	9	10	11	5	7	8	12	13	14
Father	+	−	−	−	+	−	−	−	−	−	+	+
Mother	−	+	−	−	−	+	+	−	−	+	−	−
Children:												
First	−	−	−	−	+	+	−	−	−	+	−	+
Second	−	+	−	−	+	−	+	−	−	−	−	+
Third	+	−	−	−	−	+	−	−	−	+	+	−
Fourth	+	+	−	−	−	−	+	−	−	−	+	−

	Phenotypes	Haplotypes
Father	A1, 10 / B13, 14	A1, B13 / A10, B14
Mother	A2, 11 / B5, 12	A2, B5 / A11, B12
Children:		
First	A10, 11 / B12, 14	A10, B14 / A11, B12
Second	A2, 10 / B5, 14	A10, B14 / A2, B5
Third	A1, 11 / B12, 13	A1, B13 / A11, B12
Fourth	A1, 2 / B5, 13	A1, B13 / A2, B5

uals afflicted with these diseases possess B8 compared with about 24 percent in healthy controls.

Histocompatibility Typing

There are two major methods of matching donor and recipient for tissue grafts: (1) serological (antibody) tests and (2) compatibility tests. HLA antigens of the A, B, and C regions of the human MHC react with antibodies and therefore are referred to as **serologically detectable** (SD). "Antigens" of the D region cannot be detected by antibodies. They can, however, be detected by observing the reactions of lymphocytes in tissue culture or in the intact body. These antigens are thus referred to as **lymphocyte-detectable** (LD). The LD properties of lymphocytes in tissue culture may be associated with human DR antigens since this appears to be the case with their counterparts in the mouse (Ia antigens). Some immunologists apply the term "transplantation antigens" only to preparations that can be shown to produce hypersensitivity to skin grafts or delayed cutaneous reactions (i.e., LD antigens); the term "histocompatibility antigens" is applied to substances that can be detected by *in vitro* tests (i.e., SD antigens). The latter behave as "incomplete antigens" when used in transplantations (e.g., most mammalian erythrocytes cannot provoke transplantation immunity).

If a prospective tissue graft recipient has all of the LD and SD antigens of a prospective donor, this is considered to be a "match" (a compatible situation, unlikely to lead to rejection of a graft). However, if the donor has one or more LD or SD antigens not present in the recipient, the graft is likely to be rejected. Donor and recipient must also be of the same ABO blood group because antigens of this system are on most body cells and the "natural" anti-A and/or anti-B present in the serum of the recipient could initiate a complement-mediated cytolytic attack on the incompatible graft.

SEROLOGICAL TESTS

Since HLA antigens are present on virtually all nucleated cells, it is convenient to use blood lymphocytes as a source of SD antigens in histocompatibility typing. Typing reagents are very expensive and are often polyvalent rather than monovalent (i.e., they have mixed populations of antibodies recognizing more than one antigenic specificity). The most common histocompatibility assays are cytotoxicity tests and are therefore performed using micro methods (using lambda or microliter amounts of antisera). Leukocytes may be extracted by centrifugation and removal of the buffy coat overlying the red cells. Granulocytes (neutrophils, basophils, and eosinophils) can be absorbed on glass, nylon, or cotton. The remaining cells are mostly lymphocytes. Alternatively, they can be purified by the Ficoll-Hypaque method (Figure 10.8). A lymphocyte preparation containing about 10^6 cells per milliliter is commonly used as the antigen. Microliter (lambda) amounts of the antigen are reacted in different wells of a plastic block with microliter amounts of various HLA antibodies. Rabbit or human complement (considered for this test to be superior to guinea pig complement) is added to each well. A small amount of mineral oil is then added to each well or the entire block may be covered with plastic film to prevent

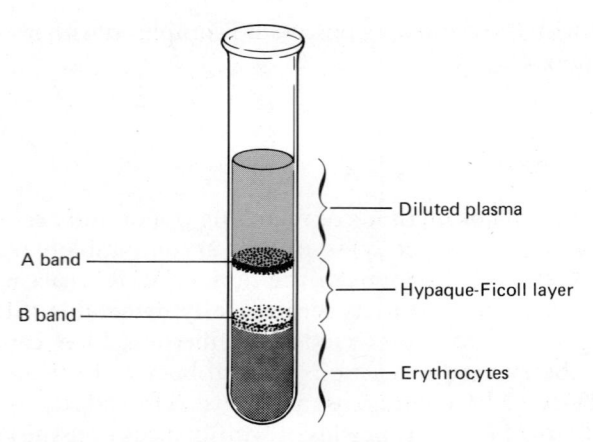

FIGURE 10.8. The Ficoll-Hypaque method for isolation of mononuclear leukocytes. Heparinized venous blood is carefully layered over Ficoll-Hypaque solution to form a sharp interface. The tubes are centrifuged and the A band is removed carefully with a pipette. Cells in this layer are washed in Hanks balanced salt solution (HBSS) and fetal calf serum (FCS). The cell pellet should then be free of platelets and erythrocytes and should contain 60 to 85 percent lymphocytes and 15 to 40 percent monocytes. The B band contains mostly mature granulocytes.

evaporation of the reagents. If a histocompatibility antigen on the lymphocyte is recognized by the IgG or IgM antibody, an antigen-antibody reaction occurs that binds complement. The bound complement kills the lymphocyte and damages its membrane so that subsequent addition of a dye (such as trypan blue or eosin) results in staining of that cell (Figure 10.9). Only dead cells become stained. Microscopic examination reveals which cells are stained and therefore possess the HLA antigen homologous with the specificity of the antibody.

At least two variations of the microcytotoxicity test just described are widely used. By briefly incubating lymphocytes with $Na_2{}^{51}CrO_4$, they become labeled with the radioactive isotope of chromium. The cells are washed to remove any unabsorbed isotope and then used as antigens for the test. If the cell membrane is damaged by the antibody-activated complement, the isotope rapidly leaks out and can easily be detected in the extracellular fluid. As with all radioimmune assays, this test is extremely sensitive. A second variation of the cytotoxicity test labels the viable lymphocyte with a fluorescein dye. Immunologically damaged cells allow the dye to leak out. Washing the cells removes the unabsorbed dye. If microscopic examination reveals unstained cells, it is used as an index of cytotoxicity. Pretreatment of lymphocytes with various enzymes renders them more sensitive to the cytotoxic effects of complement and accelerates the test reaction.

COMPATIBILITY TESTS

In contrast to the serological tests that attempt to establish the antigenic composition of potential donors and recipient, compatibility tests merely attempt to ascertain if recipient lymphocytes are reactive with cells or tissues of a potential donor. The most popular *in vivo* compatibility test is the

mixed-leukocyte (lymphocyte) culture (MLC) or **mixed-lymphocyte reaction** or response (MLR). If recipient lymphocytes in tissue culture are mixed with those of an incompatible donor, both lymphocytes would react to the foreign antigens of each other. They would change from their relatively undifferentiated condition as small lymphocytes to larger "blast cells" on the way to becoming immunologically reactive T cells. This "blast cell transformation" phenomenon involves an increase in cell size, enlargement of the nucleus, increased mitotic activity, and intensive nucleic acid synthesis. Many of these changes can be observed microscopically, but the work is tedious and fraught with subjective interpretations. A much more objective and quantitative assay technique involves the use of radioactive isotopes. Actively dividing lymphocytes exposed to tritiated (^{3}H) thymidine (a nucleotide of DNA) will incorporate the radioactive isotope into its DNA. The cells are washed to remove any unincorporated isotope and then assayed for radioactivity in a scintillation counter. This test often requires incubation for five days, but the amount of radioactive labeling does serve as a reliable index of compatibility. Results from MLC and cytoxicity tests are in close agreement for detecting nonidentity of major HLA antigens. The MLC, however, may detect some histocompatibility antigens missed by the cytotoxicity tests for lack of appropriate antibodies. Since it is possible that only the donor cells would be transformed by those of the recipient (and not vice versa), the MLC is usually performed as a "one-way MLC." This is done by treating the cells of the potential donor so that they can no longer replicate their DNA and therefore cannot incorporate the tritiated thymidine. Treatments with ionizing radiations or the chemical mitomycin

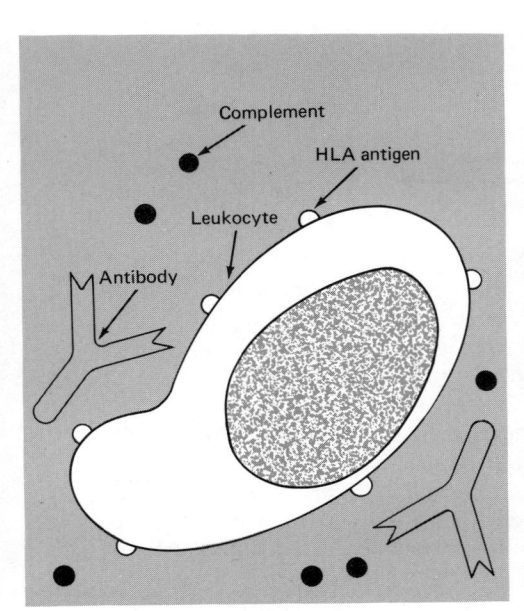

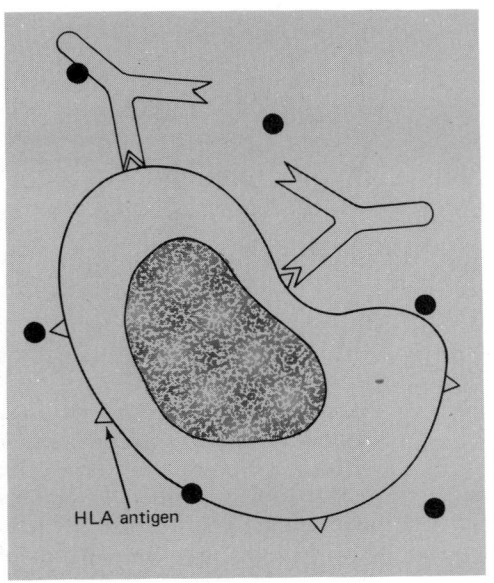

Transplantation and Onco-immunology

FIGURE 10.9. Complement-mediated cytotoxic test for an HLA antigen. In a negative test (left) antibody is not homologous with the HLA antigen on the leukocyte; complement is not activated and the cell is not stained by the dye. In a positive test (right) antigen-antibody reaction activates complement, damages the cell membrane, and the dye enters the cell.

C are commonly used for this purpose. Although the treated cells cannot undergo blast cell transformation, they still can stimulate the untreated incompatible recipient lymphocytes to do so. When only the response of recipient lymphocytes is assayed in this manner, the results are highly predictive of graft survival (Figure 10.10).

A second kind of compatibility test is the **normal lymphocyte transfer** (NLT) reaction. This test is the *in vivo* correlate of the MLC. Normal lymphocytes of the transplant recipient and unrelated volunteers (to serve as

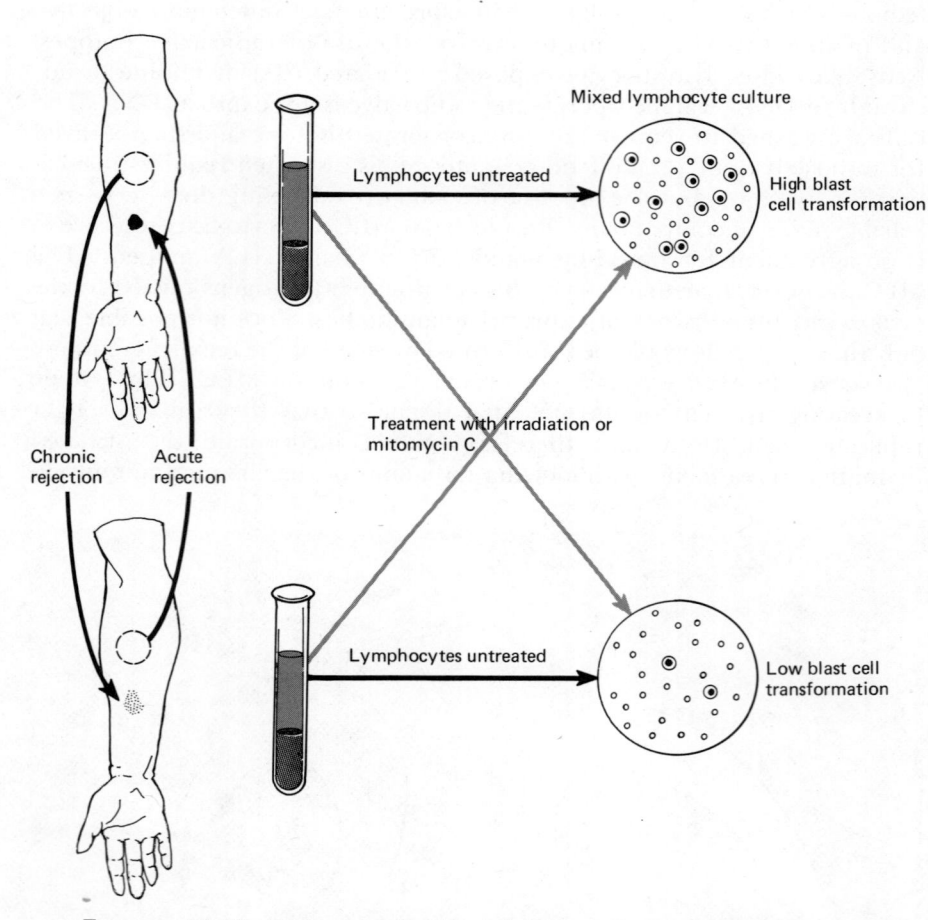

FIGURE 10.10. One-way mixed-lymphocyte culture (MLC) test. Two aliquots of lymphocytes are extracted from a pair of potential donor-recipient reciprocal graft transplants. One aliquot from each individual is treated with irradiation or mitomycin C to inhibit DNA synthesis. The other aliquot is untreated. Mixing different aliquots from different individuals results in a one-way test of the treated lymphocytes' capacity to stimulate blast cell transformation in untreated lymphocytes. If many transformations are observed, it indicates that the donated tissue would be rapidly (acutely) rejected; if few transformations are observed, it indicates that a longer time would be required for the graft to be rejected (chronic rejection). In clinical practice, reciprocal transplants are rarely performed, but the technique can be modified to accommodate one-way transplants.

controls) are collected, purified, and injected into the skin (normally containing few, if any, lymphocytes) of one or more potential donors (Figure 10.11). After one or two days the inoculation sites are observed for inflammation. The degree of incompatibility is indicated by the diameter of the reaction zone and the intensity of the erythema. The individual exhibiting the least NLT reaction in comparison with those of the controls would be the best source of tissue for the recipient among those tested. In this test, the normal lymphocytes of the recipient would recognize any incompatible histocompatibility antigens of the potential donor and elicit an inflammatory immunological skin response, the intensity of which usually would be predictive of the rate of graft rejection. However, individuals with certain diseases may have lymphocytes that exhibit little or no reactivity in the NLT. For example, patients with severe kidney diseases may have nonreactive lymphocytes in the NLT. This is unfortunate because these are the people who most need kidney transplants. There is also some risk in subjecting potential donors to lymphocytes from patients with diagnosed or potential malignancies. Because of these and other limitations, the NLT is not as widely used as the MLC, and the compatibility tests as a group are not as widely used as the serological tests.

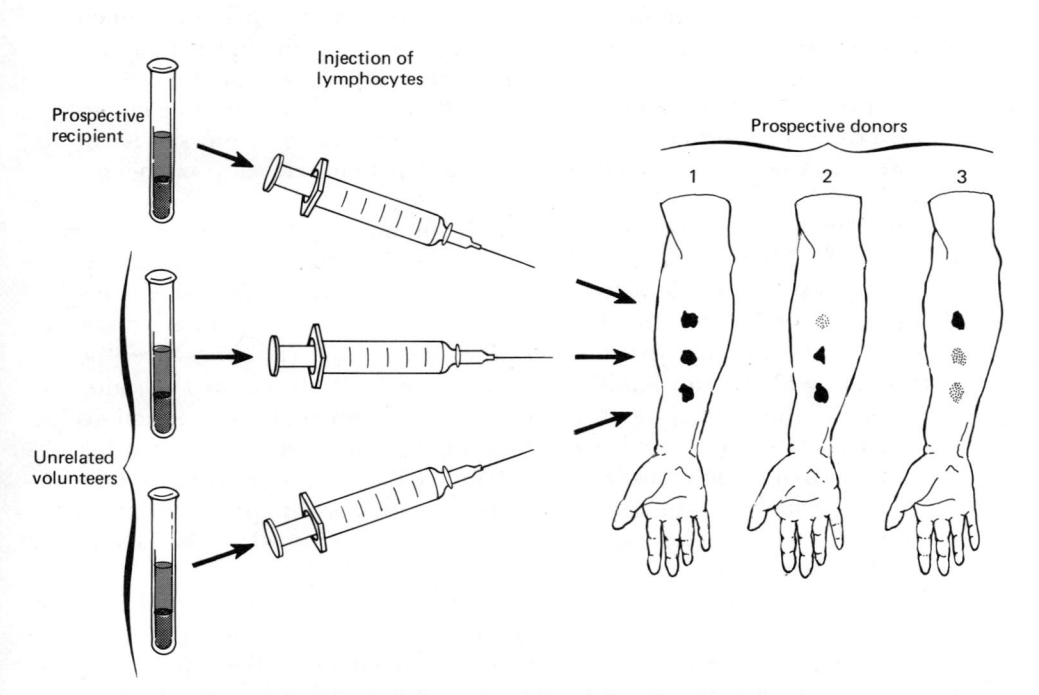

FIGURE 10.11. Normal lymphocyte transfer (NLT) test. Lymphocytes are harvested from the prospective graft recipient and from several volunteers (unrelated to the recipient, to the group of potential donors, or to each other). Each cell preparation is injected intradermally into a group of prospective donors. After about two days the skin reactions are evaluated. The best choice for donor among the tested group is the person displaying the least reaction from the prospective recipient's lymphocytes in comparison with those of the controls (unrelated volunteers) on the same person. Number 2 is the best choice in this example.

Immunosuppression

Aside from grafts between identical siblings, the only transplants with any chance of survival in humans are well-matched allografts. For reasons given previously, it is virtually impossible to find a donor with exactly the same histocompatibility antigens as that of the intended recipient. The best that can be done is to select a donor having the least number of antigenic differences with the recipient. Even grafts with only minor histoincompatibilities will be rejected eventually (chronically) unless the immune defenses of the host are somehow compromised. Therefore, virtually all human allograft recipients require **immunosuppression.** Immunosuppressive agents fall into three major categories: (1) radiation, (2) chemicals, and (3) biologicals.

Whole body radiation can nullify the immune system, but it also can interfere with mitotic activity and the replenishment of vital organs such as bone marrow. This alone is a potentially lethal condition. Localized radiation of the graft and extracorporal (outside the body) radiation of the recipient's blood aid in prolonging graft survival times. Radiation as a single agent, however, is relatively ineffective. Better results are usually obtained when it is combined with chemical and/or biological immune suppressors. During times when the immune system is suppressed, the patient is much more susceptible to pathogens and cancer. Most of the deaths of immunologically suppressed transplant patients result from bacterial, viral, and/or fungal infections. Since radiation and/or immunosuppressive chemicals are used (in addition to surgery) for the treatment of tumors, it is not surprising that about 2 percent of transplant patients develop oncogenic complications.

Many chemicals function to suppress the immune system by interfering with DNA or RNA synthesis and hence nonspecifically also retard mitotic and protein-synthesizing activities of all cells. Drugs such as 6-mercaptopurine and 5-fluorouracil are classified as base analogs of normally occurring purines and pyrimidines. Purines and pyrimidines are the basic building blocks (nucleotides) of nucleic acids. With the incorporation of analogs of the normal bases, normal template and replicative functions of nucleic acids are disrupted. Some base analogs interfere with the synthesis of the normal nucleotides from lower-molecular-weight precursors. One of the most widely used chemicals of this group is azathioprine (Imuran) whose side group (a substituted imidazole ring) is removed by the host to produce 6-mercaptopurine.

Another group of immunosuppressive chemicals contains the folic acid antagonists. Amethopterin (Methotrexate) and aminopterin inhibit tetrahydrofolic acid, which is an essential intermediate in the synthesis of purines. Nucleotide analogs and folic acid antagonists are classified as **antimetabolites.** These are synthetic compounds similar to those that nourish cells. Attempts by the cell to use these substances instead of normal metabolites result in interruption of biosynthetic pathways.

Alkylating agents such as the sulfur and nitrogen mustards can cross-link guanine-cytosine base pairs in DNA, thereby preventing dissociation of the strands during replication. Alkylation of amino groups on adenine and especially on guanine could cause misreading during transcription into mRNA and thereby produce aberrant proteins. Lymphocyte precursor cells treated with alkylating agents cannot divide, resulting in lymphocytopenia (fewer than the normal number of lymphocytes). Because the effects of these chemicals so closely parallel those seen after irradiation, they are sometimes referred to as **radiomimetic drugs.**

Corticosteroids such as cortisol and cortisone are used to treat delayed-type (T cell–mediated) hypersensitivity reactions. They generally exhibit anti-inflammatory properties by causing lymphocytolysis, depressing phagocytosis, and inhibiting cell division. These steroids also interfere with antibody production (mainly IgG of the primary response). Because steroids suppress IgG production much more than that of IgM, this has been interpreted as evidence that these two classes of antibodies are produced by different cell populations. Many other kinds of chemicals (antibiotics, enzymes, plant alkaloids, etc.) also have immunosuppressive activities. Some chemicals are most effective only when given prior to transplantation; others are more effective either at the time of or just after transplantation; still others are effective either before or after transplantation. Timing and dosage of drug administration is critical for maximal benefit to the patient.

Antilymphocyte serum (ALS), antilymphocyte globulin (ALG), and anti-T lymphocyte (antithymocyte) serum (ATS) are the most widely used biological immunosuppressive agents. ALS is usually prepared by immunizing a heterologous species with cells from spleen, thymus, lymph nodes, or blood. It contains antibodies not only to lymphocytes but to many other types of cells as well. Most of the extraneous antibodies can be removed from ALS by adsorption with homologous kidney or liver antigens. The adsorbed serum still contains many extraneous proteins that can be eliminated by purifying the globulin fraction (ALG). An even more specific antithymocyte serum can be prepared by using thoracic duct lymphocytes as the source of antigen. It can also be purified to the globulin fraction as antithymocyte globulin (ATG). The immunosuppressive effect of these preparations is most pronounced when given to the patient prior to transplantation. Larger doses result in greater immunosuppression. The exact mechanism(s) by which ALS becomes effective are not known. It seems to reduce the numbers of both B and T lymphocytes. The "blindfolding hypothesis" proposes that ALS antibodies combine with lymphocytes and the coated cells become masked from recognizing the foreign antigens of the transplant. It is also possible that both of these mechanisms, as well as others, operate in unison. Severe local hypersensitivity reactions are commonly observed in patients who receive ALS intramuscularly. If given intravenously, fever and mild systemic anaphylactic shock and serum sickness symptoms develop. These problems usually necessitate termination of ALS treatment within a few weeks after transplantation. Furthermore, precipitating antibodies soon may develop to the foreign proteins in ALS that probably reduce if not completely neutralize its effectiveness. This really leaves only the chemicals as the long-term immunosuppressive agents in practical usage. There is considerable variation in immunosuppressive action from one ALS preparation to another. It has been very difficult to assay the effectiveness of these antilymphocyte sera, and there is little agreement among immunologists as to which methods of production and assay are best for humans.

Immunological Privilege

Immunologically privileged sites are anatomical locations into which transplants from the same or different species may be made with success. Perhaps the best-known example in experimental immunology is the cheek pouch of the hamster. These saclike cavities are located along the jaw and extend to the shoulder. They serve as storage areas for food gathered during foraging excursions and transport back to the animal's den. The contents of the pouch are then disgorged by manipulation of the front legs. Although the lining of the cheek pouch is highly vascularized, it has a poor lymphatic drainage system. This seems to be the essential feature of all privileged sites. Even xenografts of human tissue can survive when transplanted to the hamster cheek pouch. Of medical interest, the cornea of the eye (and perhaps also the anterior chamber of the eye) is a privileged site. The cornea is an avascular tissue. Corneal transplants are highly successful if care is taken to avoid contact with vascular tissues. Tissues of the brain and central nervous system are also considered to be immunologically privileged sites. The so-called "blood-brain barrier" separates the brain and cerebrospinal fluid from the blood. The barrier sites in the choroid plexus, the blood vessels of the brain and subarachnoid space, and the arachnoid membrane that overlies the subarachnoid space are characterized by vascular tight junctions that normally prohibit leukocytes from entering the nervous system. T lymphocytes may enter the brain in certain viral and autoallergic diseases, but it is not clear what fraction migrates between endothelial cells and what fraction migrates through them (a process called **emperipolesis**). Relatively low levels of protein exist in CSF (0.4 percent of plasma levels). The barrier normally restricts the entry of immunoglobulins, especially the larger ones (19S, class IgM). However, in some CNS diseases, the level of immunoglobulins in CSF is elevated, presumably from stimulation of lymphocytes within the brain. Transplants of brain tissue are of little medical use at present.

Immunologically privileged tissues are those that survive as allografts or xenografts regardless of where they are transplanted. These tissues usually consist of structural elements that survive even after the cells from which they were formed have died. Dense connective tissues of extracellular fibers form the matrix of bones, cartilage, tendons, and ligaments. Looser connective tissues form the matrix of heart valves and major blood vessels. If the living components of these grafted tissues are destroyed by the immune system of the host, they may be replaced by cells of the host.

There may be no advantage in using allografts of bone or cartilage for their structural qualities over the use of stainless steel pins or plastic replacement parts. Pig hearts are about the same size as human hearts, and it is from this source that transplants are often obtained to replace human heart valves. In this instance, the flexibility of natural heart valves gives superior performance to synthetic valves. Ball-in-chamber artificial valves are noisy and damage blood cells every time they snap closed. Even though the cellular elements of privileged grafts may be dead, they still possess antigens that can sensitize the recipient. This can make it more difficult to find a compatible match if at some subsequent time the individual needs a blood transfusion or a tissue graft. Prosthetic devices are therefore often preferred over the use of privileged tissue grafts. A **prosthesis** (-ses, plural) is an artificial replacement for any part of the body.

One of the most enigmatic immunological conditions in nature is the failure of a mother to reject the foreign tissue antigens of her baby. Half of the heredity of a baby is derived from the father. Therefore, there are usually at least several strong histocompatibility differences between the fetus and its mother. The exact mechanism(s) that protects the fetus from attack by maternal T lymphocytes is incompletely known. It is believed that mucoproteins in the trophoblastic layer of the placenta act as an impermeable barrier to maternal lymphoid cells. It is of interest to note that the amount of trophoblastic mucoproteins produced by the fetus seems to increase in proportion to the degree of antigenic incompatibility with its mother. The developing fetus is an example of an immunologically privileged tissue that can survive only when orthotopically transplanted into its normal location (a "prepared" uterus).

Oncoimmunology

Cancer is second only to heart disease as the leading cause of deaths in the United States, followed by stroke and accidents (Figure 10.12). Certain parts of the body are more likely than other parts to incur cancer and be responsible for death (Figure 10.13). Everyone should know the seven warning signals of cancer.

C hange in bowel or bladder habits
A sore that does not heal
U nusual bleeding or discharge
T hickening or lumps in breast or elsewhere
I ndigestion or difficulty in swallowing
O bvious change in wart or mole
N agging cough or hoarseness

A "lump" (fourth danger sign) may be either a cyst or a tumor. A **cyst** is an abnormal collection of fluid within a sac or wall. If the duct of a gland becomes plugged and the gland continues to secrete, a retention cyst is

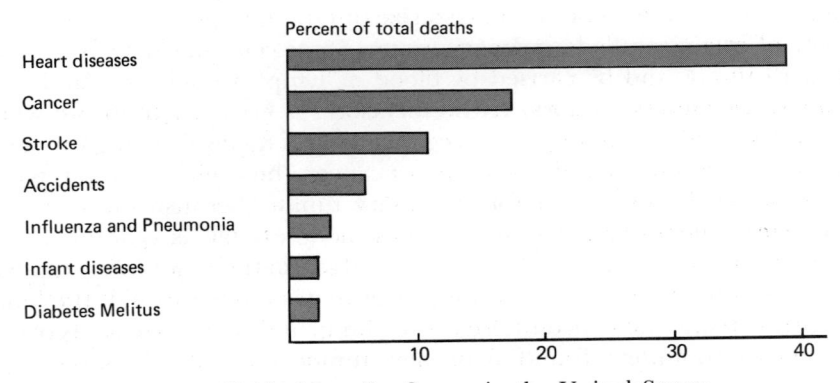

FIGURE 10.12. Mortality factors in the United States.

Serology and Immunology

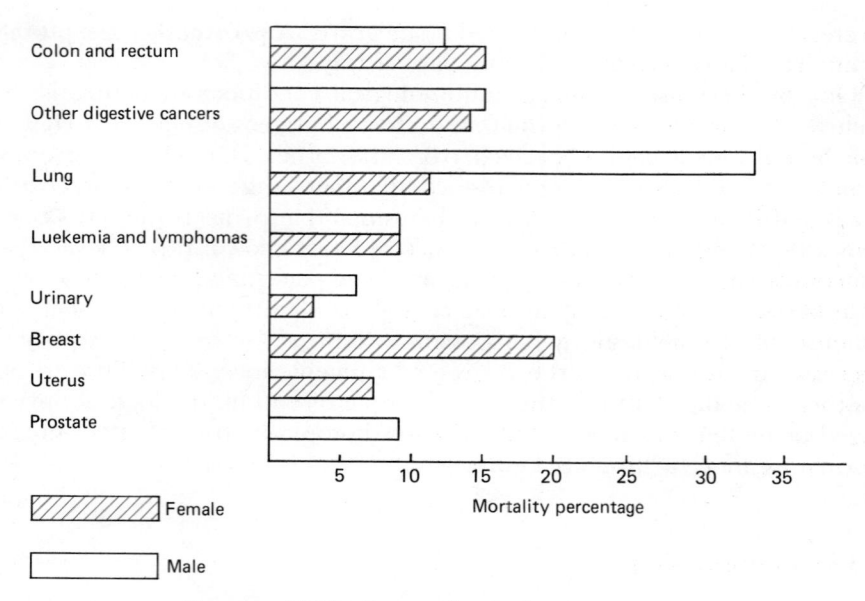

Site	
Colon and rectum	~12 (M), ~15 (F)
Other digestive cancers	~15 (M), ~14 (F)
Lung	~33 (M), ~11 (F)
Leukemia and lymphomas	~9 (M), ~9 (F)
Urinary	~6 (M), ~3 (F)
Breast	~20 (F)
Uterus	~7 (F)
Prostate	~9 (M)

FIGURE 10.13. Cancer deaths by site and sex.

formed. A common example is a sebaceous cyst. Cestodal parasites, such as *Echinococcus granulosus,* cause hydatid cysts, which are commonly found in the liver and are often of great size. A **tumor** is a "lump" of new and unusual tissue growth (**neoplasm**). **Benign** (nonmalignant) tumors may be discomforting or unsightly (e.g., "warts"), but often may be self-limiting and nonfatal. However, in some cases (e.g., benign brain tumors) they may be indirectly fatal by crowding and/or pressure effects on circulation to normal tissues. A large benign tumor of the bowel might cause a fatal obstruction. Certain brain tumors are inoperable, but most other benign tumors can be "cured" by surgical removal. **Malignant** tumors, on the other hand, are uncontrollable growths that tend to disseminate and/or tend to recur after removal and are almost always fatal without treatment. In many cases, the lifespans of patients with malignancies can be significantly prolonged through a combination of treatments with surgery, radiation, and chemotherapy.

A **cancer** is a malignant neoplasm manifesting invasiveness of surrounding tissues and a tendency to **metastasize** (migrate) to new sites. A tumor in its site of origin is called a **primary tumor.** Some cells may detach from the primary tumor and be carried by blood or lymph to new sites and there establish **secondary tumors.** If the metastasis is via the lymph, we would look for secondary tumors in the regional lymph nodes draining the site of the primary tumor. In the case of breast cancer, the axillary (armpit) lymph nodes would be examined for secondary tumors because the lymphatic drainage of the breast flows through these nodes. If cancer cells metastasize through the blood, they tend to become lodged in the first venous capillary bed encountered. Thus, if a breast cancer metastasizes through the blood, the first capillary bed encountered is the lung, and that is where secondary cancers are commonly found. A primary tumor of the abdomen is likely to be carried by the portal venous system to the liver, etc. A **sarcoma** is a cancer of nonepithelial connective tissues. Osteosarcoma (bone), lymphosarcoma (lymphoid tissue), and neurogenic sarcoma (nerve fibers) are examples. A **carcinoma** is a cancer of epithelial tissue, exemplified by skin cancer and adenocarcinoma (gland epithelium). A **leukemia** is a cancer of hematopoietic tissues that results in progressive proliferation of abnormal leukocytes, commonly detected by abnormally high white blood cell counts.

CANCER ETIOLOGY

It was pointed out earlier in this chapter that immunological surveillance against cancer is thought to be partly related to shared histocompatibility antigens of normal and cancer cells of the host. However, when normal cells become transformed into cancer cells, unusual antigens commonly appear on the neoplastic cells. A healthy immune system should be able to recognize the neoplastic antigen(s) as foreign and destroy the cancer cells before they become a recognizable tumor. It is easy to see why cancers are more prevalent in immunologically compromised individuals. It is more difficult to understand why cancers develop in individuals with apparently healthy immune systems. A partial explanation may involve the enhancing antibodies discussed earlier in this chapter. If these antibodies are unable to activate the complement system, they may occupy receptor sites on tumor cells and block recognition of their "foreignness" by cytolytic antibodies and/or T lymphocytes. It is possible for neoplastic cells to arise without the appearance of neoantigens. Many other factors must surely be involved in the escape of cancer from immune surveillance, but what they are remains a mystery.

Some mice strains have a much higher incidence of certain types of cancer than other strains. This is evidence for a genetic predisposition to develop cancer in those animals. It seems reasonable to expect that genetic predisposition to develop some cancers also occurs in humans. Indeed, some cancers display a familial tendency, i.e., affecting several members of the same family. It is now known that a translocation between a chromosome number three and a chromosome number eight is associated with a certain kind of kidney cancer.

In addition to hereditary factors, some environmental factors are also known to predispose to certain cancers. Smoking is a predisposing factor to the development of lung cancer. Excessive exposure of the skin to ultraviolet rays is a predisposing factor to skin cancer. Inhalation of asbestos fibers is a likely cause of mesothelioma (a cancer of membranes lining the chest and abdominal cavities).

Carcinogens are substances known to induce cancers. Many (if not most) of them are known to be mutagens, i.e., substances capable of causing genetic changes or mutations. There are undoubtedly many genes involved in the mitotic process and in the control of cell division. Conceptually, a mutation in several or many of these genes could result in loss of regulation over cell proliferation and permit cancerous growth.

Viruses can also cause tumors. A papovavirus is responsible in humans for the benign skin tumors called warts; a poxvirus is responsible for the benign skin tumors called molluscum contagiosum. Virally induced cancers are known in mice and other animals, and a virus is highly suspected in at least one human cancer (Burkitt's lymphoma).

Serology and Immunology

Burkitt's lymphoma is primarily a cancer of the jaw, associated facial bones, and abdominal organs of children in the mosquito belt of central Africa. Particles indistinguishable from the Epstein-Barr virus (EBV, a DNA virus of the herpes group) have been seen in electron micrographs of cultured Burkitt cells. Furthermore, high antibody titers to EBV capsid antigens and to lymphoma cell antigens have been found in both Burkitt's lymphoma patients and those suffering from infectious mononucleosis. It is unknown why EBV infections in some cases produce a relatively mild disease (infectious mononucleosis) and in other cases a severe and potentially lethal disease (Burkitt's lymphoma). It is hypothesized that some infections with EBV early in infancy might transform immature B lymphocytes so that they can continue to replicate and eventually give rise to lymphoma cells. Under primitive conditions, most primary infections with EBV occur at an early age and usually cause no significant illness unless the individual is already infected with malaria. Malarial infections are known to suppress the immune system and thereby enhance the proliferation of EBV-transformed lymphocytes. In more economically advanced societies, improved hygiene may delay primary infections with EBV until late childhood or adolescence when people are more likely to develop mononucleosis. Most American cases of Burkitt's lymphoma, however, cannot be associated with either malaria and/or EBV; neither viral-DNA positive cells nor Epstein-Barr nuclear antigen-positive cells have been detected in the tumors, and the patients have antibody profiles comparable to those of normal children. Long-term remissions have been induced in patients with Burkitt's lymphoma treated with the alkylating agent cyclophosphamide. Spontaneous remissions of tumors have been reported in patients with Burkitt's lymphoma and choriocarcinoma and probably also occur in other neoplastic diseases.

Oncogenic viruses can be thought of as supplying new nuclear nucleic acid to infected cells. When the virus enters the cell, it may shed its protein coat, and its genetic material may become integrated into the host chromosome as a **provirus.** For all practical purposes, the virus disappears because it has now become part of the host genome. Since the host genome has acquired new genetic material, it qualifies as a mutant cell. A provirus may trigger transformation of the cell into a malignant state. Some viruses, especially the RNA tumor viruses, form proviruses that are defective in part of their genome. These defective proviruses may be able to induce cancer but cannot replicate autonomously. It is also possible for a complete provirus to be released from the host chromosome (excision, deintegration) and begin replication of infective **virions** (complete virus particles). In this case, the virus would likely cause symptoms of viral disease rather than cancer.

Viruses can be serologically identified by three types of antigens. Antigens of the coat proteins are **viral antigens.** Viruses that have shed their coat proteins can no longer be detected serologically by these indicators. The virus seems to have "disappeared." The genetic material of RNA tumor viruses codes for an enzyme called RNA-dependent DNA-polymerase (reverse transciptase) that makes a DNA copy of the viral RNA. A part of the DNA copy can then become integrated into the host DNA. Murine (mice) and avian (bird) RNA tumor viruses may, in some instances, continue to replicate infectious virions within transformed cells so that viral antigens are serologically detectable. Oncogenic RNA viruses, or at least the genes that can potentially transform a normal cell into a tumor cell, may be vertically transmitted (from parents to offspring) via infected eggs or milk or while *in utero*. Since the viral antigens might be present in the offspring when self-determination occurs, these individuals would show immunological tolerance toward the tumor. DNA viruses, on the other hand, tend to become proviruses without intracellular multiplication to produce complete virions. Viral antigens would therefore seldom be found in tumors induced by DNA viruses.

Virally infected cells commonly display two new kinds of antigens not found in virions. One group of antigens associated only with certain viruses (most notably SV40 and polyoma viruses) is found in the cell nucleus and is referred to as **T antigens** (originally "tumor" antigens). Some of these T antigens may be virus-induced enzymes. The host may respond by making anti-T immunoglobulins, but these antibodies usually cannot penetrate the virally infected cells and so cannot contribute to tumor immunity. The presence of these antibodies cannot tell us if cell transformation has taken place. It is important to bear in mind that the presence of an oncogenic virus within a host does not necessarily mean that a tumor has been induced.

The second group of antigens found in virally infected cells and in most transformed cells, termed **tumor-specific antigens** (TSA) or **tumor-specific transplantation antigens** (TSTA), is located in the plasma membrane. Each kind of oncogenic virus seems to control specific host genes so that all tumors produced by that kind of virus bear the same unique antigen. B lymphocytes respond by producing anti-TSA, but the titer of these antibodies has little correlation with tumor immunity. Antitumor antibodies of all kinds seem to contribute little to tumor immunity, and some of them (enhancing antibodies) may actually favor the growth of the tumor. It is still a mystery why some tumors can escape T lymphocyte responses but cannot escape B lymphocyte responses. It is, of course, the T lymphocytes and macrophages that are primarily responsible for immunological surveillance and tumor regression. Perhaps the TSA are relatively weak antigens to a particular host and do not stimulate a strong immunity. Maybe the mutant malignant cell has a very rapid growth rate that produces new tumor cells faster than the immune system can destroy them. Tumors often develop in individuals with depressed T lymphocytic immunity, as in the very young or old or in those that are immunosuppressed.

The chemicals used to treat cancer are those that interfere with rapidly multiplying cells. Unfortunately, their action is nonspecific and thus they may interfere with cell division generally, including cells of the immune system. Therefore, anticancer drugs are also immunosuppressants. Some primary tumors can be treated by surgical removal. If the primary tumor has metastasized to various places in the body, it is not feasible to locate and remove all of the secondary growths. The situation is usually inoperable and often terminal. One reason large tumors should be removed surgically, if possible, is because **antigen overloading** (synonymous with "immunological tolerance," "acquired tolerance," and "immunological unresponsiveness") can contribute to **immunological paralysis.** This is a specific depression of immune response against only the excessive antigen(s). Removal of the excess antigen restores function to that segment of the immune system.

Serology and Immunology

The mechanism of immunological paralysis is poorly understood. If the tumor size is reduced by surgery, a stimulated immune system may be able to dispose of a few remaining cancer cells.

SEROLOGICAL INDICATORS OF CANCER

Each type of oncogenic virus induces its own unique TSA that is constant from one host to another (within the same species) regardless of the tissue in which it is expressed. On the other hand, chemically induced tumor antigens are unpredictable both within and between individuals. Regardless of the etiology of a tumor, neoplastic cells often incur a biosythetic shift from an adult to an immature (fetal) pathway of protein production. Hence, the identification of fetal proteins (antigens) in an adult patient may be indicative that an oncogenic condition exists. These antigens are variously termed **carcinofetal, carcinoembryonic,** or **regression proteins.** One of the best-known regression proteins is called **carcinoembryonic antigen** (CEA). It is a glycoprotein of molecular weight 100,000 to 200,000 containing about 50 percent carbohydrate and travels electrophoretically with the beta globulins. Its function during embryogenesis is unknown. This antigen was originally identified by immunodiffusion tests, but now is more commonly detected by a much more sensitive radioimmunoassay. It was formerly believed that CEA was diagnostic for colon cancers, but this has been proven incorrect. It appears in many types of cancerous and nonmalignant conditions (Figure 10.14). However, titers of CEA can be monitored to indicate the effectiveness of cancer therapy. If the titer of CEA drops after surgery and/or chemotherapy and then rises again, it indicates that all of

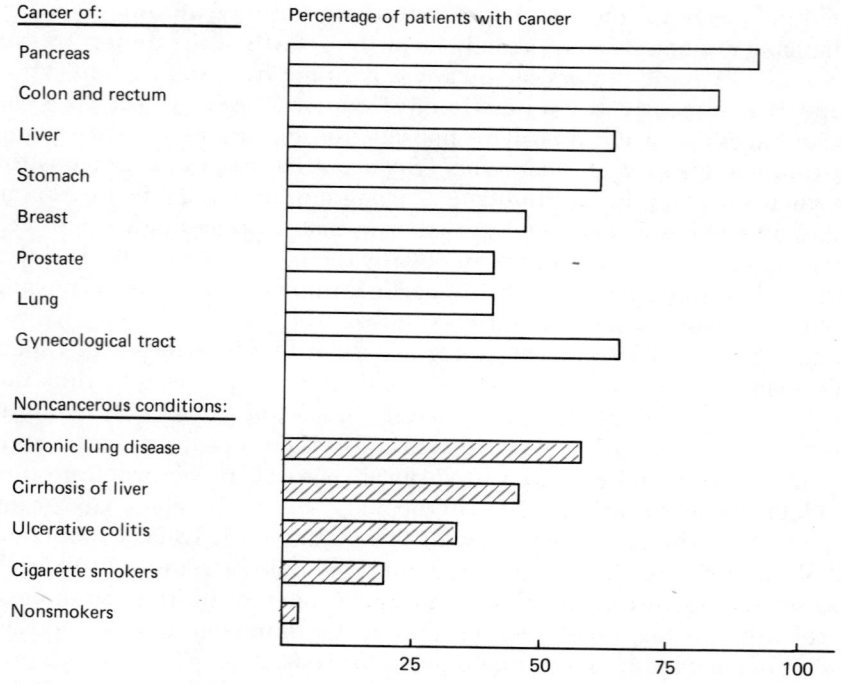

FIGURE 10.14. Incidence of carcinoembryonic antigen (CEA) in people with and without cancer.

the neoplastic cells were not removed or killed; some remained and are proliferating and synthesizing this regression protein.

Since CEA tends to be produced more by tumors than by normal tissues, it has been possible to help identify cancerous regions of the body by injecting radioactively labeled anti-CEA antibodies and monitoring the patient with a gamma scintillation camera. For example, if a lung tumor is synthesizing large amounts of CEA, the radioantibodies would mainly congregate in the vicinity of the tumor. Tumor imaging by the camera has correlated well with some X-ray diagnoses of lung tumors. There are still some problems with the technique, however. For example, brain cancer detected by computerized tomography has not been detected by radioantibody scan because the antibodies cannot pass the blood-brain barrier. Lymphocytic lymphomas are a type of cancer that do not synthesize CEA and therefore cannot be detected by this technique. Despite its limitations, it may prove to be a useful adjunct to other diagnostic tests.

Several other regression proteins are known to be produced irregularly by various cancerous and nonmalignant conditions. **Alpha fetoprotein** (AFP) is produced quite regularly in patients with hepatocarcinoma (liver cancer), but it is also found in cases of viral hepatitis, extrahepatic tumors (lung, stomach, pancreas), and ataxia telangiectasia. AFP is an α_1 globulin of about 70,000 daltons and very similar in biophysical properties to albumin, making its purification a difficult problem. As with most regression proteins, the biological function of AFP is unknown. It is produced by the yolk sac and fetal liver and can be detected in the amniotic fluid. After the fourteenth week of gestation, the amount of AFP normally decreases gradually. It may be increased, however, by as much as eight times the normal level in a fetus with a neural tube defect such as anencephaly or spina bifida. AFP is known to bind to T lymphocytes, and this union could block interaction of the lymphocyte with target cell antigens (including cancer cell antigens).

Another regression protein produced by hepatomas, other tumors, and nonmalignant diseases is alpha-2 hepatic protein (AHP), also named α_2 hepatic globulin or α_2 ferroglycoprotein. It has a high iron content and may be identical to a carcinofetal form of ferritin.

Isozymes (isoenzymes) are enzymes that catalyze the same reaction (functionally identical) but exhibit differences in some of their physicochemical properties such as electrophoretic mobility and antigenicity. Several enzymes (including alkaline phosphatase, glycogen phosphorylase, and aldolase) are known to be produced as different isozymes in fetal and adult stages. As hepatomas develop (and possibly other tumors as well), there tends to be a shift in the serum concentration from adult to fetal isozymes. All of these regression proteins are of potential diagnostic value but must be used in conjunction with other clinical findings.

Choriocarcinoma may develop after a normal pregnancy or from hydatidiform moles. These are tumors of the chorionic membrane of the placenta. A normal endocrine function of the chorion is to produce chorionic gonadotropin. Serological tests for this hormone in serum or urine are the basis of pregnancy tests. Excessive levels of this hormone could be attributed to a choriocarcinoma or a hydatidiform mole. However, elevated titers of HCG are also sometimes found in patients with diabetes and toxemia of pregnancy as well as in Rh-sensitized women.

PROPHYLACTIC POSSIBILITIES

The antiviral lymphokine interferon has been shown to be effective in preventing multiplication of certain cancer cells in mice. Perhaps further research along these lines will eventually lead to its use in preventions or cures for certain cancers in humans. One of the goals of recombinant DNA research is to incorporate the genes for human interferon production into bacterial or tissue culture cells and thereby cause these biological "factories" to manufacture it efficiently and inexpensively for routine clinical use.

It may be possible to nonspecifically elevate the activity of the entire immune system and thereby obtain greater numbers of tumor remissions. One of the most intensively studied adjuvants for this purpose is BCG (bacille Calmette-Guérin). This vaccine is an attenuated strain of *Mycobacterium bovis*. It seems to be most effective when injected into or very near the tumor. Animal experiments with BCG have often given favorable results as an antitumor vaccine. However, its effectiveness in humans has not yet been satisfactorily established. One theory proposes that BCG shares some antigens with certain tumors and therefore the vaccination stimulates a cross-reactive ("specific") immune response. Other theories propose that BCG has an adjuvant-like effect, nonspecifically activates B and/or T lymphocytes, makes macrophages "angry," or stimulates trapping of lymphocytes in regional lymph nodes draining the injection site. Experimental evidence exists to support each of these theories. In those cases where BCG has helped cancer patients, it is thought that killer T cells may have been stimulated to attack the tumors. In those cases where BCG has not helped cancer patients (or even occasionally has decreased their immune responses), it is proposed that suppressor T cells have been activated. Patients with the autoimmune disease called lupus erythematosus possess defective suppressor T cells. There is some evidence that distinctive antigens may exist on suppressor T cells. If antibodies can be produced against these antigens, it may be possible to employ them to nullify the activity of suppressor T cells in certain cancer patients, thereby allowing the killer T cells to affect tumor destruction. Such responses may, however, be accompanied by an increased incidence of autoallergic conditions.

Development of specific tumor vaccines is fraught with numerous difficulties. Even if specific vaccines could be obtained, there are so many different tumor-associated antigens that it is not feasible to immunize everyone against all of them. Use of autogenous tumor vaccines has been suggested, but it is difficult to understand how a cancer patient could benefit from additional exposure to his own tumor antigens. Injection of live tumor cells might establish secondary tumors and harm the patient. Nonetheless, experiments in mice have shown that the treatment of tumor cells with the enzyme neuraminidase produces a potent live-cell vaccine that stimulates both T lymphocytes and complement-fixing antitumor antibodies. These enzymatic treatments may remove specific and/or nonspecific blocking factors that shield some surface antigens from recognition by immune cells. Some degree of success has also been obtained with neuraminidase-treated human tumor vaccines, but more study is warranted. Immunization with dead tumor cells or antigenic cell fractions might adsorb all of the free enhancing (blocking) antibodies and leave some antigen free to stimulate aggressive lymphocytes. Uncommitted T lymphocytes could be artificially stimulated by exposure to concanavalin A or transfer factor (TF) or "immune RNA" derived from sensitized lymphocytes. Experimental results thus far with these substances have been equivocal. Nonetheless, many cancer researchers are looking to immunology for the ultimate weapons in the fight against this heterogeneous group of diseases.

SELF-EVALUATION

Terms

1. A graft between genetically dissimilar members of the same species.
2. The class of lymphokines that cause destruction of target tissues.
3. The phenomenon of an immunologically competent individual being unresponsive to one or more potentially antigenic substances (e.g., as a result of the presence of these substances during the period when immunological competency is attained) that under other circumstances would be capable of inducing an immune response. (2 words)
4. A synonym for runting disease or wasting disease, induced by injecting adult lymphocytes into newborn mice. (2 words)
5. General name for antigens involved in graft rejection phenomena.
6. The prolongation of graft survival attributed to "blocking antibodies."
7. Strains of laboratory animals that differ from one another by only one or a few selected traits.
8. The totality of antigenic products of the HLA genes transmitted by a gamete.
9. General term for immunosuppressive chemicals that are easily mistaken by cells for normal constituents (e.g., nucleotide base analogs) and interfere with normal biochemical processes (especially those involved in mitosis).
10. Fetal antigens, often produced by adults with cancers. (2 words)

Multiple Choice. Choose the one best answer.

1. Major histocompatibility antigens in the mouse are products of the H-2 genetic locus designated (a) S (b) I (c) K (d) more than one of these (e) all of these
2. The strongest correlation between a disease and an HLA antigen found to date involves (a) myasthenia gravis (b) Graves' disease (c) ankylosing spondylitis (d) glomerulonephritis (e) multiple sclerosis
3. Which of the following is not considered to be an immunosuppressant? (a) Imuran (b) antihistamines (c) corticosteroids (d) ALS (e) folic acid antagonists
4. Which of the following is not an immunologically privileged site? (a) brain (b) hamster cheek pouch (c) cornea (d) trophoblastic layer of the placenta (e) glomerulus of the kidney
5. Which of the following is not one of the seven warning signs of cancer? (a) persistent nasal discharge (b) a sore that does not heal (c) change in a wart or mole (d) change in bowel or urinary habits (e) difficulty in swallowing
6. A form of cancer that is most probably caused by a virus is (a) hepatoma (b) mesothelioma (c) Huntington's chorea (d) Burkitt's lymphoma (e) ataxia telangiectasia
7. Which of the following is a nonspecific enhancer of immune responsiveness? (a) neuraminidase (b) TF (c) alpha fetoprotein (d) BCG (e) beta microglobulin
8. The most widely used serological test for HLA typing is a form of (a) toxin neutralization (b) immune enhancement (c) complement-mediated cytotoxicity (d) leukoagglutination (e) fluorescent antibody technique
9. Which of the following grafts is most likely to be rejected by a HVG reaction? (a) heterotopic autograft (b) syngraft (c) adult lymphocytes grafted into a

neonatally thymectomized mouse (d) graft of an F_1 to an F_2 from highly inbred strains of mice (e) skin graft of a boy onto his twin sister
10. Which of the following is classified as a compatibility test for HLA antigens? (a) MLR (b) NLT (c) "third-man" test (d) more than one of these (e) all of these

True-False

1. Too much of a given antigen can overload the immune system, rendering the individual temporarily in a state of "immunological paralysis" and unresponsive to any antigenic challenge by the same or different antigens.
2. Most deaths of transplant patients are ultimately attributable to the effects of immunosuppressant treatments.
3. Antigens of the D region of the MHC in humans are lymphocyte-detectable.
4. ABO incompatibility between donor and recipient is not an important consideration as far as survival of tissue grafts is concerned.
5. Transplantation antigens of the mouse K and D regions are serologically detectable.
6. Ia antigens are products of the Ir genes in mice and found predominantly on T cells.
7. The HLA-D region of the human MHC appears to be the functional equivalent of the H-2I region of the mouse MHC.
8. HLA typing is potentially much more useful in resolving cases of disputed parentage than ABO blood typing.
9. Viral-induced TSA antigens are restricted to the host cell nucleus.
10. Anticancer drugs are also immunosuppressants.

Quality Control in Serological Testing

APPENDIX

There are at least four criteria by which the credibility of a serological test is measured: (1) sensitivity, (2) specificity, (3) accuracy, and (4) precision. The smallest amount of substance that can be detected constitutes the **sensitivity** of the test. Thus, a radioimmunoassay that can detect picogram (10^{-12}) quantities of an antigen is about a million times more sensitive than an immunodiffusion test that only measures microgram (10^{-6}) quantities of the same antigen. The concentrations of many substances have no clinical importance unless they become elevated above a critical value, called the "threshold of significance." In such cases, there is no need to employ tests with "limits of detection" below the threshold of significance. Whatever test is used should be able to discriminate between small changes in the concentrations of immune substances within a patient as a function of time. Such findings can aid the physician in diagnosing the cause of a disease and/or the patient's response to therapy. If a test fails to detect the substance in a sample that actually contains it, the result is said to be a "false negative." If the sample is known by other laboratory tests to contain the substance (or if the clinical symptoms of the patient indicate that the substance should be present), the sample is considered to be a "true positive." From these two kinds of specimens it is possible to calculate an "index of sensitivity" for each test.

$$\text{Index of sensitivity} = \frac{\text{true positives} - \text{false negatives}}{\text{true positives}} \times 100$$

False positive results may be produced by a serological test that is "out of control" with respect to such potentially manageable factors as temperature, pH, ionicity, incubation times, centrifugal forces and centrifuge times, age of specimen, the addition of substances to the specimen prior to the test (e.g., anticoagulants), the administration of drugs (therapeutic or otherwise) to the patient prior to the test, etc. In addition to these "extrinsic" factors, there may be "intrinsic" factors over which there is no potential control. The patient may possess naturally occurring immunological substances (or may have acquired them as a result of infection by a different organism than the one under test, or from the environment) that interfere with or cross-react with the serological reagents used in the test. The reactivity of a specimen due to one or more extraneous intrinsic factors is classified as a **biological false positive** (BFP). For example, there are several identical or closely related antigens shared by species of *Histoplasma, Blastomyces, Brucella,* and *Francisella* that elicit antibodies that cross-react to various degrees with all of those species possessing the corresponding antigens. As a general rule, the patient's serum tends to give stronger reactions with the organism (or antigen) that caused his disease, and in this sense the homologous antigen-antibody recognition is behaving specifically. However, to the degree that false positive results are produced, the **specificity** of the test would appear to be relatively poor. Specimens obtained from people considered by clinical symptoms or other laboratory tests to be free of the immunological substance under test constitute a pool of "true negatives." From these two kinds of specimens, an "index of specificity" can be calculated for each test.

$$\text{Index of specificity} = \frac{\text{true negatives} - \text{false positives}}{\text{true negatives}} \times 100$$

Serology and Immunology

The **accuracy** of a serological test is a reflection of how close the results are to the absolute values of immune substances in reference or control specimens. The values established for reference samples by commercial suppliers of diagnostic serological reagents are assumed to represent the true values because they have presumably been determined from numerous tests performed under ideal conditions by highly qualified personnel. National and international standards (when available) are considered to represent well-defined reference values for immunological substances.

The term **precision** is used in two ways. It can be used to denote the size of the increments used in the measure. For example, when measured by different techniques or by different kinds of instrumentation, the true protein content of a serum (6.41 gm percent) may be variously estimated at 6, 6.2, 6.37, or 5.891. All four measurements are accurate to different numbers of significant figures. The last measurement is the most precise, but the least accurate. The most **reliable** of these four measurements is 6.37 because it represents the best combination of accuracy and precision. Another way to use precision is as a synonym for **reproducibility.** If repeated tests of the same sample by the same method produce a tight pattern (small variation) of results, the test is said to be highly reproducible or to have a high degree of precision. Figure A.1 presents three patterns in which the hypothetical results of four replicate tests are displayed around the true (absolute) value.

If we could measure every person in a given population for a particular serological characteristic, we could calculate its average value for the entire population. Such values derived from data of an entire population are called **parameters.** A population can be defined as any group you want it to be, such as all patients who have shown clinical signs of a given disease or all patients who have not shown such signs. However, we seldom (if ever) have such complete data on large populations and hence do not know what the true population parameters are. The best we can do is to take random samples from the population and perform similar calculations on the sample data. The single values derived from the set of sample data are called **statistics.** If our sampling technique is adequate, the statistic should reflect (but not necessarily equal) the corresponding parameter. All other things being equal, the larger the sample size, the more accurately the statistic should represent the parameter. For any one sample there is a probability (chance) that its statistic deviates from the parameter. If we assume that such deviations are strictly due to chance (experimental error), we can make predictions concerning the limits within which the corresponding population parameter should reside.

There are two major categories of statistics: (1) measures of central tendency and (2) measures of dispersion. Measures of central tendency include the mean, median, and mode. The **mean** or **arithmetic average** of a sample is calculated by summation of the individual measurements (variables) and division by the total number of

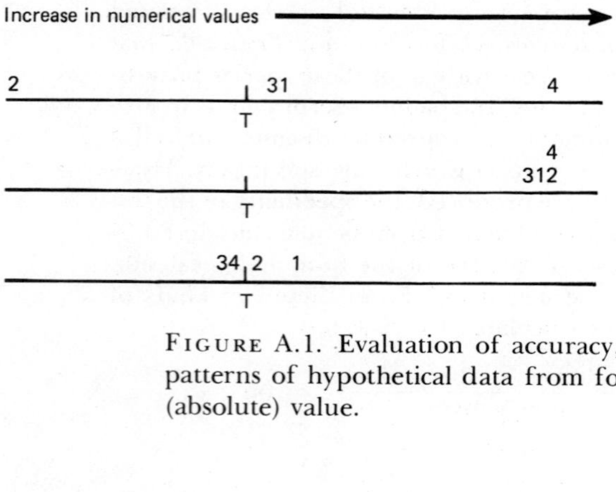

	Reliability	Average accuracy	Reproducibility (precision)
2 31 4 (T)	Fair	High	Low
4 312 (T)	Fair	Low	High
34 2 1 (T)	Good	High	High

FIGURE A.1. Evaluation of accuracy, precision, and reliability for three patterns of hypothetical data from four replicate tests (1 to 4). T = true (absolute) value.

individuals (sample size). In statistical notation, this is represented by

$$\bar{X} = \frac{\sum_{i=1}^{n} X_i}{n}$$

where $\bar{X}$ (pronounced "X bar") is the sample mean, X_i represents the measurement on the ith individual, n is the sample size, and $\sum_{i=1}^{n}$ (Sigma) indicates a summation of the X_i measurements beginning with the first individual ($i = 1$) and ending with the last (n^{th}) individual. The corresponding mean value of the entire population from which the sample was drawn (parameter) is designated by the lower-case Greek letter mu (μ).

The **median** is the middle value of a data set. It is that value above and below which an equal number of variables are distributed in the sample. If the data are ordered according to numerical value and the sample size is an odd number, the median lies in the middle of the array. If the sample size is an even number, the median is the average of the two middle values of the array.

The **mode** is the most frequently observed variable in the data set. It is possible to have more than one mode in a data set.

Measures of data dispersion around the mean include the range, standard deviation, and variance. The range of the sample data is represented by the highest and lowest values. This of course tells us nothing of the pattern of data distribution within the limits of the range and consequently is of little use for quality control. A more useful measure of dispersion within a sample is the **standard deviation** (s, or SD), calculated by the following formula.

$$s = \sqrt{\frac{\sum_{i=1}^{n} (X_i - \bar{X})^2}{n - 1}}$$

The numerator of this formula is the sum of the squared differences between each variable and the average of the entire sample. The denominator contains a correction for small samples called the **degrees of freedom** (one less than the sample size). For samples larger than about 30 it usually makes little difference if division is by n or by $n - 1$. A standard deviation (s) calculated in samples of 30 or larger usually is a very good estimate of the corresponding parameter, σ (found by substituting N, the population size, for $n - 1$ in the previous formula). Table A.1 dis-

Table A.1 CALCULATION OF STATISTICS $\bar{X}$ AND s FROM COUNTS OF DEGRANULATED BASOPHILS IN TEN HYPOTHETICAL ALLERGY PATIENTS

	\multicolumn{11}{c}{Patient Number}
	1	2	3	4	5	6	7	8	9	10	Totals (Σ)
Degranulated basophil count (X)	2	0	1	4	3	1	1	0	2	1	15
($X - \bar{X}$)	0.5	−1.5	−0.5	2.5	1.5	−0.5	−0.5	−1.5	0.5	−0.5	0
($X - \bar{X}$)^2	0.25	2.25	0.25	6.25	2.25	0.25	0.25	2.25	0.25	0.25	14.5
X^2	4	0	1	16	9	1	1	0	4	1	37

$\bar{X} = 15/10 = 1.5$; $s = \sqrt{14.5/9} = 1.27$; s (machine formula) $= \sqrt{\dfrac{37 - \dfrac{(15)^2}{10}}{9}} = 1.27$

plays some sample data and calculations of the mean and standard deviation by the above formula and also by an equivalent "machine formula" used with mechanical or electronic calculators.

$$s = \sqrt{\frac{\Sigma X^2 - \frac{(\Sigma X)^2}{n}}{n-1}}$$

If the data are closely grouped around the mean, the standard deviation will be a relatively small value; if the sample measurements are widely spread, the standard deviation will be relatively large. A relatively small standard deviation calculated from repetitive tests on the same reference standard would indicate that the test was one of high precision. The degree of accuracy would depend on how close $\bar{X}$ was to the true value of the reference sample.

If the sampling is done adequately, the sample standard deviation should reflect the dispersion of the entire population from which the sample was drawn. The lower-case Greek letter "sigma" (σ) is used to represent the standard deviation parameter. For some statistical purposes the square of the standard deviation (s^2), called the **variance,** is used; the corresponding parameter is σ^2.

As a general rule, the standard deviation tends to increase as mean values become larger. The **coefficient of variation** (CV) is useful for comparing the dispersion of two similar sets of data or for comparing one day's test results with another, etc. The coefficient of variation is the standard deviation divided by the mean.

$$CV = \frac{s}{\bar{X}}$$

For the data of Table A.1, $CV = 1.27/1.5 = 0.847$ and would commonly be expressed as a percentage (85 percent). Some measurements made in the clinical laboratory vary widely from one time to another within the same individual. For example, the preinfection vs. postinfection titers of specific microbial antibodies vary markedly; indeed, it is by a fourfold or greater rise in titer of specific antibodies between paired sera that serologically confirms infection. The serum uric acid level of a patient requires a series of measurements over a prolonged period of time in order to establish his "normal" average. Other measurements may vary widely from one individual to another, but can be relatively constant within a given individual (e.g., insulin levels determined by RIA for diabetic vs. nondiabetic patients or serum cholesterol levels in normal people). Thus, a relatively high coefficient of variation is expected for serum uric acid tests and a relatively low coefficient of variation is normal for serum cholesterol tests on the same individual.

Normal Distribution

There are two major categories of errors potentially inherent in any experimental procedure. A **systematic error** tends to produce results that deviate, on the average, in a given direction and magnitude from the true value. These systematic errors are often attributable to miscalibrated instrumentation so that readings are consistently biased on either the high or low side of the true value. If repeated measurements on the same sample progressively become more deviant in a given direction with time, a **trend** is said to exist. Among the factors that may contribute to a trend are the gradual deterioration of reagents, fading of a color standard, cumulative pipetting errors in making serial dilutions, etc. Systematic errors are potentially controllable, and every effort should be made to do so.

Random errors, on the other hand, are intrinsic variables (uncontrollable) due strictly to chance events. They do not tend to deviate from the true value in either direction or magnitude. Rather, they tend to fall within a predictable range and form what is called a **normal distribution** or Gaussian curve (Figure A.2). The mean, median, and mode are equivalent values in a normal distribution. The larger

Normal Distribution

```
                    •
                  • • •
                • • • • •
              • • • • • • •
            • • • • • • • • •
Hypothetical ┼───┼───┼───┼───┼───
  values    28  30  ↑32  34
              Mean, median, mode
```

Non-normal Distribution

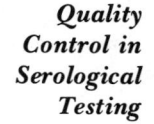

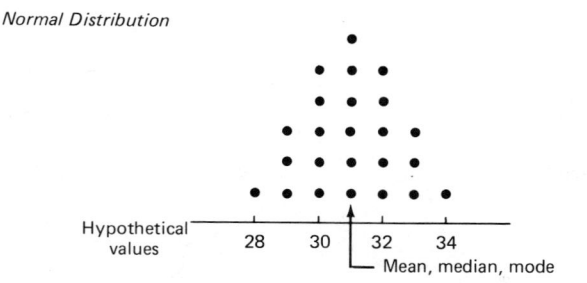

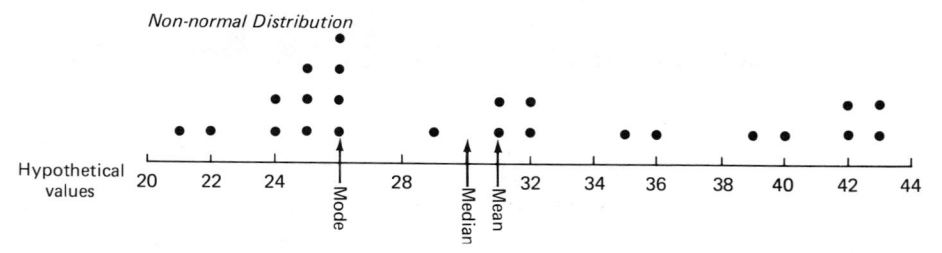

```
                •
              • •
            • • •         • •
          • •   • •     • •         • •   • •
Hypothetical ┼───┼───┼───┼───┼───┼───┼───┼───┼───┼───┼───
  values    20  22  24  ↑ 28 ↑↑32  34  36  38  40  42  44
                      Mode  Median
                            Mean
```

FIGURE A.2. Scatter diagrams of twenty-four measurements in normal and nonnormal distributions. Normal distributions typify samples from healthy people; samples from hospitalized patients are more likely to form nonnormal distributions.

the deviation of a variable from the mean, the smaller its probability of occurrence. This is the rule that causes random errors to form the symmetrical bell-shaped curve. If a perpendicular to the base line is constructed to pass through the point of maximal slope on the normal curve, the distance from the mean to that perpendicular is the standard deviation (Figure A.3). Approximately two thirds (68 percent) of the area under the curve (or two thirds of the number in the population) should be found within one standard deviation on either side of the mean ($\mu \pm 1\sigma$). Approximately 95 percent of the population should reside within two standard deviations of the mean ($\mu \pm 2\sigma$).

When reference standards are available, they should be run concurrently with the unknowns (patient's samples) using the same reagents and test procedures. Controls should be randomly interspersed among the samples rather than always being the first or last samples. Conventionally, clinical laboratory tests are considered to be **out of control** if the reference standards fall outside the limits $\bar{X} \pm 2s$. Only about 5 percent of random errors should be outside this range. When such an "outlier" value is found, the reference sample should be run again. If the repeat test is also out of control, all facets of the test (including reagents, instruments, and procedures) should be scrutinized to determine the source of the erroneous results. No determination of patient values should be made until the problem is found and corrected.

The most widely used system of quality control in the medical laboratory employs the $\bar{X}$ or Levey-Jennings chart. This is a graphic plot of day-to-day results on each reference or control specimen as shown in Figure A.4. The mean and standard deviation for the reference standard used on the chart is determined from previous tests in the same laboratory. The values established by a given laboratory should fall within the acceptable range provided by the supplier of the standard. On day 4, the plot △ was out of control. It was repeated the same day and gave the plot ⊡, again out of control. Careful examination of all aspects of the test revealed that the

Serology and Immunology

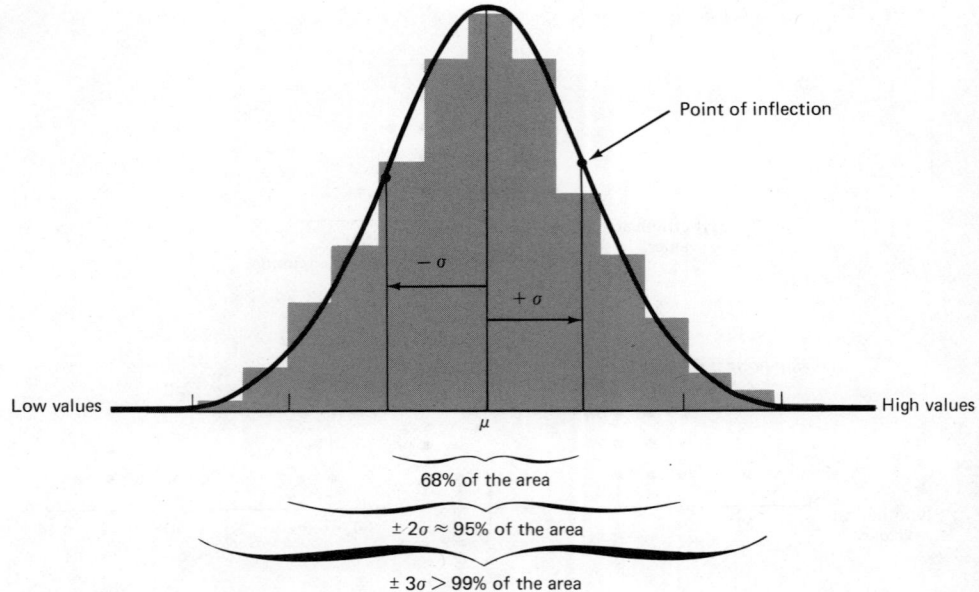

FIGURE A.3. Idealized normal distribution for an entire population. μ = population mean; σ = standard deviation.

reagents had become contaminated. These were replaced, and a third test of the reference sample (plot ⊙) indicated that the test was back in control.

As a rule of thumb, if six consecutive plots fall on the mean line or on one side of the mean line, the test is considered to be out of control. This situation is called a **shift.** Such a shift occurred in Figure A.4 from days 10 through 15. The spectrophotometer was recalibrated and the test was back in control on day 16.

If six successive plots are distributed in one general direction on the Levey-Jennings chart, it indicates that a **trend** exists. Such a trend is shown in Figure A.4 from days 19 through 24. Again the procedure was examined and the problem corrected. The test was back in control on day 26.

Weighted Average

When calculating statistics based on the past month's records, it would be inappropriate to use any data that indicated either a shift or a trend because during these intervals the test was out of control and the observed values did not represent random variations. Using only the eighteen values "in control" on Figure A.4, the monthly average is 5.11, very close to the accumulated average of 5.15 from previous months. This new statistic can be used with the accumulated average (based on 104 previous days of "in-control" data) to calculate a new weighted average.

$$\text{Weighted average} = \frac{(5.11)(18) + (5.15)(104)}{18 + 104} = \frac{91.98 + 535.6}{122} = 5.144$$

A similar weighting can be done with the new standard deviation value based on the latest eighteen days of "in-control" data.

Confidence Levels

It is conventional to accept a test result for a reference or standard as being "in control" if it lies within $\bar{X} \pm 2s$. The extreme values of this range are called the 95 percent **confidence limits,** and the range itself is the 95 percent **confidence interval.** If a 68 percent confidence level is used ($\bar{X} \pm 1s$), too many "normal" values would

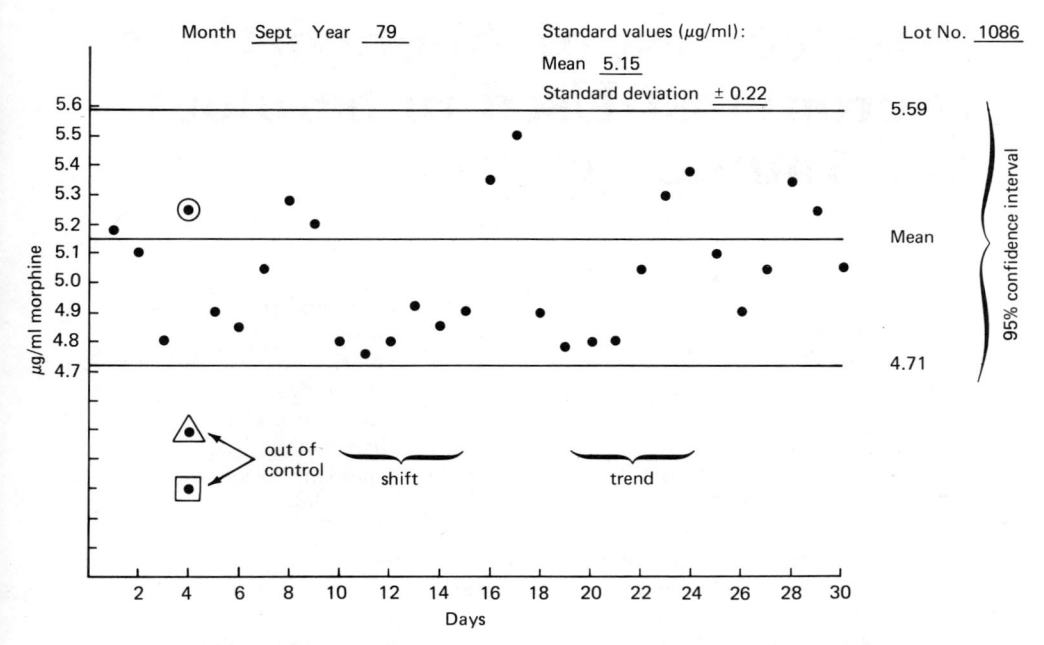

FIGURE A.4. X̄ or Levey-Jennings quality control chart on a reference standard containing 5 μg/ml morphine by immunoenzyme test.

fall outside the acceptable range. If a 99 percent confidence level is used ($\bar{X} \pm 3s$), almost any test result will be acceptable. The 95 percent confidence level seems to be the best compromise for avoiding both these problems.

Provided that a good estimate of σ is available from the sample standard deviation (s) in sample sizes over 30, the 95 percent confidence limits within which the true population mean (μ) should exist can be calculated by the following formula.

$$\mu = \bar{X} \pm 2 \left(\frac{s}{\sqrt{n}} \right)$$

For example, if the mean IgG concentration in 500 healthy adults is 1,275 mg/100 ml of blood and the sample standard deviation is ±280, we estimate that the true mean is within the values $1,275 \pm 2(280/\sqrt{500}) = 1,275 \pm 25$. Thus we take only a 5 percent chance of being wrong when we assume that the population mean lies between 1,250 and 1,300 mg percent. If some other laboratory reports their average value (sample size 500 or larger) to be less than 1,250 or greater than 1,300 mg percent, we would be forced to conclude that a different measuring technique was employed and/or a different population was being sampled (perhaps a population including babies or hospitalized adult patients).

Selected List of Abbreviations (Acronyms) Used in Serology and Immunology

aa	amino acid	ART	automated reagin test
AABB	American Association of Blood Banks	As	antiserum
		ASCP	American Society of Clinical Pathologists
AACC	American Association of Clinical Chemists	ASM	American Society for Microbiology
ab	antibody		
ABC	antigen-binding capacity	ASMT	American Society of Medical Technology
ABH	related antigens of the ABO blood group system	ASLO, ASLT, ASO, ASOT	antistreptolysin O (titration test)
ABO	ABO blood group system		
abs	absorbed, absorption; antibodies		
ACD	acid citrate dextrose (anticoagulant)	ATG	antithymocyte globulin
		ATP	adenosine triphosphate
ACTH	adrenocorticotropic hormone	ATS	antithymocyte serum
ADCC	antibody-dependent cell-mediated cytotoxicity	AuA	Australia antigen (hepatitis)
ADNase	antideoxyribonucleotidase	B cell	bursa of Fabricius derived (or equivalent) lymphocyte with antibody production potential
AED	antiepileptic drug		
AFP	alpha fetoprotein		
Ag, ag	antigen	BCG	bacille Calmette-Guérin
AGD	agar gel diffusion	BDB	bis diazotized benzidine
AGN	acute glomerulonephritis	BE	beef erythrocyte
AH	antihyaluronidase	BF	blastogenic factor
AHG	antihuman globulin; antihemophilic globulin	B/F	bound/free ratio
		BFN	biological false negative
AHP	alpha-2-hepatic protein	BFP	biological false positive
AIHA	autoimmune hemolytic anemia	BGG	bovine gamma globulin
		BGS	blood group substance
alb	albumin	B-J	Bence-Jones (protein)
A/G	albumin/globulin ratio	BM	bone marrow
ALG	antilymphocyte globulin	BOB	Bureau of Biologics
ALS	antilymphocyte serum	BSA	bovine serum albumin
Am	allotypic antigen on IgA heavy chain	C	complement (C' = obsolete); constant region of immunoglobulin polypeptide chain (C_L = constant region of light chain, C_H = constant region of heavy chain); C-carbohydrate of streptococci
ambo	amboceptor		
AMA	American Medical Association		
AML	acute myelogenous leukemia		
AMP	adenosine monophosphate		
ANA	antinuclear antibody		
ANF	antinuclear factor (ANA)		
ANS	8-anilo-1-naphthalene-sulfonic acid	CBC	complete blood count
		cc	cubic centimeter
anti-	antibody (specificity follows hyphen)	CCAT	conglutinating complement adsorption test

Selected List of Abbreviations (Acronyms) Used in Serology and Immunology

CCC	Coombs control cells	D^u	weak (incomplete) antigen of D in Rh blood group system
CDC	Centers for Disease Control (Atlanta, Georgia)	E*	complement-lysed erythrocyte
CEA	carcinoembryonic antigen	EA	egg albumin (ovalbumin); sensitized erythrocyte (E = erythrocyte, A = antibody)
CEP	counterelectrophoresis		
CF	complement fixation; chemotactic factor	EAC	erythrocyte-antibody-complement complex
CFA	complete Freund's adjuvant		
CFT	complement fixation test	EAE	experimental allergic encephalomyelitis
CGD	chronic granulomatous disease (congenital dysphagocytosis)	EBF	erythroblastosis fetalis
CIE or CIEP	counter immunoelectrophoresis	EBV	Epstein-Barr virus
CMI	cell-mediated immunity	ECF-A	eosinophilic chemotactic factor of anaphylaxis
CML	cell-mediated lympholysis; chronic myelogenous leukemia		
CMV	cytomegalovirus	ED50	50 percent effective dose; 50 percent hemolysis
CNS	central nervous system		
coag	coagulation	EDTA	ethylenediamine tetraacetic acid (anticoagulant)
con A	concanavalin A		
conj	conjugate, conjugated		
cont	control	EIA	electroimmunoassay (rocket electrophoresis); enzyme immunoassay
CPB or CPBA	competitive protein binding (assay)		
CPD	citrate, phosphate, dextrose (anticoagulant)	EID	electroimmunodiffusion
		ELISA	enzyme-linked immunosorbent assay
cpm	counts per minute		
CRP	C-reactive protein		
CSC	complement-sensitized cells	EMIT	enzyme-multiplied immunoassay technique (Syva)
CSF	cerebrospinal fluid		
CTL	cytolytic T lymphocyte	EOA	egg ovalbumin
CV	coefficient of variation	ESR	electron spin resonance; erythrocyte sedimentation rate
D	diffusion coefficient; major antigen of Rh blood group system		
DAB or DANSYL	1-dimethylaminonaphthalene-5-sulfonyl chloride	$F_1, F_2,$ etc.	first filial generation of offspring, etc.
DAT	direct antiglobulin test	FA or FAB	fluorescent antibody
D/C	direct Coombs test		
DEAE	diethylaminoethylene	Fab, F_{ab}	fragment antigen binding
DIC	disseminated intravascular coagulation		
dil, dils, diln	dilution	FADF	fluorescent-antibody dark field technique
DNA	deoxyribonucleic acid	FBS	fetal bovine serum
DNase	deoxyribonuclease	FCS	fetal calf serum
DNCB	dinitrochlorobenzene (chlorodinitrobenzene)	Fc, F_c	fragment crystallizable
DNFB	dinitrofluorobenzene	FDA	Food and Drug Administration
DNP	dinitrophenyl group		
dpm	disintegrations per minute	FDP	fibrinogen degradation products
DPT	diphtheria, pertussis, tetanus		

Serology and Immunology

FIA	Freund's incomplete adjuvant		hemagglutination protein of influenza virus
FITC	fluorescein isothiocyanate	H-2	major histocompatibility system in mouse
F_m	fragment, membrane-bound	HA	hemagglutination
		HAA	hepatitis-associated antigen
FP	false positive	HAI	hemagglutination inhibition
F:P	fluorochrome-to-protein (antibody) molar ratio	HANE	hereditary angioneurotic edema
		Hb	hemoglobin
FRAT	free radical assay technique	HB_sAg	hepatitis B surface antigen
		HCG	human chorionic gonadotropin
F_s	fragment, soluble		
FSH	follicle-stimulating hormone	HD_{50}	complement dose able to hemolyze 50 percent of red cells
FTA	fluorescent treponemal antibody test		
		H & E	hematoxylin and eosin
		HEP	high egg passage
FTA-ABS	fluorescent treponemal antibody absorption test	HGG	human gamma globulin
		HGH	human growth hormone
		HI	hemagglutination inhibition
Fy	Duffy blood group system	HLA	human leukocyte (lymphocyte) antigen; major histocompatibility system of humans
GALT	gut-associated lymphoid tissue		
		HPLC	high-pressure liquid chromatography
GBM	glomerular basement membrane		
		HSA	human serum albumin
GC	gonococcus	HTSH	human thyroid-stimulating hormone
GCFT	gonococcal complement fixation test		
		HVG	host vs. graft
GDA	glycidaldehyde	I or Ir	immune response
GDD	gel double diffusion	Ia	alloantigen on surface of mouse B lymphocytes
GGG	C3 proactivator (factor B)		
		IBR	infectious bovine rhinotracheitis
GI	gastrointestinal		
glob	globulin(s)	IC	intracardiac, intracerebral, intracutaneous
GLC	gas-liquid chromatography		
		ID	immunodiffusion; identification; intradermal
Gm	allotypic variants on gamma heavy immunoglobulin chains		
		IE or IEP	immunoelectrophoresis
		IEOP	immunoelectroosmophoresis
gm, gms	gram(s)	IF	immunofluorescence; initiating factor
GP	guinea pig		
GPK	guinea pig kidney	IFA	indirect fluorescent antibody
GVH	graft vs. host	Ig	immunoglobulin (IgG = class G, etc.)
H	histocompatibility antigens; bacterial flagellar antigens; heavy immunoglobulin chains; antigen related to ABO blood groups; horse; $H_x =$	I-K	immunoconglutinin
		IM	intramuscular; infectious mononucleosis
		IMD_{50}	antigen dose required to immunize 50 percent of a group of test animals
		Inv	allotypic variants on kappa light immunoglobulin chains

Selected List of Abbreviations (Acronyms) Used in Serology and Immunology

in vitro	"in glass" (serological)	LNPF	lymph node permeability factor
in vivo	"in life" ("immunological")	LPS	lipopolysaccharide (endotoxin)
IP	intraperitoneal	L/S	lecithin-sphingomyelin ratio
Ir	immune response	LT	lymphotoxin
isol	isolation	Lu	Lutheran blood group system
ITP	idiopathic thrombocytopenic purpura	Ly	antigenic surface markers on T lymphocytes
IU	international unit		
IV	intravenous	M	molar; myeloma protein; streptococcal surface antigen
J chain	"junction" peptide chain bound to IgM and IgA	MAA-TP	microhemagglutination test for *Treponema pallidum*
JAMA	Journal of the American Medical Association	MAF	macrophage activating factor
Jk	Kidd blood group system	MCA	mixed-cell agglutination
		MCF	mastocytolytic factor
		med	medium
K	killer cell; Kell-Cellano blood group system; antigens associated with bacterial capsules	MF	mycelial form; mitogenic factor
		Mg	magnesium
		mg	milligram(s)
KAF	conglutinogen-activating factor (obsolete); C3b inactivator	MHC	major histocompatibility complex
		MHD	minimal hemolytic dose of complement
KLH, KLHC	keyhole limpet hemocyanin	MI	myocardial infarction
		MIF	migration inhibition factor
L	light immunoglobulin chain; bacterial forms without a cell wall; L_x = dosage of toxin	mIg	membrane immunoglobulin
		ml	milliliter
		MLC	mixed-lymphcyte (leukocyte) culture (see MLR)
l	liter	MLD	minimal lethal dose of microorganism or toxin
LA	leukocyte antigen		
LAL	*Limulus* amebocyte lysate	MLR	mixed-lymphocyte reaction (see MLC)
LALI	lymphocyte-antibody-lymphocytolytic interaction		
LAT	leukocyte aggregation test	MLT	Medical Laboratory Technician
LATS	long-acting thyroid stimulator	mM	millimole(s)
LC	lymphocyte	mm	millimeter(s)
LCM	lymphocytic choriomeningitis (virus)	MRD	minimal reacting dose of toxin
LD	lymphocyte-detectable; lethal dose	mRNA	messenger ribonucleic acid
		MRT	milk ring test
LD_{50}	lethal dose of toxin (or microbe) for 50 percent of a test group	MS	multiple sclerosis
		MST	mean survival time
		MT	Medical Technologist (licensed)
LDH	lactate dehydrogenase		
LE	lupus erythematosus		
Le	Lewis blood group system	N	nonreactive; N_x = neuraminidase protein of influenza virus
LEP	low egg passage		
L_f	limit of flocculation (toxins)		
LH	luteinizing hormone	NADase	nicotinamide adenine dinucleotidase
LIF	leukocyte inhibitory factor		
LISS	low-ionic-strength saline	NBT	nitroblue tetrazolium test
LMP	last menstrual period	NeF	nephritic factor

Serology and Immunology

neg	negative	PCT	plasmacrit test
ng	nanogram	Pen	Penicillin
NHG	normal human globulin	PFC	plaque-forming cells
NHS	normal human serum	PF/dil	permeability factor/dilution
NIAD	National Institute of Allergy and Infectious Diseases	PFU	plaque-forming units
		pg	picogram
NK cells	natural killer cells (null lymphocytes)	PGN	poststreptococcal glomerulonephritis
NLT	normal lymphocytic transfer test	pH	hydrogen ion concentration
		PHA	phytohemagglutinin; passive hemagglutination
NP	nucleoprotein		
NR	nonreactive	PHC	proliferating helper cell
NRS	normal rabbit serum	P-K	Prausnitz-Küstner reaction
NSB	nonspecific binding	pI	isoelectric point
NSS	nonspecific substance	PmKO	a lipopolysaccharide antigen extracted from *Mycobacterium tuberculosis*
NT	not tested		
nu	recessive gene in mouse for nude (athymic)		
NZB	New Zealand black strain of mice	PML	polymorphonuclear leukocyte
		PMN	polymorphonuclear neutrophil, polymorphonuclear leukocyte
NZW	New Zealand white strain of mice		
O	somatic antigen (endotoxin) of gram-negative bacteria; absence of antigens A and B in ABO blood group system	PNH	paroxysmal nocturnal hemoglobinuria
		POA	pancreatic oncofetal antigen
		pos	positive
OA	ovalbumin (egg albumin)	PPD	purified protein derivative (tuberculin)
OD	optical density; outside diameter		
		ppt	precipitate
O_h	Bombay blood group	PTAP	purified diphtheria toxoid adsorbed onto hydrated aluminum phosphate
OP	optimal proportion		
OT	old tuberculin		
Oz	antigen in constant region of lambda immunoglobulin light chain	PTR	plasma transfusion reaction
		PVP	polyvinylpyrrolidone
		QC	quality control
P	properdin	R	dominant gene of the Rh blood group system (r = recessive allele); rabbit; rough bacterial colony; reactive
PA	C3 proactivator		
Pa (1, 2, 3, 4)	pokeweed mitogens obtained from *Phytolacca americana*		
PAGE	polyacrylamide gel electrophoresis	RA	rheumatoid arthritis
		RAST	radioallergosorbent test
Pap test	cytological test for cervical cancer named for George N. Papanicolaou	RB200	lissamine rhodamine
		RBC	red blood cell
		RCLAAR	red cell–linked antigen-antiglobulin reaction
PAS	periodic acid Schiff; para-aminosalicylic acid		
		RDE	receptor-destroying enzyme
PAse	C3 proactivator convertase	RES	reticuloendothelial system
PB	peripheral blood	resp	respiratory
PBD	a substituted oxadiazole for liquid scintillation	RF	rheumatoid factor
		Rh	Rhesus blood group system
PBI	protein-bound iodine	RhoGAM	purified human antibodies against D factor of Rh blood group system (Ortho Pharmaceutical Company)
PBS	phosphate-buffered saline		
PCA	passive cutaneous anaphylaxis		

Selected List of Abbreviations (Acronyms) Used in Serology and Immunology

RIA	radioimmunoassay	SSS	soluble specific substance (capsular polysaccharide of *Streptococcus pneumoniae*)
RID	radial immunodiffusion		
RIP	radioimmunoprecipitation assay	stat	Latin abbreviation for *statim* (at once, immediately)
RIST	radioimmunosorbent test	STS	serological test(s) for syphilis
RNA	ribonucleic acid	T_3, T_4	thyroid hormones
RNP	ribonucleoprotein	T antigen	viral antigen found in cell nucleus
RPA	reversed passive Arthus; reversed passive agglutination test	T cell	thymus-derived lymphocyte
		T_C	killer T lymphocyte
RPCF	Reiter protein complement fixation test	T_H	helper T lymphocyte
		T_S	suppressor T lymphocyte
RPHA	reversed passive hemagglutination	TAB	vaccine containing *Salmonella typhi* and *Salmonella paratyphi* A and B
RPR	rapid plasma reagin test (Hynson, Westcott & Dunning, Inc.)		
		TABC	TAB vaccine containing *Salmonella paratyphi* C
RRA	radioreceptor assay	TABT	TAB vaccine containing tetanus toxoid
S	Svedberg unit; site of complement activation; antigen of the MNS blood group system; smooth bacterial colony; sheep	TAF	toxoid-antitoxin floccules
		TB	tuberculosis
		TBG	thyroxine-binding globulin
		TDA	therapeutic drug assay
s	sample standard deviation; soluble antigen in early virus infection	TF	transfer factor
		TFT	tube flocculation test
		TIP	translation inhibitory protein
SACl-*n*	symbols for complement action; S = antigenic site of complement activation, A = antibody, C = complement, 1 − *n* = the first to *n* complement factors	TLC	thin-layer chromatography; "tender loving care"
		TNP	trinitrophenyl
		TP	transport piece
		TPCF	*Treponema pallidum* complement fixation test
sarc	sarcoma	TPHA	*Treponema pallidum* hemagglutination test
SC	subcutaneous		
SD	serologically detectable; Schultz-Dale test; standard deviation	TPI	*Treponema pallidum* immobilization test
		TSA	tumor-specific antigen; trypticase soy agar (culture medium)
Se	dominant gene for secretion of ABH blood group substances (*se* = recessive allele for nonsecretion)		
		TSH	thyroid-stimulating hormone
		TSTA	tumor-specific transplantation antigen
SFT	serum flocculation test		
SLE	systemic lupus erythematosus	ug	microgram (actually Greek mu, μ)
SLO	streptolysin O	USC	unsensitized cells
SLS	streptolysin S	USP	United States Pharmacopoeia
sol	soluble	V	variable region of immunoglobulin polypeptide chain (V_L = variable region of light chain; V_H = variable region of heavy chain)
SP	secretory piece		
SPIR	solid-phase immunoassay reagents		
SRBC	sheep red blood cells		
SRS-A	slow-reacting substance of anaphylaxis		
SSPE	subacute sclerosing panencephalitis		

Serology and Immunology

VDRL	Venereal Disease Research Laboratory test for syphilitic reagin	WR	Wassermann reaction; weakly reactive
Vi	surface somatic antigen of *Salmonella typhi* and *S. paratyphi* C, usually associated with *virulence*	w/v	weight-to-volume ratio
		$\bar{X}$	sample average (mean)
		Xg	sex-linked human blood group system
v/v	volume-to-volume ratio	X, Y, Z cells	various stages of maturation of immunologically competent cells
WHO	World Health Organization		

References

General Immunology Texts

ABRAMOFF, P. and M. F. LAVIA. *Biology of the Immune Response.* McGraw-Hill Book Company, New York, 1970.
ALOISI, R. M. *Principles of Immunodiagnostics.* The C. V. Mosby Co., St. Louis, 1979.
BARRETT, J. T. *Textbook of Immunology* (3rd ed.). The C. V. Mosby Co., St. Louis, 1978.
BARRETT, J. T. *Basic Immunology and Its Medical Application.* The C. V. Mosby Co., St. Louis, 1976.
BELLANTI, J. A. *Immunology.* W. B. Saunders Co., Philadelphia, 1971.
BIGLEY, N. J. *Immunologic Fundamentals.* Year Book Medical Publishers, Inc., Chicago, 1975.
CARPENTER, P. L. *Immunology and Serology* (3rd ed.). W. B. Saunders Co., Philadelphia, 1975.
CUSHING, J. E. and D. H. CAMPBELL. *Principles of Immunology.* McGraw-Hill Book Co., Inc., New York, 1957.
GORDON, B. L. and D. K. FORD. *Essentials of Immunology.* F. A. Davis Company, Philadelphia, 1971.
HALLIDAY, W. J. *Glossary of Immunological Terms.* Appleton-Century-Crofts, New York, 1971.
HERBERT, W. J. and P. C. WILKINSON (Editors). *A Dictionary of Immunology* (2nd ed.). Blackwell Scientific Publications, Oxford, England, 1977.
HOOD, L. E., I. L. WEISSMAN, and W. B. WOOD. *Immunology.* The Benjamin/Cummings Publishing Co., Inc., Menlo Park, Calif., 1978.
HUMPHREY, J. H. and R. G. WHITE. *Immunology for Students of Medicine* (3rd ed.). F. A. Davis Company, Philadelphia, 1970.
KABAT, E. A. *Structural Concepts in Immunology and Immunochemistry* (2nd ed.). Holt, Rinehart and Winston, New York, 1976.
KABAT, E. A. *Structural Concepts in Immunology and Immunochemistry.* Holt, Rinehart and Winston, Inc., New York, 1968.
LANDSTEINER, K. *The Specificity of Serological Reactions* (Revised Edition). Dover Publications, Inc., New York, 1962.
QUINN, L. Y. *Immunological Concepts.* The Iowa State University Press, Ames, 1968.
RAFFEL, S. *Immunity* (2nd ed.). Appleton-Century-Crofts, New York, 1961.
Readings from Scientific American. Immunology. W. H. Freeman and Company, San Francisco, 1976.
ROITT, I. M. *Essential Immunology* (2nd ed.). Blackwell Scientific Publications, Oxford, England, 1974.
ROSE, N. R., F. MILGROM, and C. J. VAN OSS (Editors). *Principles of Immunology.* Macmillan Publishing Co., Inc., New York, 1973.
STREILEIN, J. W. and J. D. HUGHES. *Immunology—A Programmed Text.* Little, Brown and Company, Boston, 1977.
WEIR, D. M. *Immunology; An Outline for Students of Medicine and Biology* (4th ed.). Churchill Livingstone, Edinburgh, 1977.
WEISER, R. S., Q. N. MYRVIK, and N. N. PEARSALL. *Fundamentals of Immunology for Students of Medicine and Related Sciences.* Lea & Febiger, Philadelphia, 1969.

Specific Immunological Topics

BILLINGHAM, R. and W. SILVERS. *The Immunobiology of Transplantation.* Prentice-Hall, Inc., Englewood Cliffs, N. J., 1971.
BLANKENSHIP, J. and J. B. CAMPBELL. *Laboratory Mathematics; Medical and Biological Applications.* The C. V. Mosby Co., St. Louis, 1976.

Serology and Immunology

BRATTIN, W. J. and I. SUNSHINE. *Immunological assays for drugs in biological samples.* Am. J. Med. Tec. 39(6):223–30, 1973.

BRYANT, N. J. *An Introduction to Immunohematology.* W. B. Saunders Co., Philadelphia, 1976.

BURNET, F. M. *Immunology, Aging, and Cancer.* W. H. Freeman and Company, San Francisco, 1976.

BURNET, F. M. *The Clonal Selection Theory of Acquired Immunity.* Vanderbilt University Press, Nashville, 1959.

CAPRA, J. D. and A. B. EDMUNDSON. *The antibody combining site.* Sci. Amer. 236(1):50–59, Jan. 1977.

CAWLEY, L. P. and B. MINARD. *Immunologic Reactions in Gel.* Lab-Ed, Inc., Wichita, Kansas, 1973.

CHERRY, W. B., M. GOLDMAN, and T. R. CARSKI. *Fluorescent Antibody Techniques in the Diagnosis of Communicable Diseases.* U.S. Dept. of Health, Education and Welfare, Public Health Service, Bureau of State Services, Communicable Disease Center, Atlanta, Georgia; Public Health Service Publication No. 729, 1960.

COOPER, E. L. *Comparative Immunology.* Prentice-Hall, Inc., Englewood Cliffs, N. J., 1976.

CROWLE, A. J. *Immunodiffusion* (2nd ed.). Academic Press, New York, 1973.

CUNNINGHAM, A. (Editor). *The Generation of Antibody Diversity: A New Look.* Academic Press, New York, 1976.

CUNNINGHAM, B. A. *The structure and function of histocompatibility antigens.* Sci. Amer. 237(4):96–107, Oct. 1977.

DAUSSET, J. (Editor). *Tissue Typing.* Vox Sanguinis 11(3), May-June, 1966.

ENGLE, R. L. and L. A. WALLIS. *Immunoglobulinopathies.* Charles C Thomas Publisher, Springfield, Ill., 1969.

ERSKINE, A. G. *The Principles and Practice of Blood Grouping.* The C. V. Mosby Co., St. Louis, 1973.

FEINGOLD, B. F. *Introduction to Clinical Allergy.* Charles C Thomas Publisher, Springfield, Ill., 1973.

FRASIER, C. H. *Aspects of Liquid Scintillation Counting.* Beckman Instruments, Inc., Fullerton, Calif., 1973.

FRASIER, C. H. *Introduction to Radioimmunoassay.* Beckman Instruments, Inc., Fullerton, Calif., 1973.

FRAZIER, C. A. *Insect Allergy; Allergic and Toxic Reactions to Insects and Other Arthopods.* W. H. Green, St. Louis, 1969.

GÖTZE, O. and H. J. MÜLLER-EBERHARD. *The alternative pathway of complement activation.* Advances in Immunology 24:1–35. Academic Press, New York, 1976.

HILDEMANN, W. H. *Immunogenetics.* Holden-Day, San Francisco, 1970.

HILL, R. B. and H. P. HAWLEY. *Immune Complexes and Disease.* Basic Pathology Series (S-2951). National Audiovisual Center, Washington, D.C., 1973.

HORROCKS, D. L. *Principles of Gamma Counting.* Beckman Instruments, Inc., Fullerton, Calif., 1974.

MANNING, M. J. and R. J. TURNER. *Comparative Immunology.* John Wiley and Sons, New York, 1976.

OSLER, A. G. *Complement; Mechanisms and Functions.* Prentice-Hall, Englewood Cliffs, N.J., 1976.

OTTAVIANO, P. J. and A. F. DISALVO. *Quality Control in the Clinical Laboratory: A Procedural Text.* University Park Press, Baltimore, 1977.

OUCHTERLONY, Ö. *Handbook of Immunodiffusion and Immunoelectrophoresis.* Ann Arbor Science Publishers, Inc., Ann Arbor, Mich., 1968.

PARKER, C. W. *Radioimmunoassay of Biologically Active Compounds.* Prentice-Hall, Inc., Englewood Cliffs, N.J., 1976.

RANSOM, J. P. *Practical Competitive Binding Assay Methods.* The C. V. Mosby Co., St. Louis, 1976.

SHULMAN, S. *Tissue Specificity and Autoimmunity.* Springer-Verlag, New York, 1974.
SNELL, G. D., J. DAUSSET, and S. NATHENSEN. *Histocompatibility.* Academic Press, New York, 1976.
STANWORTH, D. R. *Immediate Hypersensitivity; The Molecular Basis of Allergic Response.* American Elsevier Pub. Co., New York, 1973.
STERNBERGER, L. A. *Immunocytochemistry.* Prentice-Hall, Inc., Englewood Cliffs, N.J., 1974.
TERASAKI, P. I. (Editor). *Histocompatibility Testing 1970.* The Williams & Wilkins Company, Baltimore, 1970.
TURK, J. L. *Delayed Hypersensitivity.* American Elsevier Pub. Co., New York, 1975.
WEISS, L. *The Cells and Tissues of the Immune System; Structure, Functions, Interactions.* Prentice-Hall, Inc., Englewood Cliffs, N.J., 1972.
WILKINSON, P. C. *Chemotaxis and Inflammation.* Churchill Livingstone, Edinburgh, 1974.
WOLSTENHOLME, G. E. W. and J. KNIGHT (Editors). *Complement.* Little, Brown and Company, Boston, 1965.

Immunology Laboratory Manuals

ACKROYD, J. F. *Immunological Methods.* F. A. Davis Company, Philadelphia, 1964.
Army Technical Manual TM8-227-1: Laboratory Procedures in Clinical Serology. U.S. Govt. Printing Office, Washington, D.C., 1960.
Army Technical Manual TM8-227-3: Laboratory Procedures in Blood Banking and Immunohematology. U.S. Govt. Printing Office, Washington, D.C., 1966.
BENNETT, C. W. *Clinical Serology.* Charles C Thomas Publisher, Springfield, Ill., 1968.
BLOOM, B. R. and P. R. GLADE (Editors). *In-Vitro Methods in Cell-Mediated Immunity.* Academic Press, New York, 1971.
BURRELL, R. *Experimental Immunology* (5th ed.). Burgess Publishing Company, Minneapolis, Minn., 1979.
CAMPBELL, D. H., J. S. GARVEY, N. E. CREMER, and D. H. SUSSDORF. *Methods in Immunology; A Laboratory Text for Instruction and Research* (2nd ed.). W. A. Benjamin, Inc., New York, 1970.
CLAUSEN, J. *Immunochemical Techniques for the Identification and Estimation of Macromolecules.* North-Holland Publishing Company, Amsterdam, 1969.
CROWLE, A. J. *Immunodiffusion.* Academic Press, New York, 1961.
DUNSFORD, I. and J. GRANT. *The Anti-Globulin (Coombs) Test.* Oliver and Boyd, Edinburgh, 1959.
GOLDMAN, M. *Fluorescent Antibody Methods.* Academic Press, New York, 1968.
Hyland Laboratories: Hyland Reference Manual of Immunohematology. Hyland Laboratories, Los Angeles, 1965.
KABAT, E. and M. M. MAYER. *Experimental Immunochemistry* (2nd ed.). Charles C Thomas Publisher, Springfield, Ill., 1961.
KWAPINSKI, J. B. G. *Methodology of Immunochemical and Immunological Research.* John Wiley & Sons, New York, 1972.
NATVIG, J. B., P. PERLMANN, and H. WIGZELL (Editors). *Lymphocytes; Isolation, Fractionation and Characterization.* University Park Press, Baltimore, 1976.
NERENBERG, S. T. *Electrophoretic Screening Procedures.* Lea & Febiger, Philadelphia, 1973.
NOWOTNY, A. *Basic Exercises in Immunochemistry; A Laboratory Manual.* Springer-Verlag, New York, 1969.
Ortho Diagnostics. *Blood Group Antigens & Antibodies As Applied to Compatibility Testing.* Ortho Diagnostics, Raritan, N.J., 1967.
Ortho Diagnostics. *Blood Group Antigens & Antibodies As Applied to Hemolytic Disease of the Newborn.* Ortho Diagnostics, Raritan, N.J., 1968.

Serology and Immunology

Ortho Diagnostics. *Blood Group Antigens & Antibodies As Applied to the ABO & Rh Systems.* Ortho Diagnostics, Raritan, N.J., 1969.

Ortho Diagnostics. *Quality Control in the Blood Bank.* Ortho Diagnostics, Raritan, N.J., 1973.

Ortho Pharmaceutical Corp. *Blood Group Antigens & Antibodies as Applied to Blood Transfusion.* Ortho Pharmaceutical Corp., Raritan, N.J., 1960.

ROSE, N. R. and P. BIGAZZI (Editors). *Methods in Immunodiagnosis.* John Wiley & Sons, New York, 1973.

ROSE, N. R. and H. FRIEDMAN (Editors). *Manual of Clinical Immunology.* American Society for Microbiology, Washington, D.C., 1976.

WILLIAMS, C. A. and M. W. CHASE (Editors). *Methods in Immunology and Immunochemistry.* Academic Press, New York, 1967.

General Medical Technology References

ALTER, A. A. et al. *Medical Technology Examination Review.* Volume 1. Fourth Edition. Medical Examination Publishing Company, Inc., Flushing, N.Y., 1977.

BAUER, J. D., P. G. ACKERMANN, and G. TORO. *Clinical Laboratory Methods* (8th ed.). The C. V. Mosby Company, St. Louis, 1974.

BAUER, J. D., G. TORO, and P. G. ACKERMANN. *Bray's Clinical Laboratory Methods* (6th ed.). The C. V. Mosby Company, St. Louis, 1962.

DAVIDSOHN, I. and J. B. HENRY (Editors). *Todd-Sanford Clinical Diagnosis by Laboratory Methods* (15th ed.). W. B. Saunders Company, Philadelphia, 1974.

FRANKEL, S. and S. REITMAN (Editors). *Gradwohl's Clinical Laboratory Methods and Diagnosis.* Volumes 1 and 2. The C. V. Mosby Company, St. Louis, 1963.

GOODALE, R. H. *Clinical Interpretation of Laboratory Tests* (6th ed.). F. A. Davis Company, Philadelphia, 1969.

HARRIS, A. B. and M. B. COLEMAN (Editors). *Diagnostic Procedures and Reagents.* American Public Health Association, Inc., New York, 1963.

HELPER, O. E. *Manual of Clinical Laboratory Methods* (4th ed.). Charles C Thomas Publisher, Springfield, Ill., 1965.

LEVINSON, S. A. and R. P. MACFATE. *Clinical Laboratory Diagnosis* (6th ed.). Lea & Febiger, Philadelphia, 1961.

LYNCH, M. J. et al. *Medical Laboratory Technology and Clinical Pathology* (2nd ed.). W. B. Saunders Company, Philadelphia, 1969.

MEYER, J. S. and L. S. STEINBERG. *Review of Laboratory Medicine.* The C. V. Mosby Company, St. Louis, 1971.

MILLER, S. E. (Editor). *A Textbook of Clinical Pathology* (7th ed.). The Williams & Wilkins Company, Baltimore, 1966.

RAPHAEL, S. S. et al. *Lynch's Medical Laboratory Technology* (3rd ed.). W. B. Saunders Company, Philadelphia, 1976.

SELIGSON, D. (Editor). *CRC Handbook Series in Clinical Laboratory Science.* Section D: Blood Banking. Volume 1. CRC Press, Inc., Cleveland, Ohio, 1977.

SELIGSON, D. (Editor). *CRC Handbook Series in Clinical Laboratory Science.* Section F: Immunology. Volume 1. Part 1. CRC Press, Inc., West Palm Beach, Fla., 1978.

SEMRAD, A. M. (Editor). *Comprehensive Review for Medical Technologists.* The C. V. Mosby Company, St. Louis, 1975.

Answers

Chapter 1

TERMS	MULTIPLE CHOICE	TRUE-FALSE
1. antigen	1. b	1. F
2. serology	2. c	2. T
3. reticuloendothelial system	3. e	3. T
4. resistance	4. a	4. F
5. agglutinins	5. d	5. F
6. complement	6. d	6. F
7. opsonins	7. a	7. F
8. passive	8. c	8. F
9. bursa of Fabricius	9. e	9. F
10. (immunological) tolerance	10. b	10. T

Chapter 2

TERMS	MULTIPLE CHOICE	TRUE-FALSE
1. paraproteins	1. a	1. T
2. electrophoresis	2. a	2. F
3. isoelectric point	3. c	3. T
4. Bence-Jones proteins	4. b	4. T
5. hinge (region)	5. c	5. F
6. isotypes	6. a	6. F
7. allotypes	7. e	7. F
8. idiotypes	8. b	8. T
9. allelic exclusion	9. b	9. T
10. combinatorial association	10. d	10. T

Chapter 3

TERMS	MULTIPLE CHOICE	TRUE-FALSE
1. blood group system	1. e (b and c)	1. T
2. erythroblastosis fetalis	2. a	2. F
3. pseudoagglutination	3. d	3. T
4. reverse (serum) grouping	4. e	4. F
5. zeta potential	5. c	5. T
6. titer	6. d	6. F
7. lectins (phytohemagglutinins)	7. b	7. T
8. Bombay	8. e	8. T
9. secretor	9. e (a and d)	9. T
10. antihuman globulin (Coombs serum)	10. a	10. F

Chapter 4

TERMS	MULTIPLE CHOICE	TRUE-FALSE
1. gene dosage	1. a	1. F
2. steric hindrance (interference)	2. e	2. F
3. amorphic	3. c	3. F
4. public (high-frequency)	4. b	4. T
5. reagin	5. d	5. F

Serology and Immunology

6. jaundice (icterus)	6. d	6. T
7. stat	7. b	7. T
8. atypical (irregular)	8. e (a, c, d)	8. F
9. cold agglutinins	9. d	9. T
10. compatibility (cross-matching)	10. b	10. T

Chapter 5

TERMS	MULTIPLE CHOICE	TRUE-FALSE
1. precipitinogens	1. d	1. F
2. optimal proportion	2. b	2. T
3. prozone	3. a	3. T
4. interfacial (ring) test	4. c	4. F
5. C-reactive protein	5. d	5. T
6. Oudin	6. a	6. F
7. Ouchterlony	7. e	7. F
8. rockets	8. e (a & c)	8. F
9. electroendosmosis (endosmosis)	9. b	9. T
10. immunoelectrophoresis	10. b	10. T

Chapter 6

TERMS	MULTIPLE CHOICE	TRUE-FALSE
1. nonspecific cold hemagglutinins	1. b	1. F
2. heterophile	2. b	2. T
3. Widal	3. a	3. F
4. Weil-Felix	4. e (a,b)	4. T
5. cardiolipin	5. c	5. F
6. hemagglutination inhibition	6. d	6. F
7. antigenic (immunological) drift or shift	7. d	7. F
8. indirect (passive)	8. e (a,b)	8. T
9. reversed passive	9. a	9. T
10. dissociation (or antigenic variation)	10. c	10. T

Chapter 7

TERMS	MULTIPLE CHOICE	TRUE-FALSE
1. anaphylatoxin	1. d	1. T
2. chemotaxin	2. b	2. F
3. immune (serological) adherence	3. a	3. T
4. fixation	4. c	4. T
5. amboceptor	5. c	5. F
6. Rice (test)	6. d	6. T
7. conglutinin	7. e (b,c,d)	7. F
8. properdin	8. a	8. F
9. Danysz phenomenon	9. e	9. F
10. Schick (test)	10. b	10. F

Chapter 8

TERMS	MULTIPLE CHOICE	TRUE-FALSE
1. fluor	1. a	1. F
2. *Treponema pallidum* immobilization	2. d	2. T
3. quenching	3. c	3. F

Answers

4. ligand	4. b	4. F
5. liquid scintillation (counter)	5. c	5. F
6. homogeneous	6. e (b,c)	6. T
7. antinuclear	7. c	7. T
8. competitive protein-binding assays	8. a	8. F
9. radioallergosorbent test	9. c	9. F
10. ferritin	10. e (a,c)	10. T

Chapter 9

TERMS	MULTIPLE CHOICE	TRUE-FALSE
1. hereditary angioneurotic edema (HANE)	1. e	1. F
2. idiopathic	2. b	2. F
3. iatrogenic	3. c	3. T
4. nitroblue tetrazolium	4. d	4. F
5. anergy	5. a	5. F
6. nude	6. c	6. T
7. Prausnitz-Küstner (PK test)	7. d	7. T
8. Arthus	8. e	8. T
9. purified protein derivative (PPD)	9. a	9. F
10. transfer factor (TF)	10. b	10. T

Chapter 10

TERMS	MULTIPLE CHOICE	TRUE-FALSE
1. allograft	1. c	1. F
2. lymphotoxins	2. c	2. T
3. immunological tolerance	3. b	3. T
4. allogeneic disease	4. e	4. F
5. histocompatibility	5. a	5. T
6. enhancement	6. d	6. F
7. congenic	7. d	7. T
8. haplotype	8. c	8. T
9. antimetabolite	9. e	9. F
10. regression proteins	10. d (a,b)	10. T

Index

Page numbers in bold face type contain definitions of terms. Acronyms have been avoided in this index wherever possible. Citations for acronyms may be located by: (1) finding the correct name or term from the list of acronyms following the appendix, and (2) referring to the bold face page citation(s) for the correct name in the index.

ABO blood group system, 68–76, 168, 320–321, 329
Absorbed serum, **62**
Absorption, **62**
Accessory cell, 26–27
   dysfunction, 279–280
Accuracy (QC), 347–348
Acquired immunity
   immunity, 2, 71
   resistance, 5
Active immunization, **9**, 10
Acute serum, 64
Adenyl cyclase, 287
Adjuvant, **12**, 344
   Freund's, 12
Adoptive immunity, **320**
Adrenalin, see Epinephrine
Adrenergic drugs, **289**
Adrenocorticotropic hormone, 279
Adsorption, **62**
Affinity, 61, **63**
Agammaglobulinemia
   infantile sex-linked, 282–283
   see also Hypogammaglobulinemia
Agglutination, 168–197
   bacterial, 6, 174–181
   coagglutination, 178
   hemagglutination, 169–174, 191–193
     see also Blood groups
   indirect, 190–197
   inhibition tests, 195–197
   in vivo, 114
   mixed field, **91**
   passive, **62**, 190–197
   reversed passive, **197**
   Streptococcus MG, 180–181
   vs. precipitation, 32–33
   viral hemagglutination, 184–190
   zoning, 136
Agglutinin, **7, 168**
   adsorption, 62
   albumin, **85**
   cold, **112, 123**, 309
   complete, **85**
   febrile, **179**–180
   IgG, 14
   IgM, 14
   saline, **85**
Agglutinogen, **7, 168**

Aggressins, **3**
Agranulocytes, see Mononuclear leukocytes
Albumins, 37, 40
   bilirubin complex, 94–95
   bovine serum, q.v.
   egg, 135–138
Alexin, **200**
Alkylating agents, 334
Allelic exclusion, **57**
Allergens, **286**
Allergic encephalomyelitis, 311
Allergist, **292**
Allergy, **286**
   asthma, 287, 292
   atopy, **286**
   complement-mediated, 201
   desensitization, 291–292
   hay fever, **286**
   immunoglobulin-mediated, 52
     see also Immunoglobulin IgE
   of infection, **299**
   insect bites and stings, 236
   in vitro test, 293
   skin tests, 292
   see also Hypersensitivity
Allogeneic
   disease, **320**
   graft, **315**
Allograft, 281, **315**–316
Allosteric
   protein, 7
   site, **7**
   transformation, **201**, 207
Allotypes, **46**
   Am, 47
   Gm, 47
   Inv, 47
   Km, 46–47
Alpha fetoprotein, 158, **343**
Alpha heavy chain, 46
Alpha-2 hepatic protein, 343
Alpha procedure (precipitation), 136
Alternate complement pathway, see Properdin
Alum, 12
Am allotypes, **47**
Amboceptor, **210**
Amino acids
   hydrophobic, 59
   see also Protein structure

Index

Amniocentesis, 99
Amorphic gene, **108**
Anamnestic response, **14**
Anaphylactoid reaction, **290**–291
Anaphylatoxin, **201, 290**
Anaphylaxis, **287**–288
   eosinophilic chemotactic factor of, **290**
   IgE-mediated, 287
   IgG-mediated, 290
   induction of, 293
   insect bites (stings), 236
   in vitro, *see* Schultz-Dale test
   local, *see* Arthus reaction
   mediators, 289–290
   passive cutaneous, **292**
   slow reacting substance of, **289**
Anemia, 71, 95
Anergy, **281, 290**
Angioneurotic edema, **208,** 281
Ankylosing spondylitis, 328
Anthrax, 2, 11, 141
Antiasthmatic drugs, 273
Antibiotics, 293, 335
Antibodies, **1,** 30–65
   albumin, **85**
   antinuclear, 263–267
   antiplatlet, 10, 310–311
   antitoxins, **7,** 139, 225–236
   atypical, **71, 104, 118**
   bivalent, **34**
   blocking, **87**
   blood group, 116–117
   cold, *see* Cold hemagglutinin
   colostral, 15
   combining site, 57–61
   complete, **85**
   coproantibody, **51**
   cytophilic, **24,** 54
   cytotropic, **287**
   enhancing, 321, 339, 341
   enzyme-conjugated, *see* Enzyme immunoassay
   ferritin-conjugated, *see* Ferritin
   fluor-conjugated, *see* Fluorescent antibody test
   functions, 5, 6
   heterocytotropic, **293**
   homocytotropic, **293**
   identification, 125–129
   incomplete, **87**
   irregular, **71, 104, 118**
   labeled, *see* Labeled reagents
   monospecific, 64
   monovalent, *see* Immunoglobulin IgE
   natural, 69, 71
   nonprecipitating, 287
   purification of, 62–64
   reaginic, **52**
   source, 19
   specificity, **32**
   sperm, 312

Antibodies [*cont.*]
   structure, 42–61
   titer (titration), 8
   tumor, 341
   univalent, **87**
   valence, **34**
   viral, 7, 305
   weak, 129
   see also Immunoglobulins; specific antibodies
Antibody-dependent cell-mediated cytotoxicity, **306,** 317
Anticoagulants, 113
   ACD, 113, 174
   citrate, 113, 214
   CPD, 113
   EDTA, 113, 174, 184, 214
   heparin, 174, 184
   potassium oxalate, 174
   sodium citrate, 113, 174
   sodium oxalate, 174
Anticomplementary
   factors, 182, 217
   unit, **218**
Anticonvulsion drugs, 273
Antiepileptic drugs, 273
Antigen, **1,** 30–65
   bacterial, 174–181
   beta, 25
   Boivin, **174, 224**
   carcinoembryonic, 342–343
   carrier, 12
   characteristics, 30–32
   cognate, **22, 91**
   complete, **32**
   conjugated, 12, 26
   cross-reactive, *see* Cross reactions
   determinant sites, 30, **32**
   epitope, **32**
   factors, **32**
   flagellar, 176
   fluorescent, 247
   Forssman, 170–171
   H-type, **176**
   haptenic, **26**
   hepatitis-associated, 113
   heterophile, **170**–171
   histoincompatibility, **315**–333
   homologous, **22**
   immunodominant groups, **31**
   incomplete, **26**
   K-type, **176**
   lymphocyte-detectable, **329**
   Maxted, 142
   neoantigen, **293**
   neoplastic, 339
   O-type, **176**
   occult, **307**
   overloading, **341**
   particulate, 12
   private, **112**

Antigen [*cont.*]
  processing, 34
  public, **112**
  Rantz, 142
  serologically detectable, **329**
  shift, 176
  size of determinant, 36
  soluble, 12
    see also Precipitation
  somatic, **176**
  specificity, **32**
  strengths, 129
  synthetic, 12, 26
  theta, 25
  thymus-dependent, 26
  thymus-independent, 25
  transplantation, 315–333
  tumor, 339 *ff*
  tumor-specific transplantation, **341**
  valence, **34**
  Vi, 176
  weak 72–73
  see also specific antigens
Antigen-antibody binding forces, 36
  Antigen-antibody reactions
  primary, 339–340
  secondary, 339–340
Antigen-binding capacity, 240
Antigen dilution confirmation test, **188**
Antigenic
  determinants, **32**
  dissociation, **176**
  drift, **176, 190**
  factors, **32**
  formula (bacterial), 177
  shift, **176**
  specificities, **32**
  variation, **176**
Antigenization, **12**
Antiglobulin, **85**
  direct test, **91**, 120
  immunoenzyme test, 269
  indirect test, **120**
  see also Coombs test
Antihistamines, 236, 289
Antihuman globulin, **85**, 108
  see also Coombs test
Anti-inflammatory agents, 283, 299
Antilymphocyte serum, 21, 335
Antimetabolites, 334
Antinuclear antibody, 263–267
Antiserum, **8**
Antistreptolysin tests, 226–229
Antitoxin, **7**, 139, 225–236
Antivenom, **7**, 235–236
Appendix, 20
Arthus reaction, **295–297**
  reversed passive, **296–297**
Artificial blood, 114
Aschoff's bodies, **309**
Ascoli test, 141

Aspermatogenesis, 312
Asthma, 287, 292
Ataxia telangiectasia, **283**, 343
Atopy, **286**
Attenuation, **11**
Atypical antibody, **71, 104, 118**
  screening test, **120**
Australia antigen, *see* Hepatitis associated antigen
Auto control, 123–124
Autoallergy, *see* Autoimmune diseases
Autoantibodies, 308–311
Autoantigen, 307
Autocoupling hapten, **293**, 300
Autofluorescence, **241**–242, 247–248
Autogeneic graft, 316
Autograft, 315–316
Autoimmune disease, 306–313
  antinucleic acids, 30
  hemolytic anemia, 309–311
  immunoglobulin-associated, 308–311
  T cell-associated, 311–313
  see also specific disease
Avidity, **62**, 63
Azoproteins, 35
  see also Diazotized proteins

B cells (B lymphocytes), **19**
  deficiency diseases, 282–284
  differentiation, 56
  killer, 306
Bacille Calmette-Guérin, **344**
Bacteria
  agglutination, 174–181
  antigenic formula, **177**
  attenuated, **11**
  avirulent, **11**
  capsule, 2–4, 33, 165, **175**–176
  contaminating reagents, 129
  febrile, 179–180
  flagellar antigens, 139, 175–178
  gram negative, 7, 30, 53, 175, 224
  gram positive, 7, 175, 225
  group antigens, **177**
  iodination, 280
  motility, 53
  nonpathogenic, **11**
  phase antigens, 177–178
  pyogenic, 4, 280
  R strain, 176
  S strain, 176–178
  serotypes, 176–178
  specific antigens, 177
  toxin, 223–235
  toxin neutralization, 6, 226 *ff*
Bacteriolysins, **6**
Bacteriolysis, 6
Bacteriophage, *see* Phage
Basophile, 23–25
  cytotropic antibody, **287**

Basophile [cont.]
  degranulation test, 293
  IgE receptors, 52
  mast cell counterpart, 201
Bee sting, 235–236, 292, 293
Beef, see Cattle
Bence-Jones protein, 42, 278, 281
Bentonite, 12
Beta 2 microglobulin, see Microglobulin
Beta antigen, 25
Beta procedure (precipitation), 136
Bile pigments, 94–96, 114
Bilirubin, 94–96, 99
Biological false
  negative reactions, 65
  positive reactions, 65, 242, 347
Biopsy, 42, 278
Bivalence, 34
Blast cell transformation, 331–332
Blastogenic factor, 303
Blocking
  antibodies, 87, 182, 291, 344
  control (fluorescence), 242
  phenomenon, 33
Blood
  artificial, 114
  clotting, 3, 201
    see also Coagulation
  composition, 1, 23–25
  counts, 25
  stains, 78–80
Blood-brain barrier, 336
Blood group factors, 68
Blood group incompatibility
  maternal-fetal, 67–68
  transfusion, 67
Blood group-specific substances, 71
Blood group systems, 67, 116–117
  ABO, 68–76
  Duffy, 68, 92, 109
  Kell-Cellano, 92, 107–109
  Kidd, 92, 109–110
  Lewis, 76, 104–105
  Lutheran, 111
  major, see ABO or Rh
  minor, 103–112
  MNS, 105–107
  P-p, 110–111
  Rh, 80–100
  Xg, 111–112
Blood grouping
  direct, 69
  reverse, 69
  serum, 69
  subgrouping, 72
Blood stain tests, 68, 78–80, 142
Blood transfusion, 320
  see also Compatibility test
Blood types, see Blood group systems
Boivin antigen, 174, 224
  see also Endotoxin

Bombay blood, 75
Bone marrow, 17, 18, 23, 42–43, 283–284
Booster response, 13
  adjuvant effect on, 12
Botulism, 7, 230, 275
Bovine, see Cattle
Bovine serum albumin
  antigen carrier, 32
  blood grouping, 86–87, 89–90
  compatibility test, 114–115
  quality control, 130
Bradykinnin, 289
Brucella, 4, 299, 347
Brucellergen, 299
Brucellosis, 179, 299
Bruton's disease, 282
Burkitt's lymphoma, 340
Bursa of Fabricius, 17, 18, 19

Cl-9, see Complement components
C1 esterase inhibitor, 208
C3 activator convertase, 206–207
Cancer, 18, 337–345
  benign, 338
  carcinoma, 339
  danger signs, 337
  etiology, 339–342
  leukemia, 339
  malignant, 338
  metastasis, 338
  of plasma cell, 37, 277–278
  predisposing factors, 339
  primary, 338
  prophylaxis, 344–345
  rheumatoid factor, 193
  sarcoma, 338
  secondary, 338
  serologic indicators, 341–342
  thymoma, 282
  vaccine, 344
  virus-associated, 305
Capping phenomenon, 26, 321–322
Capsid, 184
Capsomere, 184
Capsular swelling, 165
Capsule (bacterial), see Bacteria, capsule
Carcinoembryonic antigen, 342, 343
Carcinofetal antigen, 342–343
Carcinogens, 339
Carcinoma, 339
Cardiolipin, 181, 216
Carrier
  particles, 33, 190–194
  proteins, 26, 32, 33
Casoni test, 300
Catalase, 280
Caticholamine, 289
Cattle
  corpora lutea, 261

Cattle [*cont.*]
   erythrocyte antigen, 172
   twins, 20
Cellano blood factor, *see* Kell-Cellano blood group system
Cell-mediated cytotoxicity, 306
Cell-mediated hypersensitivity, 299 *ff*
Cell-mediated immunity, **8**, 299 *ff*
   mechanisms, 20
   phylogeny, 17–18
Cellular immunity, *see* Cell-mediated immunity
Cerebrospinal fluid, 184, 336
Chancre, **181**, 242
Chédiak-Higashi syndrome, **280**
Chemotaxin, **4, 201**, 317
   complement components, 6, 201, 296
   lymphokine, 301, 304
Chicken, 2
   bronchitis virus, 13
   bursa, 17–19
   cholera, 11
   egg protein sensitivity, 10
   laryngotracheitis virus, 13
   pox, 311
   thyroiditis, 312
Cholera, 10, 68, 186, 200
   chicken, 11
Choriocarcinoma, 343
Chorionic gonadotropin, 195, 261, 343
Chronic granulomatous disease, 279–280
Chronic mucocutaneous candidiasis, 282
Class (immunoglobulin), **46**–51
Classical complement pathway, 202–205
Clonal selection theory, **21**, 22, 53, 63
Clone, 14, **20**, 315
   cancer, 43
Clostridium, 225, 275
Clotting, *see* Coagulation
Coagglutination, **178**
Coagulase, 3
Coagulation, 3, 201, 224–226, 289, 296
   disseminated intravascular, 158
Coated cells, **89**
Coccidioidin, 299
Coctoantisera, 142
Codeine, 196–197
Coefficient of variation, 258
Cognate antigen, **22**
Cognates, **91**
Cold hemagglutinins, **112, 123**, 269, 309
Collagenase, 3
Colostrum, 15
Combinatorial
   association, **47, 57**
   translocation, **57**
Compatibility test
   blood grouping, 113–119
   histocompatibility, 330–333
   see also Crossmatch test
Competitive protein-binding assays, **261**–263

Complement, **6, 200**–222
   activation of, 5, 50, 200–**201**
   alternate pathway, 205–207
   anaphylatoxins, **201, 290**
   anticomplementary factors, 217–219
   cascade, 6, **201**–207
   cell receptors for, 21
   chemotaxins, **201**, 286
   classical pathway, 201–205
   components, 200 *ff*
   deficiencies and defects, 281
   fixation, 25
   fixation tests, 209–222
   fractions, 200 *ff*
   functions, 201
   immune adhesion, 201
   immune lysis, 113, 204–206
   inactivators and inhibitors, **207**
   in invertebrates, 17
   loss of activity, 210
   lysis of cells, 203–206, 209
   opsonin, 201
   phylogeny, 17
   properdin pathway, 202, 205–207
   regulation of activity, 207–208
   role in hypersensitivity, 201, 296, 298
   role in phagocytosis, 25
   specific component assays, 208–209
   titration of, 214–216
Complement fixation tests, 209–222
   anticomplementary unit, **218**
   antigenic unit, **219**
   indirect test, 219–221
   lytic tests, 210–220
   nonlytic tests, 220–222
   Rice test, **219**–221
Complement-staining immunofluorescence test, 246–247
Complete
   antibody, 85
   antigen, **32**
Concanavalin A, 21, 345
Confidence limits, 352–353
Congenic mouse strains, 323–324
Conglutinating complement adsorption test, 220–222
Conglutinin, 208, **220**
   complement fixation, 220–222
Conglutinogen-activating factor, **208**
Conjugated antigen, 26
Conjunctival test, 236
Constant regions of immunoglobulins, 45–46
Contact dermatitis, **300**–301
Control
   auto, **123**
   quality, 129–133, 347–352
Convalescent serum, 64
Coombs test, **85**
   cold agglutinins, 310
   compatibility test, 115–118
   control cells, **91**

Index

Coombs test [*cont.*]
   direct, **91**, 98, 120
   indirect, **120**, 168
   see also Antihuman globulin
Coons test, 240
   see also Fluorescent antibody tests
Coproantibodies, **51**
Cornea transplant, 336
Corpora lutea, 261
Corticosteroids, 335
Corticosteroid-binding globulin, 261
Cortisone, 283
Corynebacterium, 232–233
   see also Diphtheria
Counterimmunoelectrophoresis, 146, 157–159
Cowpox, 9, 11
   see also Vaccination, smallpox
C-reactive protein, 65, **142**–145, 197
Cromolyn, 290
Cross-match tests, 113–119
   see also Compatibility tests
Cross reactions, 35, 64–65, 299, 307
Crossed immunoelectrophoresis, 146, 157–159
Cushing's disease, **283**
Cyclic AMP, 287, 289
Cyst, **337**
Cytolysis, 7
   see also Bacteriolysis; Hemolysis; Killer cells
Cytophilic antibody, **24, 54**
Cytotoxicity, 223–236
   in vitro tests, 226–230, 232–233, 239–331
   in vivo tests, 230–235, 330–333
Cytotropic antibody, **287**
   heterocytotropic, 293
   homocytotropic, 293

Danysz phenomenon, **231**
Darkfield microscopy, 242–243
Davidsohn's differential test, 172–173
Dean and Webb titration, **136**
Degranulation (mast cell), 201
Delayed hypersensitivities
   cellular mediators, 281, 298–303
   chemical mediators, *see* Lymphokines
   contact dermatitis, 300–301
   tuberculin reaction, 299–300
   vs. immediate hypersensitivities, 284
Delta heavy chain, 46
Densitometry, **39**
Deoxyribonucleic acid
   antibodies, 30
      see also Lupus erythematosus
   coding for antibodies, 55
   repair system, 283
   spacer, 56
   structure, 31
Dermatitis, contact, 300–301
Desensitization, 236, 291–292

Determinant, 30, 32
Development of the immune system, 18–20
Diazotized protein, 32–33
   see also Azoprotein
Dick test, **234**
Dielectric constant, **86**
Diffusion tests, *see* Precipitation, gel phase
Di George syndrome, **281**–282
Digoxin
   immunoenzyme assay, 273
   radioimmunoassay, 254–256
Dinitrochlorobenzene, 281
Dinitroflurobenzene, 191
Diphasic bacteria, **177**
Diphtheria, 7, 16, 225, 231–234
   DPT vaccine, 15
   toxoid, 11, 12
Direct blood grouping, **69**
   antiglobulin (Coombs) test, **91**, 98, 120
Direct immunoelectrophoresis, **163**
Disseminated intravascular coagulation, 158
Disulfide bridges, 44
Dog, 2, 287, 308
Domains of immunoglobulin chains, **46**
Donnan effect, **203**
Donor screening, 120–123
Dosage effect of genes, **106**, 129, 322
Double antibody technique, 252
   see also Coombs test; Antiglobulin test
Double gel diffusion test, 151–155
Drug
   abused, 196–197, 249
   adrenergic, **289**
   antiasthmatic, 273
   antibiotics, 293
   anticancer, 341
   anticonvulsant, 273
   antihistamine, 289
   immunosuppressive, 279, 334–335
   induced hemolytic anemia, 309
   induced platelet damage, 310–311
   radiomimetic, 335
   sympathomimetic, **289**
D^u antigen, **89**–93
Duffy blood group system, 68, 109
Dysgammaglobulinemia, 277–279, 283
Dysphagocytosis, congenital, 279

E rosette, 281
Echinococcus, 300, 338
Eczema, 283, **294**
Edelman, G., 44
Edema, **201**, 287, 292
   hereditary angioneurotic, **208**
Effector
   cells, 5
   functions, 8, 57
   substances, 5
Egg albumin, 135–138, 294
Ehrlich, P., 200, 210, 306

Index

Electroendosmosis, **159**
Electroimmunoassay, *see* Immunoelectrophoresis
Electron microscopy immunoassay, 275
Electron spin resonance immunoassay, 273–274
Electropherogram, **39**
Electrophoresis, **37–43**, 144
  disc, **38**
  moving (free) boundary, **37**
  serological, *see* Immunoelectrophoresis
  zone, **39**
Elek test, **232–233**
Elution technique, **63**, 191
Emperipolesis, **336**
Encephalitis, experimental allergic, 311
Endosmosis, 159
Endotoxins, **174, 224**
  characteristics of, 225
  in vitro test for, 224–225
Enhancement, immunologic, **321**, 339
Enhancing antibody, 321, 339, 341
Enterobacter, 280
Envelope, viral, **184**
Enzyme
  adenyl cyclase, 287
  aldolase, 343
  alkaline phosphatase, 343
  catalase, 280
  coagulase, 225
  collagenase, 225
  fibrinolysin (kinase), 226
  glucose-6-phosphate dehydrogenase, 280
  glucuronyl transferase, 95
  glycogen phosphorylase, 343
  hemolysin, 226
  hyaluronidase, 3, 226, 229
  isozymes, **207, 343**
  lecithinase, 225
  leukocidin, 226
  lipase, 226
  monoamine oxidase, 290
  myeloperoxidase, 280
  neuraminidase, 280
  nuclease, 226, 229
  papain, 44–45, 324, 326
  pepsin, 45
  proteases, 226
  receptor destroying, 68
  reverse transcriptase, 340
  streptokinase, 229
Enzyme immunoassays
  antiglobulin technique, 269
  enzyme-linked immunosorbent assay, 267–268
  enzyme multiplied immunoassay technique, **273**
  heterogeneous, 267–269
  homogeneous, 269–273
  immunoenzymometric test, 268–269
  sandwich technique, 268

Eosinophil, 23–25, 201, 290
Eosinophilic chemotactic factor of anaphylaxis, **201, 290**
Eosinophilia, 257
Epifluorescence, 240–241
Epileptic drugs, 273
Epinephrine, 236, 289
Epithelial cells, 49
Epitope, **32**, 62
Epsilon heavy chain, 46
Epstein-Barr virus, 169
Equivalence point or zone, **135**
Errors
  random, **350**
  systematic, **350**
Erythema, **292**
Erythroblast, **96**
Erythroblastosis fetalis, **96**
  prevention of, 97–98
Erythrocyte, **1**
  antigens, *see* Blood group systems
  carriers, 190–194
  characteristics of, 24
  use in serological tests, *see* Hemagglutination
Escherichia, 280
Etiology of disease, **64**
Evolution of the immune system, 17–18
Exchange transfusion, 99
Exclusion of parentage, **74**
Exotoxins, **223–226**
  characteristics, 225
  neutralization tests, 226–230, 234
Experimental allergic encephalomyelitis, 311

Fabricius, bursa of, 17–19
False reactions, 65
  see also Biological false negative; Biological false positive
Fc receptors, 21
Febrile agglutinins, **179–180**
Feedback inhibition, **98**
Ferritin, 275, 343
Ferritin-conjugated antibodies, **275**
Fibrinogen, 1, 158
Fibrinolysin, 3
Ficoll-Hypaque technique, 329–330
Fimbrius, 175
First set reaction, **316**
Fisher, R. A., 80
Fixation of complement, 25
  see also Complement fixation
Flagellar antigens, *see* Bacteria
Flare, 292
Flocculation
  agglutination tests, 139, 182
  flagellar antigens, 176
  precipitation tests, **139**
  toxin-antitoxin, 232
  VDRL test, 182

Index

Fluor, **239**
Fluorescence quenching, 247–248
Fluorescent antibody tests, 239–247
  antitreponemal, 65
  complement-staining, 246–247
  darkfield technique, **242–243**
  direct, 239–243
  indirect, 244–246
  inhibition, 243–244
  microcytotoxicity test, 330
  quantitative, 247–248
Fluorescent antigen, 247–248
Fluorescent treponemal antibody absorption test, 65
Fluorochemicals, as blood substitute, 114
Fluorochrome, **239**, 282
Forensic serological tests, 68, 74, 78–80
Formaldehyde
  formalinized red cells, 191
  viral inactivation, 11
Forssman heterophile system, 170–171
Fragments of immunoglobulins
  Fab, **44** *ff*
  Fab', **44**
  F(ab')$_2$, **45**
  Fc, **44** *ff*
  Fc', **45**
  Fd, **45**
Franklin's disease, 278
Free-radical assay technique, 273–274
Frei test, 299
Freund's adjuvant, 12, 311–312
Fungal immunity, 7, 299

Gamma globulin, 39
Gamma heavy chain, 46
Gammopathy
  monoclonal, **277**
  polyclonal, **278**
Gel diffusion tests, *see* Immunodiffusion techniques
Gel filtration, *see* Sephadex
Gel precipitation tests, *see* Precipitation, gel phase
Gene dosage effect, **106**
Genetics
  allergic predisposition, 52–53
  of antibody diversity, 54–57
  congenic mouse strains, 323–324
  epistasis, 76
  haplotype, 327–328
  in immune response, 31–32
  multiple alleles, 81
  recombination, 56
  sex-linked gene, 111
  translocation, 339
Globulins, 37
  alpha, 39, 40
  beta, 39, 40
  gamma, 39, 40

Globulins [*cont.*]
  see also Immunoglobulins
Glomerulonephritis
  acute, 229
  Goodpasture's disease, **309**
  Masugi, **309**
  SLE, 308
Glycoprotein
  blood group antigens, 68
  histocompatibility antigens, 324
  viral hemagglutinins, 186
Gm allotypes, **47**
Gonorrhea, 13
Goodpasture's disease, **309**
Graft
  allograft, **315**
  autograft, **315**
  heterograft, **315**
  orthotopic, **315**
  rejection, 301, 316–321
  syngraft, **315**
  xenograft, **316**
Graft-vs.-host reaction, 319–320
Gram staining, *see* Bacteria
Granulocytes, **23**–25, 303
  isolation technique, 329
Granuloma, 12, 282
Group antigens, bacterial, **177**
Guinea pig
  anaphylaxis, 288
  aspermatogenesis, 312
  kidney antigen, 170–173
  lymph node permeability factor, 303
  progesterone-binding protein, 261
  serum complement, 200, 209
  toxin assay, 231, 233
Gut-associated lymphoid tissue, **20**

H chains of immunoglobulins, *see* Heavy chain
H-2 histocompatibility complex, 322, 324–327
H substance, **74**
H type antigen, **176**
Hageman factor, **202**, 289
Haplotype, **327–328**
Haptens, **26**
  autocoupling, **293**, 300
  binding of antibody, 60–61
  characteristics, 32
  complex, **33**
  conjugated, 35
  inhibitors of passive agglutination, 191
  nonprecipitating, **33**
  precipitating, **33**
  simple, **33**
Hashimoto's hypothyroiditis, 312–313
Hay fever, 286
Heavy chain, 8, **44**, 46
  diseases, 278–279

Heavy chain [*cont.*]
  gene family, 57
Helper cells
  macrophages, *q.v.*
  T cells, 26, 279
Hemagglutination
  blood grouping tests, 67–133
  cold antibodies, 169
  direct, immune, 168–174
  heterophile, 169–174
  indirect tests, 190–197
  inhibition test, **76, 186**–190
  passive, 190–197
  viral, 184–186
Hemagglutinin
  influenza, 186
  see also Agglutinin
Hematocrit, **119**
Hematopoietic system, 17
Hemoglobin, 94–96, 114
Hemolysin, **6, 210**
  titration, 211–214
Hemolysis
  complement mediated, 202–207
  toxin-mediated, 226–229
Hemolytic diseases
  ABO disease, 100–101
  erythroblastosis fetalis, **67**
  of newborn, **67**, 93–100
  Rh disease, 67, 93–100
Hemolytic transfusion reaction, **114**
Hemophilia, 120
Hemophilus, 280
Heparin, 52, 201, 287
Hepatic globulin, 343
Hepatitis
  alpha fetoprotein, 343
  associated antigen, 113
  Australia antigen, 158, 192
  passive hemagglutination test, 192–193
  VDRL crossreaction, 183
Hereditary angioneurotic edema, **208**, 281
Heredity, *see* Genetics
Heroin, 196–197
Heterocytotropic antibody, **293**
Heterogeneous immunoassay, **267**–269
Heterograft, **316**
Heterologous
  antigen, 14
  species, 9
Heterophile
  agglutination test, 169–174
  antibodies, **170**
  differential test, 172–174
  presumptive test, 171–172
Hinge region, **44**
Hirst, J. C., 184
Histamine, 52
  functions, 201
  metabolism, 290
  role in allergy, 287, 296

Histamine [*cont.*]
  source, 24, 201, 287
Histiocyte, 4, 24
Histocompatibility
  antigens, 119, 306, **315, 321**–329
  compatibility tests, 330–333
  lymphocyte detectable antigens, 329
  serological tests, 329–331
  systems, human, 327–329
  systems, mouse, 324–327
  testing, 321, 329–333
  vs. transplantation antigens, 329
Histoplasmin, 299
Hives, 292, 294
HLA, *see* Human leukocyte antigen
Hodgkin's disease, **282**
Homocytotropic antibodies, **293**
Homogeneous immunoassay, **267**, 269–273
Homograft, **316**
Homologous
  antigen, **22**
  disease, *see* Allogeneic disease
  species, 9
Hormone
  adrenocorticotropic, 279
  corticosteroid, 261, 335
  cortisone, 283
  human chorionic gonadotropin, 195, 261, 363
  progesterone, 261
  thymosin, 305
  thyroxine, 261–263
Horror autotoxicus, 306
Horse
  erythrocyte antigen, 173–174
  precipitating serum, 139
Host-parasite relationship, 144
Human chorionic gonadotropin, 195, 261, 363
Human leukocyte antigen histocompatibility complex, 322
  disease relationship, 328–329
  genetic control, 327–328
  microglobulin, 325–326
  testing, 329–333
Humor, **1**
Humoral immunity, **6**
Hyaluronidase, 3, 226, 229
Hydatidiform mole, 343
Hydrogen peroxide, 280
Hydrophobic amino acids, 59
Hyperimmunization, 14, 283
Hypersensitivity, **1**, 284–312
  allergies, 286–295
  autoallergic diseases, 306–312
  cell-mediated, 298–306
  contact dermatitis, **300**–301
  delayed, 284, 298–306
  Gell and Coombs classification, 285
  immediate, 284–295
  immune complex diseases, 295–298

Hypersensitivity [cont.]
  immunoglobulin-mediated, 284–295
  passive immunization, 10
  tuberculin reaction, 299
  types I, II, III, IV, 285
  see also Serum sickness
Hypervariable regions of immunoglobulins, 57–60
Hypogammaglobulinemia
  ataxia telangiectasia, **283**
  Bruton type, 282–283
  nude mouse, 282
  Swiss type, **283**–284
Hypothyroiditis, 312–313

Ia antigen, 21, **327**, 329
Iatrogenic diseases, **279**, 293, 310
Icterus, 99
  see also Jaundice
Idiopathic diseases, **309**
Idiotypes, **47**, 56, 287
Ig, see Immunoglobulins
Immediate hypersensitivities, 285–295
Immobilization test, 53, 243
Immune, see Immunologic(al)
Immune adherence, **25**, 201
  rosettes, 53
Immune complex diseases
  Arthus reaction, 295–297
  glomerulonephritis, 309
  serum sickness, 297–298
Immune enhancement, see Immunologic enhancement
Immune paralysis, **97**, 341
Immune response, 1–**2**, 5
  adjuvant effect, 12
  afferent limb, **5**
  anamnestic, 14
  booster, 13
  cellular, see T lymphocytes
  central limb, **5**
  efferent limb, **5**
  factors influencing, 32
  genes (loci), **286, 327**
  humoral, 13–15
  latent period, 13–14
  memory, 14
  neonatal, 15
  primary, 13
  secondary, 14
  single cells, 53–54
Immune system, 5
  ontogeny, 18–20
  phylogeny, 17–18
Immune tolerance, see Immunologic tolerance
Immunity, **1**–2
  acquired, 2, 71
  active, **9**–10
  adoptive, **320**
  antibacterial, 6–7

Immunity [cont.]
  antifungal, 7
  antitoxin, 7
  artificial, **9**
  cell mediated, **9**
  humoral, **6**
  natural, **9**
  passive, **9**–10
  vaccine-induced, see Vaccination
  viral, 7
  see also Virus
Immunization, **12**
  recommended schedule, 16–17
Immunoadsorbent, see Sorbent
Immunoadsorption, 62
Immunoblast, 6, 14, 23
  transformation, 331–332
Immunocyte, 6
Immunocytology, 23–27
Immunodeficiency
  B cells, 282–284
  complement, 281
  immunoglobulin, 282–284
  phagocytosis, 279–280
  primary disease, 283
  secondary disease, 283
  T cells, 281–284
Immunodiffusion techniques, 144–155
  double dimension, 151–155
  Ouchterlony, 151–155
  Oudin, 146–147
  radial, 147–150
Immunodominant group, **31**, 68
Immunoelectrophoresis, **41**, 159–165
Immunoenzyme assays, see Enzyme immunoassays
Immunofixation electrophoresis, **163**–165
Immunofluorescence, see Fluorescent antibody tests
Immunogenetics
  antibody diversity, 54–57
  blood group antigens, 73 ff
  histocompatibility, 322 ff
Immunoglobulin, **1**, **37**
  allotypes, **46** ff
  characteristics, 54–55
  classes, 8, **46**–53
    IgA, 9, 11, 51–52, 135, 312
    IgD, 52
    IgE, 24, 34, 52–53, 135, 257–261, 283, 286–295
    IgG, 8, 9, 14–15, 26, 42–46, 48, 57, 135, 200, 224, 247, 291
    IgM, 8, 14, 17, 25, 34, 48–50, 112, 135, 181, 200, 216, 224, 283, 336
    "IgT," 25–27
  deficiency, 282–284
  domains, **46**
  effector functions, 57
  fragments, see Fragments of immunoglobulins

Index

Immunoglobulin [*cont.*]
  gene families, 57
  hypervariable regions, **57–59**
  isotypes, **46**
  ontogeny, 18–20
  phylogeny, 17–18
  purification, 62–64
  structure, 42–46
  subclasses, **46**
  subtypes, **46**
  switch region, 58
  synthesis, *see* Plasma cell
  types, **46**
Immunohematology, 67–133
  see also Blood groups
Immunologic(al) amplification, 20
Immunologic competence, 10, 13
Immunologic drift, **176, 190**
Immunologic enhancement, **321**, 339
Immunologic incompetence, 14, 17
Immunologic maturity, 13
Immunologic memory, 2
  lack of in passive immunity, 10
Immunologic paralysis, **97, 341**–342
Immunologic privilege, 336–337
Immunologic response, *see* Immune response
Immunologic sandwich, **245**, 258, 268
Immunologic shift, *see* Immunologic drift
Immunologic surveillance, 18, **321**
  see also Cancer
Immunologic tolerance, **20, 319**, 341
Immunologic unresponsiveness, 341
Immunologic valence, **34**
Immunology, 1 *ff*
Immunopathology, 277–313
Immunoprecipitates, **41**
  see also Precipitation
Immunoproliferative diseases, **43**, 277–279
Immunosuppression
  antilymphocyte serum, 335
  chemical agents, 334–335
  disease association, 279
  steroids, 335
Incompatibility
  blood transfusion, *see* Compatibility test
  grafts, *see* Histocompatibility
  hemolytic disease of newborn, 93–101
Incomplete antibody, **87**
  see also Blocking antibody
Incomplete antigen, *see* Hapten
Indirect tests
  agglutination, 190–194
  antiglobulin, **120**
  Coombs, **120**
  fluorescent, **244**–246
Infantile sex-linked agammaglobulinemia, **282**–283
Infection, **3**
Infectious mononucleosis
  anemia, 309
  Epstein-Barr virus, 340
  heterophile agglutinin test, 169–174
  VDRL crossreactions, 183
Inflammation, 6, 20, 23
Influenza
  cell receptor, 68
  duration of immunity, 13
  immunization, 16
  peplomeres, 186
  serotypes, 189–190
  see also Virus
Inhibition, **33**
  blocking reaction, 33
  fluorescence, 243–244
  hemagglutination, viral, **186**–190
  passive agglutination tests, 195–197
Initiation factor, 206–207
Insect bites (stings), 235–236
Integumentary system, 3
Interfacial test, *see* Ring test
Interferons, 303–306
  anti-cancer, 344
Inv allotypes, *see* Km allotypes
Invertebrate "immunity," 17–18
Ir genes, 286, 327
Irradiation, 334
Irregular antibody, **71, 104, 118**
Isoelectric focusing, **40**–41
Isoenzyme, **207, 343**
Isograft, 316
Isohemagglutinin, *see* ABO blood group system, antibodies
Isotypes, **46**
Isozyme, **207, 343**

J chain, **48**–49, 51
Jaundice, **99, 114**
Jerne plaque technique, 53
Job's syndrome, 279–280

K antigens, **176**
K cells, **306**
Kahn test, 183
Kappa immunoglobulin chain, 46
  gene family, 57
Kell-Cellano blood group system, 107–109
Kern marker, 46–47
Kernicterus, **95**
Kidd blood group system, 109–110
Kidney dialysis, 193
Killer cells, 306
Kinnins, *see* Bradykinnin
Kline test, 183
Km allotypes, **46**–47
Koch's postulates, 307
Kolmer complement fixation test, 208, 216–218
Kupffer's cell, 24
Kveim test, **282**

Index

L immunoglobulin chain, *see* Light chains
L$_X$ doses of toxin
  L$_+$ dose, **231**
  L$_0$ dose, **231**–232
  L$_r$ dose, **231**–232
L forms (bacteria), 174
Labeled reagents
  enzyme-labeled, 263–273
  ferritin-labeled, 275
  fluor-labeled, 239–248
  radioisotope-labeled, 249–263
  spin-labeled, 273–274
Lambda light immunoglobulin chain, 46
  gene family, 57
Lancefield groups, 142
Landsteiner, K., 35, 67, 80, 105, 144
Landsteiner's rules, **69**
Latent period, **13**–14
Latex particles
  antigen carrier, 12, 33
  passive agglutination test, 194–195, 229, 299
Lattice, 32, 135
Laurell technique, 155
LD$_{50}$, **230**
LE body, **264**
LE cell, 263–264, 308
  see also Lupus erythematosus
LE factors, 263–264
Lectin, **72**, 76, 108
Lepromin, 299
Leprosy, 64, 183, 193, 282, 299
Lethal dose, *see* LD$_{50}$
Leucocytes, *see* Leukocytes
Leukemia, **339**
Leukocydin, 4
Leukocyte, **1**, 23
  agranulocytes, 23–25
  characteristics, 24–25
  classification, 23–25
  granulocytes, 23–25
  histocompatibility antigens, 119
  inhibitory factor, 303
  isolation technique, 329
  mononuclear, 24–25
  polymorphonuclear, 23–25
Leukocytotoxicity test, 329–331
Leukotaxin, 297
Leukotriene, 289–290
Levey-Jennings chart, 351–353
Lewis blood group system, 76, 104–105
Ligand, 251
Light immunoglobulin chain, 8, **44**, 46
Limulus amebocyte lysate test, 224–226
Lipids
  as antigens, 30
  in precipitation tests, 143
Lipopolysaccharides
  activation of complement, 205–206
  as antigens, 30

Lipopolysaccharides [*cont.*]
  endotoxin, **174**, 205–206, **224**
  mitogen effect, 21, 25
Lock and key hypothesis, 2, 62
Low ionic strength saline, **86**
Lupus erythematosus, **263**–267
  antinuclear antibodies, *q.v.*
  LE body, **264**
  LE cell, 263–**264**, 308
  LE factor, 263–264
  reagin induction, 216
  rheumatoid factor, 193
  suppressor T cell dysfunction, 344
  VDRL crossreaction, 183
Lutheran blood group system, 111
Lygranum, 299
Lymph node
  B lymphocyte maturation, 20
  BCG effect on, 344
  cancer, 282, 338
  permeability factor, 303
Lymphocyte
  antigen stimulation, 31
  B cell, **18**
  capping, 26
  cell receptors, 63
  cellular interactions, 26–27
  characteristics, 21, 23–24
  committed, 5
  cytotoxic (killer), 306
  experienced, 14
  helper, 26, 279
  isolation technique, 329–330
  mitogens, response to, 21
  null, **25**
  primed, 5
  suppressor, 27, 344
  T cell, **20**, 185
  virgin, 14
Lymphocyte-detectable histocompatibility antigens, 329
Lymphocytic choriomeningitis virus, 284
Lymphocytotoxin, **223**, **317**
Lymphogranuloma venereum, 299
Lymphoid organs and system
  nodes, 338
  ontogeny, 18–20
  phylogeny, 17–18
  primary, 17
  secondary, 17
Lymphokines, 2, 5, **9**, **20**, **301**–306
  see also specific lymphokines
Lymphoma, 278
Lymphopenia, 282
Lymphotoxin, **223**, 282, 303, **317**
Lysis, 6
  bacteriolysis, 6
  cytolysis, 7
  hemolysis, 6, 226
  scoring reactions, 213
Lysogenic conversion, **176**

Index

Lysosomal enzymes, 23–24
Lysozyme, 3

M protein, 43, 46, **277**, 309
Macroglobulin, *see* Immunoglobulin class M
Macrophage, **24**
  activating factor, 317
  antigen processing role, 98
  cell interactions, 26–27
  functions, 4, 6
  IgG receptors, 24
  killer, 306
  migration inhibition, 301
  monocyte precursor, 23
  rosette component, 53
Major crossmatch test, **114**
Major histocompatibility complex, **322**
  human, 327–329
  mouse, 324–327
Malaria, 64, 68, 183, 340
Mancini test, 147, 149
Mantoux test, 299
Mast cell
  basophil precursor, 24
  cytotropic antibody, **287**
  degranulation test, 201
  IgE receptors, 52
  products, 201
  structure, 288
Masugi nephritis, **309**
Maternal-fetal privilege, 337
Maxted antigen, 142
Mazini test, 183
Measles, 11, 16, 311
Median, **349**
Megakaryocyte, 23
Memory cells, 2, 10, 287
Messenger RNA, 56
Metastasis, **338**, 341
Methotrexate, 334
Mice, *see* Mouse
Microcytotoxicity test, 329–330
Microdroplet technique, 53
Microglial cell, 24
Microglobulin, 325–326
Microphage, 25
Microtiter system, 187, 220
Migration inhibition factor, 301–302
Minimal reacting dose, **230**
Minimum lethal dose, **230**
Minor crossmatch test, **114**
  alternatives to, 120–123
Mitogenic factor, 303
Mitogens, 21, **26**, 27
Mixed field agglutination, **91**
Mixed leukocyte culture (MLC), 330–332
Mixed lymphocyte reaction (MLR), 330–332
MNS blood group system, 105–107
Mode, **349**
Molds, *see* Fungal immunity

Moloney test, **234**
Moniliasis, 282
Monoclonal gammopathy, **43**, **277**
Monocyte, 23–24
Mononuclear leukocyte, **24**, 301
Mononucleosis, *see* Infectious mononucleosis
Monophasic bacteria, **177**
Monospecific antibody, 64
Monovalent
  antibody, *see* Immunoglobulin class E
  antigen, **34**
Morphine, 197
Mouse
  congenic strains, 323–324
  histocompatibility system, 322–327
  inbred strains, 315, 319
  mitogen response, 21
  nude, 25, **282**
  runting disease, **320**
  SLE model, 308
  thymus, 19
Mu immunoglobulin chain, 46
Mucous membranes, 3, 291
Multiple
  germ line theory, **55**
  myeloma, 42–43, 277–278
Multivalence, **34**
Mumps, 11, 16, 311
Mutagens, 334, 339
Mutation
  immunocompetent cell, 307
  immunoglobulin, 46
  neoantigen, 307
  somatic theory, 56
  viral, 11, 15
Myasthenia gravis, 311, 328
Mycobacterium, 4, 344
  as adjuvant, 12
  see also Tuberculosis
Mycoplasma, 169, 174–175
Myeloma, 42–43, 57, 277–278
Myeloperoxidase, 280
Myocardial infarction, 142–143

Natural antibody, 69, 71, 104
Neisseria, 280
Neoantigen, 18, 293, 307, 309
Neonatal immune response, 15
Neoplasm, 18, **338**
  benign, 338
  malignant, 338
  see also Cancer
Nephalometry, 141, 225
Neufeld "Quellungreaktion," **165**
Neuraminidase, 68, 186, 344
Neutralization
  toxin, 226–230, 232–236
  viral, 186, 304–305
Neutrophil, 23–25
  dysfunction, 279–280

Neutrophil [cont.]
    inhibitory factor, 303
Nezelof syndrome, **282**
Nichols strain of treponeme, 242–244, 246
Nicotinamide dinucleotidase, 229
Nitroblue tetrazolium reduction test, 279–280
Nonsusceptibility, **2**
Normal distribution, **350–352**
Normal lymphocyte transfer reaction, 332–333
Nucleic acids
    antibodies, 263–267
    antigens, 30
Nucleoproteins, 263–264, 266
Nude mouse, 25, **282**
Null lymphocyte, **25**, 306

O antigen
    bacterial, somatic, **176**, 224
    erythrocyte, see Blood group systems, ABO
Occult antigen, **307**
Old tuberculin, 299
Oncogenic virus, 12, 339–341
Oncoimmunology, 337–345
Ontogeny of immune system, 18–20
Ophthalmia, sympathetic, 311
Opsonic index, **8**
Opsonin, **7–8**, 25, 201
Opsonization, 6
Optimal proportion, precipitation, **136**, 138
Ouchterlony technique, 151–155
Oudin technique, 146–147
Ovalbumin, 56
Overproduction diseases, 277–279, 281
Oz allotypes, 46–47

P blood group system, 110–111, 310
Packed cells, 71, 119
Paired sera, **64**, 226
Papain, 44–45, 324, 326
Parameter, **348**
Paraprotein, **37, 281**
Paraproteinemia, **37, 281**
Parasitic immunity, 23, 68, 201, 300
    see also specific organisms
Parathyroid gland, 282
Paratope, **32**, 62
Parentage exclusion, 68, 74, 328
Paroxysmal cold hemoglobinuria, **310**
Passive agglutination, **62, 190**–194
    reversed, 197
Passive cutaneous anaphylaxis, **292**, 297
Passive immunity, **9**–10, 53
Pasteur, L., 2, 11, 311
Paternity tests
    blood groups, 74
    leukocyte antigens, 328
Patient screening, 124–125

Paul-Bunnell test, 171–172
Penicillin hypersensitivity, 293
Peplomere, **185**
Peplos, **184**
Pepsin, 3, 45
Peroxide, 280
Pertussis, 15–16, 175
Peyer's patches, 20, 291
Pfeiffer phenomenon, 200
Phacoanaphylaxis, 312
Phage
    conversion, **176**
    temperate, 232
Phagocyte, **4**
    disfunction, 279–280
    see also Macrophage
Phagocytic index, **8**
Phagocytosis
    antibodies, see Opsonin
    antigen processing, 31
    cells and tissues, 3
    complement's role, 25, 201
    deficiency diseases, 279–280
    enzymes of, 4
    phylogeny, 18
    resistance to, 3, 175
Phagolysosome, **4**
Phagosome, see Phagolysosome
Phase variation, **176–177**
Phylogeny of immune system, 17–18
Phytohemagglutinin, 21, **72**, 168
Pilus, 175
Pirquet technique, 299
Placenta
    anastomosis, 20
    antibody passage, 8, 14, 50
    antigen passage, 13, 290
    chorion, 343
    fetal privilege, 337
Plaque-forming cells, **53**
Plasma, **1**
    in transfusion, 120
Plasma cell, **6**, 22–23
    antibody production, 6, 49, 53
    antigen receptor, 6
    characteristics, 21
    neoplasm, 277–278
    ontogeny, 19, 56–57
    see also B lymphocyte
Plasma expander, 120
Plasmapheresis, **120**
Plasmodium, 68
Platelet, 23–25
    Arthus reaction, 296
    EDTA damage, 113
    IgE receptors, 52
    specific component therapy, 120
    thrombocytopenia, **283**, 310–311
Pneumococcus C-polysaccharide, 142
Pneumonia, primary atypical, 169, 309
Pneumonitis (immunologic), 296

Index

Poison
  ivy, 300
  oak, 300
  sumac, 300
  see also Toxin; Venom
Pokeweed mitogen, 21
Poliomyelitis
  Sabin vaccine, 11, 13, 16
  Salk vaccine, 11, 16
Polyacrylamide gel, see Electrophoresis
Polyclonal gammopathy, **43**
Polymorphonuclear leukocyte, see Granulocyte
Polypeptides, see Proteins
Polysaccharides
  as antigens, 30–31
  bacterial capsule, 4
  blood group antigens, q.v.
  lipopolysaccharides, 30
  precipitating, 33
  structure, 31
Polyvalence, **34**, 64, 236
Porter, R., 44
Poststreptococcal glomerulonephritis, **309**
Postvaccinal encephalomyelitis, 311
Postzone, **136**
P-p blood group system, 110–111, 310
Prausnitz-Küstner reaction, 286, 292–293, 297
Precipitation, **32–34**, 135–165
  capsular, 165
  fluid phase, 135–144, 190
  forensic tests, 142
  gel phase, 144–165
  H type, 139
  inhibition, **35**
  quantitative tests, 138–139
  Quellung reaction, 165
  R type, 139
  radial immunodiffusion, 147–150
Precipitin, **135**
Precipitinogen, **135**
Precision, 347–**348**
Pregnancy tests
  agglutination inhibition test, 195, 343
  rubella, 189
Primary vs. secondary antibody response, 13
  see also Immune response
Primed lymphocyte, 5
Private antigens, **112**
Privileged sites and tissues, 336–337
Proenzyme, **201**
Progesterone-binding protein, 261
Properdin, 202, **205**–207
Prostaglandins, 289
Prosthesis, **337**
Protein
  allergens, 293–294
  as antigen, 30, 107
  autofluorescence, 248

Protein [cont.]
  carrier, 32
  chemically modified, see Azoprotein; Toxoid
  denatured, 32, 36
  diazotized, 32–33
  globular, 36
  lens, 311–312
  nucleoproteins, 263–266
  precipitating, 33
  regression, 342–343
  structural levels, 30
  transport, 261
Proteus, 175, 179–180
Protoplast, **174**
Provirus, 232, **340**
Prozone, **136**, 182
Pseudoagglutination, **69**
Public antigens, **112**
Purified protein derivative, 21, **299**
Purine and pyrimidine analogs, 334
Pyrogen test, **224**–226
Pyronin, 22

Q fever, 179, 211
Quality control
  blood banking, 129–133
  serological tests, 347–352
Quantitative precipitation, 138–139
Quellung reaction, **165**
Quenching
  fluorescence tests, **248**
  radioactive tests, 253

R strain, 176
Rabbit
  anaphylaxis, 288
  complement, 209, 329
  culturing treponemes, 183
  Pasteur vaccine, 311
  precipitating serum, 139
  pyrogen test, 224
  toxin assay, 232–234
Rabies
  active immunity, 11
  hemagglutination, 184
  Pasteur vaccine, 311
Race, R., 80
Radial immunodiffusion, 147–150
  complement assays, 208–209
  immunoglobulin assays, 282
Radiation
  cancer treatment, 334
  immune system effects, 334
Radioactive
  chromium, 330
  thymidine, 331
Radioallergosorbent test, **260**–261, 286–287

Index

Radioimmunoassay, 249–261
    digoxin, 254–256
    IgE, 257–261
    sensitivity, 65
Radioimmunoprecipitation test, **258–260**
Radioimmunosorbent test, 287
    direct, **258**
    indirect, **257–258**
Radioisotope-labeled antibodies, *see* Radioimmunoassays; Competitive protein-binding assays
Radioligand inhibition, 251
Radiomimetic drug, **335**
Radioreceptor assay, **261**
Ramon titration, **136**
Rantz antigen, 142
Rapid plasma reagin test, **183–185**
Reaction
    of identity, 152–153
    of nonidentity, 152–153
    of partial identity, 152–153
Reagent red blood cells, 69, **120**, 124–129
Reagin
    allergic, **52, 286–287**
        see also Immunoglobulin class E
    rapid plasma reagin test, 183–185
    syphilitic, **65**, 113, **181, 216**, 287
Receptor destroying enzyme, 68, **186**
Recombinant DNA technology, 305, 344
Red blood cells, *see* Erythrocytes
Regression protein, **342–343**
Reiter strain, 242–243, 245
Reliability, **348**
Reproducibility, 258, **348**
Resistance, 4–5
Response, immune, *see* Immune response
Ressler's technique, 155–157
Reticulocyte, **96**
Reticuloendothelial system, 4
Reverse blood grouping, **69**
Reversed passive
    agglutination tests, **197**
    Arthus reaction, **296–297**
Rh blood group system, 80–100
    disease, 93–100
    D^u cell, **89–93**
    genetics, 80–84
    nomenclature
        Fisher-Race, 80–81
        Rosenfeld, 80
        Wiener, 81–84
Rh disease, 93–100
Rhesus, *see* Rh blood group system
Rheumatic fever, 142–143, 309
Rheumatoid arthritis
    passive hemagglutination test, 193–194
    VDRL crossreacting, 183
Rheumatoid factor, **193**, 308
Ribonucleic acid
    antibodies, 30, 264–267
    antigens, 31, 264–267

Ribosomal RNA, 22
Rice test, **219–221**
Rickettsia, 179–180, 211
Ring test, **140–142**
Rivers' postulates, 307
Rocket electroimmunoassay, 155
Römer titration
    antitoxin, 231–232
    precipitation, 136
Rosenfeld, R., 80, 107
Rosette technique, **53**
    B cell, 282
    T cell, 281
Rubella
    hemagglutination inhibition test, 187–189
    passive hemagglutination test, 191–192
    vaccination, 17
    vaccine, 11
Rubeola, *see* Measles
Runt disease, **320**
Russell bodies, **22, 278**

S strain, 176
Sabin vaccine, 11, 13
Saline agglutinin, 139, 175–178
Salk vaccine, 11
    see also Poliomyelitis
Salmonella, 139, 175–178
    Widal test, **179**
Sarcoidosis, **282**
Sarcoma, 338
Scarlet fever, 226, 234–235
Schick test, **234**
Schlepper molecule, **32**, 181
Schultz-Charlton test, **234**
Schultz-Dale test, **294**–295
Scintillator
    cocktail, 253
    counting window, **254**
    crystal, 253
    discriminator, **254**
    liquid, 253
    scaler, 254
Screening test, **65**
SD antigens, 329
Second set reaction, **317**
Secondary disease, *see* Allogeneic disease
Secondary response, *see* Immune response, secondary
Secretor
    Lewis association, 104–105
    test, **76**
    trait, **76**
Secretory component, **49**, 51
Secretory IgA, 51
Secretory IgM, 49
Selective theory of antibody production, *see* Clonal selection
Self recognition, 2, 13, 18, 20–22
Sensitivity of test, **64**, 141, 258, **347**

Index

Sensitization
  in vitro, 89
  in vivo, 13–15
Sensitized cells, **89**
Sephadex, 257–258, 260
Sequestered antigen, 307
Sequestrene, *see* Anticoagulants, EDTA
Serogroups, **177**–178
Serologic adhesion, 201
Serologic reactions
  see also Agglutination; Complement fixation; Precipitation;
  tagged reagents, 239–275
Serologic reagents
  preparation of, 62–64
  quality control, 131–133
Serologic tests, 64–65
  accuracy, **347**–348
  false reactions, 65
  forensic, 68
  precision, 347–**348**
  reliability, **348**
  reproducibility, **348**
  screening test, **65**
  sensitivity, **64**–65, **347**
  specificity, 64–65, 347
Serologically detectable histocompatibility antigens, **329**
Serology, 1 *ff*
Serotonin, **289**
Serotypes, 176–178, 189
Serratia, 280
Serum, **1**
  absorption of, 62
  electrophoretic pattern of, 37–41, 43
  fractionation techniques, 37–41
  grouping, 69
  pared sera, **64**
Serum proteins
  albumins, 36
  chemical properties, 36–41
  functions, 36
  globulins, 36
  physical properties, 36–41
Serum sickness, **170**, 235–236, **297**–298
Shared antigens, *see* Cross reactions
Sheep
  anthrax immunity, 11
  cell agglutinins, 170
  erythrocyte rosettes, 281
  red blood cells
    complement fixation test, 210–222
    heterophile antibody test, 171–174
Shift (QC), **352**
Shock tissue (organ), **287**
Singlet oxygen, 280
Skin tests
  allergy, 292
  Casoni, 300
  fungal, 299
  toxin immunity, 234

Skin tests [*cont.*]
  tuberculin, 299
  venom immunity, 235–236
Slow reacting substance of anaphylaxis, **289**
Smallpox, 11, 13, 15, 311
Snake venom, 7, 235–236
Soluble specific substances, **165**
Somatic
  antigen, **176**
  mutation theory, **56**
Sorbent, **242**
Spacer DNA, 57
Specific antigens, bacterial, **177**
Specific component therapy, 119–120
Specific resistance, 5
Specificity, 61
  antibody, **32**, 62
  antigen, **32**
  serological test, **64**, **347**
Spider bites, 7, 235
Spleen, 17, 283
Spur (immunoprecipitate), 152–153, 163
S-R variation, **176**
Standard deviation, **349**–350
Staphylococci, 4, 178, 225, 280
Statistic, **348**
Stem cells, 17, 18, 23
Steric hindrance, 7, 35, 207
Steric interference, *see* Steric hindrance
Steroids, 299, 335
Streptococci, 4, 142, 165, 176, 178, 226, 229, 234, 280, 309
Streptococcus MG agglutination test, 180–181
Streptokinase, 229
Streptolysin, 226–229, 309
Subclasses of immunoglobulins, **46**
Subgroups of blood types, 72
Subtypes of immunoglobulins, **46**
Superoxide radical, 4
Suppression of immune response, 334–335
Suppressor cell, 27, 344
  dysfunction, 279, 283, 308, 312
Surveillance, immunologic, **18**, **321**
Sutter blood factors, 128
Swiss type agammaglobulinemia, 283–284
Switch region of immunoglobulin, 58
Sympathetic ophthalmia, 311
Sympathomimetic drug, **289**
Syngeneic graft, 315–316
Syngraft, 315–316
Syphilis
  fluorescent antibody tests, 242–246
  immobilization test, 243
  Kolmer complement fixation test, 216–219
  rapid plasma reagin test, 183–185
  reagin, **181**
  rheumatic factor, 193
  serological tests for, 181–184
  vaccine, 13
  VDRL test, 64–65, 182–183
  Wasserman test, 216–218

Syphilis [cont.]
  see also Treponema pallidum
Syphilitic reagin, **65**, 113, **181**
  complement fixation tests, 216–217
Systemic lupus erythematosus, **263**–267, 308–309
  see also Lupus erythematosus

T antigens, **341**
T cell-B cell interactions, 26–27, 279
T cell-T cell interactions, 279
T cells, **20**
  amplifier, 27
  antiviral, 185–186, 341
  cell receptors, 63
  characteristics, 21
  deficiencies, 281–284
  delayed hypersensitivity, role in, 27, 284–285
  helper effect, 26, 279
  killer, 27, 285, 306, 321, 344
  suppressor dysfunction, 279, 283, 308, 312
  suppressor effect, 27, 344
T lymphocytes, see T cells
T3, T4, 261–263
Tagged reagents, 239–275
  see also Labeled reagents
Tanned erythrocyte, 191
Tetanus, 7
  DPT, 15
  immunization against, 10, 16
  susceptible species, 230
  toxoid, 11–12
Theophylline, 273, 289
Thermoprecipitation test, 141, 142
Theta antigen, 25
Third man (person) test, **317**–318
Thrombocytopenia purpura, 283, **310**–311
Thymectomy, 19, 282, 285, 312
Thymocyte, 19
Thymosin, 305
Thymus
  alymphoplasia, 283
  cancer, 282
  congenital absence, 25
    see also Nude mouse
  deficiency disease, 281
  dependent antigen, 26
  dysplasia, 283
  hormones, 19, 305
  independent antigens, 25
  ontogeny, 19–20
  phylogeny, 17–18
  primary lymphoid organ, 283
  transplants, 284
Thyroglobulin, 312
Thyroiditis, 312–313
Thyroxine (T₄), 261–263
Thyroxine-binding globulin, 261–263
Tine test, 299

Tiselius, A., 37
Tissue transplantation
  graft rejection, 316–321
  graft vs. host reaction, 319–320
  histocompatibility antigens, **315**, 329
  suppression of immune response against, 334–335
  terminology, 316
  see also Histocompatibility; Graft(s)
Titer, 8, **64, 72**
Titration test, **71**
Todd unit, **228**
Tolerance, immunologic, **20, 319**, 341
Tonsil, 20, 291
Toxin, **223**
  diphtheria, 11
  Elek test, **232**–233
  endotoxin, **224**–225
  exotoxin, **223**–225
  flocculation test, 232
  LD₅₀, **230**
  minimal lethal dose, **230**
  minimal reacting dose, **230**
  neutralization, 6, 231
  tetanus, 11, q.v.
Toxoid, **11**, 139
Transfer factor, 303, 345
Transfer RNA, 56
Transformation
  lymphocyte, 21, 301, 331–332
  oncogenic, 339–340
Transfusion reaction
  exchange, 99
  specific component therapy, 119–120
Translation inhibitory protein, **303**–304
Transplantation, see Tissue transplantation
Transplantation antigen, 329
  see also Histocompatibility antigens
Transport piece, see Secretory component
Trend (QC), **352**
Treponema pallidum
  complement fixation test, 181, 216–218
  fluorescent treponemal antibody absorption tests, 181, 242–245
  hemagglutination test, 181
  immobilization test, 243, 246
  Nichols strain, 243–244, 246
  Reiter strain, 242–243, 245
  VDRL test, 64
  see also Syphilis
Trichinosis, 300
Triiodothronine (t₃), 262–263
Triple response, 292
Trophoblast, 337
Trypanosomiasis, 183
Tuberculin, 21
  old, **299**
  purified protein derivative, **299**
  reaction, 299
Tuberculosis, 193
Tularemia, 179

Tumor immunology, 337–345
  antigens, 341–342
  immunity, 341
  vaccines, 344
  see also Cancer
Tumor specific transplantation antigens, 341
Twins
  dizygotic, **20**, 316
  fraternal, **316**
  monozygotic, **315**
Type of light chain, 46
Typhoid fever, 176, 179–180
Typhus, 179, 183

Ultracentrifugation, 144
Univalent antibody, 87
Universal donor, **71**, 73
Universal recipient, **71**
Urticaria, **292**, 294
Urushiol, 300

Vaccination, 11–12, 15
  attenuated virus, 11
  bacille Calmette-Guérin, 344
  DPT, 15
  inactivated virus, 11
  influenza, 13
  measles, 11
  mumps, 11
  pertussis, 15–16
  poliomyelitis, 11, 13
  rabies, 11, 311
  rubella, 11, 187–189
  Sabin, 11
  Salk, 11
  smallpox, 9, 11, 15
  tetanus, 10, 16
  whooping cough, 15–16
  yellow fever, 11
Vaccinia, see Virus
Vaccines, **11**
  see also Vaccination
Valence, 34
Variable regions of immunoglobulins, 45–46
Variance, **350**
Variation, coefficient of, **350**
Variola, see Virus
Vasoactive amines, 289
VDRL test, 64–65, 182–183
Venereal disease, 13
  lymphogranuloma venereum, 299
  syphilis, q.v.
Venom, **235**–236, 292
Versene, see Anticoagulants, EDTA
Vi antigen, 176
Vibrio cholerae, 68
Virgin lymphocytes, 14, 21
Virion, **184**, **340**

Virus
  antibodies, 1
  antigens, 1, 340
  bacteriophage, 232
  cancer-related, 339–341
  capsid, **184**
  capsomere, **184**
  cell-mediated immunity against, 341
  Coxsackie group, 184
  diseases, see specific diseases
  ECHO group, 184
  envelope, **184**
  Epstein-Barr, 169, **340**
  hemagglutination, 184–186
  hemagglutination inhibition test, 186–190
  hepatitis, 113, 158, 192–193
  Herpes group, 185, 305
  immunity mechanisms, 304–305, 321
  influenza, 68, 186, 189–190
  interferon, effects on, 2, 303–306
  LCM, 284
  measles, 11, 16, 311
  mumps, 184, 311
  neurotropic, 311
  oncogenic, 339–341
  papovavirus, 339
  parainfluenza, 184
  peplomere, **185**
  peplos, **184**
  phage, 53
  polyoma, 341
  pox, 339
  provirus, 232, 311, **340**
  rabies, 184
  rubella, 11, 17, 187–189, 191–192
  serotypes, 189–190
  smallpox, 9, 15
  SV40, 341
  tumor virus, 340
  vaccines, 10
  vaccinia, 9, 184
  variola, 9, 15, 184
Vollmer patch test, 299

Waldenström's macroglobulinemia, **278**
Warm antibody (37°C), 90, 116–117
Wassermann test, 216–218
Wasting disease, **320**
Weak
  antigens, 72–73
  chemical bonds, 59–60
Weighted mean, **352**
Weil-Felix test, **179**–180
Wharton's jelly, 112
Wheal and flare reaction, 292, 300
White blood cells, see Leukocytes
Whooping cough, see Pertussis
Widal test, **179**
Wiener, A., 80–81
Wiskott-Aldrich syndrome, **283**

Index

Witebsky's postulates, **307**
Witebsky's substances, **71**
World Health Organization, 15
Wright's stain, 24

Xenogeneic graft, 316
Xenograft, **316**
Xg blood group system, 111–112
X-Y-Z cells, 22

Yeast, 7
Yellow fever, 11

Zeta potential, **86**
Zone electrophoresis, **39**
Zoning phenomenon, **136,** 144, 190